Radiology Pathology Correlations of Breast Lesions

Malini Harigopal • Liva Andrejeva
Kamaljeet Singh • John Lewin
Editors

Radiology Pathology Correlations of Breast Lesions

Springer

Editors
Malini Harigopal
Department of Pathology
Yale University
New Haven, CT, USA

Kamaljeet Singh
Department of Pathology and
Laboratory Medicine
Brown University and Women and
Infants Hospital of RI
Providence, RI, USA

Liva Andrejeva
Department of Radiology
and Biomedical Imaging
Yale School of Medicine
New Haven, CT, USA

John Lewin
Department of Radiology and
Biomedical Imaging
Yale School of Medicine
New Haven, CT, USA

ISBN 978-3-031-65710-8 ISBN 978-3-031-65711-5 (eBook)
https://doi.org/10.1007/978-3-031-65711-5

This Springer imprint is published by the registered company Springer Nature Switzerland AG
The registered company address is: Gewerbestrasse 11, 6330 Cham, Switzerland

Preface

This radiology–pathology correlation book is an ambitious attempt to consolidate the radiology and pathologic findings of breast entities into a single book written in an atlas format. Despite a rather inauspicious beginning, with delays caused by the COVID-19 pandemic, the first edition of this book has been completed. The importance of image-guided percutaneous biopsy (i.e., core needle and vacuum-assisted biopsy) in the first line management of patients with both benign and malignant breast diseases is well-established. More recently, the breakthrough discoveries in immunohistochemistry, molecular techniques, and genomics in pathology have helped to narrow our knowledge gaps. It is imperative we use this knowledge judiciously in our daily practice to optimize patient management. The pathologist has traditionally utilized recognition criteria in diagnostic histopathology; these have not changed significantly with time. However, advancements in molecular profiling of tumor have contributed unique opportunities in understanding the molecular biology of breast cancers for identifying targets for therapy. The pathology report has evolved from a mere two-line diagnosis to include important details such as biomarker and molecular signatures which are now an integral part of the histological workup.

The dominance of percutaneous biopsy as the major modality for obtaining tissue diagnosis has magnified the importance of interaction between the radiologist and pathologist in the diagnosis and management of breast diseases. The aim of this first edition is to introduce to the readers the multidisciplinary team approach required for optimal management of breast diseases in the setting of percutaneous biopsy.

Since its introduction in the 1990s, image-guided biopsy has undergone continual improvements in both ease of performance and diagnostic accuracy. These improvements are the result of advances in both imaging technology and biopsy devices. Ultrasound is the most common modality used for guiding biopsies, and ultrasound images today are superior to those of the past decades in both lesion detail and visualization of the needle itself. Mammography has benefitted from advances in digital technology that enabled the development of digital breast tomosynthesis, a 3D technique that both speeds up biopsy procedures and, more importantly, allows biopsy of subtle areas of architectural distortion. Similarly, MRI is continually improving in terms of both image quality and speed.

Biopsy devices have undergone fewer improvements over the past 2 decades than have imaging technologies. Automated large-core needle biopsy devices, the mainstay of ultrasound-guided needle biopsies, are little changed from those that were used 30 years ago. These are typically 14-gauge devices that function using a spring-loaded action to capture tissue in a trough and then cut it off in either a single motion or a two-stage operation ("open-trough"). Mammographic procedures, whether stereotactic or tomosynthesis-guided, and MRI-guided procedures are really only practical, thanks to the development of vacuum-assisted biopsy devices. These devices are larger gauge, ranging from 10 gauge to 7 gauge, and use suction to capture a large amount of tissue than what can otherwise be obtained. Just as importantly, many of the devices can obtain an essentially unlimited number of samples with a single-needle insertion. When vacuum-assisted devices were first introduced more than 20 years ago, they represented a major advancement over the spring-loaded devices, but, as with those devices, improvements since that time have been incremental.

Even with the most accurate targeting and the most reliable biopsy devices, the diagnostic challenges arising from the limited sampling of percutaneous biopsy is self-evident, as the specimen may not be representative of all the pathology. A chance of undersampling introduces the potential for differential diagnostic problems, including, at times, distinguishing between benign and malignant entities.

The diagnostic accuracy and clarity of reporting in pathology is mandatory in the era of breast conservation and neoadjuvant treatment for breast cancers. Brené Brown a well-known author once said, "Clear is Kind and Unclear is Unkind," a sentiment particularly relevant to pathology and radiology reports. The pathology report should be concise and clear and communicate to the clinician in an unambiguous manner detailing not only the relevant findings but also include relevant negative findings that would help the clinician with therapeutic decisions for patient care.

In this book, we attempt to bring together the clinical expertise of radiologists and pathologists in resolving difficult breast lesions detected on imaging. Our aim for this book is to create an easy-to-use reference for radiology and pathology residents and fellows, as well as practicing pathologists, radiologists, and surgeons.

As the two disciplines of radiology and pathology are interrelated, the scope of the text is to provide and inform readers of not only typical examples of breast lesions that correlate with imaging findings (that may or may not require surgical excision) but also to resolve problematic lesions that are discordant with imaging findings.

This book has 14 chapters with over 250 illustrations with key references. Some newer entities that have been described are included but with the understanding that this book is not an all-inclusive text. The readers are advised to seek out standard textbooks in radiology and pathology for an in-depth knowledge of imaging and pathology of breast entities.

Each chapter includes an outline with a systematic approach to each disease entity punctuated by various imaging techniques, key diagnostic points seen on imaging, and pathology followed by differential diagnostic considerations.

Finally, a summary of concordant and discordant findings is provided at the end of each section. We have included a cast of authors with expertise and experience in the major subspecialty fields of radiology and pathology with valuable input from our surgical colleagues in managing patients with breast diseases.

New Haven, CT, USA — Malini Harigopal
New Haven, CT, USA — Liva Andrejeva
Providence, RI, USA — Kamaljeet Singh
New Haven, CT, USA — John Lewin

The original version of the book has been revised. A correction to this book can be found at https://doi.org/10.1007/978-3-031-65711-5_15

Acknowledgements

We would like to acknowledge our mentors who have instilled in us an unquenchable interest and commitment to our understanding the complex specialized field of breast imaging and pathology. Our special thanks to our dedicated team of co-authors who have contributed their time and talent to accomplish this exciting endeavor in creation of the radiology–pathology correlation book. We are especially indebted to the patients whose material forms the basis for this book. Finally, this book would not have been possible without the support of our families.

Contents

1 Introduction and General Consideration of Radiology-Pathology Correlation

Malini Harigopal, Liva Andrejeva, Peter Podany, John Lewin, Madhavi Raghu, and Kamaljeet Singh

Introduction

Breast cancer is the most common cause of cancer-related death worldwide and accounts for more than 25% of newly diagnosed cancers annually [1]. The role of the pathologist in breast cancer care has evolved from merely documenting the tumor characteristics such as tumor size, histologic grade, histologic type, margin assessment, presence of lymphovascular invasion (LVI), focality, and biomarker status in surgical specimens to a more challenging one, evaluating small tissue samples obtained by needle core biopsy from palpable and non-palpable lesions detected by mammography or ultrasound.

With the advent of conservative surgeries for breast lesions, the pathologist's role has shifted to evaluating margins and sentinel lymph node biopsy at the time of excision. The emergence of core needle biopsy in the 1980s has posed new challenges for the pathologists who have to make a diagnosis from limited amounts of tissue [2]. Percutaneous image-guided biopsy is preferred over surgical biopsies with numerous advantages. The cost effectiveness and proven benefit of core needle biopsy over surgical biopsy is best illustrated in the evaluation of non-palpable indeterminate breast lesions. Ultrasound-guided interventional breast procedures, including fine-needle aspiration (FNA), core needle biopsy (CNB), and preoperative wire localization are safe, accurate, and routinely performed for lesions visualized on US [3–5]. Ultrasound guidance is usually preferred over mammography and magnetic resonance imaging (MRI) because of shorter procedure times, real-time visualization, increased patient comfort, easy access to all parts of the breast including the axilla, and lack of ionizing radiation or intravenous contrast [3–6].

Stereotactic core needle biopsy including tomosynthesis-guided biopsy is relatively quick and accurate, allowing patients to avoid surgery for benign, concordant findings. Tomosynthesis-

M. Harigopal (✉) · P. Podany
Department of Pathology, Yale University, New Haven, CT, USA
e-mail: malini.harigopal@yale.edu; peter.podany@yale.edu

L. Andrejeva · J. Lewin
Department of Radiology and Biomedical Imaging, Yale School of Medicine, New Haven, CT, USA
e-mail: liva.andrejeva@yale.edu; john.lewin@yale.edu

M. Raghu
Department of Radiology and Biomedical Imaging, Yale University, New Haven, CT, USA

Section of Breast Imaging, Nuvance Health, Danbury, CT, USA
e-mail: madhavi.raghu@gmail.com

K. Singh
Department of Pathology and Laboratory Medicine, Brown University and Women and Infants Hospital of RI, Providence, RI, USA

M. Harigopal et al. (eds.), *Radiology Pathology Correlations of Breast Lesions*,
https://doi.org/10.1007/978-3-031-65711-5_1

guided core biopsy facilitates tissue diagnosis for mammographic abnormalities seen on 2D and 3D mammograms including asymmetries, focal asymmetries, masses, architectural distortions, and calcifications (Figs. 1.1 and 1.2).

The widespread implementation of mammographic screening programs has increased the detection of numerous entities including benign and high-risk lesions. The optimal management of some of these lesions, based on the wide range of reported upgrade rates, is still under debate. Therefore, different institutions should perform a practice audit to determine their rates of upgrade before deciding management protocols for several high-risk lesions. The radiologist must adequately sample the target lesion to ensure that the histologic findings are an accurate representation of the imaging target. The responsibility of deciding the best management for the patient, such as routine screening versus follow-up imaging, repeat biopsy, or referral to a surgeon, lies with the radiologist. Although the American College of Radiologist's guidelines require that the radiologists perform a radiology-pathology correlation and submit an amended report, some cases are best performed and discussed in a multidisciplinary conference setting [7]. The radiology-pathology correlation addresses whether or not the histologic diagnosis correlates with the lesion seen on imaging. Some studies have shown that the discordance rates with needle core biopsies range from 1% to 8% [8–10]. Discordances are problematic as this may lead to a delay in diagnosis and unnecessary surgeries. The pathologists need to understand the value of correlation with imaging findings. For example, when obtaining additional deeper H&E levels in cases where calcifications seen on radiology are not readily explained by those seen on pathology (Figs. 1.3 and 1.4).

The pathologist cannot work in isolation when reviewing tissue from needle core biopsy specimens to generate a diagnosis. The pathologist

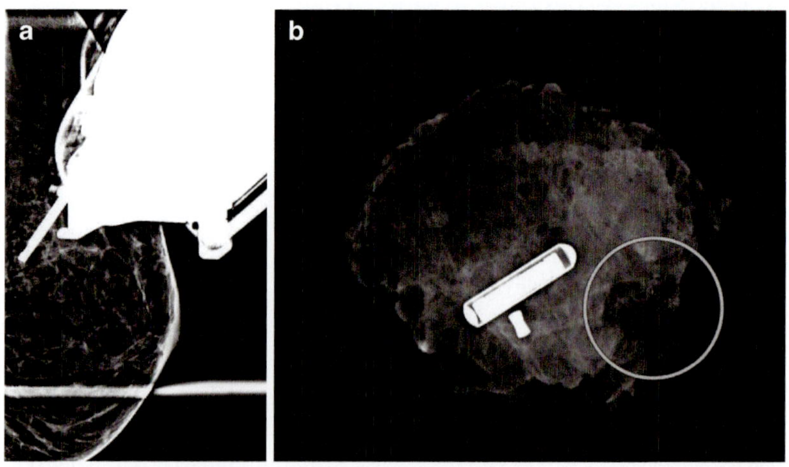

Fig. 1.1 An image of a stereotactic biopsy for calcifications (**a**), and a radiograph (**b**) of a surgical specimen with calcifications on the edge (white circle)

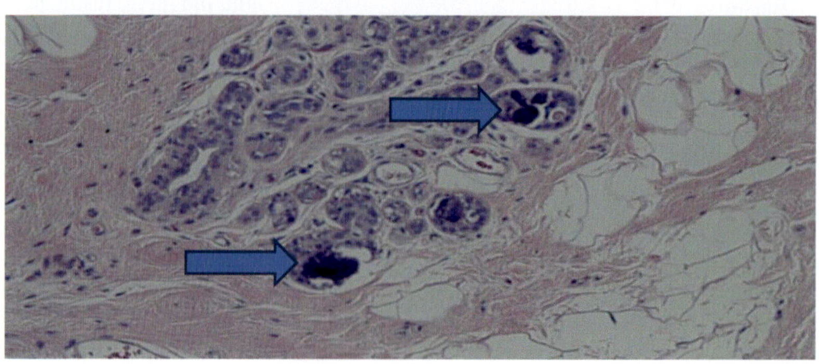

Fig. 1.2 An example of calcifications in a benign breast on H&E which appear dark purple (blue arrows)

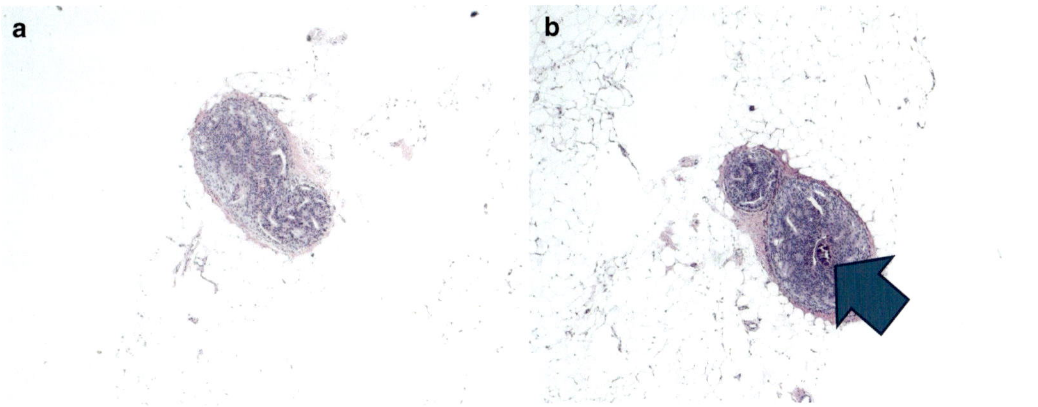

Fig. 1.3 An example of a biopsy in which calcifications were seen on radiology, but the initial H&E histological levels had no calcifications even on level 8 (**a**). On level 9 (**b**) the calcifications (blue arrow) became apparent highlighting the importance of cutting deeper levels to correlate the pathology with the radiology

and radiologist must have a means of communication either through individual discussions or a multidisciplinary conference as appropriate. This dialogue between the radiologist and pathologist is essential to resolve discrepant cases. Several studies have demonstrated the utility of radiologic-pathologic correlation in managing patients with breast disease [9–11]. Despite the benefit of a regular multidisciplinary conference in addressing discrepancies in radiologic and pathologic correlations in many major academic centers, the practice is not universal and may not be feasible in some community-based centers.

The pathologist should be familiar with breast imaging modalities such as mammography, ultrasound, MRI, as well as breast interventional methods (including US, mammography or MRI). The American College of Radiology has established the Breast Imaging Reporting and Data System (BI-RADS®), a standard reporting lexicon utilized by radiologists around the world to describe and assess findings on screening and diagnostic imaging [7]. The pathologist can make a conclusive diagnosis in a majority of lesions by taking into consideration imaging characteristics that correlate with a likelihood of malignancy and include features such as size, shape (e.g., round or oval versus irregular) and margin type (e.g., circumscribed versus indistinct or spiculated). The radiologists should have a good understanding if the biopsy report issued by the pathologist explains the imaging characteristics. For example, if the mass is resolved after the biopsy, the pathology report should reflect remnants of a cyst wall or calcifications to explain the imaging findings. At our institution, if the initial histology of three H&E slides did not show calcifications, we traditionally cut deeper H&E levels in an attempt to find calcifications. An x-ray of the paraffin block should be performed if calcifications are still not present on deeper H&E levels (Fig. 1.5).

Needle core biopsy poses unique challenges partly because the sample is not representative of the entire lesion. Some tumors are heterogeneous such as papillary and fibroepithelial tumors, both benign and malignant. False-negative results, albeit rare, range between 1.6% and 2.4% and occur due to under sampling, which occurs at all needle sizes, but is more common with biopsy devices smaller than 14 gauge such as those sometimes used in ultrasound-guided procedures [3, 4]. Radiologic-pathologic discordance rates range from 2% to 7.7% for US-guided CNBs [8–10]. The American College of Radiology practice guidelines recommend performing concordance with pathology and imaging findings after every procedure as part of the post-procedure follow-up communication with the referring provider [7]. There are five categories for designating breast CNB outcomes per Parikh *et al.*: concordant malignancy, in which a radiologically

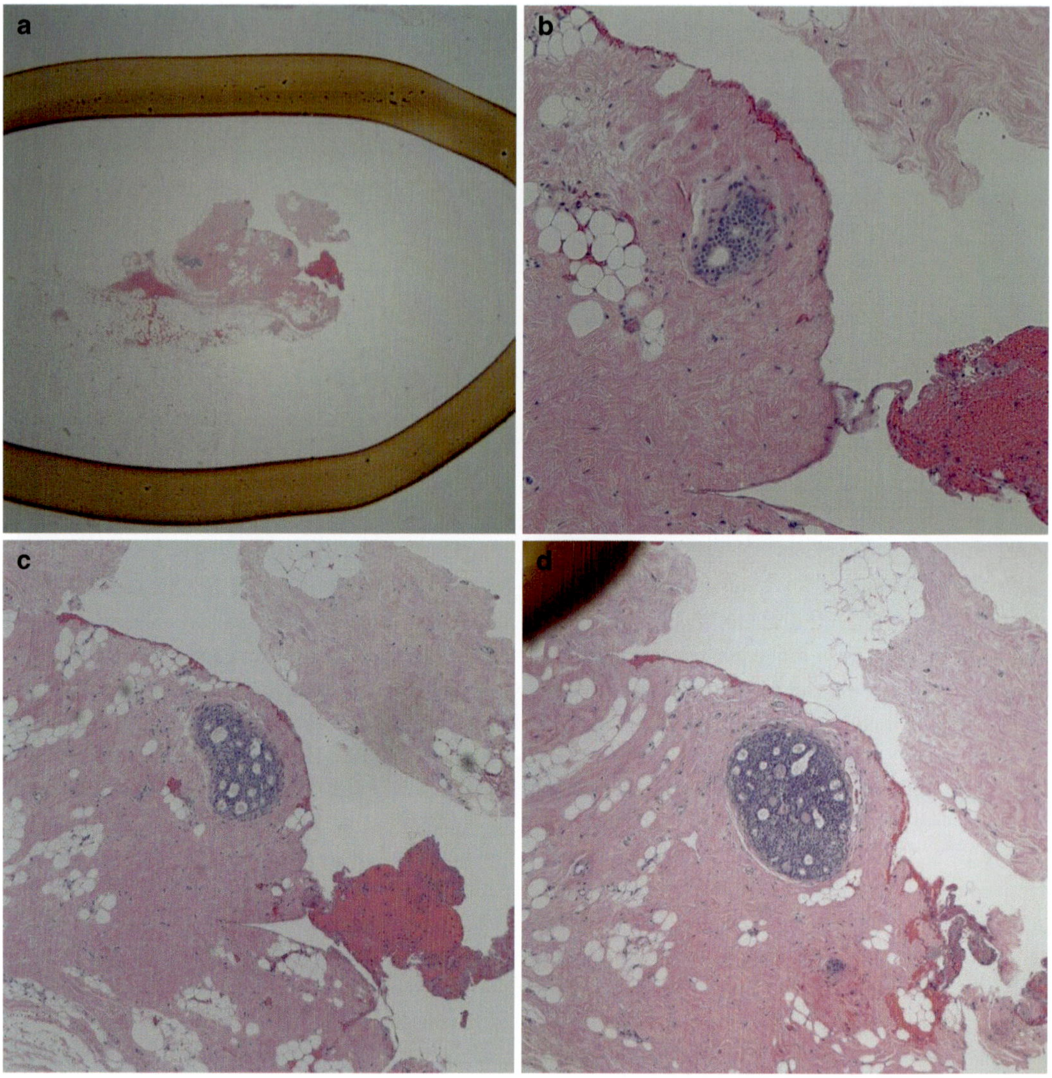

Fig. 1.4 A core needle biopsy which was found to have ADH on H&E deeper sections. On level 1 (**a**) there is only a small focus not diagnostic for ADH which becomes larger on level 4 (**b**). In levels 5 (**c**) and 7 (**d**) the lesion became even larger with architectural atypia and cribriform spaces involving a single duct space, diagnostic for ADH

suspicious lesion is diagnosed as cancer on CNB; concordant benign, in which a radiologically low suspicion lesion is diagnosed as benign; discordant malignancy in which a radiologically low suspicion lesion such a well-circumscribed homogeneous oval mass comes back as malignant on histopathology; discordant benign where a radiologically suspicious lesion comes back benign on histopathology; and high-risk borderline [9]. A high-risk lesion seen in pathology requires correlation with the target lesion seen on imaging [9]. If it was an incidental finding, then the imaging should be re-reviewed. It is a valuable exercise to document the extent of the lesion seen on histology. High-risk borderline lesions include atypia and lobular neoplasia, which increase the lifetime risk of cancer and may be upgraded to cancer on excision [9] (Fig. 1.6). From the pathology perspective, our understanding of the biology of breast cancer and its precursors has evolved with molecular profiling of tumors. We now know that not all patients diag-

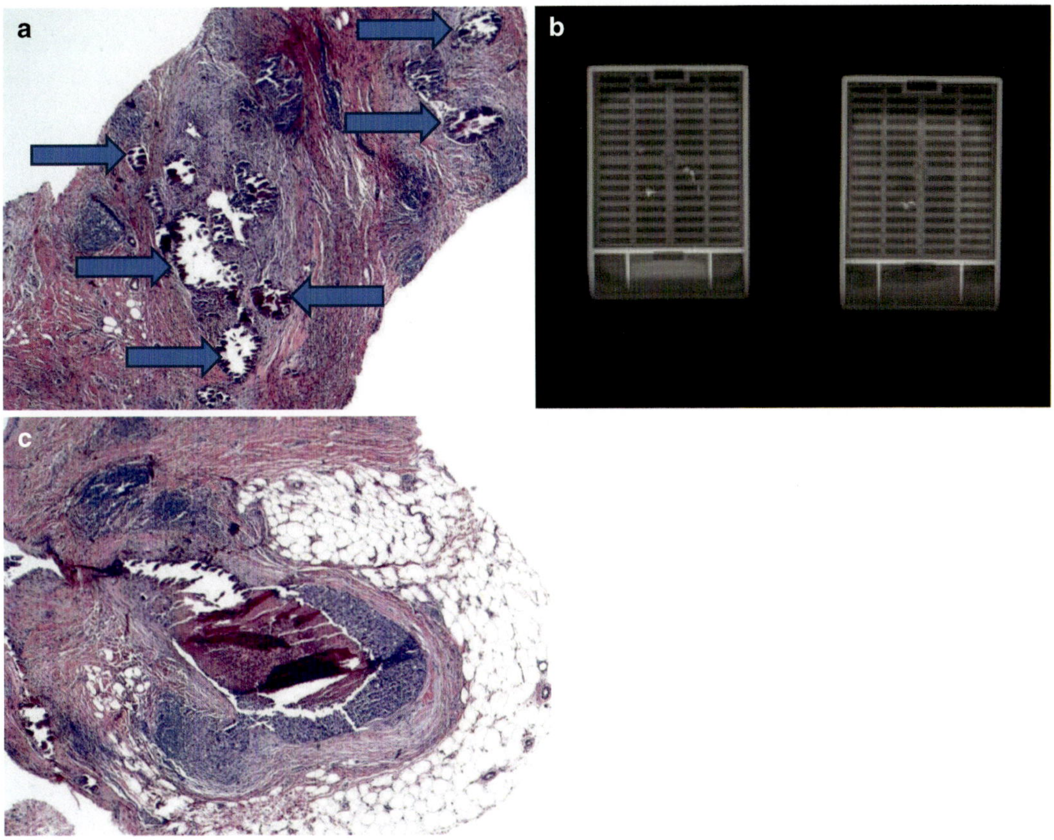

Fig. 1.5 A core needle biopsy specimen with ductal carcinoma in situ (DCIS), associated pleomorphic calcifications (blue arrows) and necrosis on H&E (**a**). X-ray imaging of the paraffin-embedded tissue blocks (**b**) highlights and correlates with the calcifications seen on initial H&E as well as on deeper levels (**c**)

nosed with high-risk breast lesions on image-guided core biopsy such as a papilloma, radial scar, atypical lobular hyperplasia, lobular carcinoma in situ (classic type), columnar cell lesions with FEA, and mucocele-like lesions require surgical excision. With additional data on long-term outcomes, it is now recognized that every high-risk lesion does not need to be excised. The management of high-risk lesions has changed over the years with numerous peer-reviewed literature supporting the follow-up of these benign concordant core biopsy results if they have been adequately sampled [8, 11]. Furthermore, management decisions in these patients need to be based on a correlation between radiological and pathological findings, further increasing the importance of communication between the radiologist and the pathologist. The upgrade rates for these high-risk lesions are variable based on the study population, definition of upgrade, methodology used for sampling, the devices used (e.g., 16- or 14-gauge automated core biopsy versus 11- or 9-gauge vacuum-assisted biopsy) and the number of cores sampled. The American Society of Breast Surgeons (ASBrS) put forth a consensus statement on high-risk breast lesions in 2016 that outlines their management of these borderline and high-risk lesions identified on core needle biopsy [12]. Since that time however, the management of these lesions has continued to evolve.

A diagnosis of ADH on core biopsy requires surgical excision with some exceptions for minimal volume ADH [13] (Fig. 1.7). Classic-type LCIS or ALH can be excised or followed clinically and by imaging workup [13]. However,

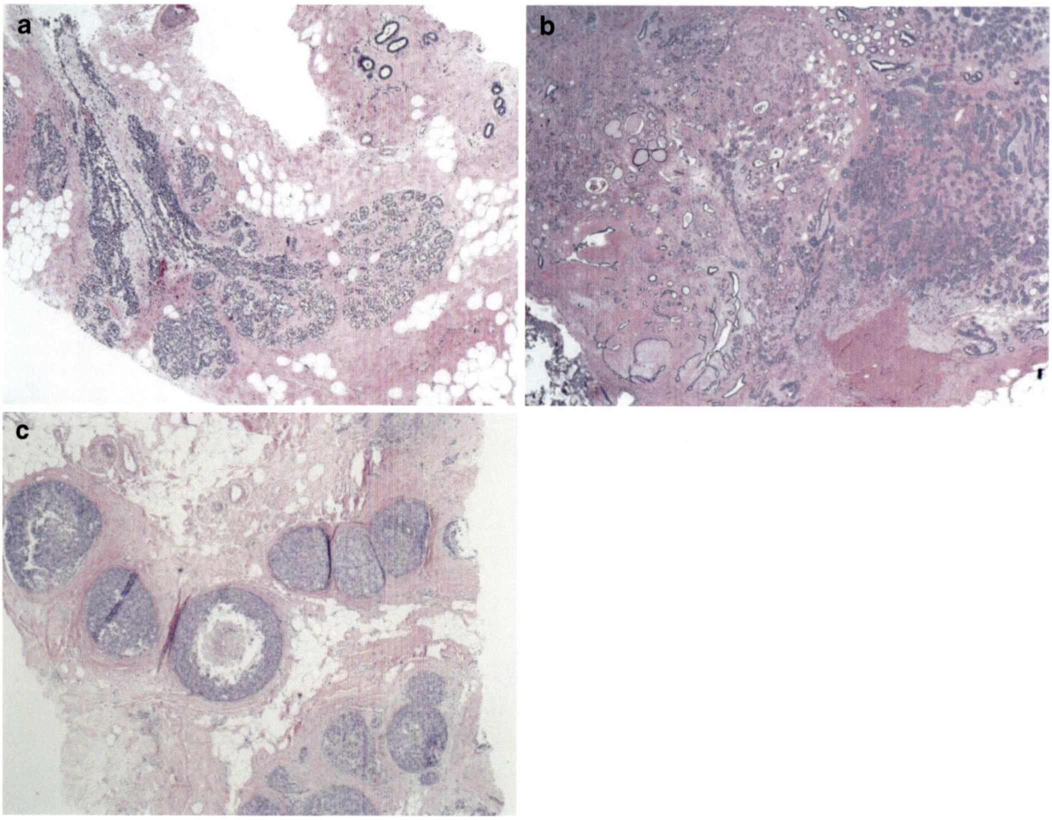

Fig. 1.6 Low power of terminal ductal lobular units (TDLU's) demonstrating proliferation of discohesive, monotonous cells with low-grade features leading to some distention of the lobules with enough involvement to be at the border of atypical lobular hyperplasia and lobular carcinoma in situ (**a**). A fibroadenoma with stromal expansion and compressed glandular component with involvement by lobular carcinoma in situ, classic type. The lobular cells are monotonous with similar nuclei and little variability and are distending the lobules of the terminal ductal lobular units, with involvement of greater than 50% of the unit. In addition, they demonstrate a discohesive appearance characteristic of lobular neoplasias (**b**). A core biopsy with marked distension of lobules by a discohesive cell population, the hallmark of lobular carcinoma in situ (**c**)

excision is warranted for discordant pathology and inadequate sampling. In cases of pleomorphic LCIS and florid LCIS an excisional biopsy is recommended [13].

In cases of pure flat epithelial atypia or columnar cell lesions, observation with clinical and imaging follow-up is required with excision for those cases associated with ADH [13]. Papillary lesions require excision or clinical follow-up depending on whether they are palpable lesions or those with atypia [13] (Fig. 1.8). Incidental microscopic benign papillomas can be followed. Similarly, radial scars with atypia and complex sclerosing lesions require excision except for small and adequately sampled lesions [13, 14] (Fig. 1.9). Again, this is based on meticulous radiology and pathology concordance.

Fibroepithelial lesions with concern for phyllodes tumor require surgical excision with adequate margins [13]. Mucocele-like lesions can be excised or followed-up if completely benign with 6-month imaging and clinical follow-up as the upgrade rates are low (<5%) [13]. Desmoid-type fibromatosis requires wide local excision [13].

Knowledge of the typical imaging features of these and newly recognized histological entities is a must for practicing pathologists and trainees. The most recent edition of the WHO classifica-

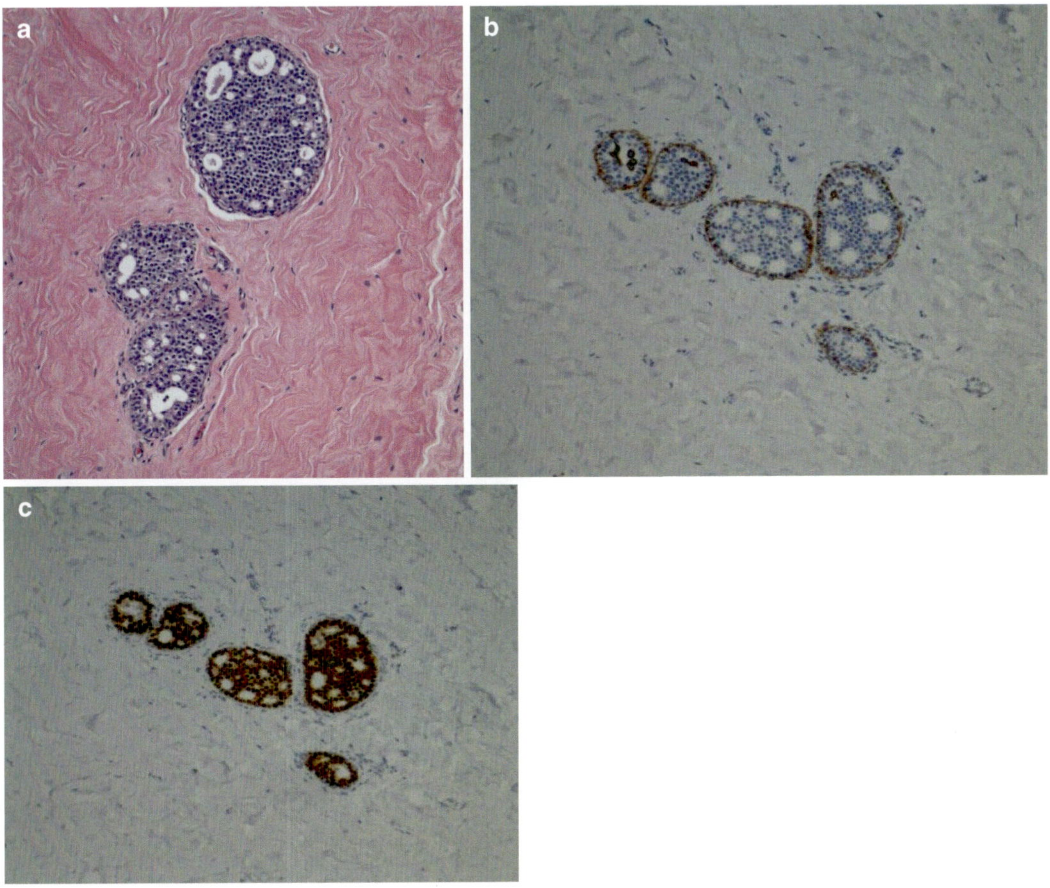

Fig. 1.7 An example of ADH versus UDH (**a**) on H&E in a breast specimen. Immunohistochemical stains for CK5/6 (**b**) highlight myoepithelial cells lining the periphery of the duct while ER (**c**) shows strong uniform staining throughout the lesion supporting a clonal process such as ADH. Abnormal proliferation of the lumenal cells of the breast leading to the formation of rigid bridging, and "punched out" holes as well as nuclei that appear monotonous with little variability further support ADH. The low-grade features of this lesion and small size less than 2 mm support the diagnosis of ADH over ductal carcinoma in situ

Fig. 1.8 A core needle biopsy with fragments of tissue demonstrating fibrovascular cores and papillary architecture involved by low-grade atypia and luminal cell proliferation diagnostic of a papillary lesion involved by atypical ductal hyperplasia

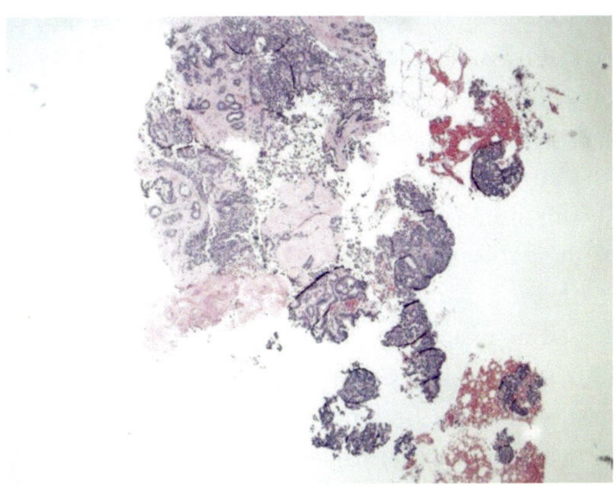

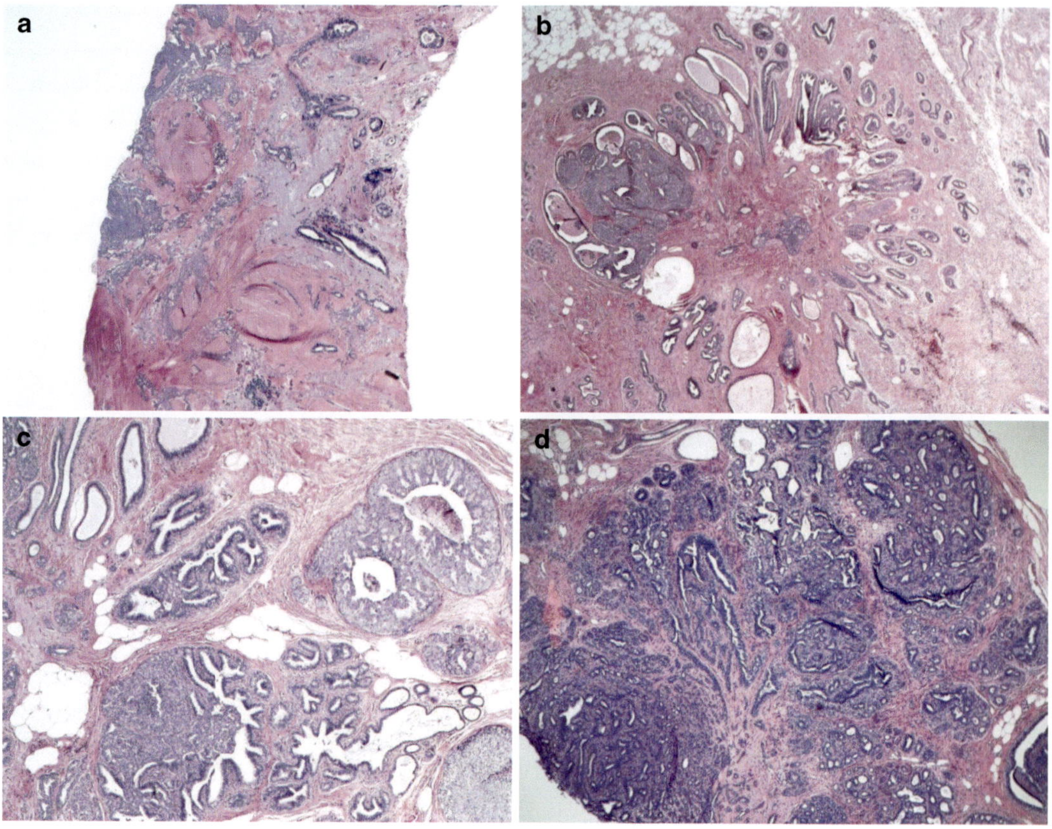

Fig. 1.9 A core needle biopsy demonstrating central sclerosis with fibroelastotic stroma and entrapped glands radiating outward in a portion of radial scar (**a**). A core needle biopsy with a radial scar with areas involved by usual ductal hyperplasia (**b**). A radial scar with involvement by DCIS (**c**). A complex sclerosing lesion with similar features to a radial scar with intermingling areas of sclerosis, entrapped and distorted glands and fibrocystic changes, but is larger in size, typically >1 cm. In this example the complex sclerosing lesion has papillary areas making it a complex sclerosing papillary lesion (**d**)

tion of breast tumors (Jan 2020) describes many new histological entities like florid lobular carcinoma in situ, and tall cell carcinoma with reverse polarity [15]. In this book, we aim to include radiologic and pathologic findings of these newer histological entities.

In summary breast pathologists have adapted to the evolving radiology field. Pathologists utilize various strategies to work up the tissue samples. For example, an X-ray of tissue blocks to find calcifications, performing multiple deeper tissue levels to find a mass lesion correlate, and X-rays of the fresh tissue to find metal clips are standard. In this book, we will share these simple but essential steps that are needed for the optimal workup of the breast tissue samples.

Radiologic-pathologic correlations are becoming a norm in academic and community practices with weekly dedicated multidisciplinary consensus conferences involving radiologists, pathologists, and surgeons involved in care of patients diagnosed with breast lesions on CNB. The consensus review followed by management suggestions, with change in a recommendation to repeat biopsy or follow-up imaging, is expected to improve the quality of care.

This radiology-pathology correlation book will be a helpful reference book with numerous case scenarios that will discuss examples of concordant and discordant cases with suggestions for a management plan.

Case presentations of concordant and discordant scenarios with relevant text and images are presented. Furthermore, management decisions in these patients need to be based on a correlation between radiological and pathological findings in a multidisciplinary setting. Knowledge of typical radiological findings of these histological entities is a must for practicing pathologists and trainees.

While there are several separate resources available for radiology residents to study imaging modalities, there are few if any books illustrating simultaneous radiology pathology correlates. Similarly, pathology residents and fellows are exposed to several textbooks on the pathology of breast biopsies. This textbook is expected to be a useful reference for residents, fellows, and practicing attendings in both disciplines. As the two disciplines of radiology and pathology are interrelated, the scope of the text is to provide and inform readers of not only typical examples of breast lesions that correlate with imaging findings that may or may not require surgical excision but also to resolve problematic lesions that are discordant with imaging findings. Our aim for this book is to create an easy-to-use simple and concise reference for radiology and pathology residents and fellows and practicing pathologists and radiologists, which would integrate the radiologic and pathologic appearance of relatively common breast lesions side-by-side, with easy-to-understand descriptions and illustrations.

Each chapter will outline a systematic approach to each disease entity punctuated by various imaging techniques, key diagnostic points seen on imaging and pathology followed by diagnostic considerations.

References

1. Cancer of the Breast (Female)—Cancer Stat Facts. *SEER*, https://seer.cancer.gov/statfacts/html/breast.html.
2. Corben AD, Edelweiss M, Brogi E. Challenges in the interpretation of breast core biopsies. Breast J. 2010;16:S5–9.
3. Youk JH, Kim EK, Kim MJ, et al. Sonographically guided14-gauge core needle biopsy of breast masses: a review of 2,420 cases with long term follow up. AJR Am J Roentgenol. 2008;190:202–7.
4. Schueller G, Jaromi S, Ponhold L, et al. Ultrasound guided 14-gauge core needle breast biopsy: results of a validation study in 1352 cases. Radiology. 2008;248:406–13.
5. Loberman L. Percutaneous image-guided core biopsy. Radiol Clin North Am. 2002;40:483–500.
6. Basset LW, Mahoney MC, Apple SK. Interventional breast imaging: current procedures and assessing for concordance with pathology. Radiol Clin North Am. 2007;45:881–94.
7. American College of Radiology. ACR practice guideline for the performance of ultrasound-guided percutaneous breast interventional procedures. Available at: http://www.acr.org/secondarymainmenucategories/quality_safety/guidelines/breast/us_guided_breast.aspx
8. Liberman L, Drotman M, Morris EA. Eta Imaging-histologic discordance at percutaneous breast biopsy: an indicator of missed cancer. Cancer. 2000;89:2538–46.
9. Parikh J, Tickman R. Image-guided tissue sampling: where radiology meets pathology. Breast J. 2005;11:403–9.
10. Idowu MO, Hardy LB, Souers RJ, et al. Pathologic diagnosis correlation with imaging findings: a College of American Pathologists Q-probes study of 48 institutions. Arch Pathol Lab Med. 2012;136:53–60.
11. Bleiweiss IJ, Jaffer S, Drossman SR. Breast core biopsy: a pathologic-radiologic correlative approach. Elsevier; 2008. ISBN:978-1-4160-0026-6
12. Youk JH, Kim EK, Kim MJ, Ko KH, Kwak JY, Son EJ, Choi J, Kang HY. Concordant or discordant? Imaging-pathology correlation in a sonography-guided core needle biopsy of a breast lesion. Korean J Radiol. 2011;12(2):232–40.
13. The American Society of Breast Surgeons; Consensus guideline on concordance assessment of image-guided breast biopsies and management of borderline or high-risk lesions: https://www.breastsurgeons.org/docs/statements/Consensus-Guideline-on-Concordance-Assessment-of-Image-Guided-Breast-Biopsies.pdf, 2016.
14. Weisman PS, Sutton BJ, Siziiopikou KP, et al. Non-mass- associated intraductal papillomas: is excision necessary? Hum Pathol. 2014;45:583–8.
15. WHO. Classification of tumors editorial board. In: Breast tumours. WHO classification of tumors. 5th ed. Lyon, France: IARC; 2019.

2 Circumscribed Masses

Malini Harigopal, Madhavi Raghu, Ramya Pham, Alexander Rende, Peter Podany, and Liva Andrejeva

Homogeneous Benign

Lactating Adenoma

Lactating Adenoma: Commonly referred to as nodular lactational hyperplasia, lactating adenomas are seen during the third trimester of pregnancy or postpartum [1]. They can be seen in fibroadenomas from nonpregnant or non-lactating women [1, 2]. These circumscribed lesions composed of compact enlarged glands with hyperplasia of lobules and secretory or lactational changes with scant intervening stroma. They may be multiple or bilateral and can undergo infarction.

M. Harigopal (✉) · P. Podany
Department of Pathology, Yale University, New Haven, CT, USA
e-mail: malini.harigopal@yale.edu; peter.podany@yale.edu

M. Raghu · A. Rende
Department of Radiology, Yale University, New Haven, CT, USA
e-mail: alexander.rende@yale.edu

R. Pham
Department of Radiology, Case Western Reserve University, Cleveland, OH, USA

L. Andrejeva
Department of Radiology and Biomedical Imaging, Yale School of Medicine, New Haven, CT, USA
e-mail: liva.andrejeva@yale.edu

- **Clinical Presentation**: Lactating adenomas can present as a palpable mass during pregnancy and lactation.
- **Imaging Findings**:
  - **Mammography**: Typically presents as a circumscribed oval or gently lobulated mass (Fig. 2.1).

    May manifest as a spiculated mass, in which case biopsy is recommended.
  - **MRI**: Similar to fibroadenoma; although rarely imaged with MRI.
  - **US**: Ultrasound is usually the initial modality for evaluation as these masses present in pregnant and lactating patients.

    These tumors closely resemble fibroadenomas in that they also appear as circumscribed oval or gently lobulated, hypo- to isoechoic masses, but are usually more vascular than fibroadenomas (Fig. 2.2).

    Rarely, this may appear as a complex cystic and solid mass.
  - **BI-RADS**: 3.
  - **Differential Diagnosis**: Benign: fibroadenoma, tubular adenoma. Malignant: circumscribed cancer, particularly high-grade IDC (invasive ductal carcinoma).
- **Pathology Findings**:
  - **Microscopic Histology**: The hyperplasia of the lobules results from increase in the number of acini which exhibit secretory changes [3] (Fig. 2.3).

M. Harigopal et al. (eds.), *Radiology Pathology Correlations of Breast Lesions*,
https://doi.org/10.1007/978-3-031-65711-5_2

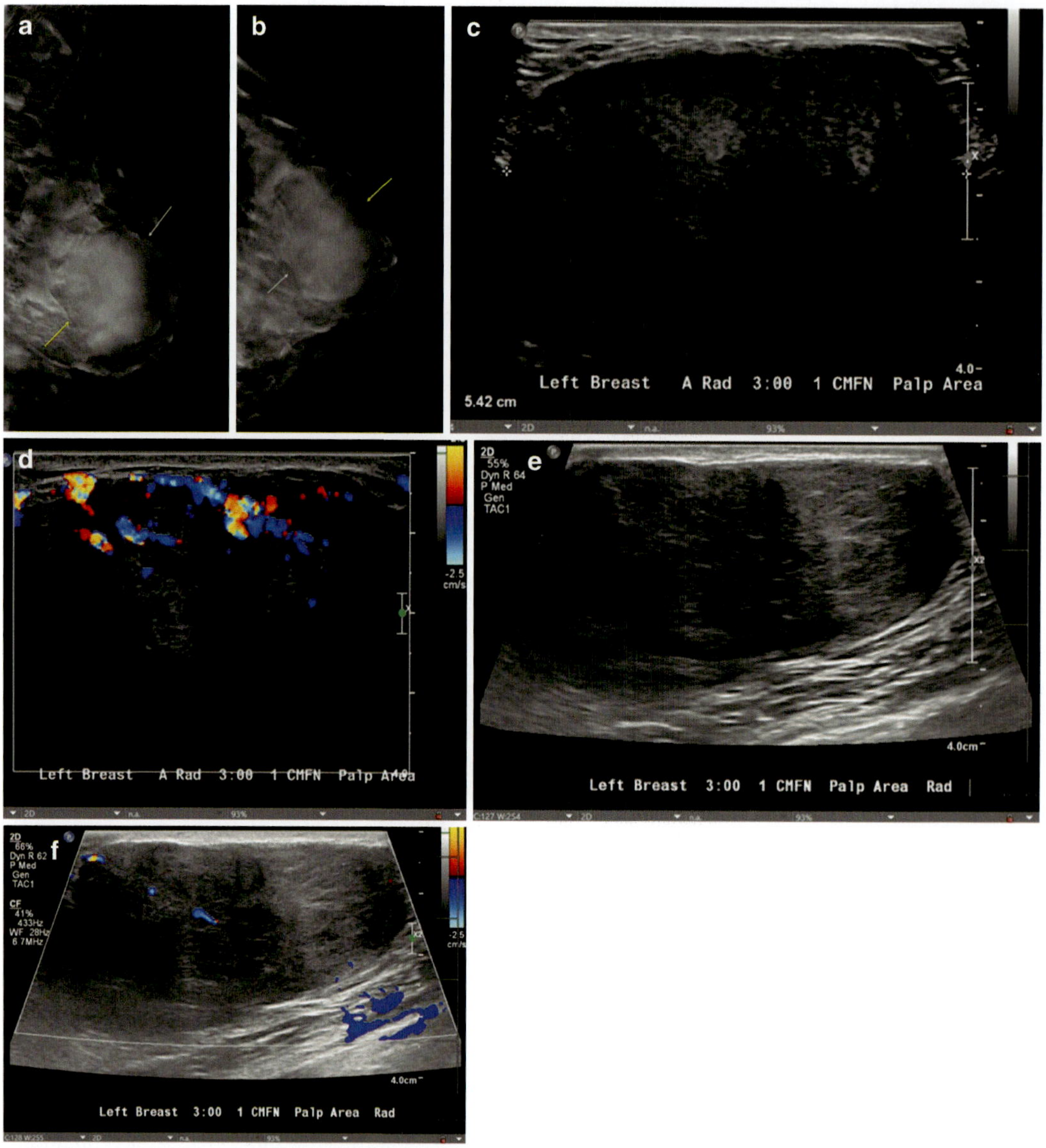

Fig. 2.1 A 23-year-old lactating woman presented with a palpable left breast mass. Mammography (**a**, **b**) and ultrasound (**c**, **d**) revealed a lobulated, hypoechoic mass. Biopsy revealed a lactational adenoma. The same patient presented for follow-up 2 years later due to persistence of the left breast mass which was once again seen on ultrasound (**e**, **f**). Excisional biopsy now showed a fibroadenoma with the prior biopsy clip identified

Lactating adenomas are regarded as hyperplasia of normal lactational breast tissue rather than a neoplasia.
On low power magnification, histologic examination shows nodules of hyperplastic breast tissue with circumscribed margins.

On higher power examination, nuclear enlargement with cytoplasmic vacuolization and hobnail appearance is evident.
The lesion is completely benign and eventually resolves spontaneously [3].

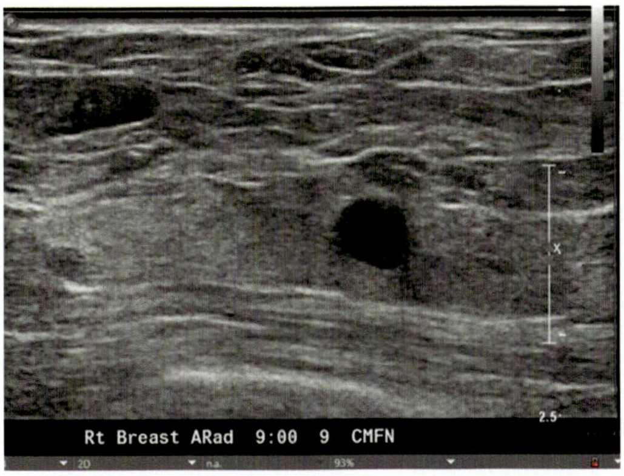

Fig. 2.2 A 34-year-old breastfeeding woman presented for early screening due to high-risk genetics. Mammography was negative but ultrasound revealed a circumscribed, hypoechoic lesion that was biopsied and found to be a lactating adenoma

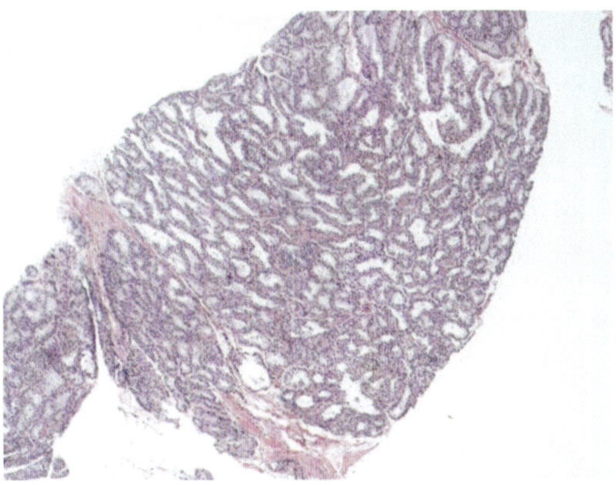

Fig. 2.3 A 34-year-old woman presented for biopsy of a possible mass versus cyst to evaluate for atypia or malignancy. On imaging the lesion was moderately suspicious/ BI-RADS 4. Ultrasound-guided biopsy was performed. The lesion showed a circumscribed border composed of hyperplastic lobules lined by cuboidal epithelium with vacuolated cytoplasm and some lumen containing eosinophilic secretions indicative of a lactating adenoma

- **Differential Diagnosis**: Fibroadenoma, fibrocystic changes, abscess, galactocele.
- **Management**: Benign imaging findings do not require biopsy. Occasionally suspicious findings on sonography with irregular shape or margins may need active intervention to exclude malignancy. Diagnosis on core needle biopsy requires no further workup or follow-up by imaging.

Adenomyoepithelioma

Adenomyoepithelioma: Seen in women with an age range of 26–82 years old [4]. It is considered a variant of intraductal papillomas. Adenomyoepitheliomas are rare and considered to be benign, but may demonstrate malignant transformation, especially when larger than 2 cm [5].

- **Clinical Presentation**: Adenomyoepitheliomas can present as solitary painless masses. Smaller lesions may be detected on screening imaging.
- **Imaging Findings**:
  - **Mammography**: Variable appearance: oval, circumscribed mass, irregular mass with indistinct margins, or a focal asymmetry (Fig. 2.4).
  - **US**: Variable appearance: oval, circumscribed mass, irregular mass, complex cystic and solid mass.
  - **BI-RADS**: 3 or 4 depending on presentation and imaging appearance.
  - **Differential Diagnosis**: Fibroadenoma, phyllodes, pseudoangiomatous stromal hyperplasia (PASH), papilloma, papillary carcinoma, IDC.
- **Pathology Findings**:
  - **Microscopic Histology**: Histology shows nodular aggregates composed of a compact proliferation of inner epithelial and outer myoepithelial cells [6, 7] (Fig. 2.5).

    The myoepithelial cells can have clear cytoplasm which contrasts with the darkly stained epithelial cells that may undergo apocrine, sebaceous, squamous or mucoepidermoid metaplastic changes. Margins are generally well circumscribed.

    The three variants described by Tavassoli are spindle, tubular, and lobulated types based on the architectural patterns [4].
  - **Differential Diagnosis**: Sclerosing adenosis, intraductal papilloma, tubular adenoma, invasive ductal carcinoma.
  - **Management**: When diagnosed on core needle biopsy, an excisional biopsy with adequate margins is recommended to avoid recurrences [4, 6].

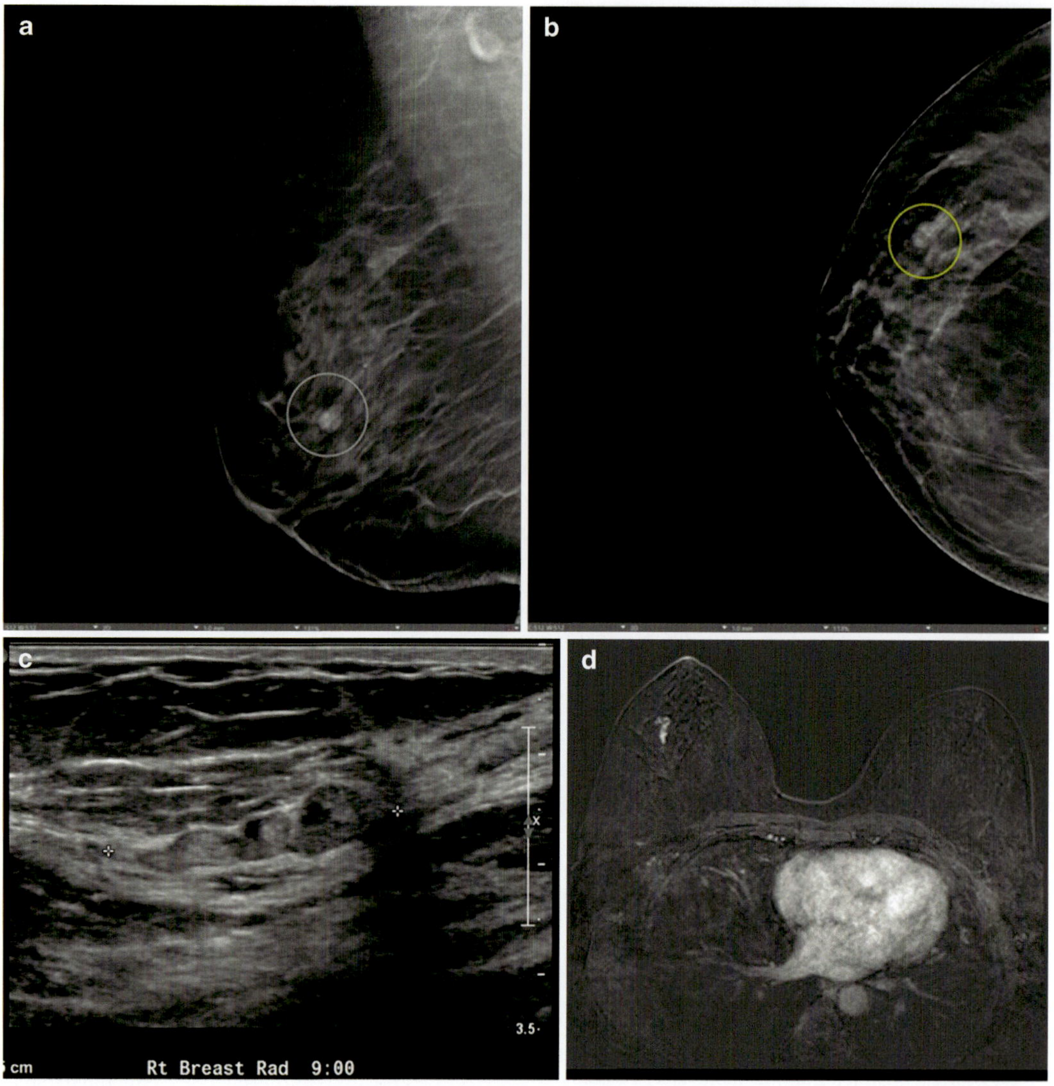

Fig. 2.4 A 60-year-old woman with a left breast mass presented for diagnostic evaluation. An incidental right breast mass was seen on mammography (**a**, **b**), ultrasound (**c**), and MRI (**d**). She underwent core needle biopsy of both the left breast mass and the incidental right breast mass revealing poorly differentiated invasive ductal carcinoma in the left breast and a papillary adenomyoepithelioma in the right breast

Intraductal Papilloma

See Chap. 3.

Galactocele

See Chap. 3.

Fibroadenoma

Fibroadenoma: Fibroepithelial lesions are composed of stromal and epithelial components admixed in varying proportions. A fibroadenoma (FA) is a benign circumscribed mass of the terminal ductal lobular unit. The stroma therefore resembles the connective tissue of

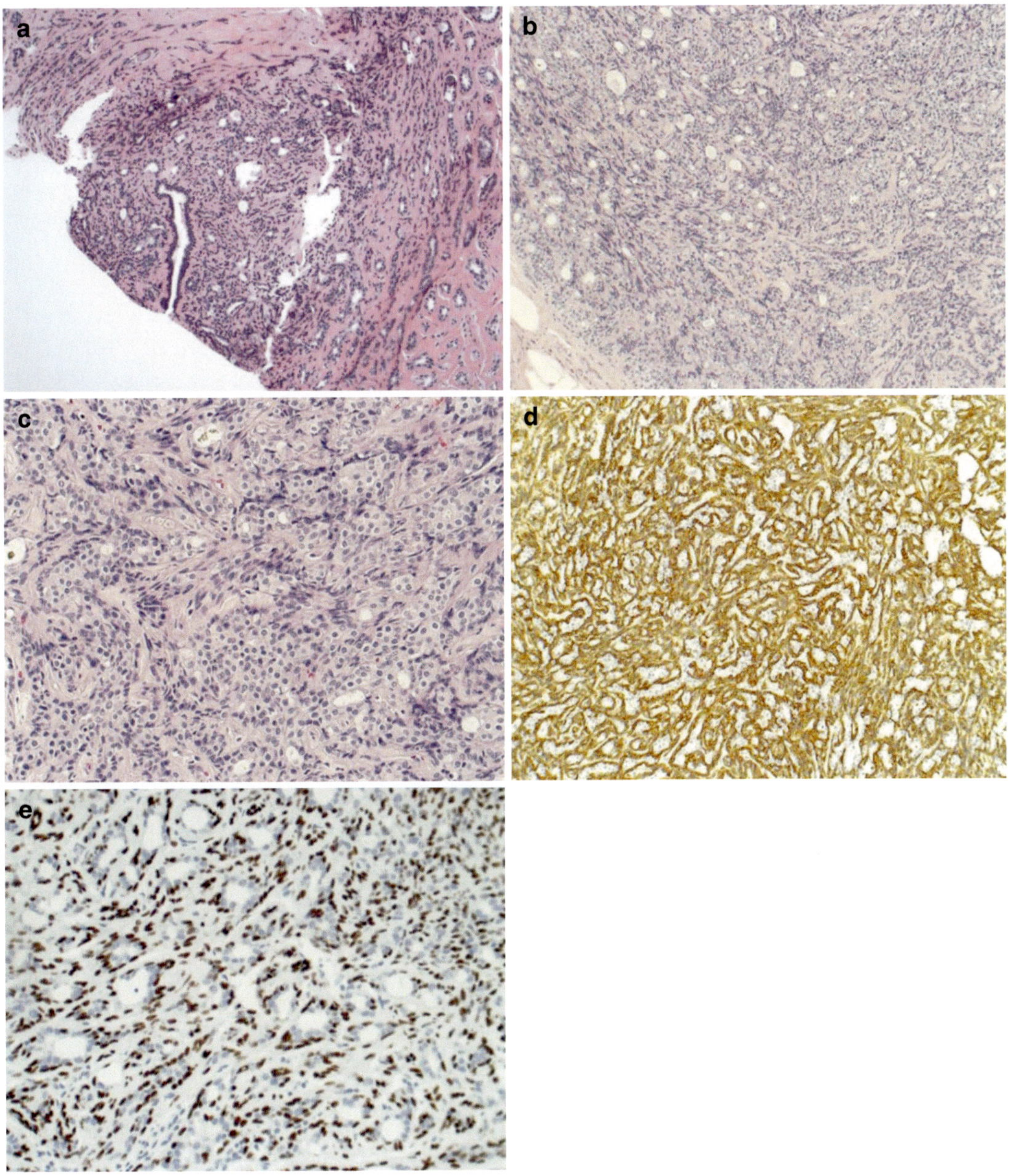

Fig. 2.5 A 25-year-old woman was found to have a 3.9 cm lobulated mass with amorphous calcifications in her right breast, suspicious for a fibroadenomatous lesion. US-guided biopsy was performed which revealed a complex sclerosing lesion involved by sclerosing adenosis and calcifications (**a**). Biphasic growth with glandular epithelial cells and spindled myoepithelial cells highlighted by CK5/6 and p63 raised the possibility of adenomyoeithelioma. The lesion was subsequently excised and found to be an adenomyoepithelioma with circumscribed lobulated margins (**b**). In this biphasic tumor the myoepithelial cells are prominent and spindled, compressing glands as well as epithelial cells (**c**). CK 5/6 and p63 staining on the resection specimen highlights the spindled myoepithelial cells (**d** and **e** respectively)

normal perilobular stroma. The stroma may contain benign heterologous elements such as mature adipose and smooth muscle tissue [8, 9]. The epithelial component is usually composed of well-defined ductal or glandular structures lined by benign columnar cells that may undergo hyperplastic changes in the form of usual ductal hyperplasia [9]. The stroma can compress the glands creating slit-like spaces referred to as an "intracanalicular" pattern. Alternatively, when the glandular components maintain their rounded contour it is referred to as a "pericanalicular" pattern [8, 9]. There is no clinical significance in making this distinction as both patterns can be seen in FA. The term complex FA is used when the FA is composed of cysts >3 mm, papillary apocrine changes, calcifications and sclerosing adenosis (Figs. 2.6 and 2.7). Cellular FA are composed of increased stromal cellularity without stromal atypia or increased mitoses (Figs. 2.8 and 2.9). Occasionally FA seen predominantly in younger women and in adolescents can grow rapidly with increased stromal cellularity and glandular epithelial proliferation concerning for atypical ductal hyperplasia or carcinoma in situ, raising concern for phyllodes tumor [10, 11] (Fig. 2.10). Giant FA are similar to FA histologically but are very large. Phyllodes tumors on the other hand have increased stromal cellularity in combination with an enhanced intracanalicular growth pattern forming cleft-like or leaf-like spaces into which the epithelium protrudes [9].

Radiology-pathology correlation is critical in some situations where the distinction between FA and phyllodes tumor cannot be readily made on core needle biopsy due to overlapping features.

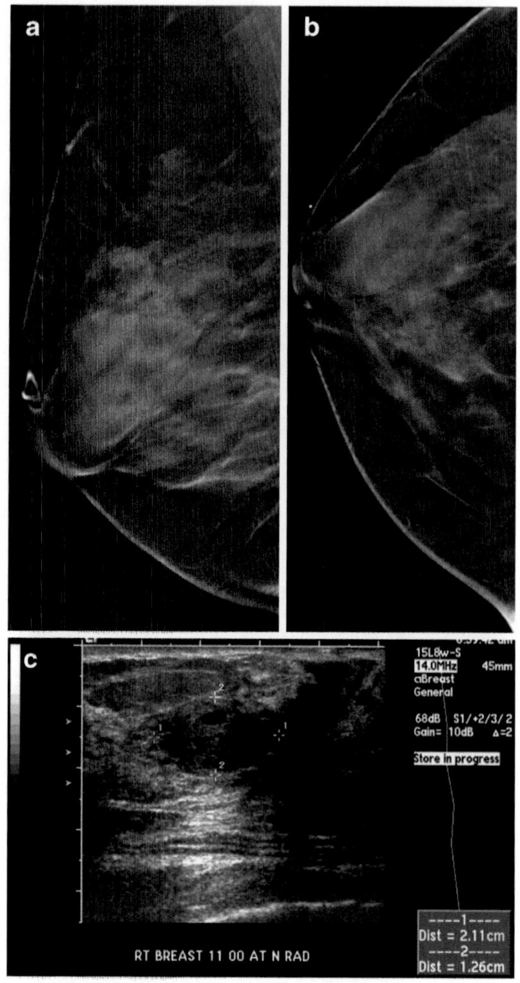

Fig. 2.6 A 35-year-old woman presents with a palpable abnormality. On mammography a 2-cm circumscribed mass is noted just posterior to the nipple (**a**, **b**). Ultrasounds show that at the 11 o'clock axis at the nipple, corresponding to the palpable abnormality, there is a 2.3-cm oval well-circumscribed hypoechoic mass with a few cystic areas (**c**). This appears to represent an interval change from the prior study and is indeterminate. On biopsy the lesion is diagnosed as a complex fibroadenoma

- **Clinical Presentation**: Usually seen in younger women <35 years, with complex FA occurring older patients [8]. Presents as solitary, mobile masses that are slow growing and are generally painless.
- **Imaging Findings**:
  - **Mammography**: A classic mammographic appearance of a fibroadenoma is a circumscribed, oval mass with 2–3 gentle lobulations, isodense to the breast parenchyma (Fig. 2.11).

    When degenerating, fibroadenomas may contain coarse calcifications, often described as "popcorn" calcifications.

    Fibroadenomas that have a classic appearance are one of the originally described BI-RADS 3 lesions.

    A growth of >20% in 6 months prompts a biopsy recommendation, as circumscribed cancers and phyllodes tumors may mimic benign fibroadenomas.

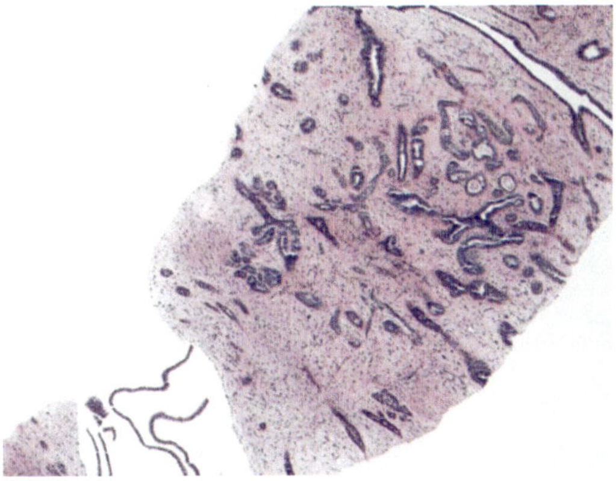

Fig. 2.7 A patient presented with a suspicious right breast mass at 10:00. On imaging the lesion was moderately suspicious, BI-RADS 4, evaluate for malignancy. Ultrasound-guided biopsy was performed and showed a biphasic fibroepithelial tumor with cysts and adenosis, diagnosed as a complex fibroadenoma

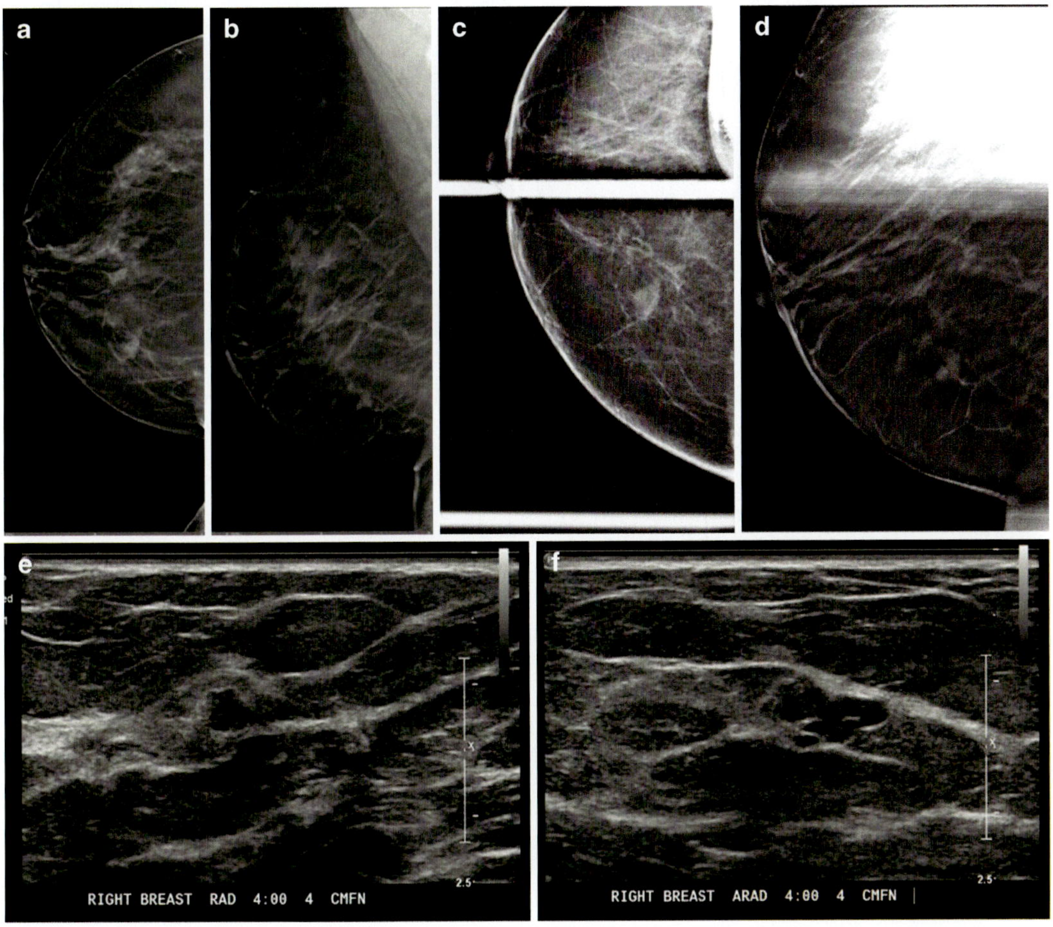

Fig. 2.8 A 48-year-old woman presents with a 1 cm mass with a circumscribed margin in the right breast at 4 o'clock middle depth noted on screening mammogram (**a**, **b**). Spot compression views again demonstrate similar findings (**c**, **d**). On ultrasound a complex cystic mass with a 0.5 cm × 0.4 cm × 0.4 cm solid component in the right breast at 4 o'clock middle depth 4 cm from the nipple is seen (**e**, **f**). This lobulated mass is hypoechoic with a hyperechoic rim and correlates to the mammographic finding. This was subsequently biopsied and found to be a cellular fibroadenoma with adjacent apocrine cysts

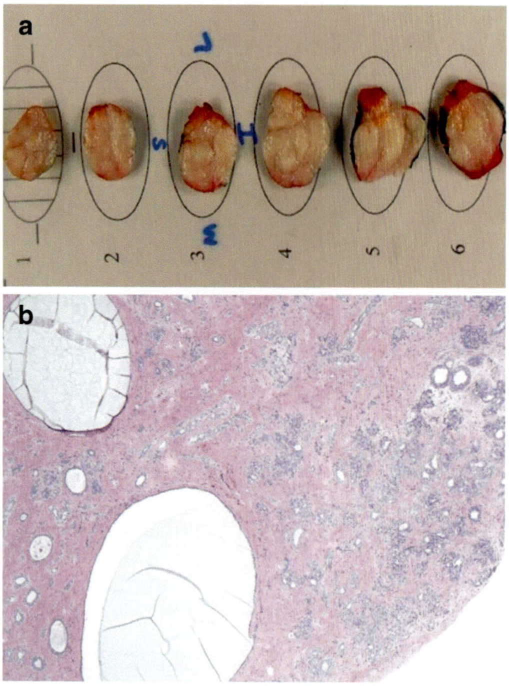

Fig. 2.9 A 45-year-old woman presents with a 1.5 cm mass with a circumscribed margin in the left breast at 7 o'clock middle depth noted on screening mammogram. On ultrasound a complex cystic mass with a 0.7 cm × 0.5 cm × 0.4 cm solid component in the left breast at 7 o'clock middle depth is seen. The lesion was subsequently biopsied. On gross examination the lesion was firm, smooth, tan-white, with well circumscribed, lobulated margins (**a**). Histology demonstrated a cellular fibroadenoma with adjacent clustered apocrine cysts (**b**)

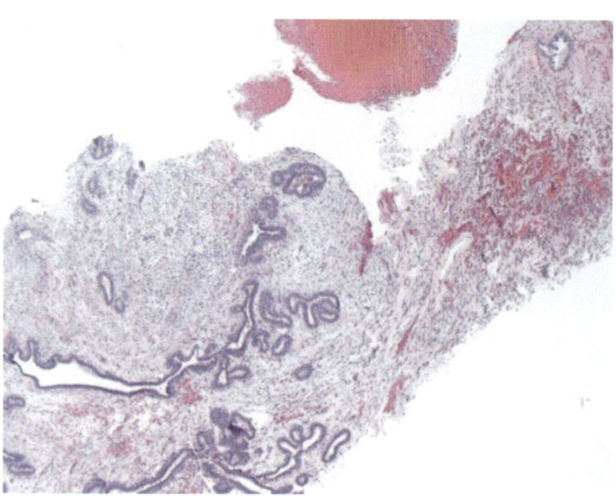

Fig. 2.10 A 37-year-old woman presents with a left breast retroareolar mass. Ultrasound is moderately suspicious, BI-RADS 4. Biopsy showed a fibroepithelial lesion. The fibroepithelial lesion showed a mild increase in stromal cellularity and mild cytological atypia. Rare mitoses are seen within the stroma. On excision a borderline phyllodes tumor is diagnosed

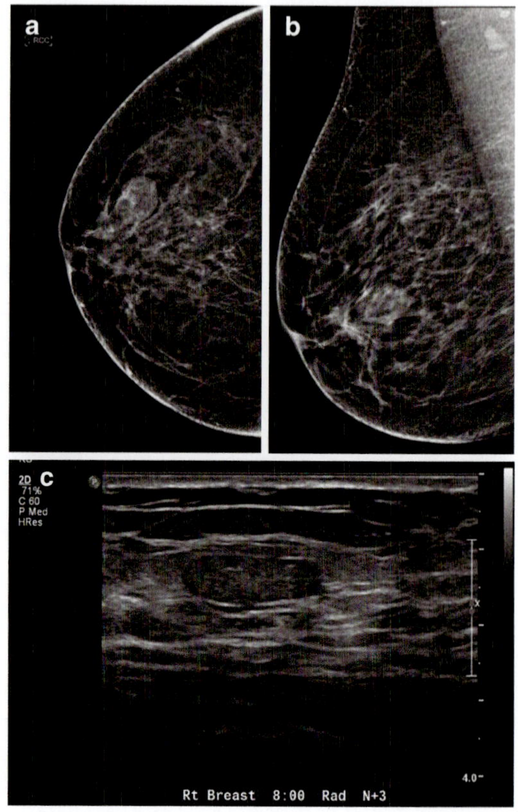

Fig. 2.11 A 63-year-old woman presented for screening mammogram. The dominate finding was a stable circumscribed equal density mass measuring 2.8 cm, central to the nipple, as well as a new focal asymmetry posteriorly (**a**, **b**). She was then called back for an ultrasound for further investigation of the focal asymmetry (**c**). Ultrasound showed a stable mass with a circumscribed margin in the right breast at 8 o'clock middle depth. This oval mass is isoechoic with circumscribed margins, and no internal flow on color doppler noted, 3 cm from the nipple. The lesion was later biopsied and found to be a fibroadenoma

- **MRI**: Hyperintense on T2 images and classically contains non-enhancing internal septations. Postcontrast: Progressively enhancing, oval, circumscribed mass.
- **US**: Circumscribed, oval or gently lobulated, hypoechoic mass. Internal vascularity may be present.
- **BI-RADS**: 3.
- **Differential Diagnosis**: Benign: lactating adenoma, papilloma, PASH, tubular adenoma, benign phyllodes. Malignant: IDC, including TNBC, DCIS, malignant phyllodes, metastases.

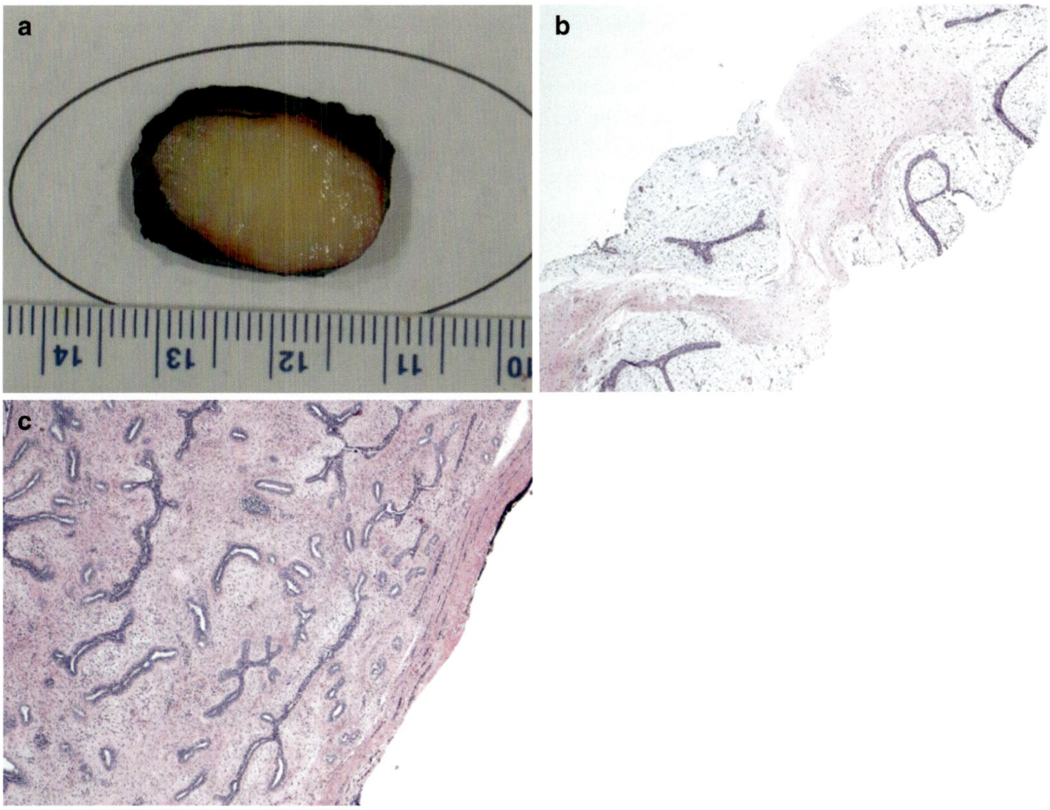

Fig. 2.12 A fibroadenoma exhibiting a firm smooth gray-white bulging cut surface (**a**). On core biopsy the tumor is biphasic with stromal and glandular elements (**b**). On excision the specimen shows peripheral circumscription with homogeneous stroma and glands arranged in an intracanalicular growth pattern with elongated slit-like lumen (**c**)

- **Pathology Findings**:
  - **Gross Description**: Smooth, lobulated, yellow with circumscribed margins that can be easily shelled out (Fig. 2.12).
  - **Microscopic Histology**: Biphasic pattern with epithelial and stromal components. Stroma may be hyalinized with calcifications in older patients which can be visualized on imaging (Fig. 2.13).
  - **Differential Diagnosis**: Complex FA, juvenile FA, phyllodes tumor.
  - **Management**: Most fibroadenomas are best treated conservatively with observation in the form of imaging surveillance.

    However, surgical excision for definitive diagnosis is recommended in patients when the lesion is symptomatic or rapidly growing in order to rule out malignancy [12, 13].

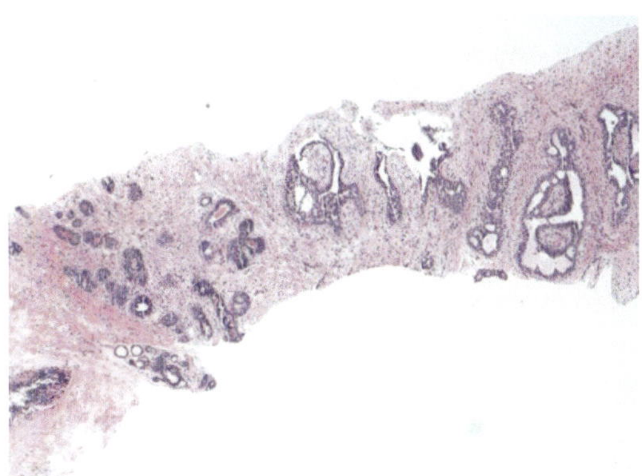

Fig. 2.13 A 39-year-old woman presented with a right breast mass. Ultrasound was moderately suspicious, BIRADS 4, rule out atypia or malignancy. Core needle biopsy showed a fibroadenoma with biphasic proliferation of epithelial and stromal components with circumscribed borders. The fibroadenoma also demonstrated involvement by usual ductal hyperplasia

Large fibroadenomas are often resected surgically due to patient symptoms or concern for sampling error on core needle biopsy. Emotional distress in the setting of a breast mass and aesthetic concerns are patient-driven reasons why surgical removal of fibroadenomas may be performed.

Given the exceptionally low likelihood of malignancy, surgical excision should be used judiciously and offered only after thorough patient education [11–13].

Alternative management suitable for smaller (<4 cm diameter), biopsy-proven fibroadenomas are cryoablation and percutaneous excision [13].

Phyllodes Tumor

Phyllodes Tumor: Phyllodes tumors of the breast are rare fibroepithelial neoplasms, representing up to 0.3–1% of breast tumors [6, 14]. They may occur within a wide age range (12–87), but usually occur in the 40–50 age group [6, 14]. Most phyllodes tumors are benign, with borderline and malignant tumors occurring less frequently. Larger tumors have a higher likelihood of malignancy, however, even benign tumors may recur after wide local excision. Malignant phyllodes are distinguished from benign phyllodes by invasive borders, high stromal cellularity, and extensive stromal overgrowth [6, 15, 16]. The risk of recurrence increases with increasing tumor size and if the patient had a lumpectomy instead of mastectomy [17]. Borderline and malignant phyllodes metastasize hematogeneously to lung and bone in 10% of cases [6]. The ten-year survival is 87%, no different from the age-adjusted population [6].

- **Clinical Presentation**: They often present as a fast-growing, circumscribed, large mass without calcifications [14]. Most patients present in their 40s [6, 14]. They may also be screening detected.
- **Imaging Findings**:
  - **Mammography**: Large, high density, round or oval, rapidly growing mass with circumscribed or indistinct margins (Fig. 2.14).

    Rarely contains calcifications.

    Malignant tumors may be irregular (Fig. 2.15).
  - **US**: Benign tumors may mimic fibroadenomas, with uniform echotexture.

    Borderline and malignant lesions are more likely to be heterogeneous, complex cystic and solid masses with fluid-filled spaces, with vascularity present [18].
  - **MRI**: Multilobulated mass that enhances rapidly and intensely without washout.

    May have internal non-enhancing septations similar to fibroadenomas [19].

    Solid enhancing areas within cystic blood-filled spaces can be seen.
  - **BI-RADS**: 4, suspicious, but may be mistaken for probably benign lesions.
  - **Differential Diagnosis**: Fibroadenoma, metaplastic carcinoma, sarcoma.
- **Pathology Findings**:
  - **Gross Description**: Circumscribed fleshy masses with well-defined margins that can be easily shelled out when benign.

    Cleft or leaf-like spaces present.

    Hemorrhage, necrosis, and ill-defined margins may be seen in borderline and malignant phyllodes tumors.
  - **Microscopic Histology**: Biphasic pattern with epithelial and stromal components and an exaggerated intracanalicular growth pattern forming leaf-like spaces (Fig. 2.16).

    Phyllodes tumors are a spectrum of tumors that encompass lesions from benign to malignant.

    In benign phyllodes tumors, the stroma tends to be more cellular than FA with periductal stromal condensation. Stroma may be hyalinized with myxoid changes resulting in stromal heterogeneity and

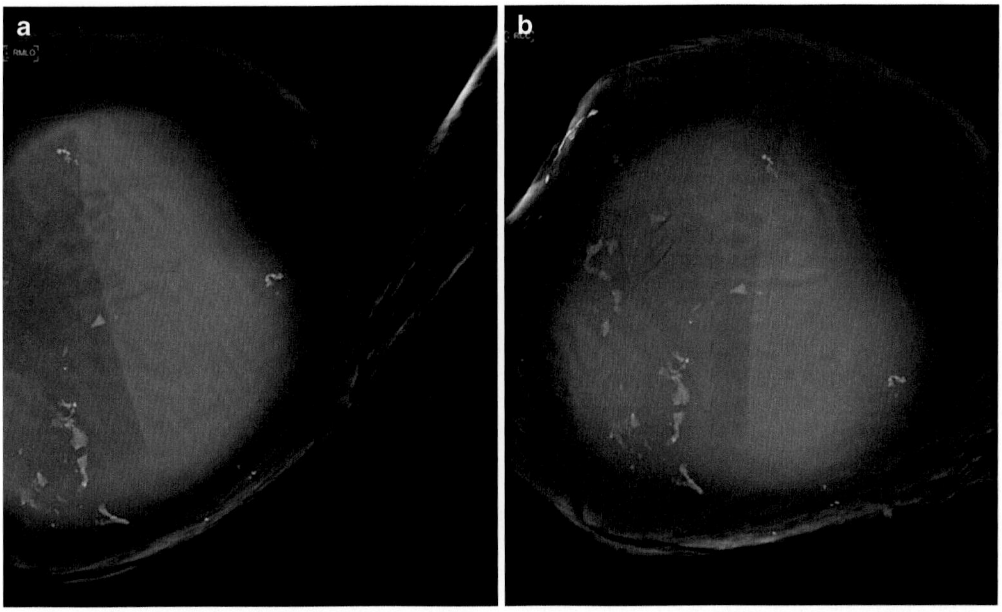

Fig. 2.14 A 43-year-old woman with severe agoraphobia who does not routinely receive medical treatment, presents with bleeding from an ulcer in a severely enlarged right breast. A chart review reveals that the patient presented with a palpable right breast mass 6 years ago, but declined further evaluation or treatment. At the hospital, a pressure dressing was placed on the ulcerated area to manage the bleeding. The dressing was removed 3 days later in order to perform diagnostic mammography, and uncontrollable bleeding from the ulcerated area ensued. The patient was taken to the operating room for an emergency mastectomy. On mammography a large, round mass with an indistinct margin within a severely distorted breast is seen (**a**, **b**). Coarse calcifications are present. Ultrasound was not performed due to bleeding. The mass is called BI-RADS: 4, suspicious. Mastectomy was performed. Due to the malignant nature of this phyllodes tumor, a chest CT was obtained to exclude pulmonary metastases, and was negative

resemblance to FA on core needle biopsy. Margins are usually well defined. Stromal atypia is minimal or absent with stromal mitosis averaging <2–5 mf (mitotic figures) per 10 hpf (high power fields) [19]. Multinucleated stromal giant cells, adipose and osseous metaplasia can be seen in benign phyllodes tumors (Fig. 2.17).

In borderline phyllodes tumors the margins can be focally infiltrative and stromal cellularity may be moderate with mild to moderate stromal atypia and stromal mitosis averaging 5–9 mf per 10 hpf [19] (Fig. 2.18).

In malignant phyllodes tumors there is increased stromal cellularity, stromal overgrowth (stroma occupies a low power microscopic field without epithelial components), marked stromal atypia and stromal mitosis averages >10 per 10 hpf. The margins are usually infiltrative (Fig. 2.19).

The presence of malignant heterologous mesenchymal components such as chondroid or lipomatous elements even in the absence of other stromal features is used as a diagnostic criterion for malignancy (with the exception of well-differentiated liposarcoma as the only heterologous component) [19, 20].

- **Differential Diagnosis**: Benign phyllodes tumors should be distinguished from cellular FA, and juvenile FA. Malignant phyllodes tumors should be distinguished from frankly malignant spindle cell sarcomas and metaplastic carcinomas.
- **Management**: Complete excision to prevent local recurrence is the main treatment [14]. Addition of radiation therapy for large tumors can aid in decreasing recurrence [14]. Chemotherapy is not beneficial.

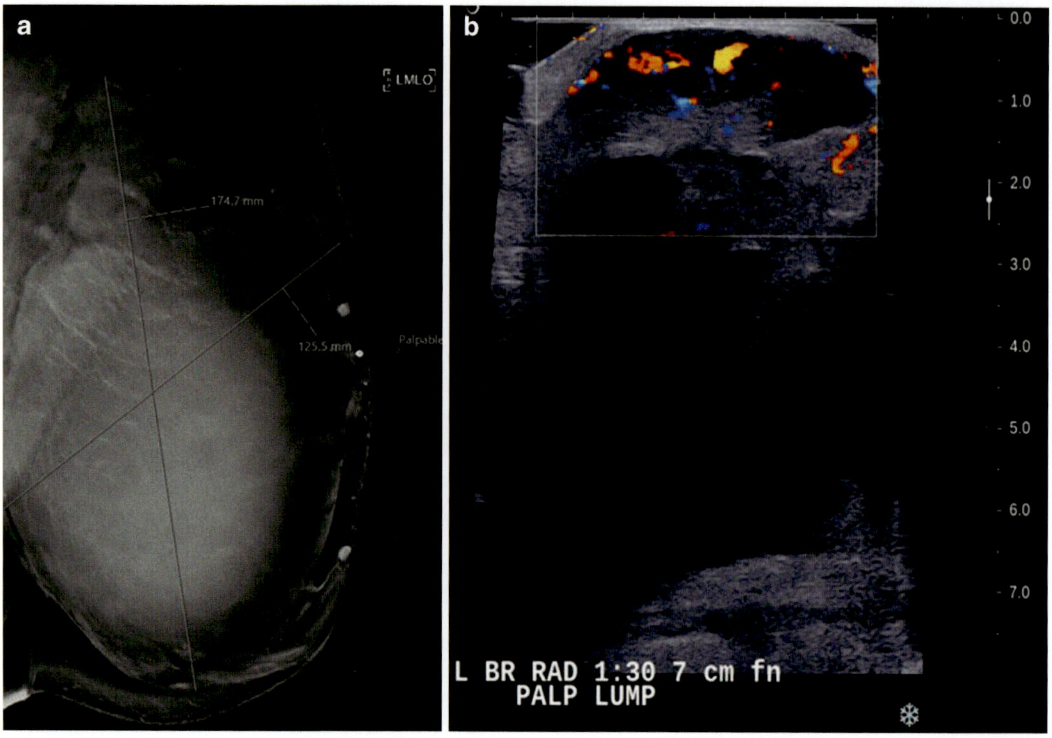

Fig. 2.15 A 55-year-old woman presented with a palpable lump on her left breast. Mammography demonstrates an irregular, partially circumscribed, increased density mass measuring 17.5 cm (**a**). Ultrasound demonstrates an irregular complex cystic and solid mass with internal vascularity and posterior enhancement (**b**). A biopsy is taken, and the pathology revealed a malignant phyllodes tumor

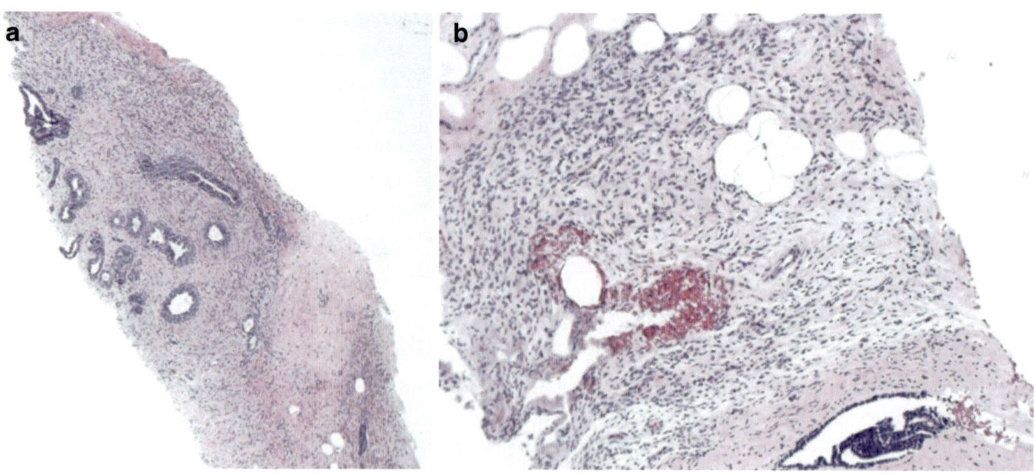

Fig. 2.16 A 55-year-old woman with multiple solid masses in the right breast presented for biopsy to rule out cancer. Biopsy showed a fibroepithelial tumor (**a**) with infiltrative margins (**b**) suggestive of a possible phyllodes tumor

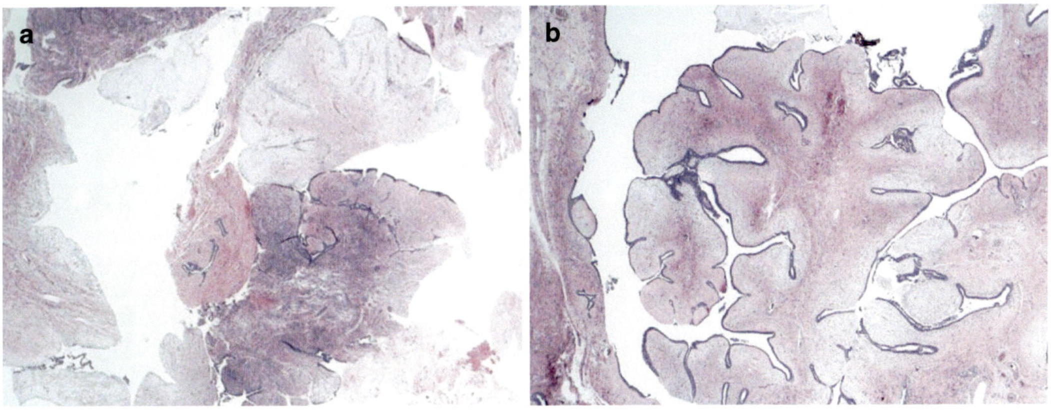

Fig. 2.17 A 45-year-old female presents with a palpable breast mass. Core needle biopsy shows a biphasic tumor with heterogeneous appearance with areas of increased stroma cellularity alternating with hypocellular areas (**a**). The patient then undergoes a lumpectomy which reveals a well-circumscribed mass with bulging firm cut surface with foci of hemorrhage and cystic degeneration. On histology a benign phyllodes tumor with well-defined border and leaf-like projections into cystic spaces can be seen (**b**). Note the condensation of stroma adjacent to the elongated epithelial-lined clefts

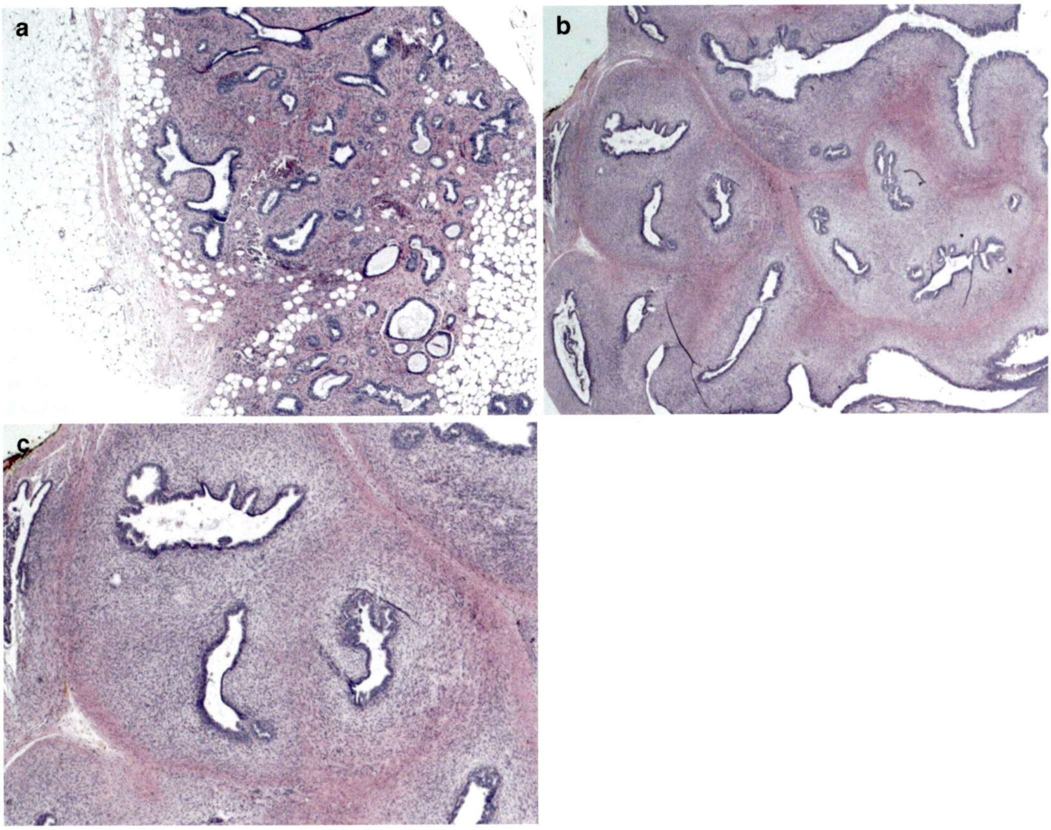

Fig. 2.18 A 38-year-old woman presents with a palpable mass in her left breast and underwent core needle biopsy which shows a biphasic tumor with moderately cellular stroma and infiltration into fat (**a**). She then undergoes excisional biopsy and grossly the tumor exhibits a predominantly well-defined border except for a focal area grossly infiltrative into adjacent fat in the inferior aspect. Histology from the excision shows moderately cellular stroma with mild to moderate stromal atypia (**b**, **c**). The tumor margins are focally infiltrative

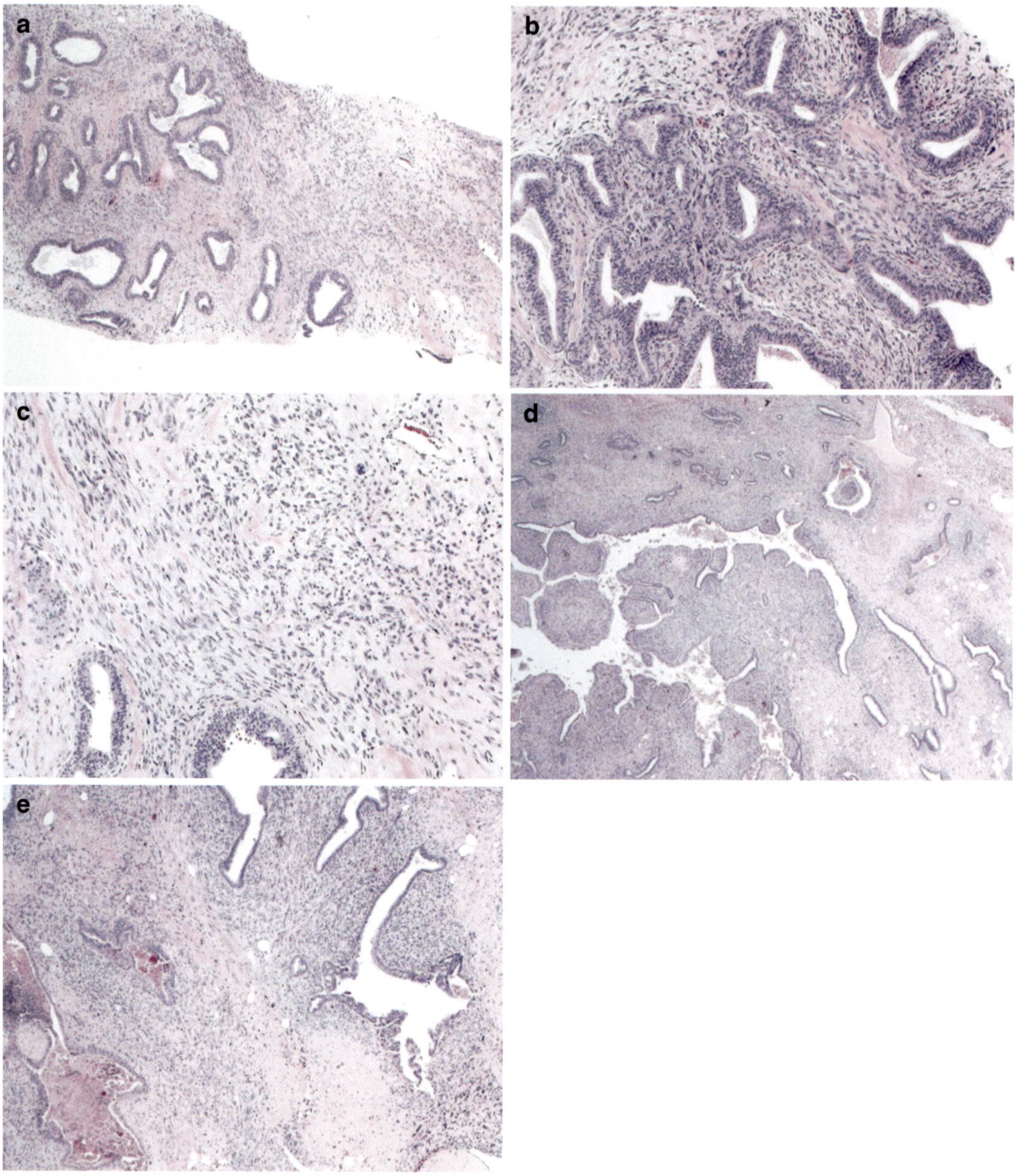

Fig. 2.19 Core biopsy demonstrating a fibroepithelial lesion with cellular stroma, marked stromal atypia, and increased mitoses raising concern for a malignant phyllodes tumor (**a** 50×, **b** 100×, **c** 200×). Excision showed a malignant phyllodes tumor with marked stromal cellularity and cellular atypia (**d** 100×, **e** 200×)

Nodular Fibrocystic Changes

Nodular Fibrocystic Changes: Fibrocystic changes are a common finding in women of reproductive age, with decreased incidence in postmenopausal women. Exposure of breast tissue to excess estrogen and decreased progesterone results in hyperproliferation of connective tissue leading to fibrosis [21]. This is followed by proliferation of the terminal ductal lobular units. Obstruction of the ducts may then lead to cyst formation characteristic of fibrocystic change.

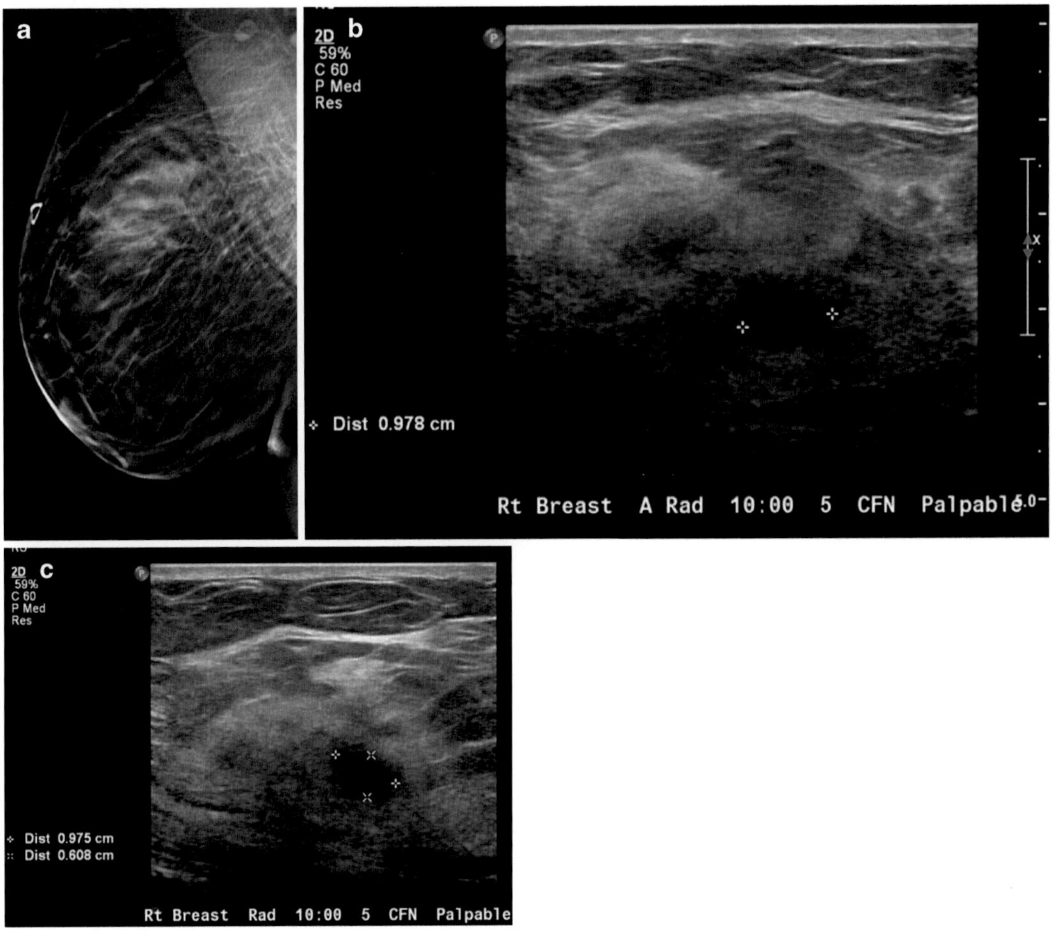

Fig. 2.20 A 53-year-old woman presented with a palpable abnormality in her right breast. Mammography showed a 4-cm irregular focal asymmetry with an indistinct margin and clustered punctate calcifications in the right breast at 10 o'clock middle depth which correlated with the palpated mass (**a**). Diffuse trabecular thickening involving the upper outer quadrant of the right breast was also noted. Ultrasound showed there are several 1 to 2.5 cm irregular lesions with indistinct margins in the right breast superior lateral quadrant middle depth which are hypoechoic (**b**, **c**). These lesions correlate with mammography findings. Biopsy later showed benign nodular fibrocystic changes

- **Clinical Presentation**: The patient may present with breast pain, tenderness or a palpable mass which may be cyclic with their menstrual cycle. Involvement is usually bilateral [21, 22]. The condition is not considered a disease but rather a normal variation in breast tissue that can fluctuate with the menstrual cycle.
- **Imaging Findings**:
  - **Mammography**: Nodular fibrocystic changes may appear as an oval, round, or lobular mass without calcifications (Fig. 2.20).

    The margins of the mass may be partially circumscribed with at least partially indistinct margins.

    Satellite nodules may also be noted.
  - **US**: On ultrasound, nodular fibrocystic changes present as an oval, round, or lobulated hypoechoic mass with mostly circumscribed, partially indistinct margins.

    Microlobulated margins may be observed due to the presence of ductal carcinoma in situ (DCIS).

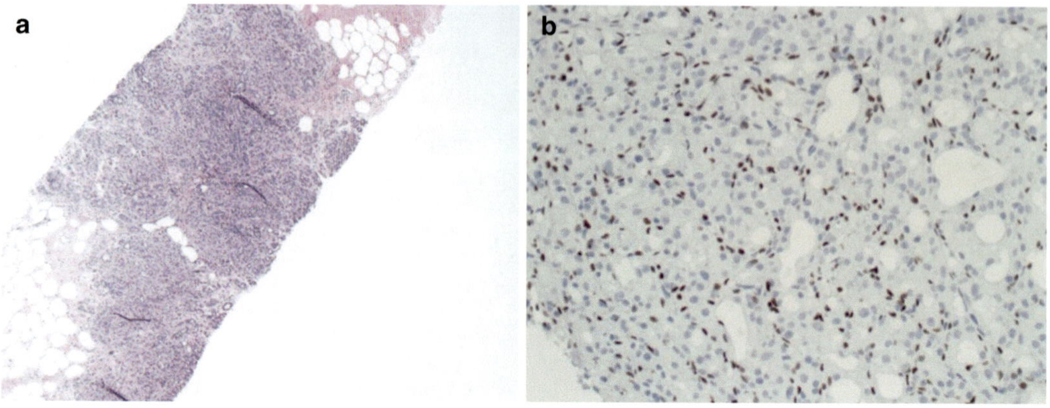

Fig. 2.21 A patient presented with a suspicious left breast mass at 4:00. Imaging was moderately suspicious/ BI-RADS 4 rule out carcinoma versus fibrocystic changes. Ultrasound-guided biopsy was performed and showed nodular sclerosing adenosis (**a**), with p63 highlighting retained myoepithelial cells (**b**) and supporting the diagnosis

Internal cystic areas from necrosis and posterior enhancement can be present, giving a "pseudo-cystic" appearance.

There is no flow on color Doppler, and the wall and surrounding tissue may appear stiff on elastography.

- **BI-RADS**: 2, 3, 4.
- **Differential Diagnosis**: Fibroadenoma: Another common benign breast tumor characterized by localized proliferation of breast ducts and stroma [23].

  Invasive Ductal Carcinoma (poorly differentiated): A subtype of breast cancer.

  Phyllodes tumor: A rare tumor that can be benign, borderline, or malignant and arises from the stroma of the breast [23].

  Non-Hodgkin's lymphomas: Lymphomas that can involve the breast tissue [23].

• **Pathology Findings**:

- **Microscopic Histology**: Nodular fibrocystic changes demonstrate cystically dilated ducts and lobules with retained myoepithelial cells (Fig. 2.21).

  Stromal fibrosis is present leading to the nodular or mass-like appearance of the lesion.

  May be associated with other benign breast changes such as adenosis, apocrine metaplasia or columnar cell changes.
- **Differential Diagnosis**: Usual ductal hyperplasia, sclerosing adenosis, cystic fibroadenoma.
- **Management**: If suspicious on imaging findings a core needle biopsy to rule out a malignant process is warranted. Otherwise, medical management of fibrocystic disease with low-estrogen oral contraceptives can be considered [21].

Homogeneous Malignant Breast Masses

Homogeneous malignant breast masses share many similar features on imaging. Specifically, they are more likely to present as oval masses with partially circumscribed margins. However, there are differences and some unique identifiable features, albeit subtle. This is described below in more detail.

Poorly Differentiated Invasive Ductal Carcinoma

Poorly Differentiated Invasive Ductal Carcinoma: Poorly differentiated invasive ductal carcinoma (IDC) is defined as a grade 3 IDC not otherwise specified (NOS). IDC NOS make up 70–80% breast cancers of which 45% are grade 3 poorly differentiated [14]. They tend to be estrogen receptor (ER) negative, HER2 positive, or triple negative [14]. Approximately 10% of invasive carcinomas can present as circumscribed

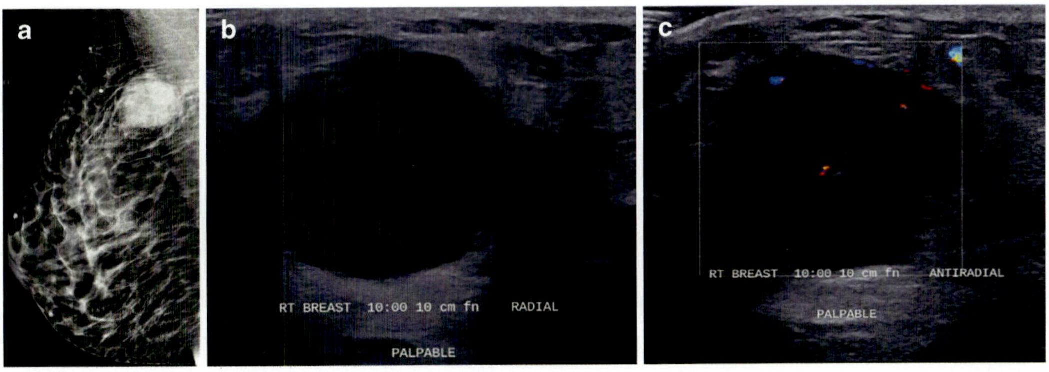

Fig. 2.22 A 26-year-old woman presents with a palpable lump. On mammogram, 2D MLO view shows an oval mass with indistinct margins and increased density (**a**). A metallic BB marker is noted near the mass. Ultrasound (**b**) demonstrates an irregular, hypoechoic mass with partially circumscribed margins and posterior enhancement. Ultrasound with Doppler (**c**) demonstrates an irregular, hypoechoic mass with internal vascularity. The mass is biopsied, and pathology demonstrates IDC grade 3, triple negative

masses. The majority are grade 3 invasive ductal carcinomas with well-defined circumscribed margins on gross and microscopic examination.

- **Clinical Presentation**: Often present as a large, firm palpable mass. They are more frequent in African American women who have a higher death rate from the disease than other groups [6].
- **Imaging Findings**:
  - **Mammography**: New or enlarging focal or global asymmetry or circumscribed, dense mass.

    If it presents as a mass, higher likelihood of circumscribed margins (36% for grade 3 versus 18% for grade 1 tumors) [18, 24].

    Associated calcifications may be noted in 37% of grade 3 tumors [18, 24].
  - **US**: Irregular, hypoechoic mass with circumscribed or partially circumscribed margins (Fig. 2.22).

    Posterior enhancement noted in 45% of grade 3 tumors [25].

    Internal vascularity and stiffness on elastography may be noted.
  - **MRI**: Irregular mass with circumscribed or indistinct margins which can be T2 bright from central necrosis.

    May demonstrate rim enhancement.

    Washout or plateau delayed enhancement in >90% of IDC [19].
  - **BI-RADS**: 4 or 5.
  - **Differential Diagnosis**: Mucinous (colloid), medullary, encapsulated or invasive papillary carcinomas.
- **Pathology Findings**:
  - **Microscopic Histology**: The tumors exhibit syncytial or solid growth pattern with absence of gland or tubule formation [26] (Fig. 2.23).

    The nuclei are high grade with prominent nucleoli.

    Mitoses are easily identified with frequent lymphocytic infiltrate.

    Stromal fibrosis and necrosis are seen centrally.

    These tumors are usually triple negative [20, 26].
  - **Differential Diagnosis**: Invasive lobular carcinoma and metastases to the breast.
  - **Management**: Standard treatment is surgery +/-radiation with consideration for chemotherapy and hormonal therapy if applicable [14]. In decreasing order, prognosis is based on nodal status > histologic grade > tumor size. Grade 3 tumors tend to be larger and more likely to be node positive at presentation [14]. While they respond better to chemotherapy, they also have higher risk of early relapse, metastasis, and death [14].

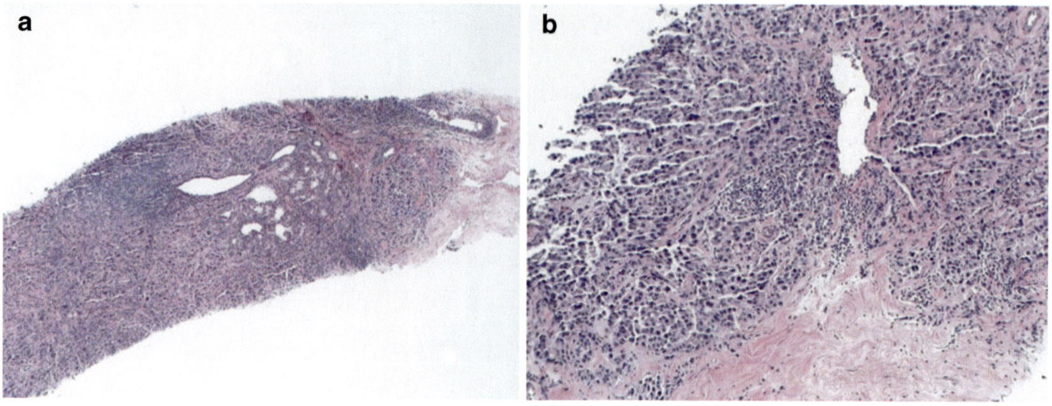

Fig. 2.23 A 32-year-old woman presented with a palpable abnormality at 11:00 on her left breast. The patient was breast-feeding at the time but had a family history of breast cancer (mother age 56). Imaging showed a hypoechoic mass. On biopsy the patient was found to have poorly differentiated invasive ductal carcinoma associated with lactational changes (**a**, **b**)

Carcinoma with Medullary Features

Medullary carcinoma is a rare subtype of invasive ductal carcinoma (IDC). It accounts for less than 5% of malignant breast tumors and 10% of malignant tumors in women 35 years of age or less [27, 28]. It has been defined as "well circumscribed carcinoma composed of poorly differentiated cells with scant stroma and prominent lymphoid infiltration" [26]. Five-year survival is 89–95%, better than for IDC NOS [14]. High recurrence rates occur in patients with tumor size greater than 3 cm with four or more involved nodes [14]. When recurrences occur, they happen early and are rare 5 years or more after diagnosis [14]. The relatively good prognosis is attributed to the presence of tumor infiltrating lymphocytes in these tumors.

- **Clinical Presentation**: Presents as an enlarging, soft, palpable mass with enlarged ipsilateral axillary nodes, even when there are no nodal metastases [14, 27]. Mean patient age is 45–54 years [14].
- **Imaging Findings**:
  - **Mammography**: Oval, round, or lobular mass without calcifications (Fig. 2.24).
    Margins are partially circumscribed with at least partially indistinct margins.
    Satellite nodules are commonly noted.
  - **US**: Oval, round, or lobulated hypoechoic mass with mostly circumscribed, partially indistinct margins (Fig. 2.25).
    Microlobulated margins due to the presence of DCIS may be noted [18].
    Internal cystic areas from necrosis and posterior enhancement can be present, causing a "pseudo-cystic" appearance.
    No flow on color or power Doppler.
    Wall and surrounding tissue are stiff on elastography.
  - **MRI**: Oval, round or lobulated mass with smooth margins, rapid initial contrast uptake and washout or plateau delayed enhancement [19].
    Cystic areas will be bright on T2 weighted images.
    Key distinguishing feature is that the internal architecture is heterogeneous.
  - **BI-RADS**: 2, 3, or 4.
  - **Differential Diagnosis**: Fibroadenoma, IDC poorly differentiated, phyllodes tumor, non-Hodgkin's lymphomas.
- **Pathology Findings**:
  - **Microscopic Histology**: These tumors exhibit high histologic grade, solid architecture (lack tubule formation) with syncytial growth pattern, and high mitotic rate (Figs. 2.26 and 2.27).
    Tumors are associated with tumor infiltrating lymphocyte-rich stroma with pushing margins and areas of geographic necrosis.

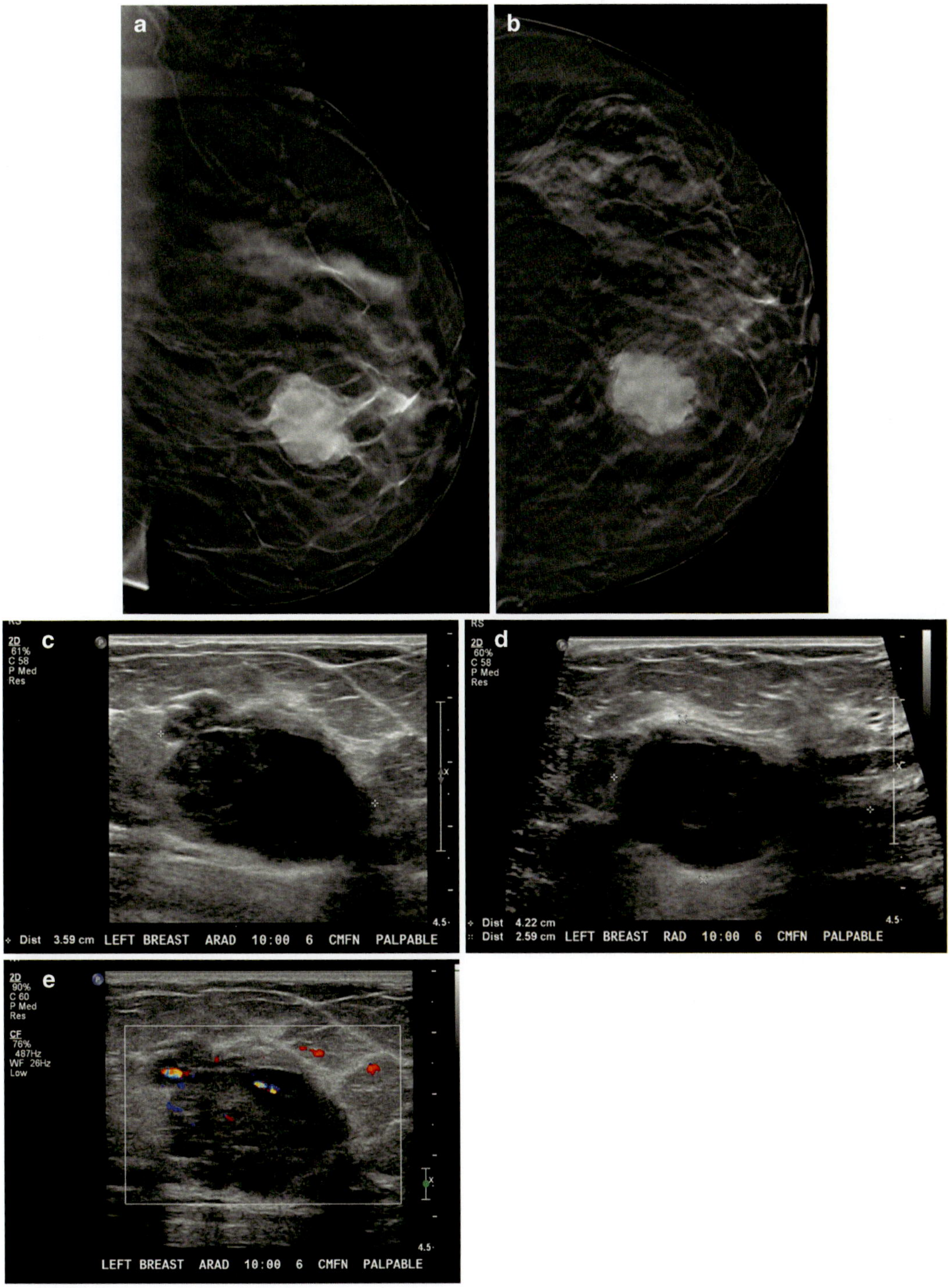

Fig. 2.24 A 73-year-old woman presents with a new palpable left breast mass. Mammography shows a 3.8-cm irregular high-density mass with a microlobulated margin in the left breast at 10 o'clock middle depth 5 cm from the nipple (**a**, **b**). There is adjacent focal asymmetry along its anterior aspect that may correspond to possible intraductal extension seen on ultrasound. On ultrasound there is a 4.2 cm × 3.6 cm × 2.6 cm irregular mass with a microlobulated margin in the left breast at 10 o'clock middle depth, 6 cm from the nipple (**c**, **d**). This irregular mass is hypoechoic. Color flow imaging demonstrates that there is vascularity present (**e**). There may be subtle intraductal extension anteriorly. This correlates with mammographic findings. The patient undergoes core needle biopsy which revealed a medullary carcinoma

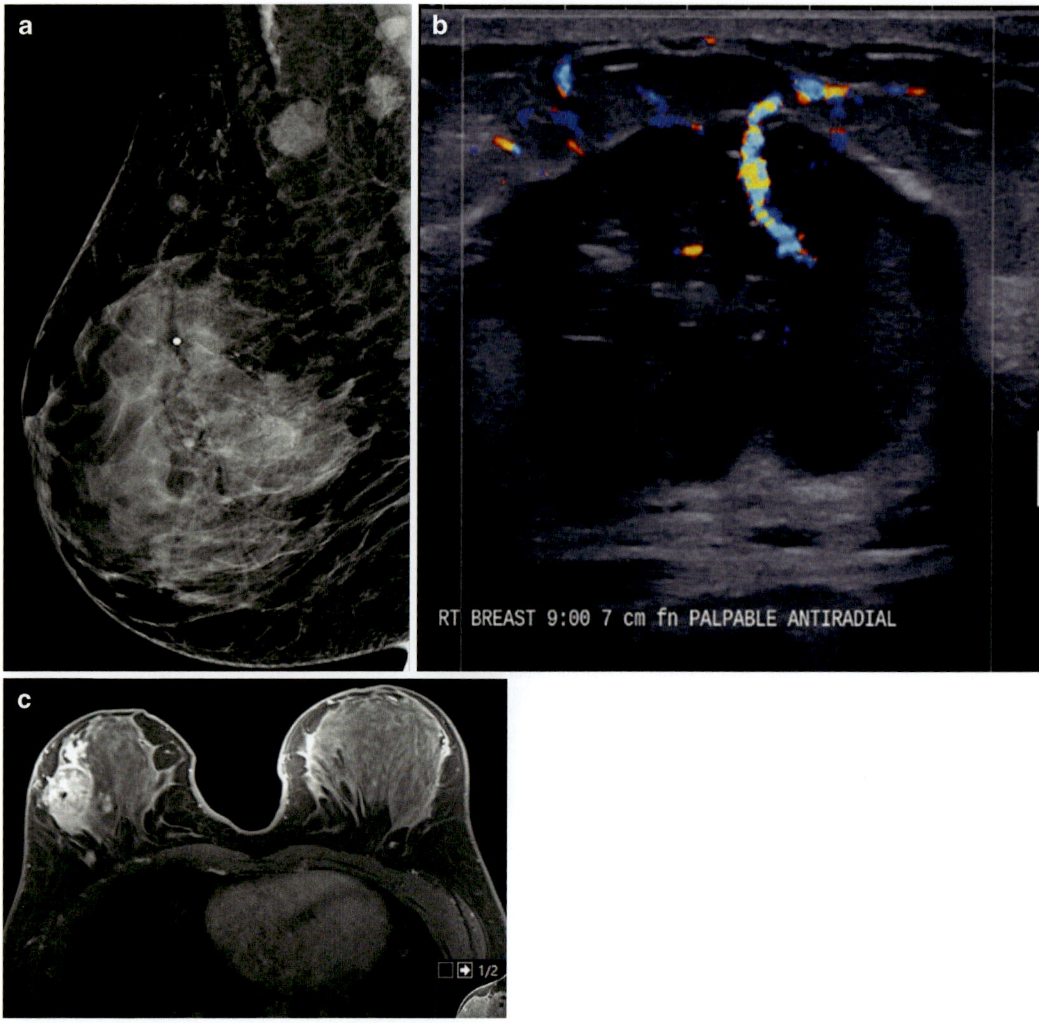

Fig. 2.25 A 26-year-old woman presents with a palpable lump in her right breast. Mammography shows an asymmetry in the central breast at posterior depth and axillary adenopathy (**a**). A metallic BB marker denoting the palpable lump is noted superior to the asymmetry. Ultrasound demonstrates an irregular, hypoechoic mass with partially circumscribed margins and marked internal vascularity (**b**). MRI (Axial postcontrast T1 weighted image with fat suppression) demonstrates an irregular, avidly enhancing mass laterally in the right breast with central signal void from a biopsy clip (**c**). The lesion is biopsied to show medullary carcinoma with lymphohistiocytic infiltrate and spread to lymph nodes

They have an ER-, PR-, HER2-negative (triple negative) biomarker profile.

They variably express basal keratin (CK5/6, EGFR).

– **Differential Diagnosis**: Includes other circumscribed breast cancers (IDC NOS, mucinous carcinoma, papillary carcinoma), non-Hodgkin's lymphoma, classic fibroadenoma, and phyllodes tumor [20].
– **Management**: Standard treatment includes lumpectomy with radiation therapy (and mastectomy when needed) and sentinel lymph node biopsy [14]. Chemotherapy may be indicated based on the size of the tumor and nodal status [14].

Mucinous Carcinoma

Mucinous Carcinoma: Mucinous carcinoma is a rare subtype of IDC also known as colloid, mucous, mucoid, or gelatinous carcinoma. It is a highly differentiated cancer that accounts for about 4% of malignant breast tumors [14]. There are two types: pure type (greater than 90% of tumor shows mucin production), and mixed type (less than 90% of tumor shows mucin production) [18, 29]. Ten-year survival for pure type is 90% (better than for IDC NOS) and mixed type is same as for IDC NOS [14]. Tumor size is not predictive of survival given that the mucinous component may compose a large part of the mass.

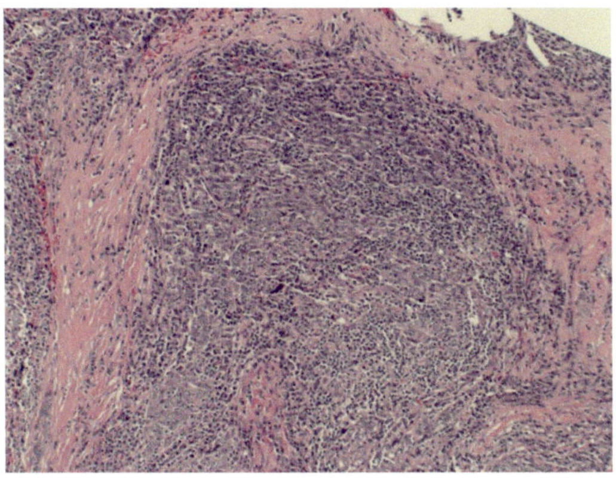

Fig. 2.26 A 30-year-old woman presents with a palpable lump in her right breast. Mammography showed asymmetry. Ultrasound showed an irregular, hypoechoic mass with partially circumscribed margins and marked internal vascularity. A biopsy was performed revealing a medullary carcinoma with poorly differentiated cells, and a prominent lymphohistiocytic infiltrate. The tumor is ER 90%, PR 60%, Her2 positive

It is not unusual to have systemic recurrences after 10 years [14]. Unusual metastases with mucin emboli causing fatal cerebral infarcts and pseudomyxoma peritonei can occur [14].

- **Clinical Presentation**: Presents as a palpable, slow-growing mass in 50% of patients [14]. The remaining patients present with nonpalpable masses on screening mammography. Mean age of presentation is in the seventh or eighth decade [18].
- **Imaging Findings**:
  - **Mammography**: Oval, round, or irregular mass of increased density with indistinct margins and rare calcifications (Figs. 2.28 and 2.29).

    Irregular shape and speculated margins seen more commonly in the mixed type. The more circumscribed the margins are, the lower the grade.

    Calcifications are rare and when present are associated with mixed type.
  - **US**: Oval, round, or irregular isoechoic mass with partially circumscribed or microlobulated margins.

    Posterior enhancement noted in more than 50% cases.

    The pure types appear more homogeneous, and the mixed types appear more as complex cystic and solid masses [18].

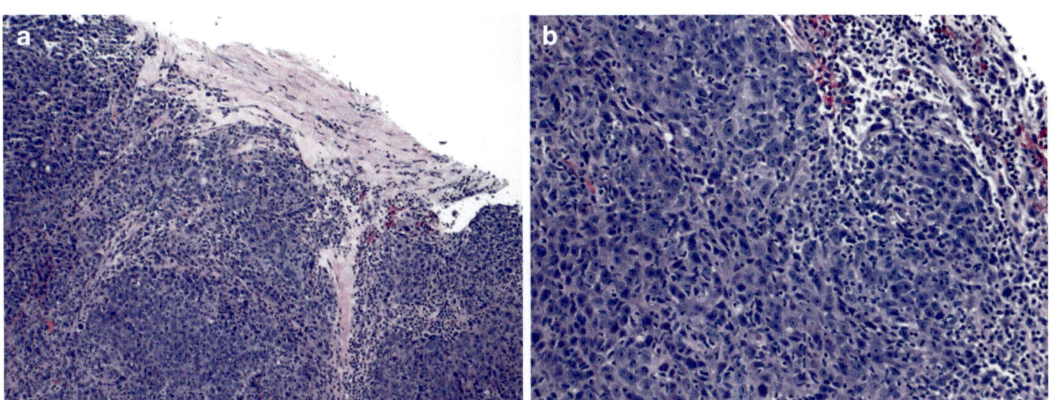

Fig. 2.27 A 77-year-old woman presents with a new palpable right breast mass. Mammography shows a 2.5-cm irregular high-density mass with a microlobulated margin. The patient undergoes core needle biopsy which revealed a circumscribed, poorly differentiated carcinoma with large lymphocytic infiltrate consistent with invasive ductal carcinoma with medullary features (**a**, **b**)

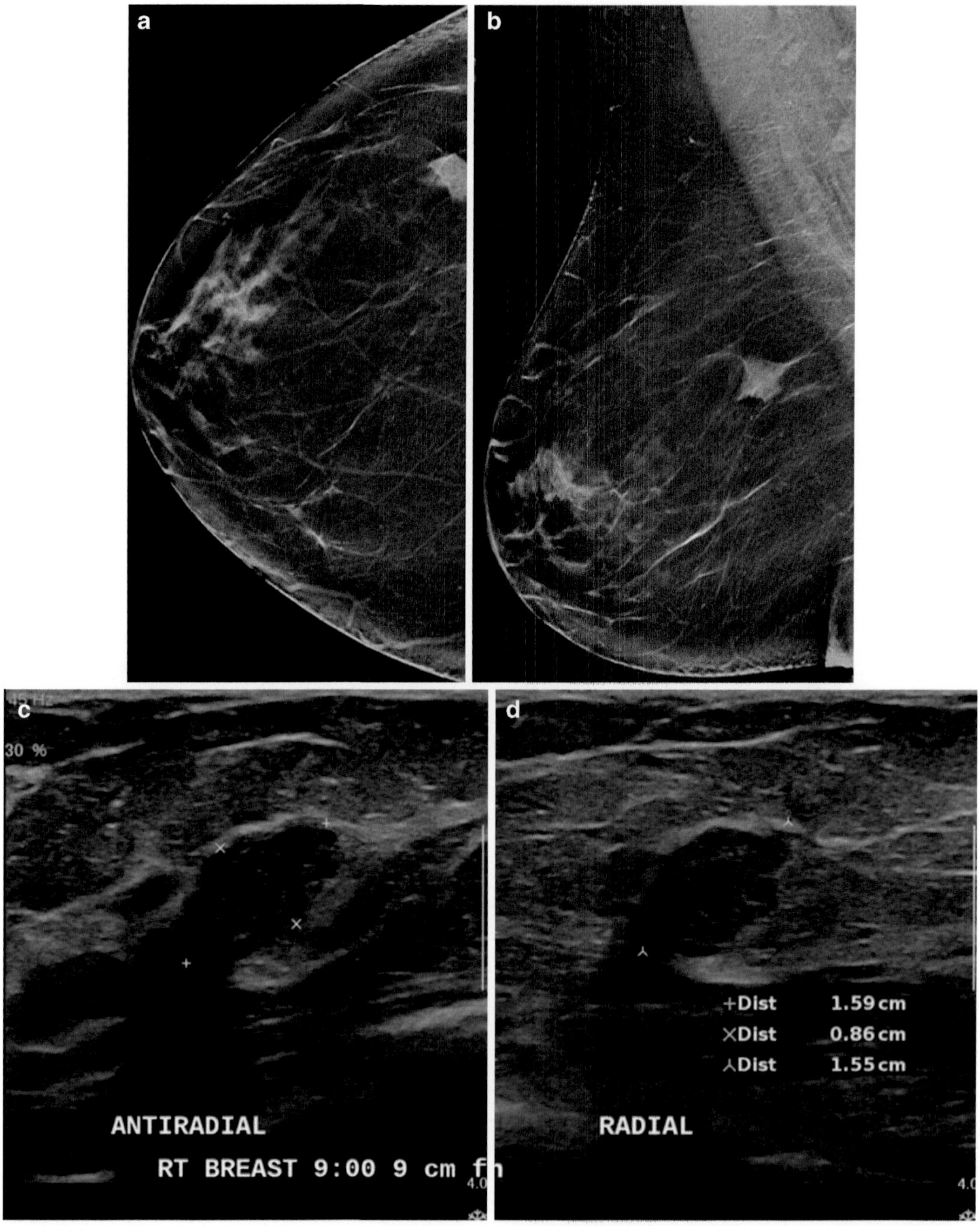

Fig. 2.28 A 65-year-old woman presents with a mass seen on screening mammogram. Mammography demonstrates a focal asymmetry centrally at posterior depth (**a**, **b**). Ultrasound demonstrates an oval, circumscribed hypoechoic mass (**c**, **d**). The lesion was biopsied revealing a mucinous carcinoma

Given that they are isoechoic to fat, they can be hard to identify and possibly overlooked by the sonographer.

Vascularity is seen in about a third of the tumors and they are usually soft on elastography [18].

– **MRI**: Oval, round, or lobulated mass with smooth, microlobulated, or indistinct margins.

The level of enhancement depends on the amount of solid component versus mucinous component [19].

The larger the solid component, the more rapid and intense the enhancement.
Some masses contain predominantly mucin with a thin rim of peripheral enhancement.
The areas of the tumor with mucin are very hyperintense on the T2 weighted images.

- **BI-RADS**: 3 or 4.
- **Differential Diagnosis**: Fibroadenoma, lipoma, poorly differentiated ductal carcinoma, fat lobule, mucocele-like tumor.

• **Pathology Findings**:
  - **Microscopic Histology**: Small clusters of tumor cells are seen floating in extracellular pools of mucin (Fig. 2.30).
    Nuclei are low to intermediate grade.

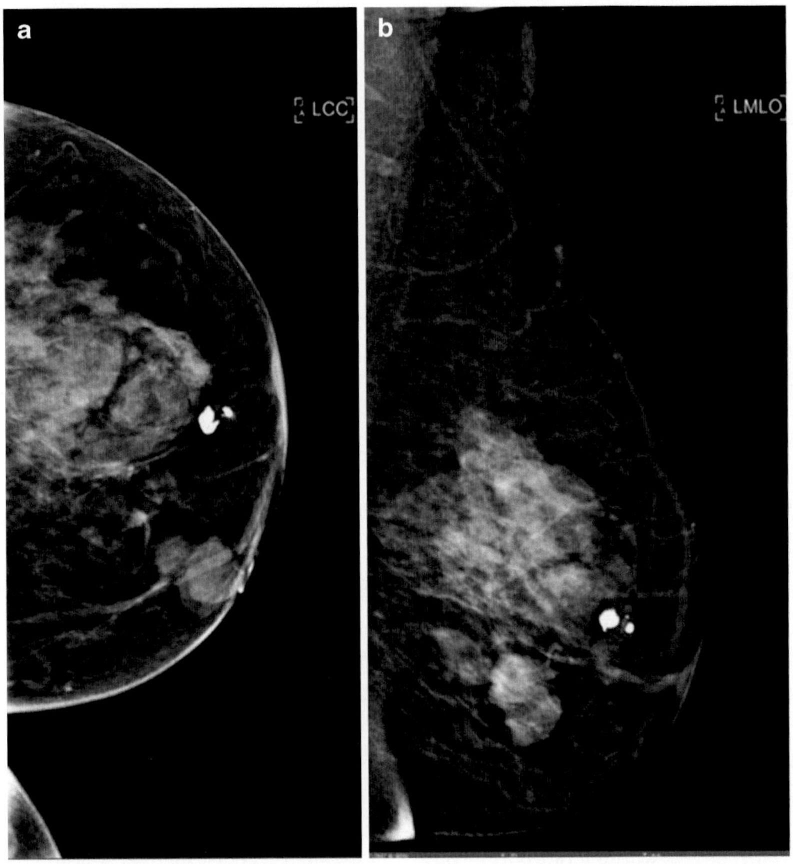

Fig. 2.29 A 60-year-old woman presented with a new palpable left breast mass. Mammography showed a cluster of masses in the left breast at 9 o'clock middle depth measuring a total span of 2.5 cm which correlated with the palpable mass (**a**, **b**). On ultrasound there is a cluster of masses with an indistinct and circumscribed margin in the left breast at 9 o'clock posterior depth (**c**, **d**). This cluster of masses is hypoechoic. This correlates as palpated and with mammography findings. Color flow imaging demonstrates that there is increased vascularity (**e**). The largest mass within this cluster measures 1.4 cm in greatest dimension. The mass is biopsied to reveal an invasive ductal carcinoma with extensive mucinous differentiation

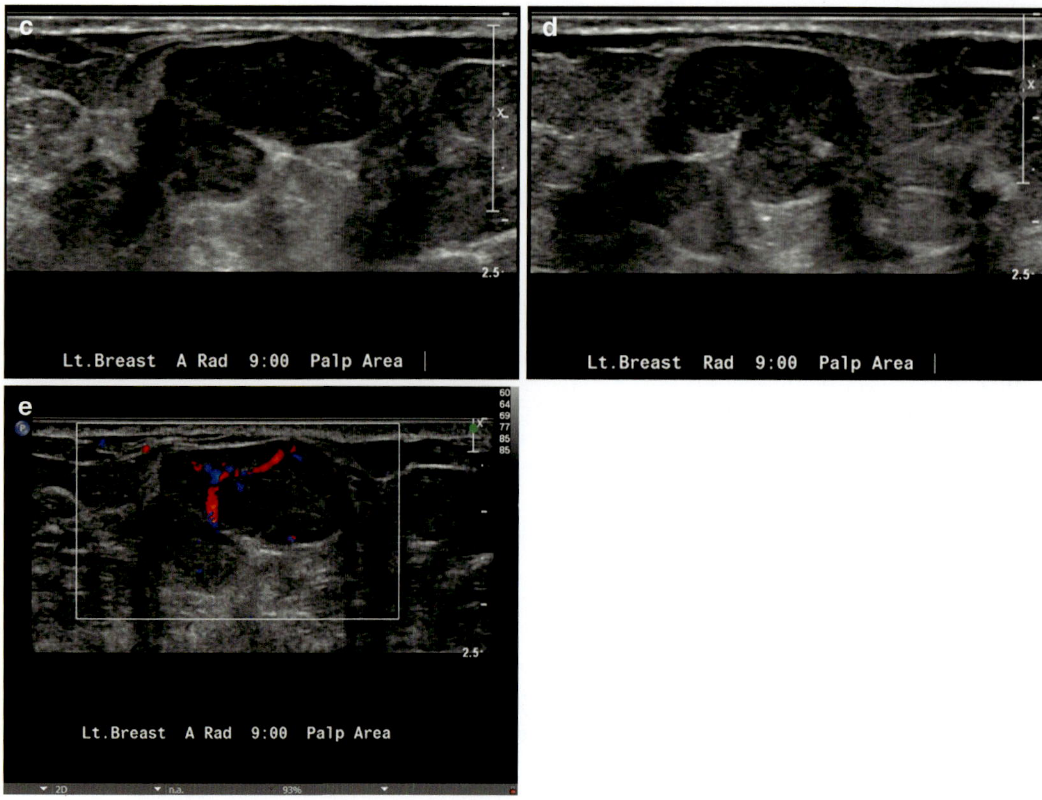

Fig. 2.29 (continued)

>90% of the tumor should show classic histology to qualify for mucinous carcinoma [20].

Two histologic types: Type A (paucicellular) and Type B (hypercellular) variants are described.

Tumors with high nuclear grade are excluded from mucinous type and are called IDC-NST.

Mucinous tumors are luminal A molecular subtype and show a biomarker profile of ER and PR positive, HER2 negative.

- **Differential Diagnosis**: Benign mucocele-like lesions and myxoid fibroadenoma.
- **Management**: Standard treatment includes lumpectomy with radiation therapy (mastectomy when needed) and sentinel lymph node biopsy [14]. Chemotherapy may be indicated based on the size of the tumor and nodal status [14]. There is a question of whether radiation therapy can be omitted for the pure type, given the overall good prognosis [26].

Metaplastic Carcinoma

Metaplastic Carcinoma: Metaplastic carcinomas make up a heterogeneous group of invasive breast cancers where a portion of the glandular epithelial cells have transformed to a nonglandular epithelial cell type (e.g., squamous cell), a mesenchymal cell type (e.g., spindle cell, chondroid, osseous, or myoid differentiation), or both [6]. They are uncommon and represent less than 5% of all breast cancers [6, 14]. They are usually negative for estrogen receptor, progesterone receptor, and HER2 [6, 14, 30]. Studies that report survival data are difficult to assess given a relatively small number of patients that have different types of metaplastic carcinoma, then undergo different

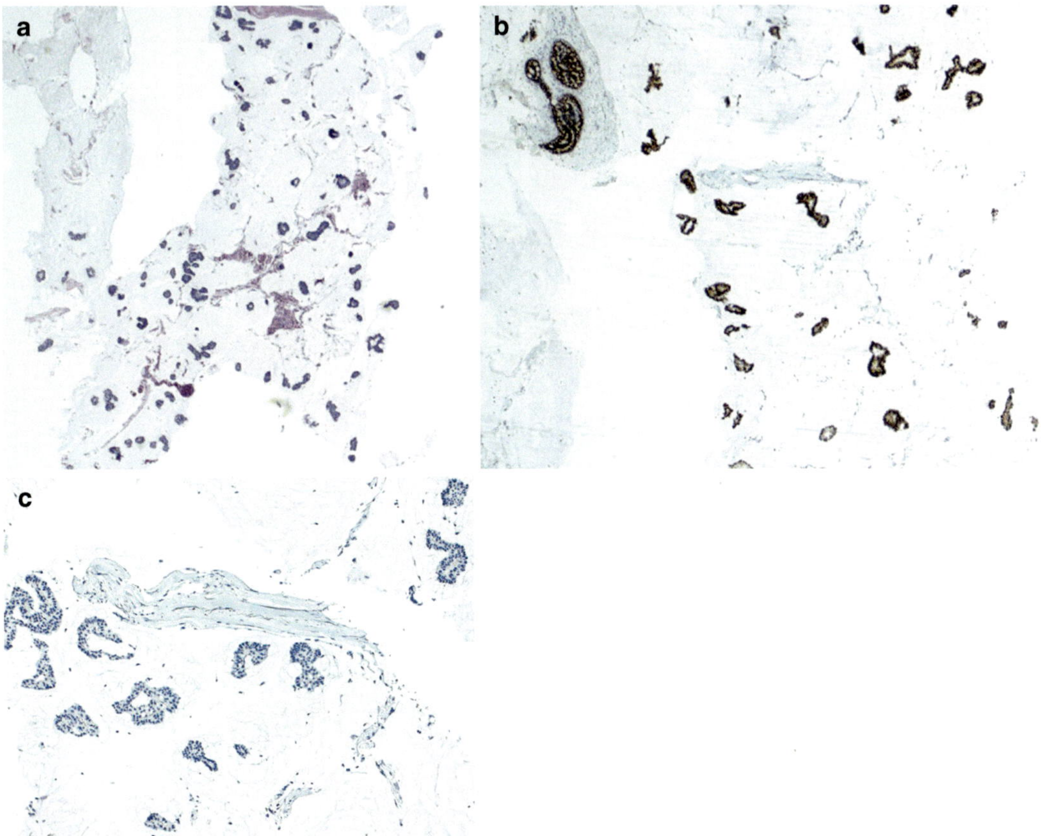

Fig. 2.30 A 56-year-old woman presents with a mass seen on screening mammogram. Mammography demonstrates a focal asymmetry. Ultrasound demonstrates an oval, circumscribed hypoechoic mass. The lesion was biopsied, and on histologic examination the mass was relatively paucicellular with abundant mucinous pools with small clusters of malignant cells floating in the mucin (**a**). On immunohistochemistry the tumor cells were strongly ER positive (**b**) and negative for HER2 (**c**)

treatments, have variable amount of follow-up, and are not clearly stratified by stage [31]. In general, these patients have lower chemotherapy response and worse outcome compared to patients with other triple-negative breast cancers [31]. Berg and Yang report a 5-year stage-specific survival of 100% for stage 1, 83% for stage 2, and 53% for stage 3 [18]. Metaplastic carcinoma can metastasize to lung and liver primarily via hematogenous spread [6].

- **Clinical Presentation**: Presents as a palpable mass that rapidly grows in a short time, usually in women older than 50 years old [6, 14, 30]. The age at diagnosis and clinical features are otherwise similar to invasive breast cancer [14].
- **Imaging Findings**:
  - **Mammography**: These can have a variable appearance on mammography depending on the type:

    They can be round, dense, circumscribed, and noncalcified.

    They can be partially circumscribed and partially spiculated if they have metaplastic and invasive components [18] (Fig. 2.31).

    Internal calcifications if present can be osteoid-like or linear and pleomorphic [32] (Figs. 2.32 and 2.33).

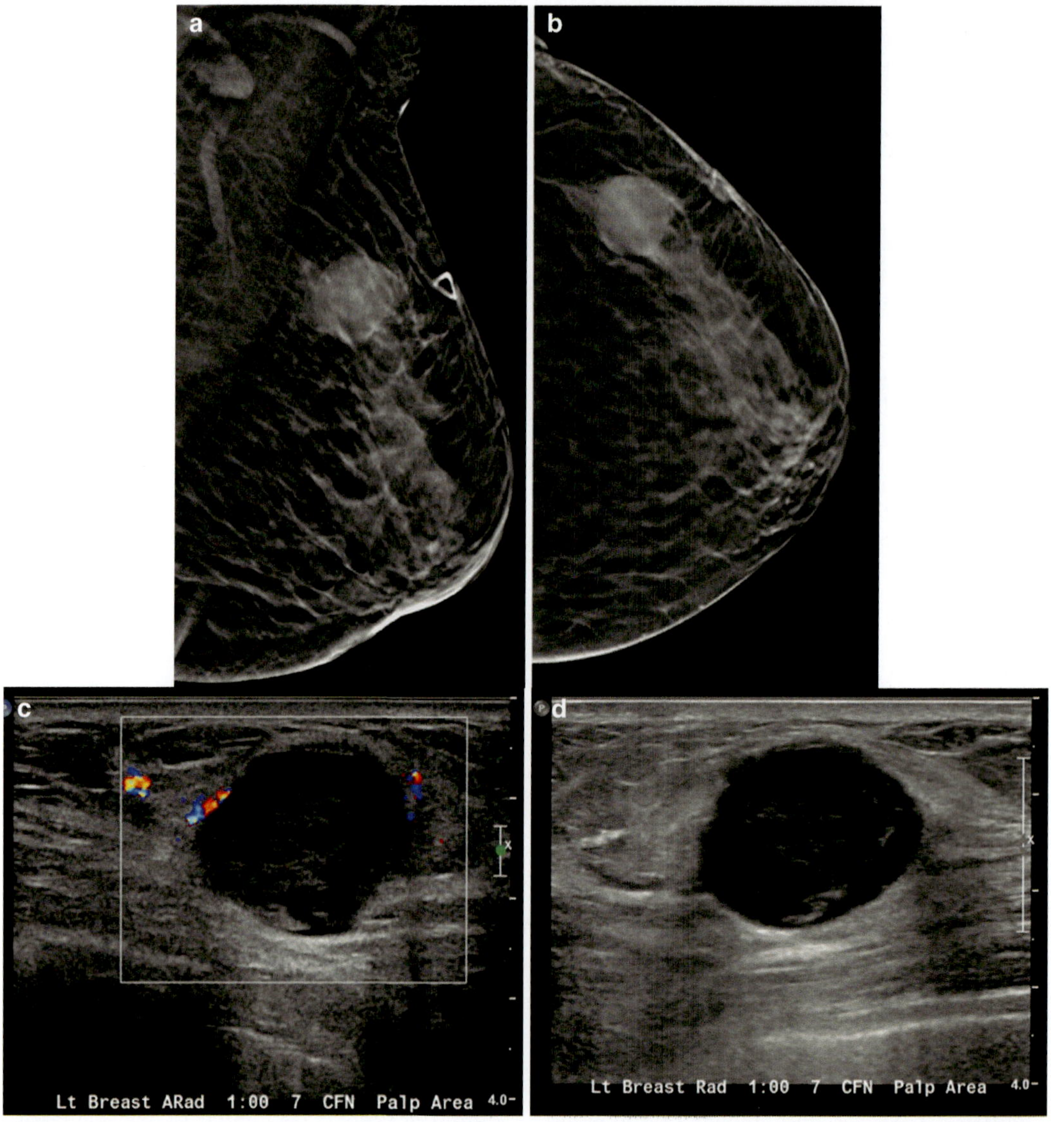

Fig. 2.31 A 67-year-old female presented with a palpable left breast mass. Mammography revealed a partially circumscribed mass, with partially indistinct margins (**a**, **b**). Ultrasound showed a complex cystic and solid mass with posterior acoustic enhancement and adjacent vascularity (**c**, **d**). The mass was considered BI-RADS 4. Ultrasound-guided aspiration of the cystic component and core biopsy of the solid component were recommended and performed revealing a metaplastic carcinoma

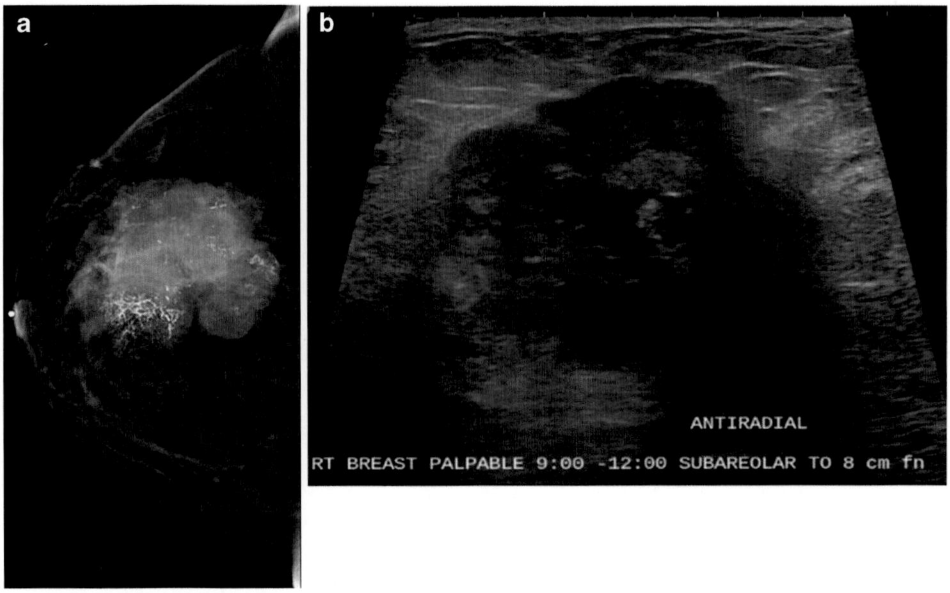

Fig. 2.32 A 66-year-old female was found to have a 6.8-cm dense lobulated mass with calcifications. Mammography demonstrates an irregular, poorly circumscribed, dense mass with fine, linear, branching, and pleomorphic calcifications (**a**). Ultrasound demonstrates an irregular hypoechoic mass with central calcifications and some posterior shadowing (**b**). A biopsy is taken and pathology revealed metaplastic carcinoma

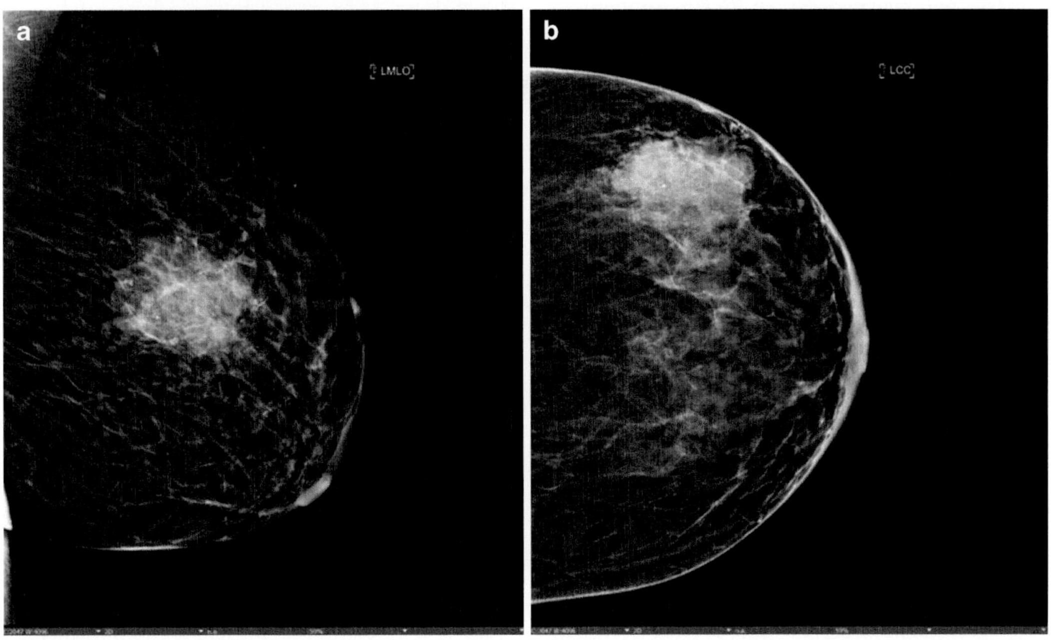

Fig. 2.33 A 65-year-old female palpated a left breast mass. Her prior screening mammogram 16 months ago was negative. Mammography now showed a large, irregular mass with a microlobulated margin and associated coarse heterogeneous calcifications (**a**, **b**). Enlarged left axillary lymph nodes were also noted. On ultrasound there was an irregular mass with a microlobulated margin, with internal vascularity and a hyperechoic rim (**c**, **d**). Enlarged left axillary lymph nodes were once again noted. The lesion was called BI-RADS 5, highly suspicious of malignancy; an US-guided biopsy of the mass and representative axillary lymph node were performed demonstrating metaplastic carcinoma

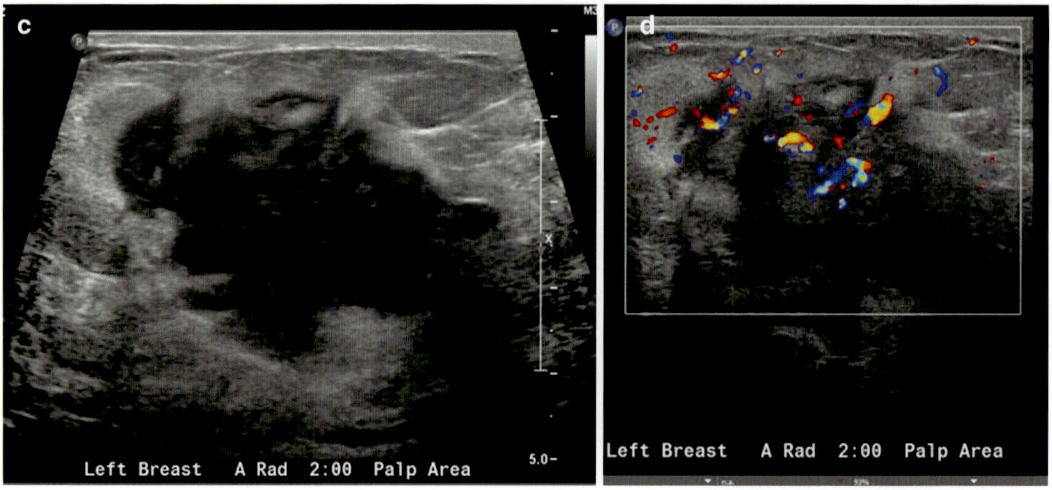

Fig. 2.33 (continued)

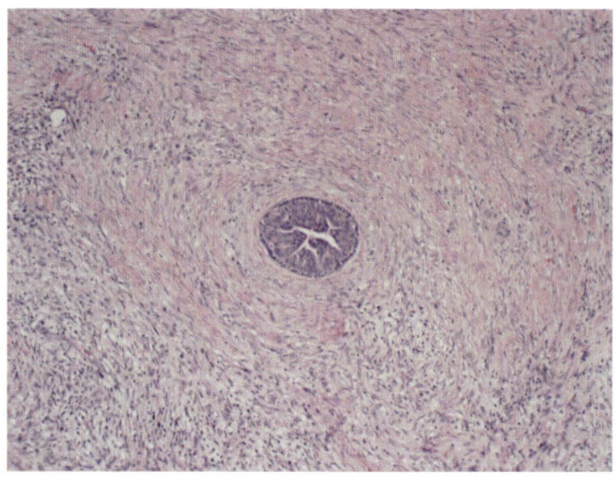

Fig. 2.34 A 59-year-old female presented with a palpable right breast mass. Mammography showed an irregular mass with a microlobulated margin which was also seen in ultrasound. The mass was biopsied demonstrating metaplastic carcinoma of the breast with a monophasic population of spindle cells surrounding focal glandular components

- **US**: The shape can be oval, round, or irregular with partially circumscribed margins.

  The echotexture can be hypoechoic and may have areas of hyperechogenicity depending on the extent of internal calcifications.

  Internal cystic areas may be present with cystic degeneration.

  Hypervascularity may be present, usually in the rim.
- **MRI**: Large round or irregular mass that is hypointense on the T1 weighted images and heterogeneously hyperintense on the T2 weighted images depending on the extent of internal necrosis and secondary cystic areas [19].

  On postcontrast images, there is intense rapid enhancement with a prominent rim enhancing component.
- **BI-RADS**: 3 or 4.
- **Differential Diagnosis**: Differential diagnosis includes primary breast sarcoma, malignant phyllodes tumor, invasive ductal carcinoma NOS without metaplasia, mucinous carcinoma, and breast metastasis (from squamous carcinoma or sarcoma).

• **Pathology Findings**:
  - **Microscopic Histology**: Adenocarcinoma is admixed with spindle, squamous or heterologous elements (cartilage, bone, benign or malignant) [26] (Fig. 2.34).

Spindle cell carcinomas with purely spindle cells may be low grade or high grade with lymphocytic infiltrate.

Myoepithelial markers p63, SMA, and a broad spectrum of keratins are required to distinguish metaplastic carcinoma from sarcomas [20].

Squamous cell carcinomas are usually cystic and can be well to poorly differentiated.

Low-grade adenosquamous carcinomas have bland spindle cells admixed with adenocarcinoma.

Often associated with a benign sclerosing lesion (papillary) [33].

Infiltrative glands arranged in solid cords and clusters with focal squamous differentiation are seen within desmoplastic stroma.

Fibromatosis-like metaplastic carcinomas are composed of bland spindle cells predominantly with slender nuclei and pale cytoplasm in a collagenized stroma. Cords of spindled tumor cells are admixed with epithelioid cells.

Metaplastic carcinomas with heterologous mesenchymal differentiation have carcinomatous areas with gland formation and transition to areas of mesenchymal differentiation with chondroid matrix or bone with or without intervening spindle cell areas.

Extensive sampling is required to find the carcinomatous areas to distinguish them from chondrosarcomas or osteosarcomas [34].

Immunostains for high molecular weight keratins are particularly helpful to demonstrate the carcinomatous areas.

Most metaplastic carcinomas are ER- and PR-negative [26].

HER2 overexpression is uncommon (<5%) [26].

- **Differential Diagnosis**: Phyllodes, pure sarcomas and other spindle cell tumors.
- **Management**: Treatment is mainly surgical excision with adjuvant radiation therapy for breast conservation [6]. Preoperative radiation therapy may be beneficial in some cases. Chemotherapy can be used with limited response [6].

Lymphoma

See Chap. 3 for additional information.

Lymphoma: Primary breast non-Hodgkin's lymphoma (NHL) is diagnosed in patients who don't have concurrent or previous history of systemic lymphoma or leukemia [18, 20]. They account for 1.7–2.2% of extranodal NHLs, 0.4–0.7% of all NHLs, and less than 1% of malignant breast tumors [26]. Bilateral lymphoma is noted in 10% of patients [14].

- **Clinical Presentation**: Patients often present with a solitary, palpable, painless, rapidly enlarging mass in the upper outer quadrant [18, 20]. They can be multiple masses or singular, and demonstrate diffuse infiltration [20]. Associated axillary adenopathy is present in 30–50% of patients at presentation [18]. The average age at presentation is 55 years old, but can range from 13 to 90 years [20]. The histologic subtype is the most important factor in prognosis [18]. Prognosis is worse in younger patients, with tumor size >5 cm, synchronous bilateral disease, or axillary nodal metastases [18]. Overall disease-free survival at 5 years is 39–70% [18].

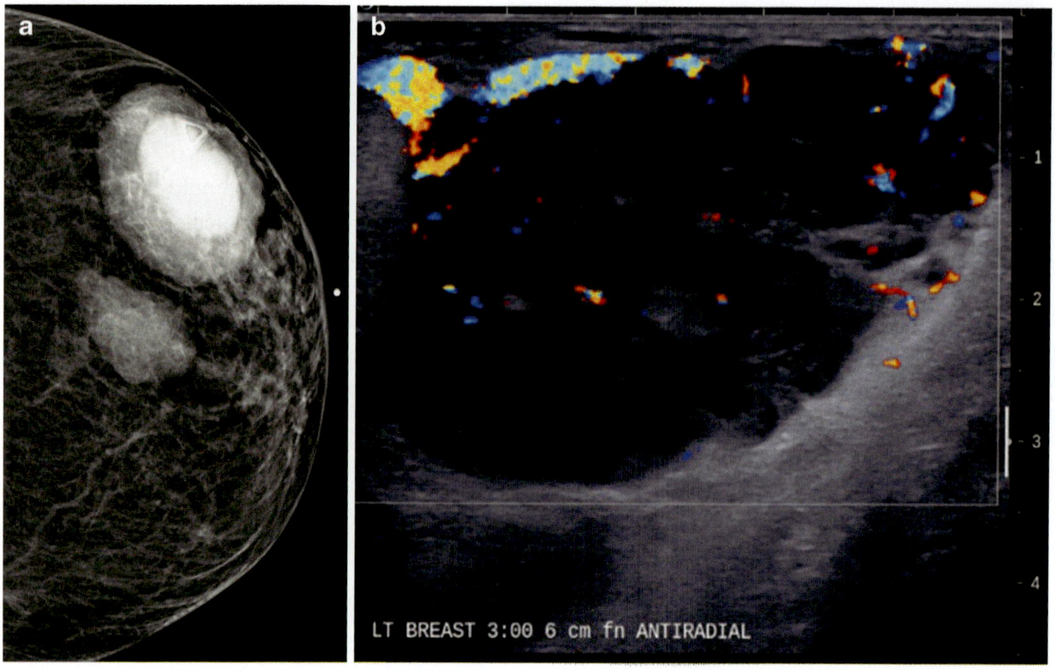

Fig. 2.35 A 74-year-old woman presents with a palpable lump in her left breast. Mammography shows an oval, dense mass deep to a triangular palpable marker in the lateral left breast with a smaller similar mass noted centrally (**a**). Ultrasound demonstrates a lobulated heterogeneously hypoechoic mass with marked internal vascularity (**b**). The lesion is biopsied, and the pathology revealed diffuse large B-cell lymphoma

- **Imaging Findings**:
  - **Mammography**: Noncalcified oval or lobulated mass with circumscribed or indistinct margins (Figs. 2.35 and 2.36).

    It can also have an infiltrative pattern and appear as a global asymmetry with skin and trabecular thickening [18].
  - **US**: Oval, lobulated, or irregular mass with variable internal echogenicity (hyper- and hypoechoic), variable posterior features, often has a thick echogenic rim, and is hypervascular.

    Associated axillary adenopathy is well assessed by ultrasound [18].
  - **MRI**: Ill-defined masses that are T1 hypointense with rapid intense enhancement with washout kinetics on postcontrast images [18, 19].

    They can demonstrate rim enhancement [19].
  - **BI-RADS**: 4, suspicious of malignancy. However, primary breast lymphoma may be mistaken for a benign lesion such as a fibroadenoma, phyllodes, cyst or clustered cysts, or a fluid collection such as an abscess.
  - **Differential Diagnosis**: Primary breast cancer, particularly mucinous, papillary, medullary, poorly differentiated IDC, TNBC, inflammatory breast cancer (particularly when presenting with breast edema and global asymmetry), secondary lymphoma, benign processes such as: fibroadenoma, phyllodes, abscess, granulomatous mastitis, diabetic mastopathy, benign-dependent edema (due to heart failure or venous obstruction).
- **Pathology Findings**:
  - **Microscopic Histology**: Variable depending on the type of lymphoma/leukemia present. See Chap. 3 for microscopic histology of different subtypes (Fig. 2.37).

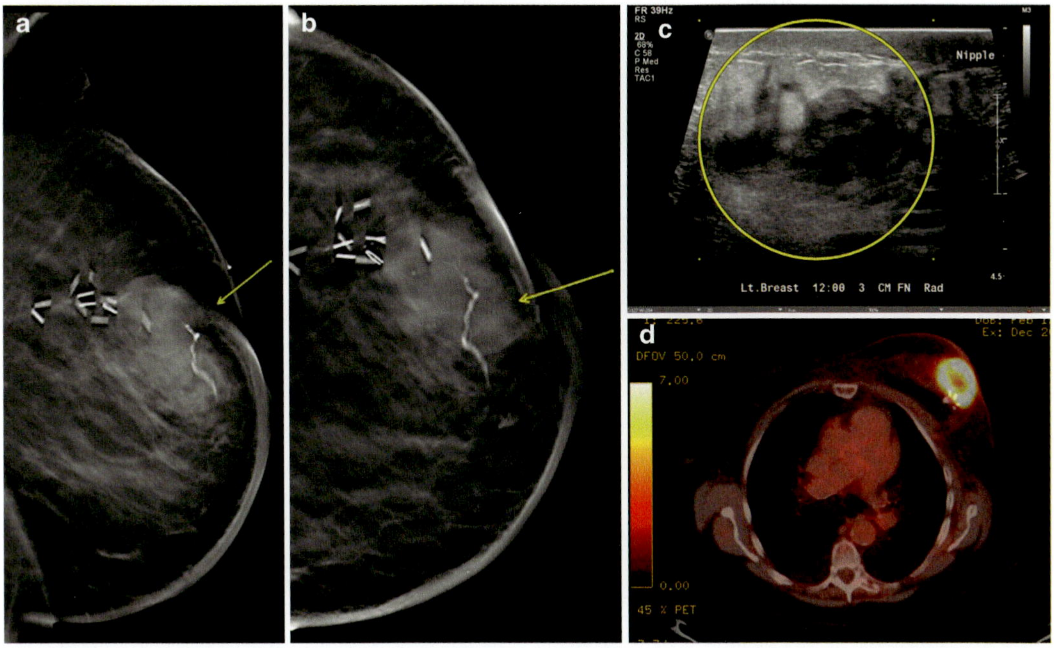

Fig. 2.36 An 83-year-old female with history of left breast IDC status post-lumpectomy and radiation therapy 7 years ago presents with a palpable lump and skin thickening of the left breast. Mammogram showed an oval left breast mass with an indistinct margin that correlates with the palpable finding (**a**, **b**). Ultrasound showed an irregular mass with an indistinct margin, and heterogeneous echotexture without increased internal vascularity (**c**). The lesion was graded BI-RADS 4, suspicious of malignancy. An US-guided biopsy was recommended and performed, yielding diffuse large cell lymphoma. As part of follow-up the patient underwent a body PET/CT scan for staging, which demonstrated the large hypermetabolic left breast mass, but no additional suspicious lesions (**d**)

- **Differential Diagnosis**: Primary breast cancer, leukemia, plasmacytoma, myeloma, metastases from extramammary lymphoma or other malignancies, and other infiltrative processes such as inflammatory breast cancer, idiopathic granulomatous mastitis, benign breast masses such as fibroadenoma, phyllodes, and breast abscess [3, 18].
- **Management**: Largely treated with chemotherapy depending on histologic type, with immunosuppression being increasingly used. Surgical treatment does not play a significant role. B-cell lymphoma can metastasize to the CNS in 5% of cases, and intrathecal methotrexate is frequently recommended for prophylaxis [26].

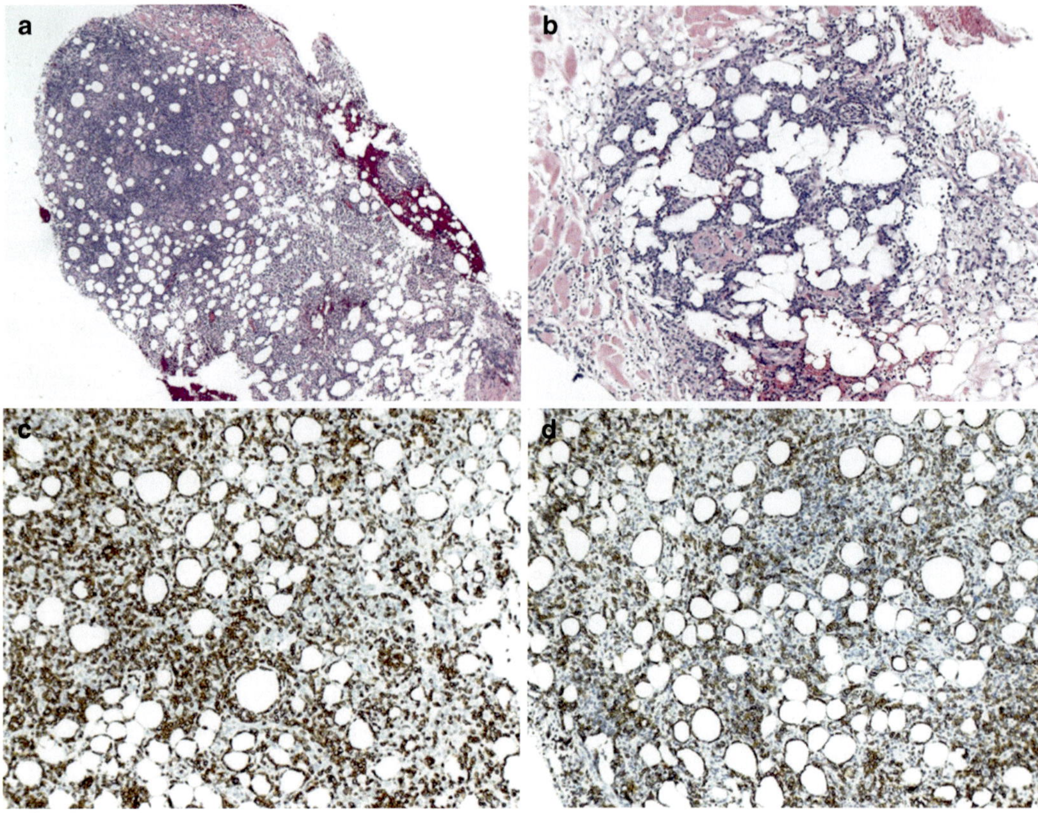

Fig. 2.37 A 33-year-old woman presented with skin thinking. On ultrasound she was found to have a nodular-like pattern of skin thickening. Biopsy showed a subcutaneous panniculitis-like T-cell lymphoma (**a**, **b**) with strong diffuse CD3 (**c**) and CD8 (**d**) staining on immunohistochemistry supporting the diagnosis of a T-cell lymphoma

Heterogeneous Benign

Hamartoma

Hamartoma: A hamartoma is a fat containing mass within breast surrounded by a pseudo capsule and typically described as a breast within a breast [35]. They have also been termed as fibroadenolipomas or adenolipomas [35]. These lesions are challenging to diagnose on core needle biopsy due to the resemblance to normal breast tissue microscopically.

- **Clinical Presentation**: May present as a palpable mass or be discovered incidentally on imaging.
- **Imaging Findings**:
  - **Mammography**: On mammogram they have an oval or round shape containing fat and soft tissue surrounded by a pseudo capsule [35] (Fig. 2.38).
  - **US**: On ultrasound they are visualized as a circumscribed mass with heterogeneous internal echo containing fat [35, 36].
  - **BI-RADS**: 2.
  - **Differential Diagnosis**: Benign: fat necrosis, galactocele, fibrosis, PASH, focally asymmetric breast tissue.
- **Pathology Findings**:
  - **Microscopic Histology**: A hamartoma is a circumscribed mass composed of a mix of ducts, lobules, fat, and collagenized stroma in varying proportions (Fig. 2.39).

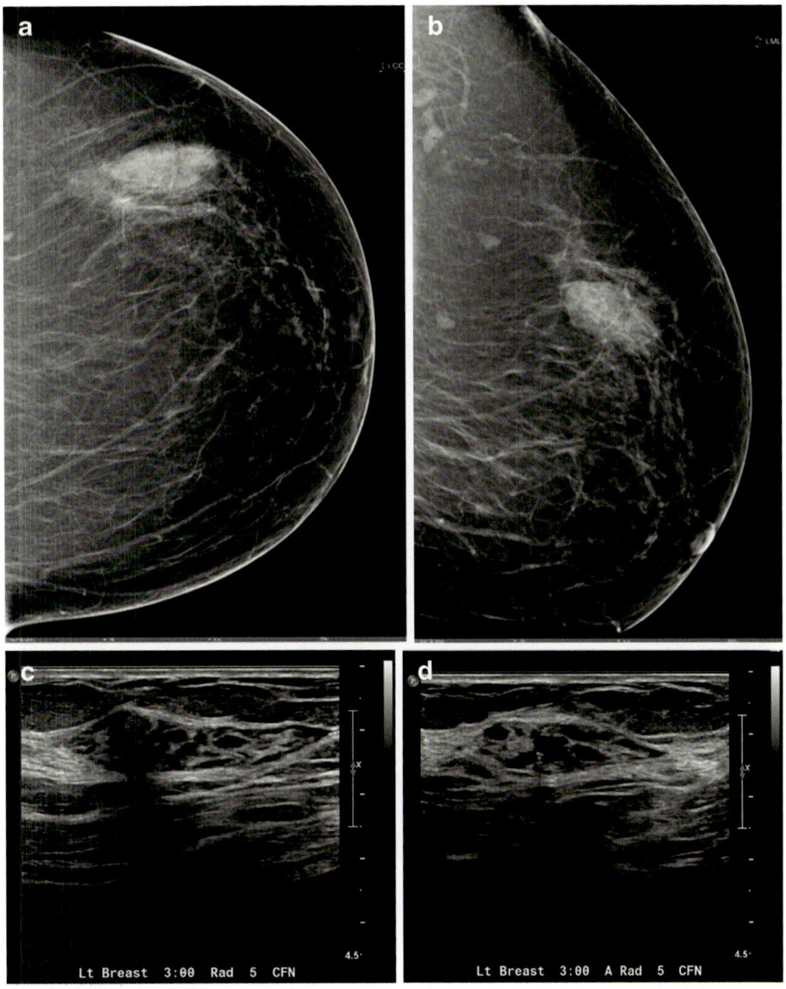

Fig. 2.38 A 41-year-old woman presented for screening mammography. On mammography, there is a focal asymmetry in the left upper outer quadrant (**a**, **b**). No suspicious calcifications are seen in the left breast. No suspicious mass or suspicious calcifications are seen in the right breast. Ultrasound was performed on the left breast in its entirety (**c**, **d**). In the 3:00 axis, 5 cm from the nipple, a heterogeneous mass with angular margin measures 3.0 × 3.4 × 1.2 cm, corresponding to focal asymmetry on mammography. The lesion is ultimately excised to reveal a hamartoma

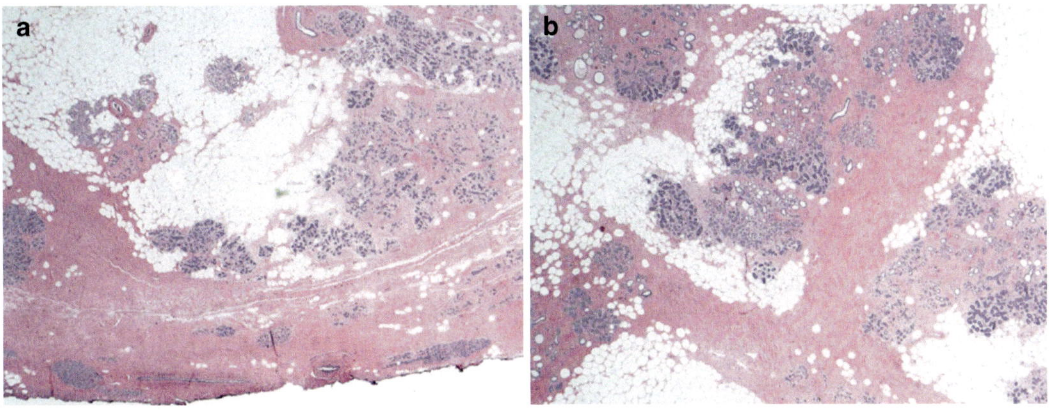

Fig. 2.39 A 31-year-old woman presented for screening mammography on which there is a focal asymmetry in the right breast. Ultrasound detected a 2.9 × 2.5 × 0.9 cm heterogeneous mass. The lesion was excised to reveal a hamartoma with well-circumscribed border with admixture of fibrous stroma, adipose tissue, and mammary glandular tissue (**a**) with nodular aggregates of breast lobules (**b**)

Some lesions consist predominantly of adipose tissue while others show an increase in stroma with smooth muscle hyperplasia called "myxoid hyperplasia" [3].

Occasionally chondroid differentiation within the fat may be seen in which case the term chondrolipoma is used [3, 37, 38].

Clinical and radiological correlation is needed due to the nonspecific histologic findings.

- **Differential Diagnosis**: Lipoma, fat necrosis/oil cysts, and intramammary lymph node.
- **Management**: When classic findings of hamartoma are seen on imaging no further workup is necessary. However, any atypical features in a fat containing mass would require surgical excision to rule out rare liposarcomas in the beast.

Benign Intramammary Lymph Node

Benign Intramammary Lymph Node: Intramammary lymph nodes are commonly found in the upper outer quadrant of the breast in the mid axillary line. They typically measure 3 mm to 1 cm.

- **Clinical Presentation**: May be clinically palpable especially in thin patients.
- **Imaging Findings**:
  - **Mammography**: Circumscribed, oval, or reniform mass with hilar fat that is frequently more easily visualized on tomosynthesis (Fig. 2.40).

    Presence of calcifications within intramammary lymph nodes may signal granulomatous disease or, in the appropriate clinical setting, metastasis.

    Intramammary lymph nodes may become enlarged in the setting of infection/inflammation, systemic neoplastic disease, or breast cancer.
  - **MRI**: Circumscribed oval or reniform mass, with hilar fat best visualized on T1 nonfat-saturated imaging.

    Intramammary lymph nodes demonstrate washout kinetics on postcontrast imaging.
  - **US**: Circumscribed, oval, or reniform mass with a hypoechoic cortex and a fatty hilum.

    Venous and arterial flow may be seen in the hilum.

    Increased vascularity within the cortex may be seen in the setting of infection/inflammation or involvement by malignancy.

    Round shape and loss of the fatty hilum are worrisome in the setting of malignancy.
  - **BI-RADS**: 2.
  - **Differential Diagnosis**: Cysts, small fibroadenomas, galactocele, lipoma, and low-grade lymphomas and metastatic disease (multiple masses).
- **Pathology Findings**:
  - **Microscopic Histology**: The histology findings on core needle biopsy consist of normal lymphoid tissue with a fibrous capsule (Fig. 2.41).

    Although, distinction from a high-grade lymphoproliferative disorder can be made on core needle biopsy, the distinction from a low-grade lymphoma is not always easy [3].

    Extension of the lymphoid tissue beyond the fibrous capsule is regarded as suspicious and will require immunohistochemical workup with a lymphoma panel of antibody stains [3].

    Intramammary lymph nodes may represent a completely replaced lymph node. Additionally, on core biopsy it may be challenging to distinguish a germinal center from medullary carcinoma which has a rich lymphoplasmacytic infiltrate with germinal center formation [3].
  - **Differential Diagnosis**: Cysts, small fibroadenomas, galactocele, lipoma, and low-grade lymphomas and metastatic disease (multiple masses).
  - **Management**: Additional management for benign lymph nodes is not needed.

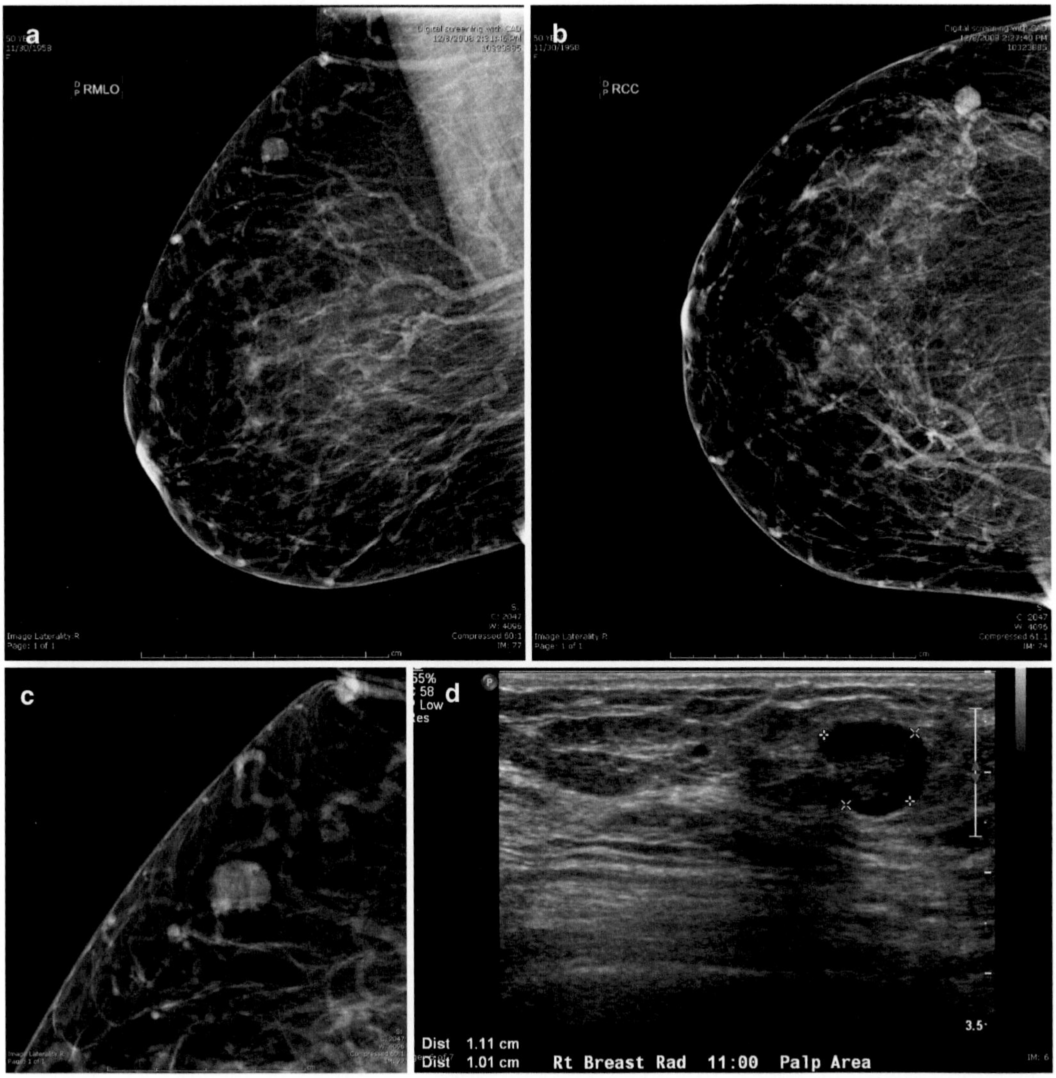

Fig. 2.40 A 45-year-old woman presents for screening. On mammography a well-circumscribed, oval lesion is noted (**a**, **b**, **c**). The lesion is also seen on ultrasound with a hypoechoic rim (**d**). Biopsy confirms the lesion is a benign intramammary lymph node

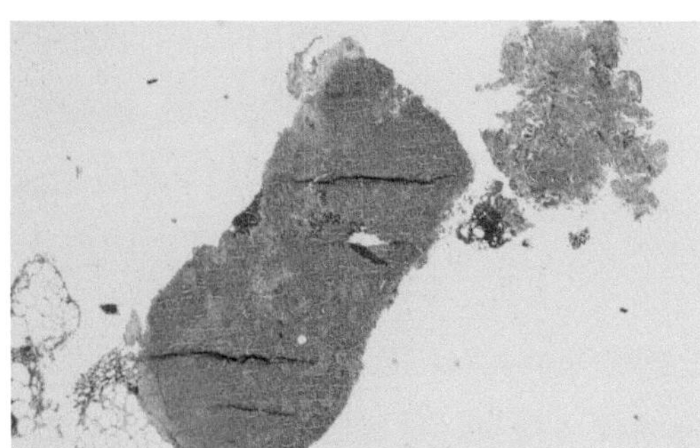

Fig. 2.41 A 36-year-old woman was found to have a lesion on mammography and ultrasound. A biopsy was performed revealing a portion of benign lymph node with a heterogeneous population of lymphocytes and portion of a fibrous capsule

Fat Necrosis

See Chap. 3

Pseudoangiomatous Stromal Hyperplasia (PASH)

See Chap. 7 for additional information.

Pseudoangiomatous Stromal Hyperplasia (PASH): Pseudoangiomatous stromal hyperplasia (PASH) is an uncommon, benign disease of the breast with unclear etiology and no association with malignancy [33]. The proposed pathophysiology of PASH is the response of myofibroblasts to hormonal stimuli, corresponding to its increased prevalence in premenopausal women and postmenopausal women on hormonal therapy [33].

- **Clinical Presentation**: PASH may present as a suspicious appearing mass with indistinct margins, which prompts a biopsy and eventual excision. Patients may report a palpable mass, but asymptomatic presentation is also common.
- **Imaging Findings**:
  - **Mammography**: A classic mammographic presentation of PASH is a mass with circumscribed or indistinct margin (Fig. 2.42).

    It may also present as a focal asymmetry.

    Associated punctate calcifications may be present.
  - **US**: A typical sonographic appearance of PASH is a round or oval hypoechoic mass with a circumscribed margin (Fig. 2.43).
  - **MRI**: PASH on MRI exhibits nonspecific features, most commonly appearing as a circumscribed oval or round, persistently enhancing mass with internal areas of increased T2 signal, or clumped non-mass enhancement with persistent kinetics [18].
  - **BI-RADS**: Variable, may range from 3 to 5.
  - **Differential Diagnosis**: Benign: fibroadenoma, adenosis, fibrocystic changes, phylloides tumor. Malignant: breast cancer, low-grade angiosarcoma.
- **Pathology Findings**:
  - **Microscopic Histology**: On histology the most characteristic appearance is complex anastomosing slit-like spaces in the intralobular stroma (Fig. 2.44).

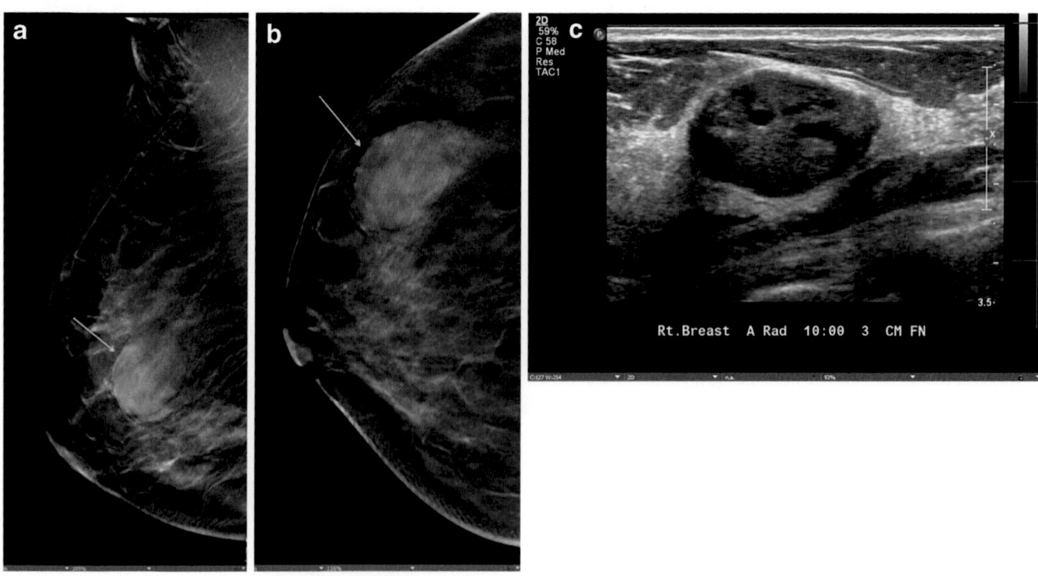

Fig. 2.42 A 41-year-old woman is called back from screening mammography for a mass. On diagnostic mammography focal asymmetry with a nodular mass in the left breast is seen (**a**, **b**). The mass is also seen on ultrasound (**c**). The lesion is graded as BI-RADS 4. A core needle biopsy was performed and revealed nodular PASH

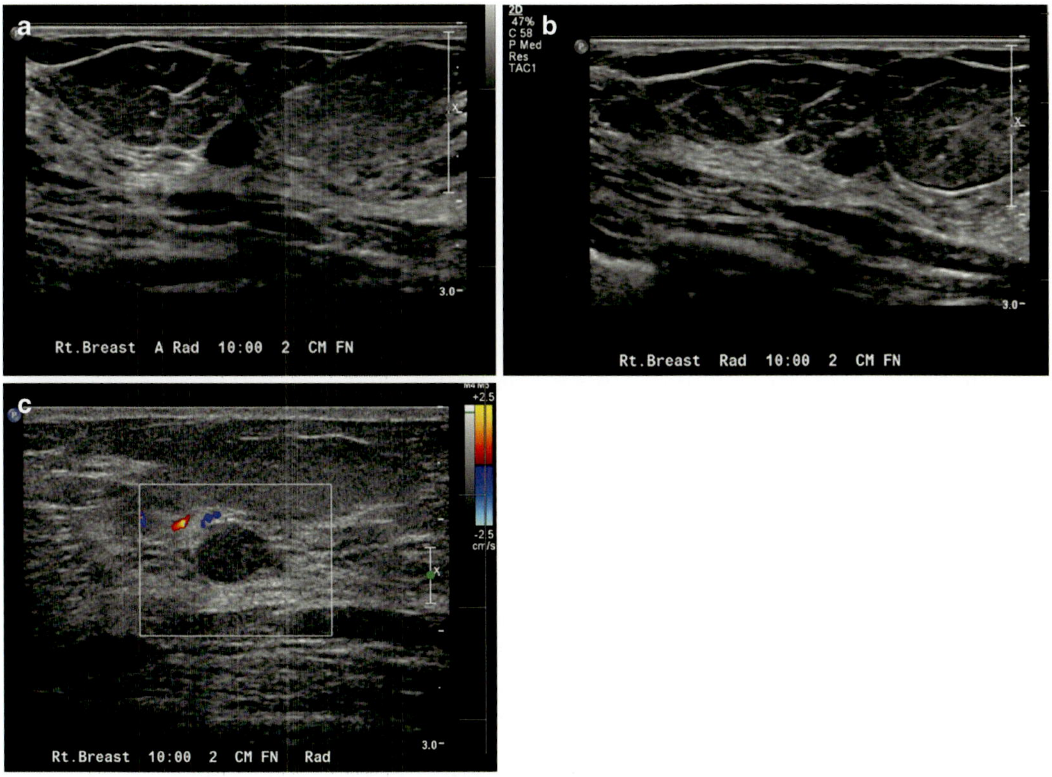

Fig. 2.43 A 47-year-old woman presented for screening mammogram (not shown). On ultrasound there is a 0.7 cm × 0.5 cm × 0.7 cm oval mass with an indistinct and circumscribed margin in the right breast at 10 o'clock anterior depth (**a**, **b**). This oval mass is hypoechoic. Color flow imaging demonstrates that there is an adjacent vascularity (**c**). On biopsy the lesion is found to be nodular PASH

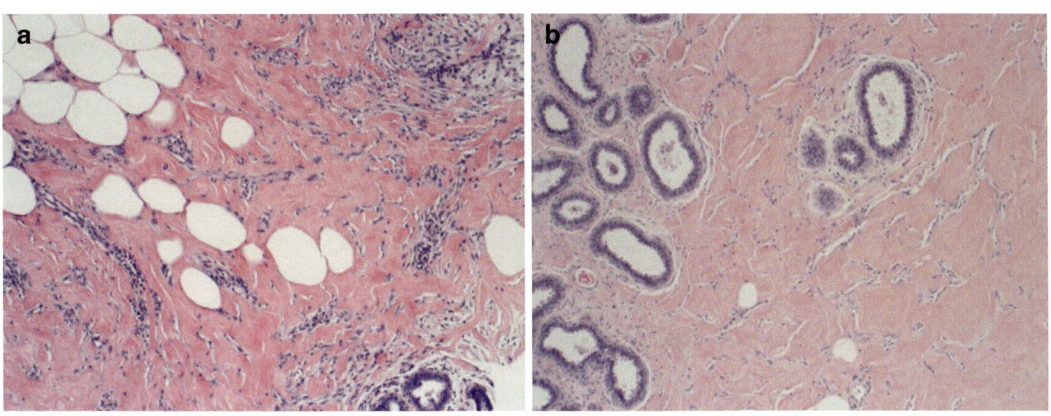

Fig. 2.44 Pseudoangiomatous stromal hyperplasia with slit-like anastamosing spaces lined by myofibroblasts in a background of dense collagenous stroma on core needle biopsy (**a**) and excision (**b**)

Myofibroblasts line these spaces which are highlighted by CD34 and vimentin [3].

They can show reactivity for PR but stain negatively or weakly by ER immunostaining.

The nuclei of the myofibroblasts are bland, without atypia or mitosis, though occasionally can be enlarged, hyperchromatic, and multinucleated.

- **Differential Diagnosis**: On a core needle biopsy the most important differential diagnosis is a well-differentiated angiosarcoma. This distinction can be readily made by prudent use of immunostains for myofibroblasts and vascular markers as PASH should be negative for the endothelial markers CD31, ERG, and D2-40 [3].

  PASH on needle core biopsy may be inconspicuous or pronounced with bundles or fascicles of myofibroblasts resulting in a cellular or fascicular form of PASH. Myofibroblastoma can then enter the differential diagnosis of fascicular PASH. This distinction may be difficult as myofibroblastoma and PASH are related lesions with proliferation of myofibroblasts.

  Rare examples of atypical PASH have been described with atypical hyperchromatic nuclei and other rare examples of PASH that show cytoplasmic inclusions as those seen in digital fibromas.
- **Management**: Although PASH demonstrates no association with malignancy, its imaging appearance may mimic malignant lesions and a biopsy is frequently necessary for confirmation [33, 39]. Although most lesions remain stable, some may exhibit growth or be symptomatic; these lesions are usually excised.

Invasive Ductal Carcinoma

See Chaps. 3, 5, and 7.

Metastatic Findings

Metastatic Findings: Metastatic breast lesions from a non-primary breast tumor are infrequent and account for <3% of breast malignancies [3, 33]. When present they are bilateral more commonly than primary breast cancer [3, 33, 40]. The location of the tumor in the subcutaneous fat may be a helpful clue as most primary tumors involve the breast parenchyma.

While any tumor can present with metastases in the breast, carcinomas are the most common with lung adenocarcinoma, ovarian carcinoma (high-grade serous carcinoma), and carcinomas of gastrointestinal and genitourinary origin being most common [3, 41, 42]. Melanomas are the second most common followed by carcinoid, sarcomas, and especially in young adolescent girls, rhabdomyosarcomas [3, 43]. Occasionally, in approximately 10–20% of cases breast metastases may be the initial manifestation of carcinoma elsewhere [33].

- **Clinical Presentation**: Metastases to the breast maybe found on workup in patients with a diagnosed primary cancer or may incidentally be discovered as the first sign of malignancy requiring further workup to find the site of origin.
- **Imaging Findings**:
  - **Mammography**: The mammographic findings are variable, and may present as a round, oval, or irregular mass with either a circumscribed or indistinct margin [18] (Figs. 2.45, 2.46 and 2.47).

    Architectural distortion or calcifications may also be observed in association.
  - **US**: Sonographic features of metastatic carcinoma are also nonspecific. They are often hypoechoic and may present as oval, round, or irregular masses with circumscribed or indistinct margins and hypervascularity [18].
  - **BI-RADS**: 4 to 5.
  - **Differential Diagnosis**: Benign: abscess, PASH. Malignant: IDC and other types of breast carcinoma.

- **Pathology Findings**:
  - **Microscopic Histology**:

    Lung adenocarcinoma: Lung adenocarcinomas metastatic to breast are seen as small tubules or glands which lack ER and PR immunoreactivity and express nuclear staining for thyroid transcription factor (TTF-1).

    Rare breast carcinomas (around 2%) express TTF-1 [33].

    ER and PR expression in lung cancers have been reported in a small percentage of cases depending on the clone [42].

    Breast-specific markers like GATA3, mammaglobin, and GCDFP-15 are useful to favor breast over lung origin as they are expressed in 80–85% of primary breast cancers [33].

    Ovarian serous carcinoma: Greater than 95% of these tumors express PAX8. However, depending on the clone used PAX8 may cross-react with breast tissue [33] (Fig. 2.48).

    Gynecologic cancers metastatic to breast are positive for WT1, another useful marker positive in 85% of cases [33, 40].

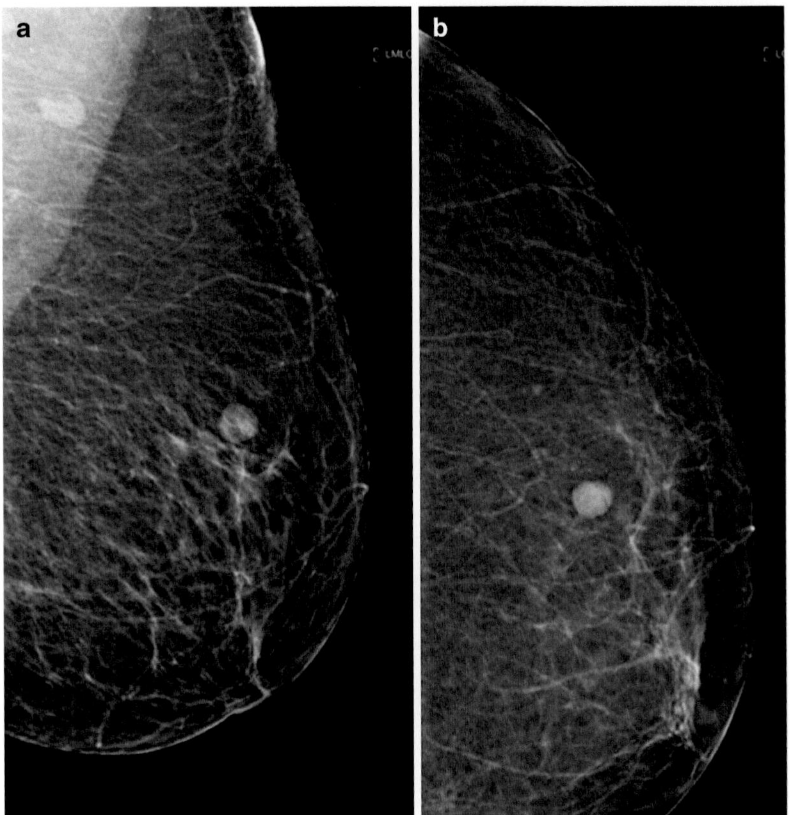

Fig. 2.45 A 69-year-old woman presented for screening which detected an oval left breast mass with distinct margins on mammography (**a**, **b**). A vascular hyperechoic mass is seen on ultrasound corresponding to the mass seen on mammography (**c**, **d**). MRI reveals that the patient also has a lung mass concerning for malignancy (**e**). Biopsy of the breast mass revealed a poorly differentiated carcinoma. Biopsy of the lung revealed a poorly differentiated non-small cell carcinoma

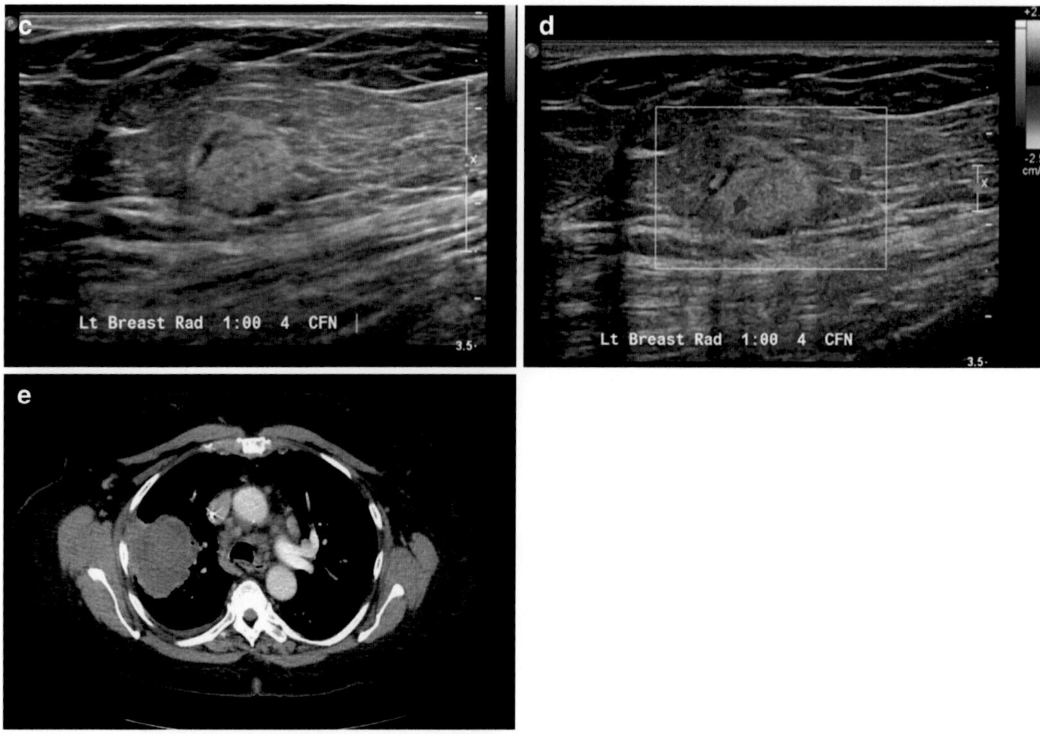

Fig. 2.45 (continued)

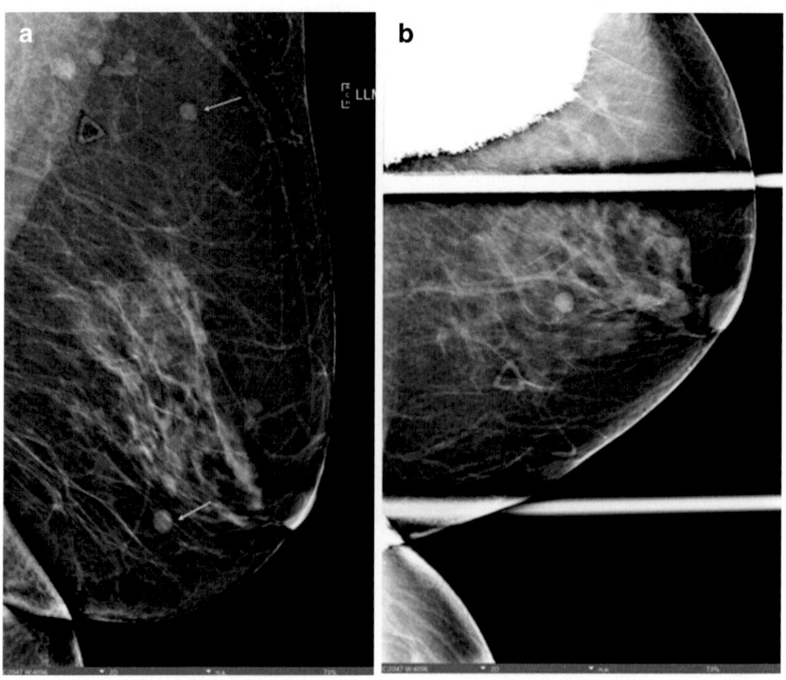

Fig. 2.46 A 65-year-old woman with a history of melanoma now presents with multiple palpable breast masses which are seen on mammography (**a**, **b**). The lesions are also seen on ultrasound as oval, hypoechoic masses with distinct margins (**c**, **d**). The lesions are biopsied to reveal metastatic melanoma

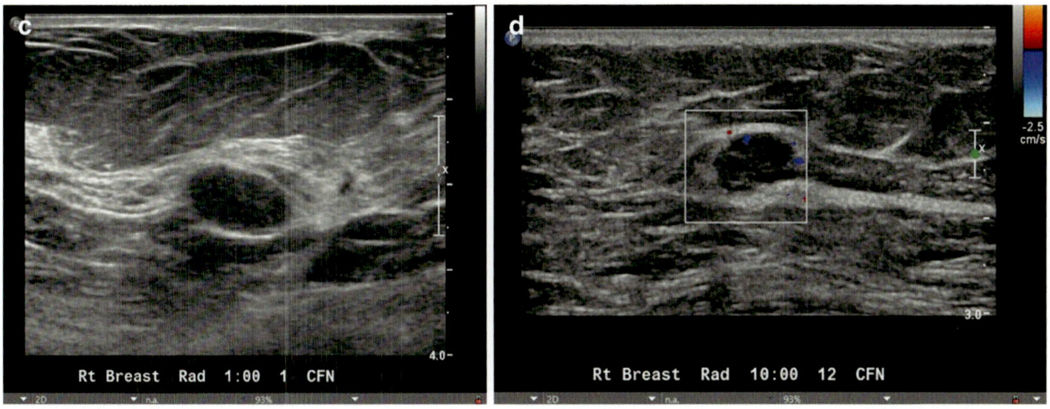

Fig. 2.46 (continued)

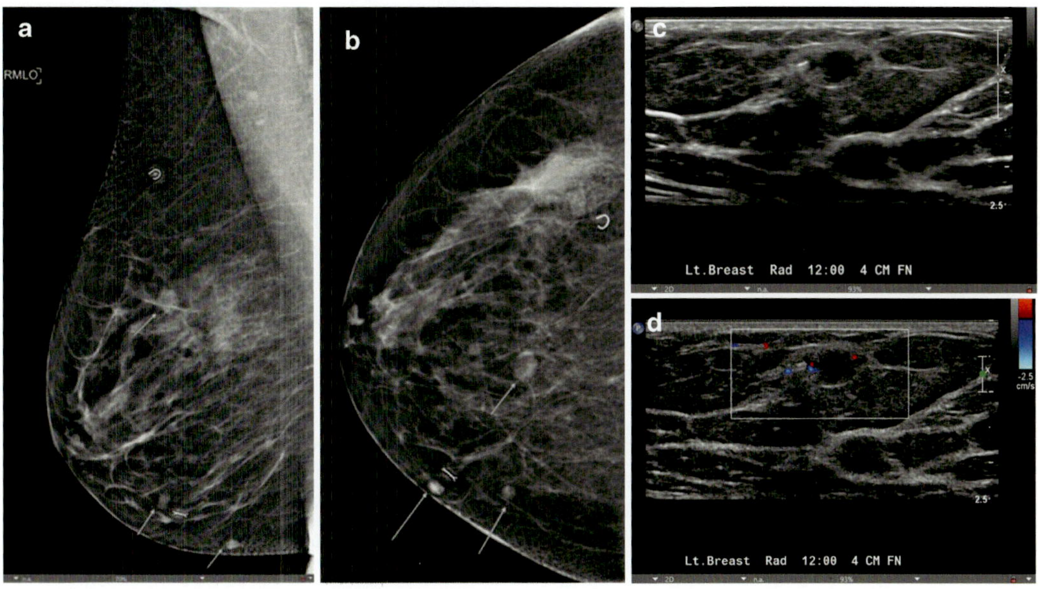

Fig. 2.47 A 59-year-old female with a history of systemic lymphoma presented with multiple breast masses seen on mammography (**a**, **b**). Ultrasound shows oval, hypoechoic masses corresponding to those seen on mammography (**c**, **d**). The patient undergoes core needle biopsy to reveal follicular lymphoma involving the breast

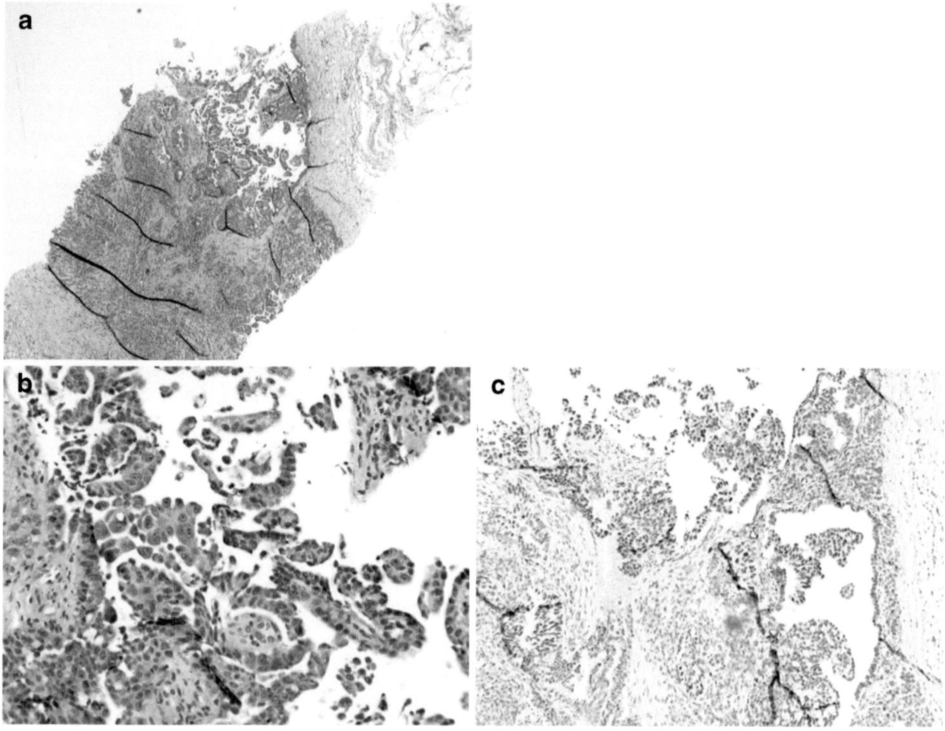

Fig. 2.48 A 63-year-old woman with a history of ovarian serous papillary carcinoma presented with a new breast mass. Biopsy was performed demonstrating a papillary lesion with occasional hobnail cells (**a**, **b**). The tumor cells showed immunoreactivity for WT1 (**c**) supporting the diagnosis of metastatic serous papillary carcinoma

Melanoma: Melanomas have a spindled or epithelioid appearance with prominent nucleoli and discohesive growth [43] (Fig. 2.49).

They are cytokeratin and ER negative, but positive for melanoma-specific markers like S100, HMB45, and melanin A.

Prostate cancer: Rarely men with prostate cancer who undergo hormonal treatment are at increased risk for primary breast cancer.

Metastases from a prostate cancer can closely mimic primary breast cancer, especially low-grade primary breast cancer.

Immunohistochemical stains that are useful to confirm prostate primary are PAP and PSA.

Carcinoid tumors: Metastases from lung and gastrointestinal primaries should be suspected if the tumor exhibits a nested growth pattern, and lacks hormone receptor expression (ER and PR).

Tumor cells show diffuse positivity for the neuroendocrine markers synaptophysin and chromogranin and should be negative for cytokeratin 7.

Although some breast cancers can show neuroendocrine differentiation.

Absence of an in-situ carcinoma can be helpful to exclude a breast primary.

Carcinoid tumors have a low-grade appearance with small uniform cells arranged in cords and trabeculae.

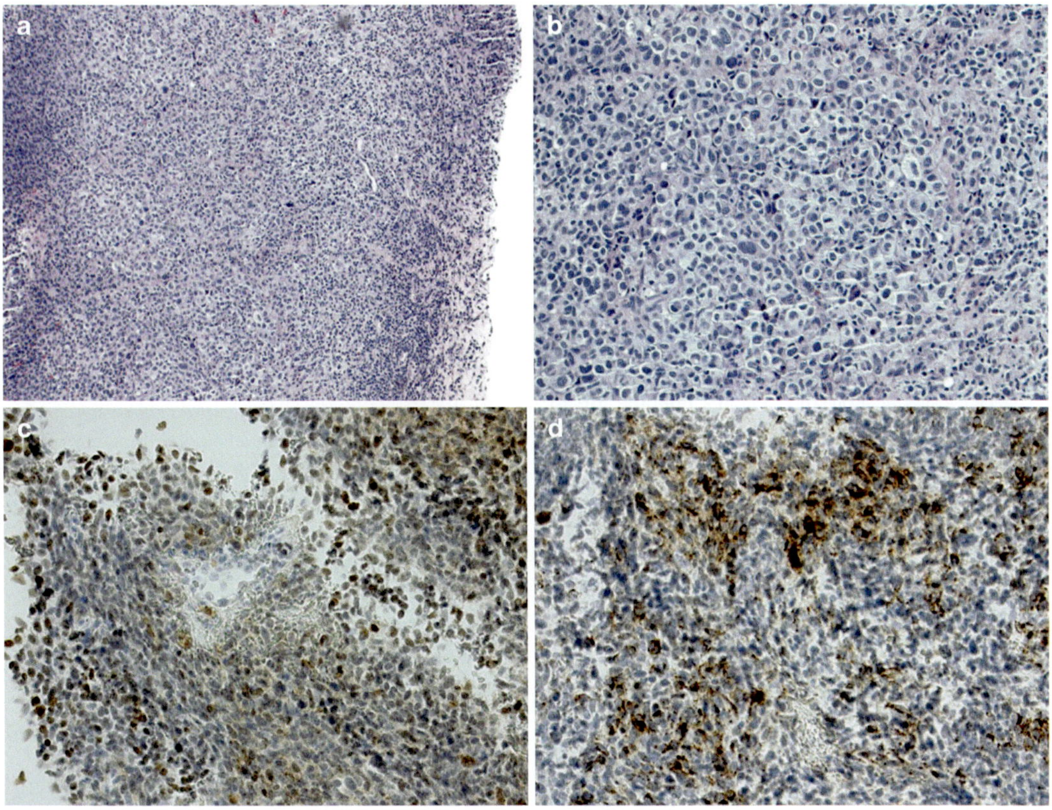

Fig. 2.49 A 71-year-old woman with a history of melanoma now presents with multiple palpable breast masses which are seen on mammography and ultrasound. The lesions are biopsied to reveal a pleomorphic population of discohesive cells with prominent nucleoli (**a**, **b**). Immunostains for S100 (**c**) and HMB45 (**d**) are positive supporting the diagnosis of metastatic melanoma

Gastric carcinoma: Signet-ring cell carcinoma can mimic primary invasive lobular carcinoma.

Since both tumors have germline mutations of E-cadherin gene, additional immunohistochemical workup is required to exclude a gastric primary.

Immunohistochemical stains for CDX2 and CK20 are positive in gastric carcinoma.

Lymphoma: High-grade lymphomas can mimic a breast primary and therefore in the appropriate clinical context, immunohistochemical staining with lymphoma markers is prudent.

GATA 3 and cytokeratin should be included in the panel which should be negative in lymphomas; however, high-grade breast cancers may also be negative.

- **Differential Diagnosis**: Lung adenocarcinoma, ovarian serous carcinoma, melanoma, prostate cancer, carcinoid tumors, gastric carcinoma, lymphoma, invasive ductal carcinoma, and primary breast carcinoma.
- **Management**: Proven metastatic carcinoma to the breast does not require excision as surgery to remove metastasis does not improve outcomes. It is therefore critical to diagnose metastatic tumors to the breast to avoid unnecessary surgery.

References

1. Hertel BF, Zaloudek C, Kempson RL. Breast adenomas. Cancer. 1976;37(6):2891–905.
2. O'Hara MF, Page DL. Adenomas of the breast and ectopic breast under lactational influences. Hum Pathol. 1985;16(7):707–12.
3. Schnitt SJ, Collins LC. Biopsy interpretation of the breast. 3rd ed. Wolter Kluwer Health; 2018.
4. Rosen PP. Adenomyoepithelioma of the breast. Hum Pathol. 1987;18(12):1232–7.
5. Hayes MM. Asenomyoepithelioma of the breast: a review stressing its propensity for malignant transformation. J Clin Pathol. 1022;64(6):477–84.
6. WHO Classification of Tumours Editorial Board. Breast tumours. In: WHO classification of tumour series, 5th ed., vol. 2. Lyon (France): International Agency for Research on Cancer; 2019.
7. Trojani M, Guiu M, Trouette H, et al. Malignant adenomyoepithelioma of the breast: an immunohistochemical, cytomorphological, and ultrastructural study of a case with lung metastases. Am J Clin Pathol. 1992;98(6):598–602.
8. Pike AM, Oberman HA. Juvenile (cellular) adenofibromas: a clinicopathologic study. Am J Surg Pathol. 1985;9(10):730–6.
9. Mrogan JM, Douglas-Jones AG, Gupta SK. Analysis of histological features in needle core biopsy of breast useful in preoperative distinction between fibroadenoma and phyllodes tumor. Histopathology. 2010;56(4):489–500.
10. Nassar A, Visscher DW, Degnim AC, et al. Complex fibroadenoma and breast cancer risk: a Mayo Clinic benign breast disease cohort study. Breast Cancer Res Treat. 2015;153(2):397–405.
11. Diaz NM, Palmer JO, McDivitt RW. Carcinoma arising within fibroadenomas of the breast: a clinicopathologic study of 105 pateints. Am J Clin Pathol. 1991;95(5):614–22.
12. Dupont WD, Page DL, Parl FF, et al. Long term risk of breast cancer in women with fibroadenoma. N Engl J Med. 1994;331(1):10–5.
13. American Society Breast Surgeons. Consensus guideline on concordance assessment of image-guided breast biopsies and management of borderline or high-risk lesions. 2023.
14. Harris JR, Lippman ME, Morrow M, Osborne CK. Diseases of the breast. 5th ed. Wolters Kluwer Health; 2014.
15. Tan BY, Acs G, Apple SK, et al. Phyllodes tumours of the breast: a consensus review. Histopathology. 2016;68(1):5–21.
16. Kalambo M, Adrada BE, Adeyefa MM, et al. Phyllodes tumor of the breast: ultrasound-pathology correlation. AJR. 2018;210:W173–9.
17. Lee JS, Chang J, Hagemann IS, Bennett DL. Radiologic-pathologic correlation: malignant Phyllodes tumor: imaging features with histopathologic correlation. J Breast Imaging. 2021:703–11.
18. Berg WA, Yang WT. Diagnostic imaging breast. 2nd ed. Amirsys, Inc; 2014.
19. Morris EA, Liberman L. Breast MRI diagnosis and intervention. Springer; 2005.
20. Rosen PP, Hoda SA. Breast pathology: diagnosis by needle Core biopsy. 3rd ed. Wolters Kluwer Health and Lippincott Williams and Wilkins; 2010.
21. Vorherr H. Fibrocystic breast disease: pathophysiology, pathomorphology, clinical picture, and management. Am J Obstet Gynecol. 1986;154(1):161–79. https://doi.org/10.1016/0002-9378(86)90421-7.
22. Stachs A, Stubert J, Reimer T, Hartmann S. Benign breast disease in women. Dtsch Arztebl Int. 2019;116(33-34):565–74. https://doi.org/10.3238/arztebl.2019.0565. PMID: 31554551; PMCID: PMC6794703
23. Malherbe K, Khan M, Fatima S. Fibrocystic breast disease. [updated 2022 Aug 8]. In: StatPearls [internet]. Treasure Island (FL): StatPearls Publishing; 2023.
24. Tabar L, Dean PB. Teaching atlas of mammography. 3rd ed. Georg Thieme Verlag; 2001.
25. Madjar H, Mendelson EB. The practice of breast ultrasound. 2nd ed. Georg Thieme Verlag; 2008.
26. World Health Organization. Histological typing of breast tumors. Tumori. 1982;68:181–98.
27. Ridolfi RL, Rosen PP, Port A, et al. Medullary carcinoma of the breast: a clinicopathologic study with 10 year follow-up. Cancer. 1977;40(4):1365–85.
28. Pedersen L, Zedeler K, Holck S, et al. Medullary carcinoma of the breast: prevalence and prognostic importance of classical risk factors in breast cancer. Eur J Cancer. 1995;31A(13-14):2289–95.
29. Cardenosa G, Doudna C, Eklund GW. Mucinous (colloid) breast cancer: clinical and mammographic findings in 10 patients. AJR Am J Roentgenol. 1994;162(5):1077–9.
30. Gunhan-Bilgen I, Memis A, Ustun EE, et al. Metaplastic carcinoma of the breast: clinical, mammographic and sonographic findings with histopathologic correlation. AJR. 2002;178:1311–571.
31. Pezzi CM, Patel-Parekh L, Cole K, et al. Characteristics and treatment of metaplastic breast cancer: analysis of 892 cases from the National Cancer Data Base. Ann Surg Oncol. 2007;14(1):166–73.
32. Choi BB, Shu KS. Metaplastic carcinoma of the breast: multimodality imaging and histopathologic assessment. Acta Radiol. 2012;53(1):5–11.
33. Rosen PP. Rosen's breast pathology. 3rd ed. Philadelphia, PA: Lippincott Williams & Wilkins; 2009.
34. Chhieng C, Cranor M, Lesser ME, et al. Metaplastic carcinoma of the breasr with osteocartilaginous heterologous elements. Am J Surg Pathol. 1998;22(2):188–94.
35. Tse GM, Law BK, Ma TK, et al. Hamartomas of the breast: a clinicopathologic review. J Clin Pathol. 2002;55(12):951–4.
36. Daya D, Trus T, D'Souza TJ, et al. Hamartoma of the breast, an underrecognized breast lesion: a clinico-

pathologic and radiographic study of 25 cases. Am J Clin Pathol. 1995;103(6):685–9.
37. Overman HA. Hamartomas and hamartoma variants of the breast. Semin Diagn Pathol. 1989;6(2): 135–45.
38. Linell F, Ostberg G, Soderstrom J, et al. Breast hamartomas: an important entity in mammary pathology. Virchows Arch A Pathol Anat Histol. 1979;383(3):253–64.
39. Degnim AC, Frost MH, Radisky DC, et al. Pseudoangiomatous stromal hyperplasia and breast cancer risk. Ann Surg Oncol. 2010;17(12):3269–77.
40. DeLAir DF, Corben AD, Catalano JP, et al. Non-mammary metastases to the breast and axilla: a study of 85 cases. Mod Pathol. 2013;26(3):343–9.
41. Khoury R, Bucau M, Bizot A, Khalil A. Breast metastasis of a lung carcinoma. BJR Case Rep. 2021;8(2):20210142.
42. Ramwani R, Wernberg J. Three cases of atypical breast metastasis from lung adenocarcinoma. Clin Med Res. 2022;20(4):231–5.
43. Barnett C, Mehta N, Towne WS, Babagbemi K, Sales RM. Metastatic melanoma in the breast and axilla: a case report. Clin Imaging. 2022;85:78–82.

3 Complex Cystic and Solid Masses

Malini Harigopal, Kimberly Cole, Peter Podany,
Anuj Verma, and Liva Andrejeva

Benign

Fat Necrosis

See Chap. 5 for additional information and microscopic images.

Fat Necrosis: Fat necrosis frequently is encountered after breast surgery: lumpectomy, mastectomy, excisional biopsy, breast reduction, and breast reconstruction. However, it may also be encountered in asymptomatic patients on screening exams.

- **Clinical Presentation**: The patient may present for diagnostic mammography and/or ultrasound with a palpable mass, and s/he may recall an episode of trauma to the breast.
- **Imaging Findings**:
  - **Mammography**: Variable appearance depending on chronicity.

    Acute lesions may be oval or round with circumscribed or indistinct margins, sometimes containing visible "bubbles" of fat (Fig. 3.1).
  - **US**: Variable appearance depending on chronicity.

    May range from ill-defined hyperechoic regions within fat lobules, to complex cystic masses without internal vascularity [1].
  - **MRI**: May manifest as oval, round or irregular masses with peripheral irregular ring enhancement with variable kinetics [2].

    Contain fat as manifested on T1 nonfat suppressed sequences [2].
  - **BI-RADS**: 2, 3, or 4 depending on imaging appearance, clinical history, and ability to correlate with clinical history of trauma to the area.
  - **Differential Diagnosis**: Abscess, complicated cyst, invasive ductal carcinoma, invasive lobular carcinoma.
- **Pathology Findings**:
  - **Microscopic Histology**: Core needle biopsy shows infarction of fat cells and hemorrhage initially, followed by histiocytes along with foreign body material and multinucleated giant cells depending on the etiology. A variable infiltrate of plasma cells, lymphocytes, and eosinophils is also often present [3, 4].

M. Harigopal · P. Podany · A. Verma
Department of Pathology, Yale University,
New Haven, CT, USA
e-mail: malini.harigopal@yale.edu;
peter.podany@yale.edu; anuj.verma@yale.edu

K. Cole
Department of Pathology, University of Chicago,
Chicago, IL, USA
e-mail: cbm7353@uchicago.edu

L. Andrejeva (✉)
Department of Radiology and Biomedical Imaging,
Yale School of Medicine, New Haven, CT, USA
e-mail: liva.andrejeva@yale.edu

M. Harigopal et al. (eds.), *Radiology Pathology Correlations of Breast Lesions*,
https://doi.org/10.1007/978-3-031-65711-5_3

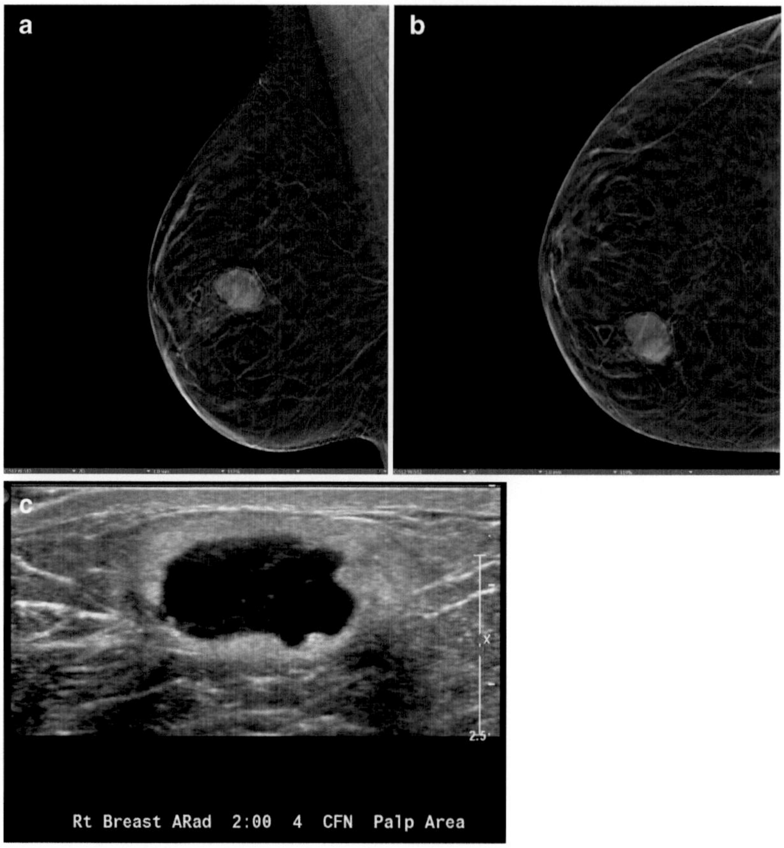

Fig. 3.1 A 43-year-old female palpated a right breast mass. She did not recall a history of trauma to the breast. Mammography revealed an oval, hyper-dense mass with an indistinct margin (**a**, **b**). Ultrasound showed a lobulated mass with internal septations, possible mural nodularity, and an echogenic rim (**c**). The lesion was classified as BI-RADS 4, suspicious; and an US-guided core needle biopsy was recommended and performed. On needle core biopsy there were cystic spaces with multinucleated histiocytes, fibrosis, and granulomatous reaction indicative of fat necrosis

As the lesion evolves with cavitation of fat, fibrosis is evident around the focus of fat necrosis with scar formation and calcifications [3].

Surrounding ducts and lobules may develop squamous metaplasia [3].

Even in older lesions, a few histiocytes persist and may be highlighted by CD68.

Additional deeper H&E levels may be useful for clinically and mammographically concerning lesions for definitive diagnosis.

- **Differential Diagnosis**: Cystically dilated ducts, duct ectasia, granulomatous inflammation.
- **Management**: Fat necrosis can be managed by observation when concordant with imaging findings. Due to the relatively rapid evolution of fat necrosis, the patient may be asked to return in as little as 6 weeks for repeat imaging to confirm that the area is changing as would be expected for fat necrosis.

Smaller areas of fat necrosis may resolve completely.
Larger areas will gradually become more cystic and assume the typical oil cyst appearance on mammography.
At times, fat necrosis may be indistinguishable from malignant lesions, such as breast cancers, particularly in patients who have been treated for breast cancer in the past. In such cases, a needle biopsy may be necessary and can be virtually diagnostic of fat necrosis.
Excision is usually not indicated and may result in additional fat necrosis.

Abscess

Abscess: A precipitating cause for an abscess could be mastitis, and both mastitis and abscess can be puerperal or nonpuerperal. Puerperal mastitis and abscesses are more common within 3 months of childbirth and may be precipitated by blocked ducts, latching difficulty, and cracked nipples [5]. Nonpuerperal infections are correlated with smoking, diabetes, obesity, and black race [5]. Abscesses may occasionally occur after oncologic or elective breast surgery. Patients who smoke may develop subareolar abscesses that become chronic as well as fistulae to the periareolar skin. These abscesses are thought to be due to squamous metaplasia of lactiferous ducts (SMOLD) [5].

- **Clinical Presentation**: The patient usually presents for diagnostic mammography and/or ultrasound with a painful, palpable mass. The breast may also be erythematous and edematous, and the patient may be febrile.
- **Imaging Findings**:
  - **Mammography**: Appearance can vary based on chronicity.
    In acute cases, abscesses may appear as round or oval masses, with margins that can range from circumscribed to indistinct [5] (Fig. 3.2).
      Associated overlying skin thickening or nipple areolar complex thickening may be present.
      Axillary adenopathy may be present.
    In chronic cases, the mammographic appearance may be indistinguishable from that of a locally advanced breast cancer.
      The abscess may appear as a spiculated mass, usually subareolar in location, with associated skin thickening and nipple retraction [5].
      Axillary adenopathy may be present.
  - **US**: In the acute setting, abscesses may be oval, round or irregular cystic masses with mobile internal echoes. The cyst wall may be thick, and increased peripheral vascularity may be present [5].
    Chronic abscesses may be irregular, difficult to distinguish from solid masses, and may have visible fistulae extending to the overlying skin.
  - **BI-RADS**: 2, 3, 4, or 5 depending on correlation with clinical history and symptoms.
  - **Differential Diagnosis**: In the chronic setting: granulomatous mastitis, inflammatory breast cancer, locally advanced breast cancer.
- **Pathology Findings**:
  - **Microscopic Histology**: Core needle biopsy shows mixed acute and chronic inflammation depending on chronicity and may progress to fistula formation [4] (Fig. 3.3).
    Surrounding breast shows typical lactational changes with vacuolated epithelial cells in puerperal mastitis.
  - **Differential Diagnosis**: Squamous metaplasia of lactiferous ducts (SMOLD),

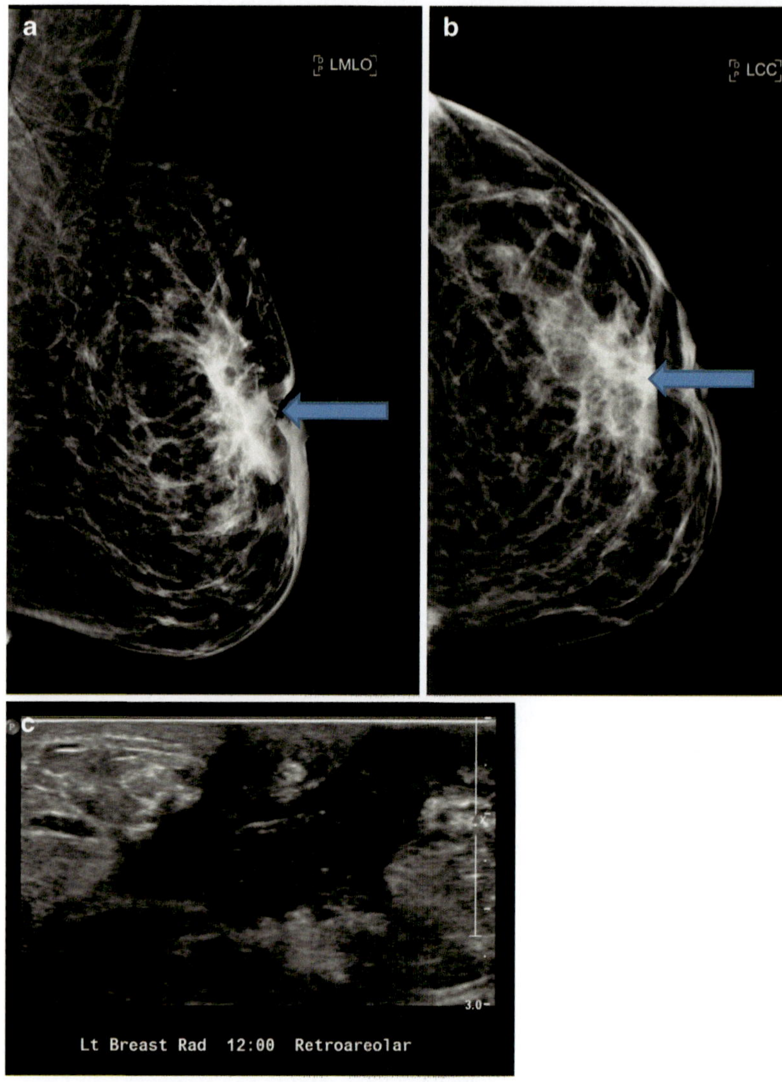

Fig. 3.2 A 46-year-old long time heavy smoker, presented with a painful, waxing and waning mass in her left breast with drainage of purulent material via several small periareolar fistulae. She had been intermittently treated for this condition with antibiotic therapy, with intermittent incomplete improvement. She had been advised to stop smoking, but was not able to quit. Mammography showed an irregular, spiculated left retroareolar mass with nipple retraction and skin thickening (**a, b**). On ultrasound there was an irregular, partially cystic mass with internal echoes, adjacent vascularity and fistula tract leading to the skin surface (**c**). The imaging findings were considered BI-RADS 2, benign findings

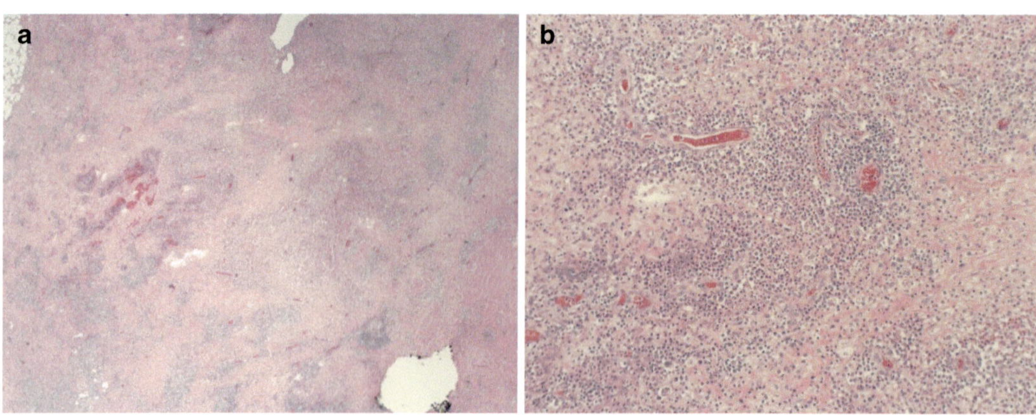

Fig. 3.3 A 63-year-old female underwent a mastectomy for invasive ductal carcinoma. On resection the background breast tissue was found to have marked mixed inflammation and abscess formation (**a**, **b**)

idiopathic granulomatous lobular mastitis, cystic neutrophilic granulomatous mastitis.

Squamous metaplasia of lactiferous ducts "SMOLD": presents as a painful retroareolar mass.

Histology shows squamous metaplasia of ducts, keratin debris and giant cells.

Idiopathic granulomatous lobular mastitis: The etiology is unknown as no microorganisms are routinely isolated and histochemical stains for organisms such as acid fast bacilli and fungi are negative; however, *Corynebacterium* have been reported in some studies [6].

Histology shows lobular inflammation with lymphocytes, multinucleated histiocytes, plasma cells, and occasional eosinophils.

Cystic neutrophilic granulomatous mastitis: A relatively new entity which has clinical and histologic features similar to idiopathic granulomatous mastitis.

Histology shows lobulocentric granulomas with associated neutrophils lining cystic spaces.

The cysts are thought to be formed by dissolution of lipid from degenerating cells during histologic processing [7].

Although, special stains for organisms are negative, culture studies have demonstrated *Corynebacterium* species [7].

- **Management**: Abscess formation in the breast is often seen associated with lactation, usually as a result of infection by *Staphylococcus aureus*. Surgical treatment is usually not required. They are usually managed by aspiration, with fluid sent for culture, followed by antibiotic therapy. Occasionally, repeat aspiration may be necessary, as purulent fluid may re-accumulate. If fluid cannot be aspirated, a surgical incision and drainage may be necessary. Chronic breast abscesses resulting from SMOLD can be refractory to conservative therapy (antibiotics and aspiration), and definitive treatment includes broad spectrum antibiotics, excision of the affected tissue and fistulae, as well as smoking cessation [5].

Mammary Duct Ectasia

Mammary Duct Ectasia: The term "duct ectasia" refers to a benign dilatation of mammary ducts filled with fluid. It is usually seen in postmenopausal women but can be seen in younger women and children [8]. The etiology of duct ectasia is thought to be due to loss of elasticity and weakening of the duct wall [4, 9, 10]. The secretions within the duct may cause obstruction of the duct with extravasation of duct contents into the surrounding stroma. Acute and chronic inflammation results in eventual fibrosis. When multiple ducts are involved bilaterally by duct ectasia, further evaluation may not be done as the likelihood of finding DCIS unassociated with microcalcifications is higher in solitary dilated ducts [11].

- **Clinical Presentation**: Patients with duct ectasia can present with a palpable mass in the subareolar location with extrusion of thick nipple discharge. The majority of patients are asymptomatic and may be detected on screening mammography [8–10]. However, occasionally patients may present with nipple discharge which is yellow, brown or green, but generally not clear or bloody. Rarely duct ectasia can present with nipple distortion or inversion due to fibrotic and scarred ducts from chronic inflammation.
- **Imaging Findings**:
  - **Mammography**: Dilated ducts with an associated irregular mass and or calcifications (Fig. 3.4).
  - **US**: Dilated ducts.
  - **BI-RADS**: 2.
  - **Differential Diagnosis**: Benign papilloma, periductal mastitis, DCIS in a dilated duct.

- **Pathology Findings**:
  - **Microscopic Histology**: Ductal dilatation with associated chronic inflammation consisting of lymphocytes and plasma cells are seen surrounding ducts (Fig. 3.5)

    Macrophages with hemosiderin and lipid can be seen within ducts and in the duct walls along with lymphocytes.

    When the duct contents extrude outside, periductal chronic inflammation can be seen.

    On core needle biopsies the diagnosis of duct ectasia can be suggested when dilated ducts are seen with periductal chronic inflammation [4, 12].

    This histologic finding is not specific to duct ectasia and can be seen in other inflammatory diseases of the breast [4].

    A diagnosis of duct ectasia usually generates a radiologic pathologic correlation in a rad path conference to ensure that that the target lesion was biopsied.
  - **Differential Diagnosis**: Cysts, SMOLD, plasma cell mastitis, and lymphoma.
  - **Management**: Asymptomatic bilateral duct ectasia is a benign finding without need for additional diagnostic workup. However, a dilated solitary duct is a rare presentation for duct ectasia and therefore requires additional workup with diagnostic workup to rule out intraductal masses such as intraductal papilloma or DCIS [11].

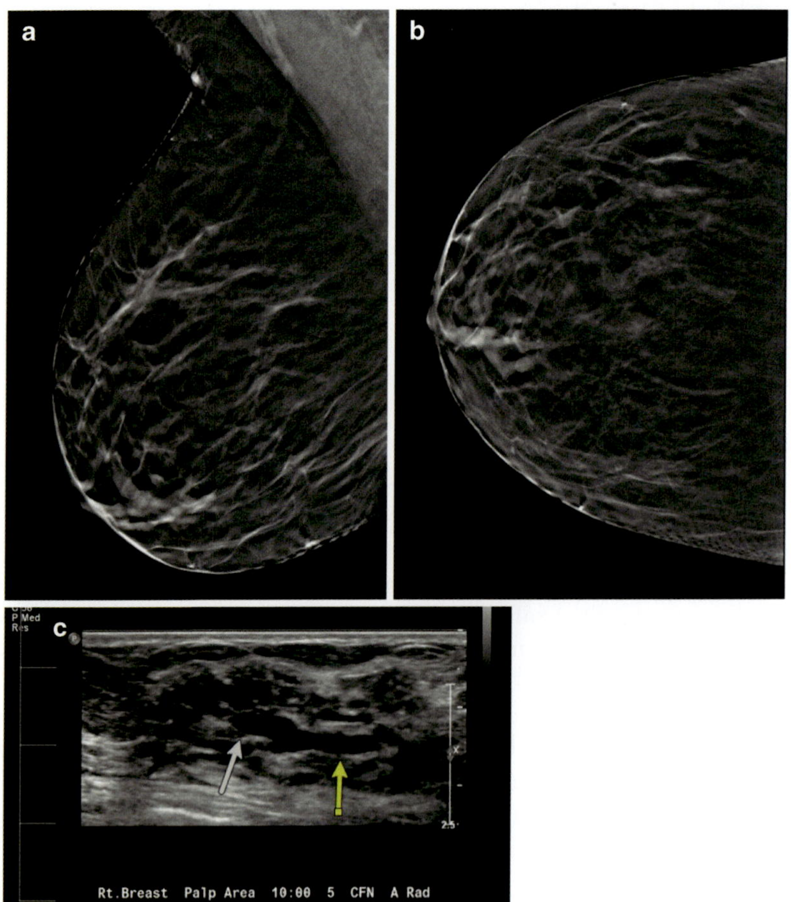

Fig. 3.4 A 45-year-old woman presented with a palpable lesion on her right breast. On mammography (**a, b**) dilated ducts were seen, which correlated with the palpable lesion and dilated ducts seen on ultrasound (**c**). These findings were also present on T1, STIR, and postcontrast subtracted MRI which highlighted the marked chronic duct ectasia (**d–f**)

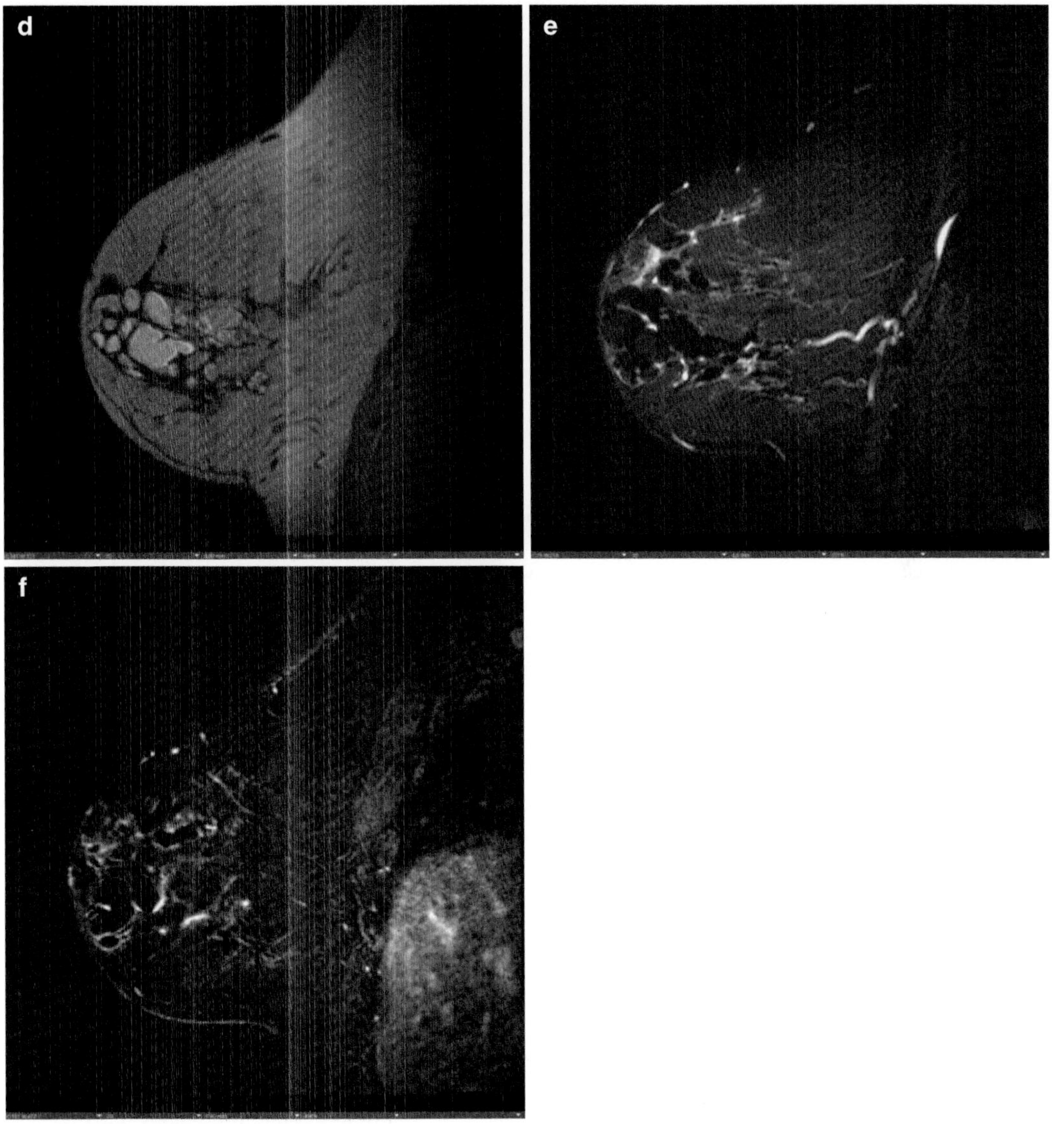

Fig. 3.4 (continued)

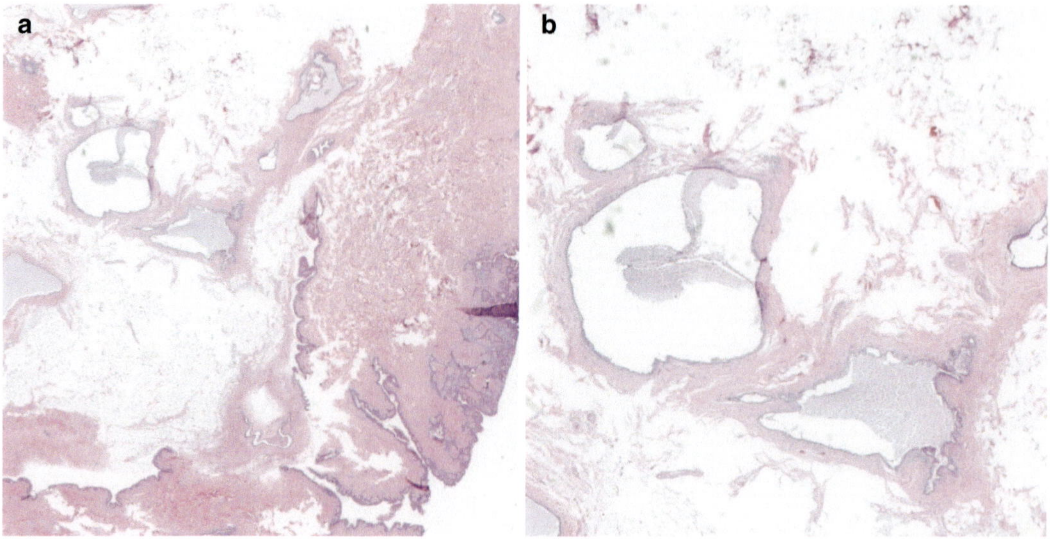

Fig. 3.5 A 74-year-old woman presented for right mastectomy due to biopsy proven invasive ductal carcinoma. Incidentally on resection ductal ectasia of the nipple with enlarged, dilated ducts was seen (**a**, **b**)

Sclerosing Adenosis

See Chaps. 5 and 7 for additional information and images.

Sclerosing Adenosis: Sclerosing adenosis is a benign lesion of the terminal duct lobular unit commonly mistaken for invasive carcinoma. It is associated with a 1.5–2.0× increased risk for subsequent development of invasive carcinoma in either breast [13, 14].

- **Clinical Presentation**: Sclerosing adenosis can present with a lobulocentric growth/mass.
- **Imaging Findings**:
  - **Mammography**: Incidentally seen as a mammographic abnormality with clustered amorphous calcifications. It can also present as a lobulated mass or when nodular as a palpable mass.
- **Pathology Findings**:
  - **Microscopic Histology**: Sclerosing adenosis can be best appreciated under low power examination as a circumscribed proliferation with lobulocentric growth around a duct.

    On higher magnification the glands are enlarged with aggregates of tubules or acini distorted or compressed by sclerotic stroma.

    The adenosis glands are lined by luminal cells with a prominent myoepithelial layer which can be spindled. However, the myoepithelial layer may be partially obscured by the surrounding sclerotic stroma [4].

    The clusters of distorted acini usually "respect" the fat but rarely can be seen to infiltrate into the surrounding fat [4].

    Perineural invasion can be seen rarely.

    Adenosis glands can become confluent forming nodular aggregates with associated microcalcifications.

    The term apocrine adenosis is used when sclerosing adenosis is involved by apocrine metaplasia of the luminal epithelium [15].

    These lesions can be particularly challenging as they can mimic carcinoma due to the nuclear enlargement and uniform appearance of the metaplastic cells.

    Similarly, in situ or invasive carcinoma (LCIS or DCIS) can involve sclerosing adenosis.

Sclerosing adenosis is frequently associated with other proliferative breast lesions like usual ductal hyperplasia, fibrocystic changes and sclerosing papillary lesions. Fibroadenomas may be involved by sclerosing adenosis [4].

Core needle biopsy of sclerosing adenosis can be difficult when the entire lesion including the periphery cannot be visualized due to the limited nature of the CNB.

- **Differential Diagnosis**: Physiologic adenosis seen during pregnancy, involution of lobules with age, invasive ductal carcinoma, microglandular adenosis, adenomyoepithlioma, and tubular adenosis.
- **Atypical Apocrine Adenosis**:

  Atypical apocrine adenosis is defined as nodular sclerosing adenosis involved by apocrine atypia. It is a rare entity with a prevalence of about 0.4% [15, 16].

  Apocrine cells show threefold variation in nuclear size and prominent nucleoli [15].

  Distinction from apocrine DCIS is not clear cut.

  Differential Diagnosis: Apocrine DCIS, invasive sclerosing adenosis, pleomorphic LCIS.

  Management: Limited data on management, surgical excision [16].
- **Microglandular Adenosis**:

  Uncommon breast lesion (prevalence of 0.2%) found incidentally or as a mass forming lesion [17, 18].

  Diagnostically challenging small glandular proliferations seen on core needle biopsy.

  Most important is to distinguish benign versus malignant.

  Noninvasive or invasive.

  Orderly or haphazard.

  Infiltrative and non-lobulocentric, small round uniform glands lined by a single layer of cuboidal epithelium. Open lumens contain PAS-positive eosinophilic secretions [18].

  The basement membrane is present but lacks myoepithelial cells.

  IHC: S100 positive, p63 negative, collagen IV positive, ER negative [18].

  Benign lesion but can be associated with invasive carcinoma in up to 27% of cases (non-obligate precursor) [19]. Similar clonal alterations between microglandular adenosis, atypical microglandular adenosis, and carcinoma [19].

  Differential Diagnosis: Tubular carcinoma, acinic cell carcinoma, tubular adenosis, sclerosing adenosis.

  Management: Microglandular adenosis diagnosed on biopsy requires an excision. Negative margins are not always feasible.

Galactocele

Galactocele:

- **Clinical Presentation**: Patients usually presents for imaging with a palpable, occasionally painful mass in the lactational or post-lactational period [20].
- **Imaging Findings**:
  - **Mammography**: May be performed if US findings are not typical.

    Circumscribed mass containing fatty material.

    Occasionally may see a fat-fluid level on a lateral view [20].
  - **US**: The initial exam of choice in a lactating woman.

    Demonstrates an oval, circumscribed mass of variable echogenicity, with hyperechoic material, sometimes mobile (the fat in the milk) within the nondependent aspect of the mass [21] (Fig. 3.6).
  - **BI-RADS**: 2, 3, 4 depending on the clinical presentation and imaging findings.
  - **Differential Diagnosis**: Simple or complicated cyst, abscess, papilloma, fibroadenoma, lactating adenoma, breast carcinoma.

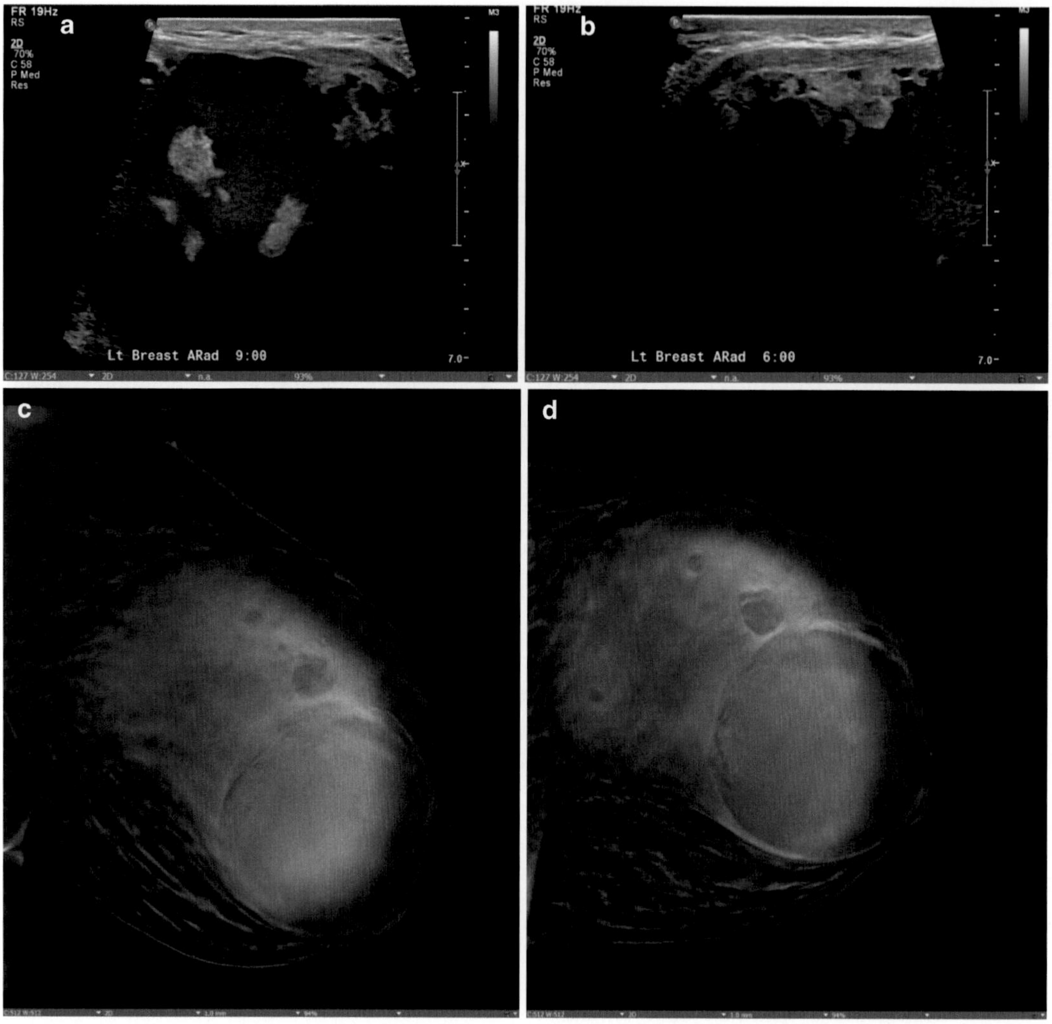

Fig. 3.6 A 25-year-old lactating female, 4 months postpartum, palpates a large mass in her left breast. While she can continue breastfeeding from her left breast, milk production is lower from the left compared to the right. Ultrasound showed a very large, oval complex cystic and solid mass (**a**, **b**). Mammogram was performed because the US appearance of the mass was not typical for a galactocele. This demonstrated a large, hyperdense oval mass that appears to contain bubbles of fat (**c**, **d**). The mass was scored BI-RADS 4a, low suspicion of malignancy. A diagnostic US-guided aspiration was recommended and performed

- **Pathology Findings**:
  - **Microscopic Histology**: Histology shows a cystically dilated duct or fragment of duct wall containing proteinaceous debris [4, 22] (Fig. 3.7).

    Surrounding breast may show secondary acute and chronic inflammation.

    Galactoceles are rarely biopsied.
  - **Management**: If painful or bothersome, a galactocele can be aspirated with US guidance. An US-guided biopsy may be necessary if findings are not typical.

    Smaller galactoceles will resolve without intervention over time [21].

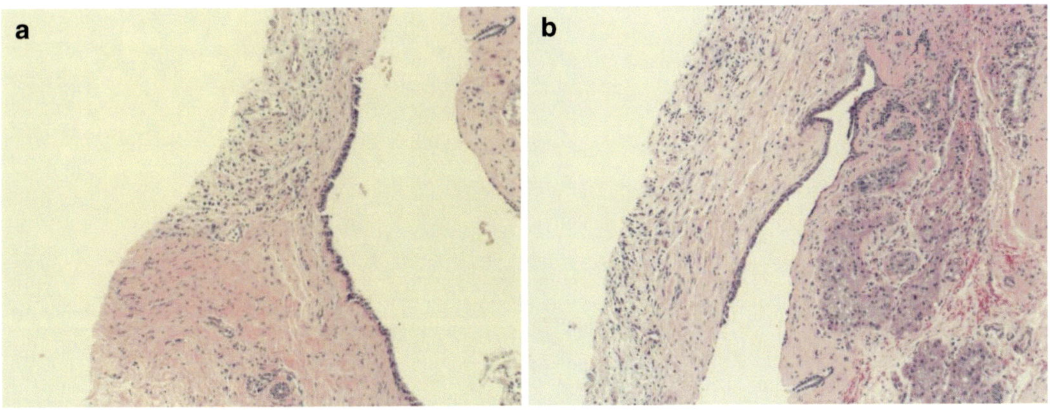

Fig. 3.7 A 40-year-old lactating woman presented with a left breast mass at 2:00. An ultrasound-guided core biopsy of the mass was performed revealing chronic inflammation, duct ectasia, and abundant acellular debris consistent with a galactocele (**a**, **b**)

Epidermal Inclusion Cyst

Epidermal Inclusion Cyst: An epidermal inclusion cyst of the breast develops due to the implantation and proliferation of epidermal elements within the dermis, with subsequent growth due to the accumulation of epithelial and keratinous debris, resulting in a lamellated keratin-filled cyst [23]. Epidermal inclusion cysts may develop due to obstructed hair follicles or pores, or possibly as a result of surgery [23]. Although these lesions are considered benign, squamous cell carcinoma within a previously benign appearing epidermal inclusion cyst has been reported [23].

- **Clinical Presentation**: These may occur anywhere within the body, but when presenting in the breast, these are usually in the axillary, parasternal, periareolar or inframammary fold region [23]. The patient usually presents for diagnostic imaging with a palpable, occasionally painful, firm mass close to the skin surface. If inflamed, the overlying skin may be erythematous [24].
- **Imaging Findings**:
  - **Mammography**: Circumscribed, iso- to hyperdense oval mass in a superficial location (Fig. 3.8).
  - **US**: Circumscribed, hypoechoic complex cystic and solid mass within the dermis [25].

    Occasionally, a hypoechoic track can be seen extending to the skin that represents the obstructed hair follicle.

    Increased adjacent vascularity may be present in cases of inflammation.
  - **BI-RADS**: 2, 3, or 4 depending on clinical and imaging findings.
  - **Differential Diagnosis**: Sebaceous cyst, complicated cyst with debris, fat necrosis, fibroadenoma, phyllodes tumor, circumscribed breast cancer.
- **Pathology Findings**:
  - **Microscopic Histology**: A cyst wall lined by squamous epithelium (Fig. 3.9).

    Includes a granular layer in the squamous epithelium.

    Keratinous debris is often present in the cyst.

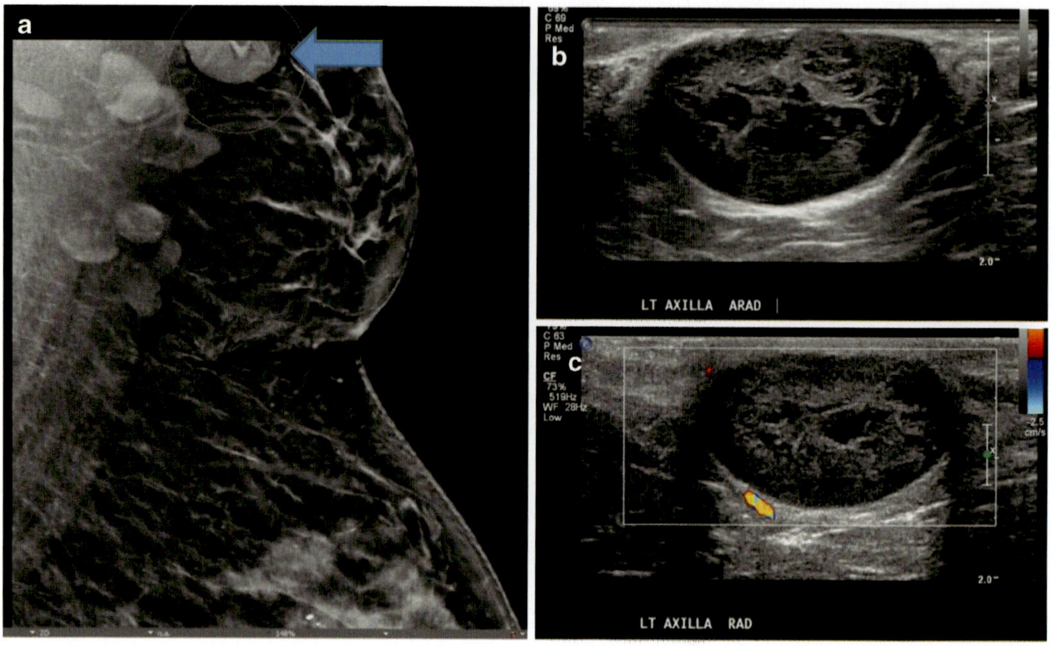

Fig. 3.8 A 51-year-old female palpated a firm mass in her left axillary accessory breast tissue. Mammography partially visualized a circumscribed oval hyperdense mass within an area of accessory breast tissue amidst benign appearing lymph nodes (**a**). On ultrasound there was an oval, circumscribed complex cystic and solid mass with adjacent increased vascularity (**b**, **c**). The mass was graded as BI-RADS 4, suspicious, and an ultrasound-guided core needle biopsy was recommended as this was thought to be concerning for an abnormal lymph node. After the biopsy, the patient developed severe pain and discharge from the biopsy site, which slowly improved over the course of 2 months, without significant response to antibiotic therapy. This was likely due to chemical cellulitis due to spillage of irritant cyst contents into the surrounding tissue secondary to the biopsy

If ruptured mixed inflammation with foreign body giant cells may be present.

- **Differential Diagnosis**: Dermoid cyst, pilar cyst, squamous cell carcinoma.
- **Management**: If not painful, these can be left alone.

  If persistently painful, these may need to be excised surgically.

  A needle biopsy is not recommended due to the risk of chemical cellulitis.

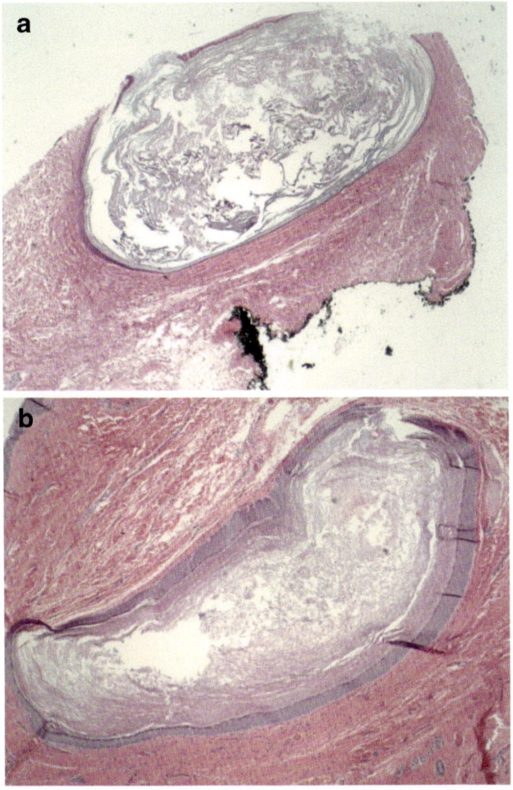

Fig. 3.9 A 41-year-old woman with a history of invasive ductal carcinoma post simple mastectomy presented for breast reconstruction surgery. During the procedure a small cyst was identified in her right breast and excised. On histology the cyst (**a**) demonstrated a squamous lining with a granular layer (**b**) and abundant keratinous debris

Postoperative Hematoma/Seroma

Postoperative Hematoma/Seroma: Seromas are not uncommon due to the rich lymphatic drainage of the breast, with lymphatic fluid accumulating in any closed space resulting from breast surgery [26, 27]. Although more common after mastectomy, up to 20% of patients may experience seromas after lumpectomy [26, 28].

- **Clinical Presentation**: Patients often present for diagnostic imaging with a palpable, sometimes painful mass in the area of bruising/prior surgery.
- **Imaging Findings**:
  - **Mammography**: Oval mass with circumscribed, obscured or indistinct margins at the surgical site (Fig. 3.10).
    Due to the surgery, associated architectural distortion may be present.
  - **US**: Oval, circumscribed avascular mass, which may be anechoic or complex cystic and solid.
  - **BI-RADS**: 2, if clinical presentation correlates with imaging findings and the finding occurs after oncologic surgery with the margins negative.
  - **Differential Diagnosis**: Fat necrosis, complicated cyst, epidermoid inclusion cyst, recurrent malignancy.
- **Pathology Findings**:
  - **Microscopic Histology**: A capsule composed of fibrous tissue (Fig. 3.11).
    May have hyaline degeneration.
    May be associated with inflammation.
  - **Differential Diagnosis**: Implant associated anaplastic large-cell lymphoma.
  - **Management**: If painful, these can be aspirated with US guidance for symptomatic relief.
    Small, asymptomatic hematomas/seromas do not need to be treated.

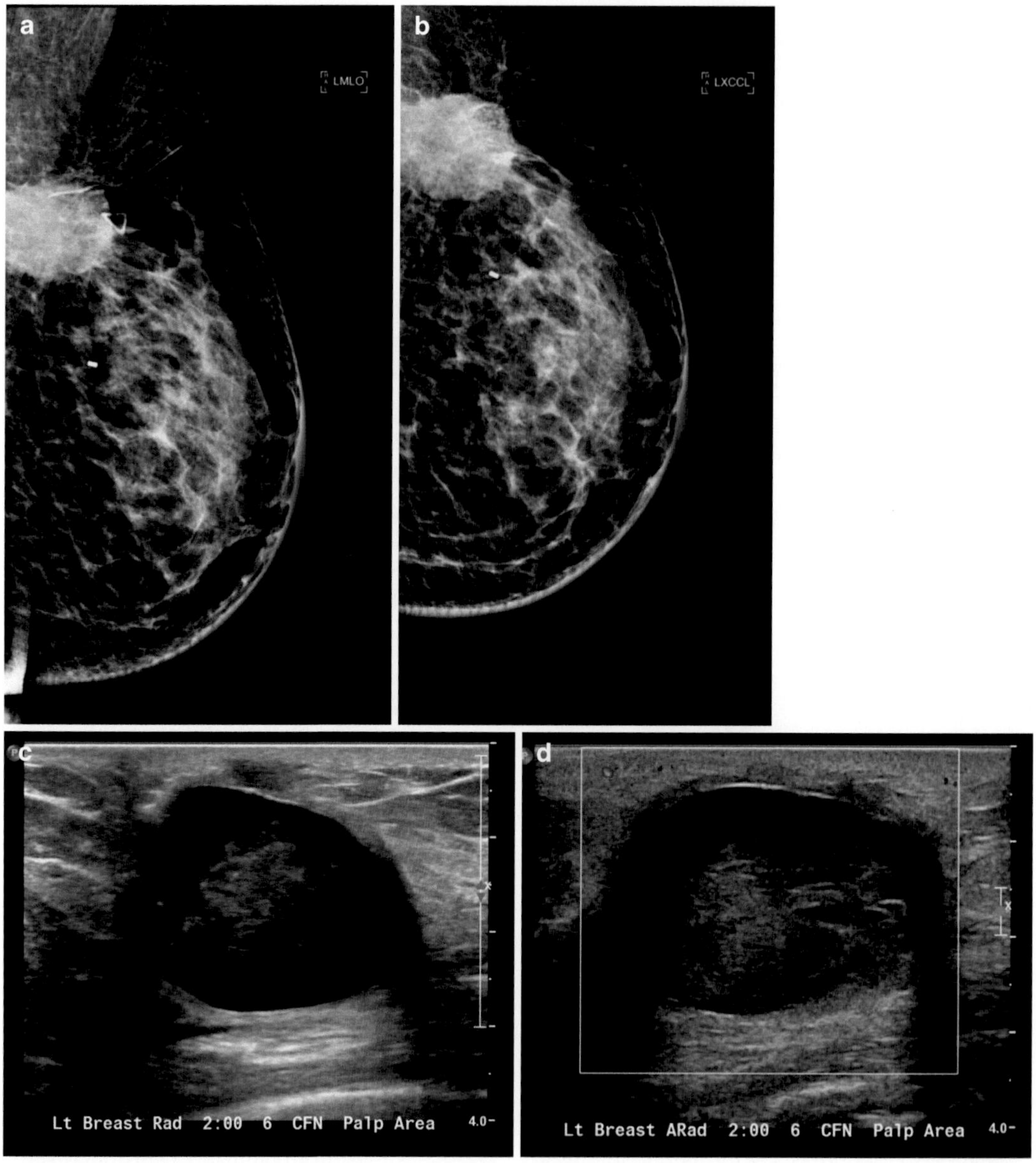

Fig. 3.10 A 54-year-old female presents with a painful, palpable mass in a left axillary tail surgical site, 11 months after left breast lumpectomy for grade 2 DCIS. On mammography there is an oval, hyperdense circumscribed mass (**a**, **b**). Ultrasound shows an oval, complex cystic and solid avascular mass (**c**, **d**). The mass is considered BI-RADS, 2, a benign finding, but US-guided aspiration was requested by the patient and surgeon for symptomatic relief

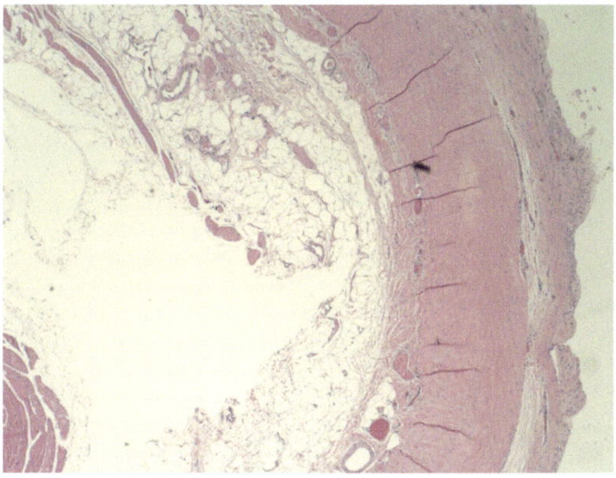

Fig. 3.11 A 43-year-old woman with breast implants underwent bilateral implant removal. During the process a seroma pocket was identified intraoperatively and excised. On histology the tissue demonstrated a strip of dense fibro-connective tissue consistent with a seroma pseudocyst wall

Lymphangioma

Lymphangioma: Lymphangiomas are rare and result due to congenital malformations of the lymphatic system. They grow slowly and may be associated with chromosomal abnormalities if congenital [29].

- **Clinical Presentation**: Most manifest before age 2, and generally occur in the axilla or neck [30]. In the breast they may present as an enlarging palpable breast mass.
- **Imaging Findings**:
  - **Mammography**: Lobulated mass or focal asymmetry (Figs. 3.12).

    May have associated calcifications if large.

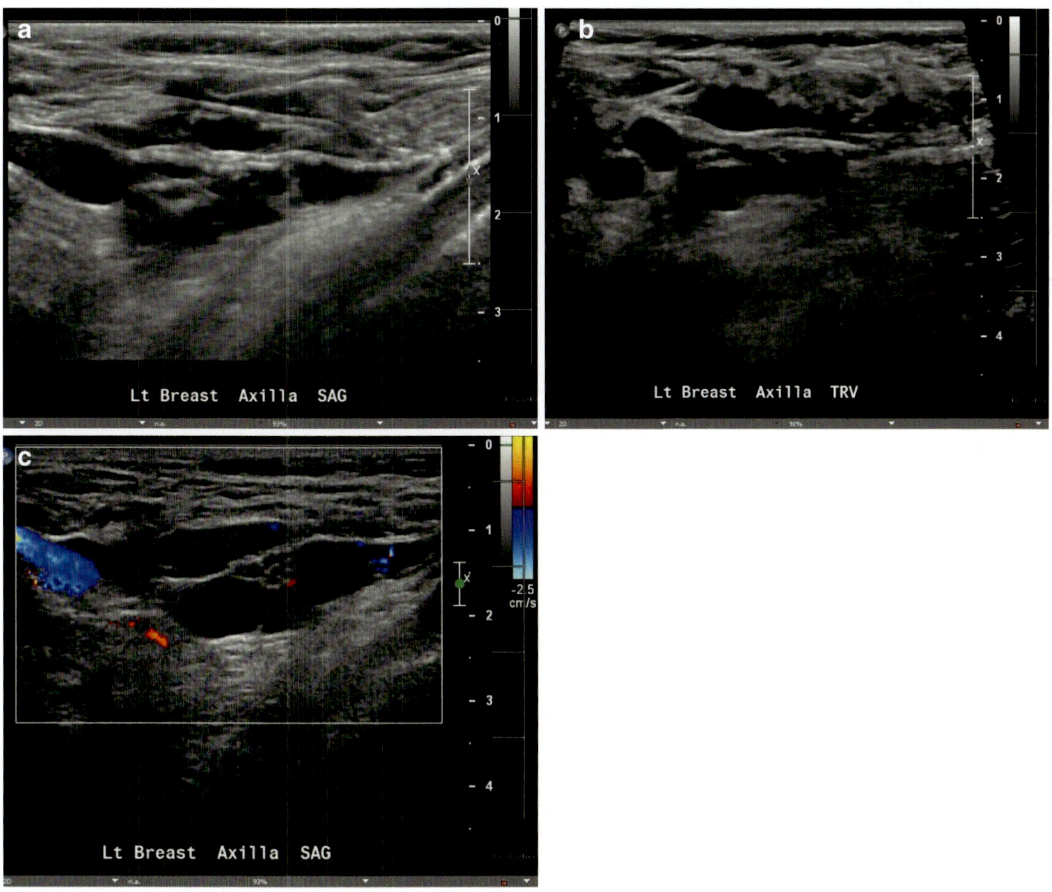

Fig. 3.12 A 46-year-old premenopausal female with family history of breast cancer and with silicone breast implants presented with an enlarging left axillary mass. Mammography was normal but the area of interest could not be included in the field of view due to its location. On ultrasound there was a multiloculated, cystic mass with septations of varying thickness in the left axilla (**a**, **b**, **c**). The mass was called BI-RADS 4, suspicious for malignancy. An US-guided aspiration and biopsy was recommended and performed, yielding atypical vascular structures consistent with a vascular malformation. A subsequent excision yielded a vascular malformation

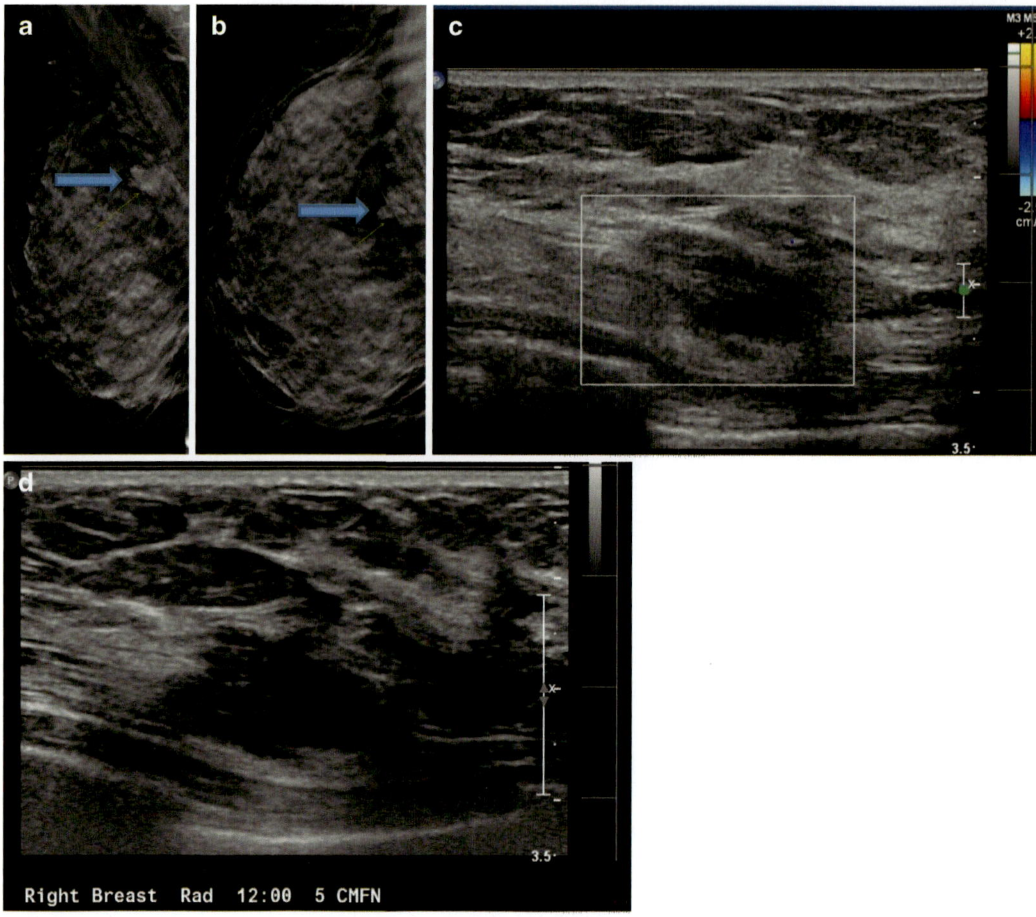

Fig. 3.13 A 41-year-old female presented for screening mammography which showed an irregular mass with a microlobulated margin in the right breast, upper outer quadrant, posterior depth (**a**, **b**). Ultrasound demonstrated a multiloculated cystic mass with septations, and no internal vascularity (**c**, **d**). The lesion was called BI-RADS 4, suspicious of malignancy. An US-guided biopsy was recommended and performed, yielding a lymphangioma

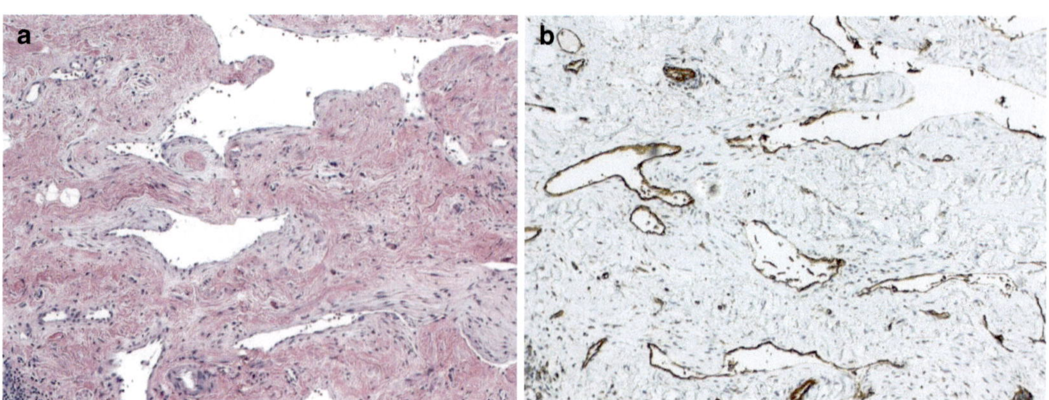

Fig. 3.14 A 38-year-old female underwent core needle biopsy after mammogram demonstrated an irregular mass in her left breast which appeared as a multiloculated cyst on ultrasound. The biopsy demonstrated a lymphangioma with numerous large, irregular endothelial-lined lymphatic channels seen on H&E (**a**). D2-40 highlights the endothelial lining and supports the lymphatic nature of these channels (**b**)

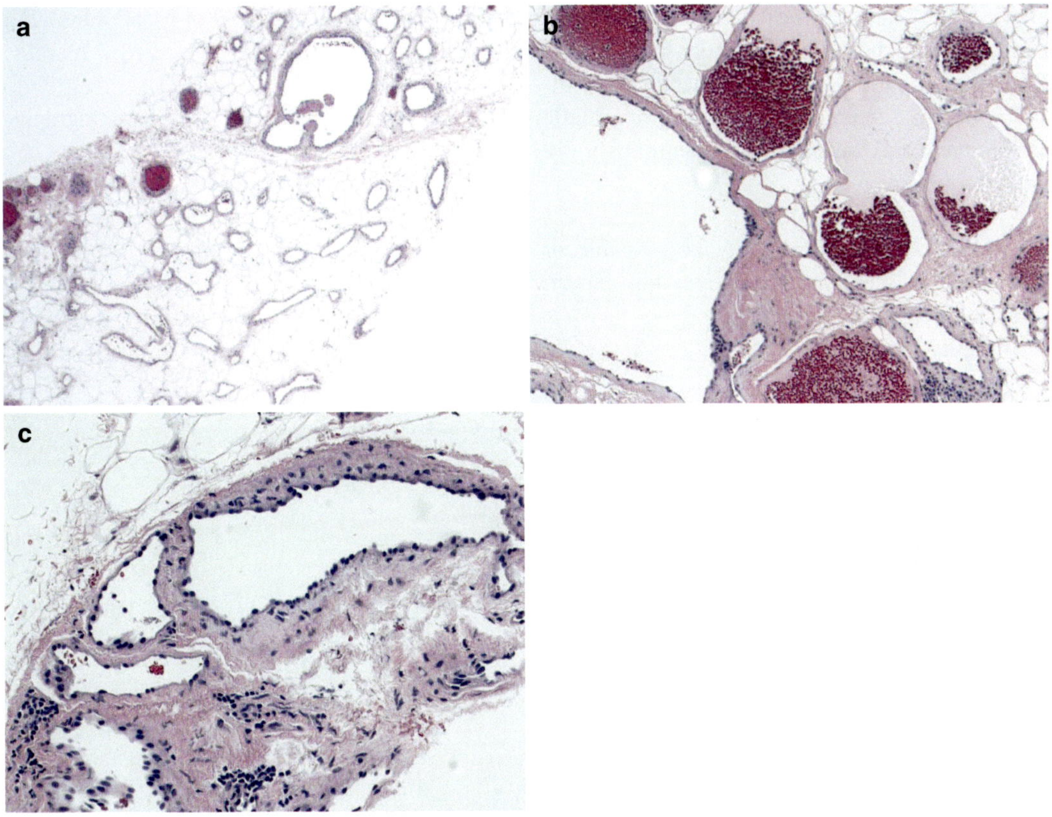

Fig. 3.15 Core needle biopsy demonstrating abundant lymphatic channels within the adipose tissue of the breast (**a**) including some dilated channels (**b**). On higher power the single cell endothelial lining can be better visualized (**c**)

- **US**: Cystic, multiloculated mass with septations of varying thickness (Figs. 3.13).
- **BI-RADS**: 2, 3, or 4.
- **Differential Diagnosis**: Clustered cysts, seroma, vascular malformation, papillary lesion, papillary carcinoma.

  In the presence of breast implants, an implant-associated anaplastic large cell lymphoma should also be considered.

• **Pathology Findings**:
- **Microscopic Histology**: Enlarged, dilated, thin-walled lymphatic channels with a flattened endothelial lining (Figs. 3.14 and 3.15).

  Often associated with lymphoid inflammation.

  May contain eosinophilic proteinaceous fluid, mast cells, and hemosiderin.

  May be associated with fibrosis if long standing [29].
- **Differential Diagnosis**: Vascular malformation, atypical vascular lesions, hemangioma.
- **Management**: No surgical excision is needed if aspiration/biopsy yields benign findings without atypia. Surgical excision is indicated if atypia is present, or if the lesion is causing adverse symptoms for the patient.

Papilloma

Papilloma: Papillomas may be subareolar or peripheral; peripheral lesions are more likely to harbor atypical cells and be associated with an increased risk of carcinoma [31]. Intraductal papillomas are benign papillary lesions most often arising from lactiferous ducts in the center of the breast and can be solitary or multiple. Papillomas are most commonly observed in perimenopausal patients, but with increasing utilization of screening US, asymptomatic papillomas are detected serendipitously in younger patients.

- **Clinical Presentation**: May be palpable or detected on screening; the patient may experience bloody nipple discharge.
- **Imaging Findings**:
  - **Mammography**: Oval or round mass with circumscribed or obscured margins (Fig. 3.16).

    Small lesions may be mammographically occult [32].

    Papillomas may have associated coarse heterogeneous or amorphous calcifications.
  - **US**: Oval or round complex cystic mass, frequently with internal vascularity, sometimes intraductal origin can be determined [32].

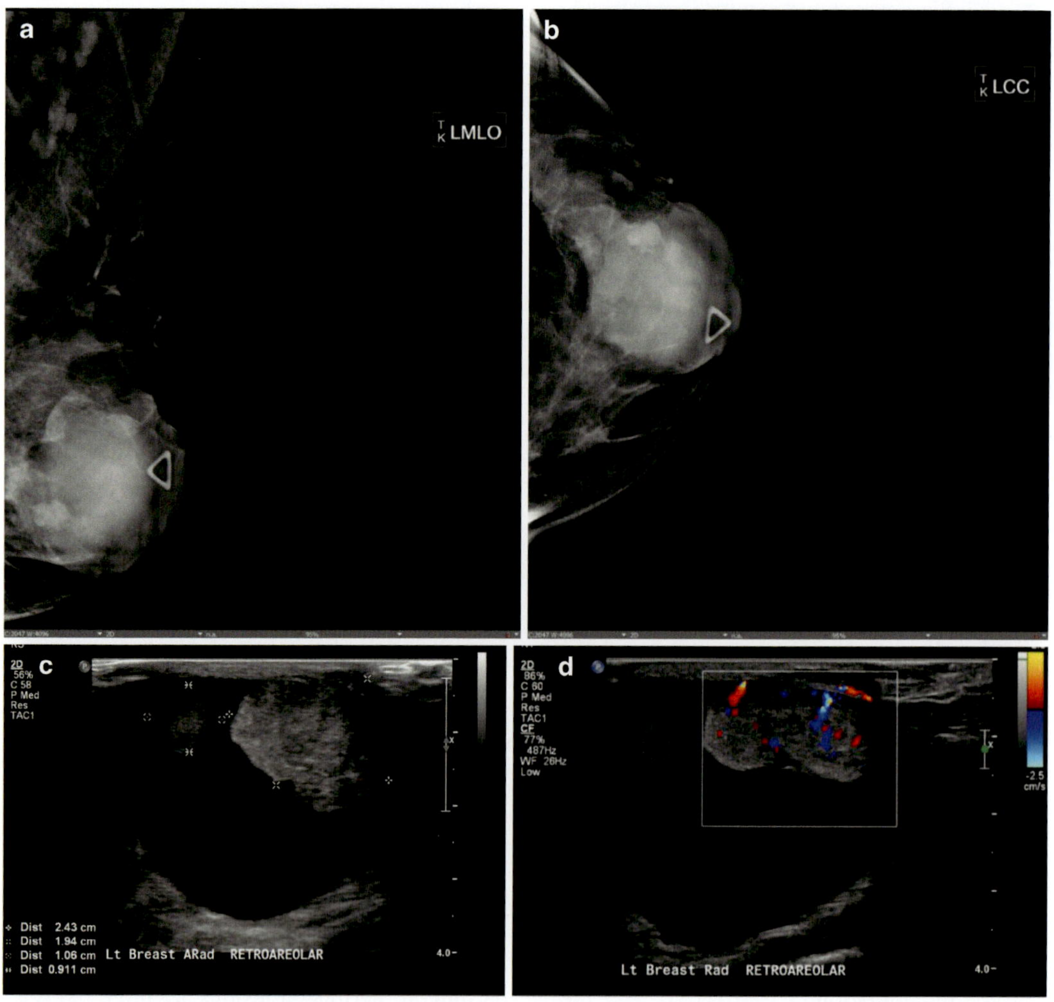

Fig. 3.16 A 36-year-old female presented with a painful, palpable left breast mass. She denies nipple discharge. On mammography there is a round, hyperdense mass with an indistinct margin (**a**, **b**) and ultrasound shows a round, complex cystic and solid mass with increased vascularity (**c**, **d**). The mass is considered BI-RADS 4, suspicious. An ultrasound-guided diagnostic aspiration of the cystic component and an ultrasound-guided needle biopsy of the solid component was recommended and performed. Aspiration of the liquid component yielded frank blood. Core needle biopsy of the solid component revealed a papilloma without atypia

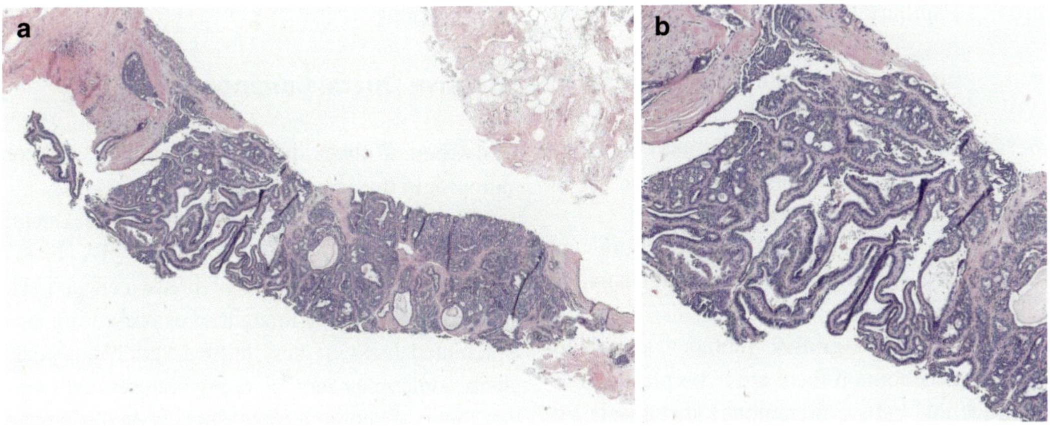

Fig. 3.17 A 76-year-old woman presented with a palpable mass at 4:00 in her right breast. The lesion was biopsied to reveal the papillary fronds and fibrovascular cores of an intraductal papilloma with involvement by usual ductal hyperplasia (**a**, **b**)

Upon aspiration, the cystic component may yield frankly bloody fluid.

- **BI-RADS**: 4, suspicious when symptomatic (palpable mass and/or suspicious nipple discharge).
- **Differential Diagnosis**: Encapsulated papillary carcinoma, phyllodes, abscess, fat necrosis, hematoma.
- **Pathology Findings**:
  - **Microscopic Histology**: Core needle biopsies of papillary lesions may be orderly with branching fronds of fibrovascular cores lined by cuboidal to columnar epithelium and myoepithelial cells (Fig. 3.17).

    The epithelium lining the fronds may become hyperplastic forming more complex architecture with secondary lumen formation and entrapped glands in the stroma.

    Solid intraductal papillomas are composed of florid epithelial hyperplasia.

    Apocrine metaplastic changes in a papillary lesion is indicative of a benign papilloma [33, 34].

    Similarly, presence of histiocytes within broad fibrovascular stroma favor a benign process [33, 34].

    Core needle biopsy may show detached fragments of papillary epithelium without a cyst wall which may be obtained from a cystic papilloma.

    Occasionally, only fragments of the cyst wall are visualized without the epithelium which results in a descriptive diagnosis suggestive of a papillary lesion.

  When the core needle biopsy sample shows papillary fronds lined by epithelial and myoepithelial layers projecting from a cystically dilated duct the diagnosis of a papilloma can be confidently made.

  Immunostains are particularly useful in demonstrating myoepithelial cells especially in sclerosing papillary lesions with distortion of the epithelial elements entrapped in the sclerotic stroma.

    In florid proliferation of the epithelium with bridging and architectural complexity, immunostains for epithelial differentiation such as CK5/6 and estrogen receptor will help distinguish atypical epithelial proliferation from usual ductal hyperplasia [35].

    Some papillomas can exhibit hyperplastic myoepithelial cells with epithelioid phenotype. Immunostains for myoepithelial markers (p63, calponin, and smooth muscle actin) can help establish the myoepithelial origin of these cells [35].

Papillary lesions involved by florid adenosis with compact proliferation of adenosis glands without lumen formation can pose a diagnostic challenge.

Infarction of a papilloma can occur spontaneously or as a result of needle biopsy procedures.

Degeneration of the epithelium can result in hyperchromasia suggestive of cytologic atypia.

- **Differential Diagnosis**: Includes an adenomyoepithelioma if there are hyperplastic myoepithelial cells. Squamous metaplasia of papillomas with or without infarction can raise concern for metaplastic carcinoma especially a low-grade adenosquamous carcinoma.
- **Management**: Symptomatic papillomas should be surgically excised.
  - Due to variable upgrade rates to carcinoma on biopsies diagnosed as papillary lesions the general management has traditionally been excisional biopsy.
  - More recently, numerous follow-up studies of papillomas confirm a low malignant potential with <5% upgrade rate, supporting more conservative management [36, 37].

Malignant

Invasive Ductal Carcinoma

See Chap. 7 for additional information and for pathologic findings and management.

Invasive Ductal Carcinoma: Invasive Ductal Carcinoma, Not Otherwise Specified (IDC NOS) is the most common type of breast cancer [31]. Although classically thought of as presenting as a spiculated mass, it may have a variable appearance, sometimes demonstrating features that overlap those of benign lesions, such as an oval shape and a circumscribed margin. In some instances it can present with a complex cystic and solid appearance on imaging (Figs. 3.18 and 3.19).

- **Clinical Presentation**: May be palpable or detected on screening mammography.
- **Imaging Findings**:
  - **Mammography**: Irregular, spiculated mass, or round mass with indistinct margins.

    May contain or be associated with pleomorphic calcifications.
  - **US**: Appearance is variable, but frequently presents as an irregular, spiculated,

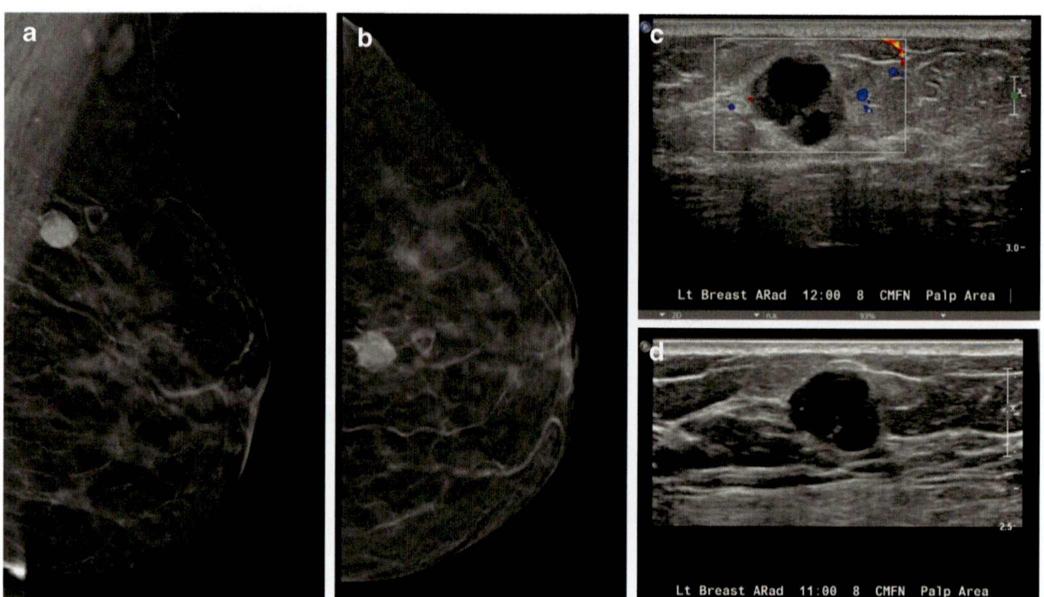

Fig. 3.18 A 64-year-old female without significant family history of breast cancer presents with a palpable mass in the left breast. Mammography showed a new oval hyperdense mass with a largely circumscribed margin (**a**, **b**), while ultrasound showed an oval, complex cystic and solid mass with internal vascularity (**c**, **d**). The mass was considered BI-RADS 4. An US-guided core needle biopsy was recommended and performed revealing invasive ductal carcinoma

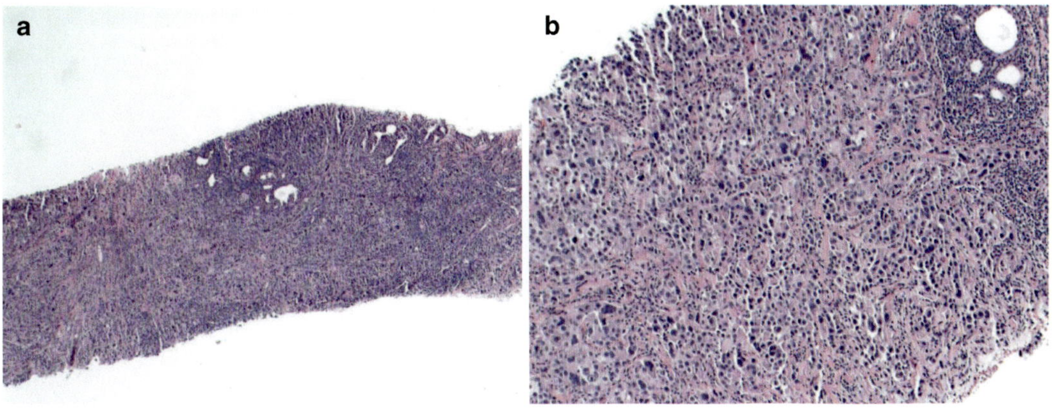

Fig. 3.19 A 55-year-old female underwent an US-guided core needle biopsy for a 1.8-cm oval mass seen on mammography. On biopsy there were diffuse sheets of highly irregular, pleomorphic tumor cells diagnosed as poorly differentiated invasive ductal carcinoma (**a**, **b**)

hypoechoic anti-parallel mass with posterior shadowing, with or without visible internal vascularity [38].

May also present as a complex cystic and solid mass.

- **BI-RADS**: 4 or 5. Although appearance may overlap with that of benign-appearing lesions and result in a BI-RADS 3 designation.
- **Differential Diagnosis**: (if presenting as a complex cystic, solid mass): papillary lesion, fat necrosis, encapsulated papillary carcinoma, phyllodes, abscess.

• **Pathology Findings/Management**: See Chap. 7.

Invasive Lobular Carcinoma

See Chap. 7.

Malignant Adenomyoepithelioma

Malignant Adenomyoepithelioma: Adenomyoepitheliomas are rare and considered to be benign but may demonstrate malignant transformation, especially when larger than 2 cm [39, 40]. Malignant adenomyoepitheliomas may metastasize to the lungs, liver, and brain [39, 40]. Axillary lymph node metastases are rare [39].

• **Clinical Presentation**: These lesions are usually screening detected but may be palpable.
• **Imaging Findings**:
  - **Mammography**: Variable appearance: oval, circumscribed mass, irregular mass with indistinct margins, or focal asymmetry (Fig. 3.20).
  - **US**: Variable appearance: oval, circumscribed mass, irregular mass, complex cystic and solid mass.
  - **BI-RADS**: 3 or 4 depending on presentation and imaging appearance.
  - **Differential Diagnosis**: Fibroadenoma, phyllodes, PASH, papilloma, papillary carcinoma, IDC.
• **Pathology Findings**:
  - **Microscopic Histology**: Histology show nodular aggregates composed of a compact proliferation of inner epithelial and outer myoepithelial cells (Fig. 3.21).

    The myoepithelial cells can have clear cytoplasm which contrasts with the darkly stained epithelial cells that can undergo apocrine, sebaceous, squamous, or mucoepidermoid metaplastic changes [41].

    Margins are generally well circumscribed.

    The three variants described by Tavassoli are spindle, tubular, and lobu-

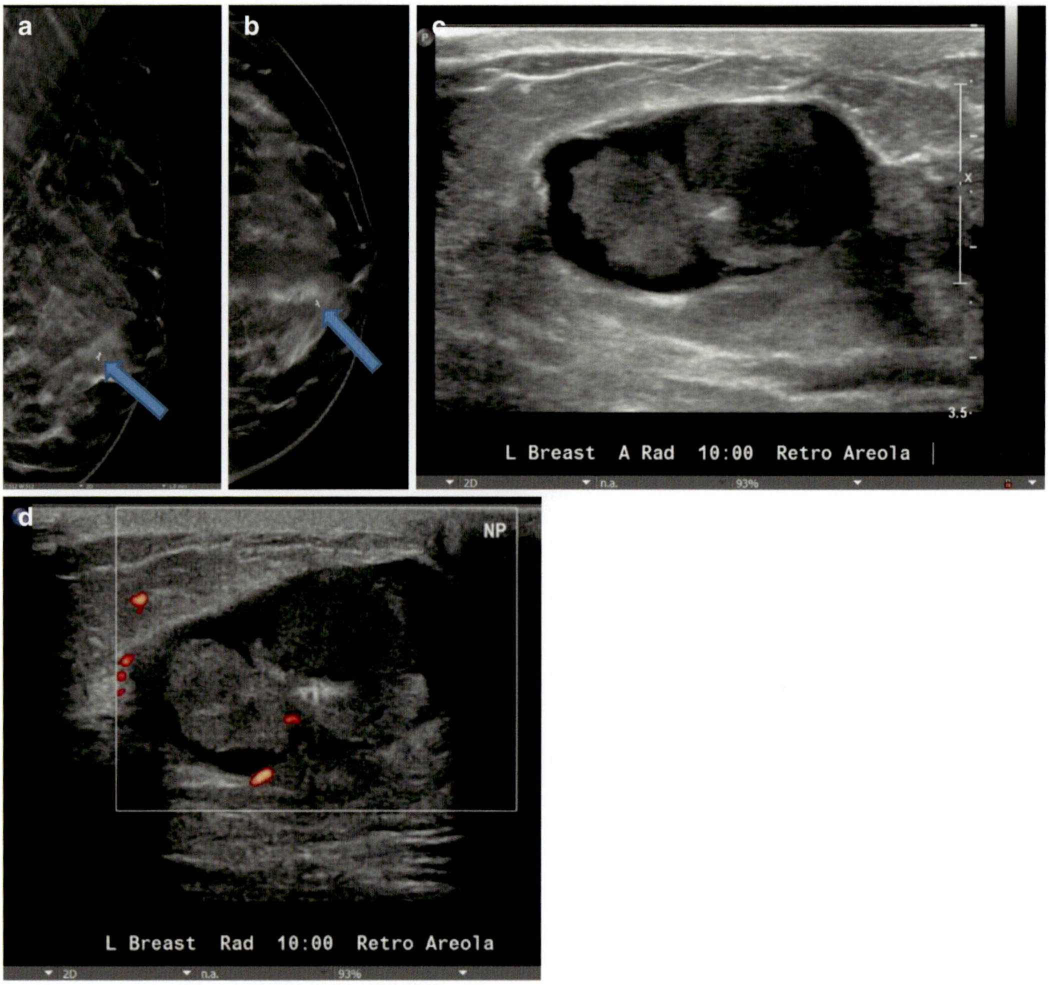

Fig. 3.20 A 46-year-old female presented with a palpable left breast mass while pregnant in 2019. The mass was biopsied with US guidance and found to be a papilloma. Due to the pregnancy, the patient did not undergo excision. However, the patient miscarried and subsequently underwent IVF treatment and became pregnant again. The patient then noted that the mass was enlarging and repeat imaging was obtained at which point the mammogram showed an oval, isodense mass with an obscured margin containing a biopsy marking clip (**a**, **b**). Ultrasound revealed an oval, complex cystic and solid mass with a prominent vascular stalk (**c**, **d**). The mass was considered BI-RADS 4, suspicious. A surgical excision was recommended and performed and diagnosed as adenomyoepithelioma

lated types based on the architectural patterns [42].

Malignant adenomyoepitheliomas may demonstrate marked cytologic atypia, mitosis, and necrosis. They can arise either in the epithelial or myoepithelial component or in both.

Extension of the intraductal component into adjacent ducts may be responsible for local recurrences [39].

- **Differential Diagnosis**: Sclerosing adenosis, intraductal papilloma, tubular adenoma, invasive ductal carcinoma.
- **Management**: Complete excision of both benign and malignant adenomyoepitheliomas is recommended, as it is difficult to differentiate between the two [43]. It is unclear if axillary lymph node sampling is beneficial in benign lesions, if the lymph nodes appear normal on imaging.

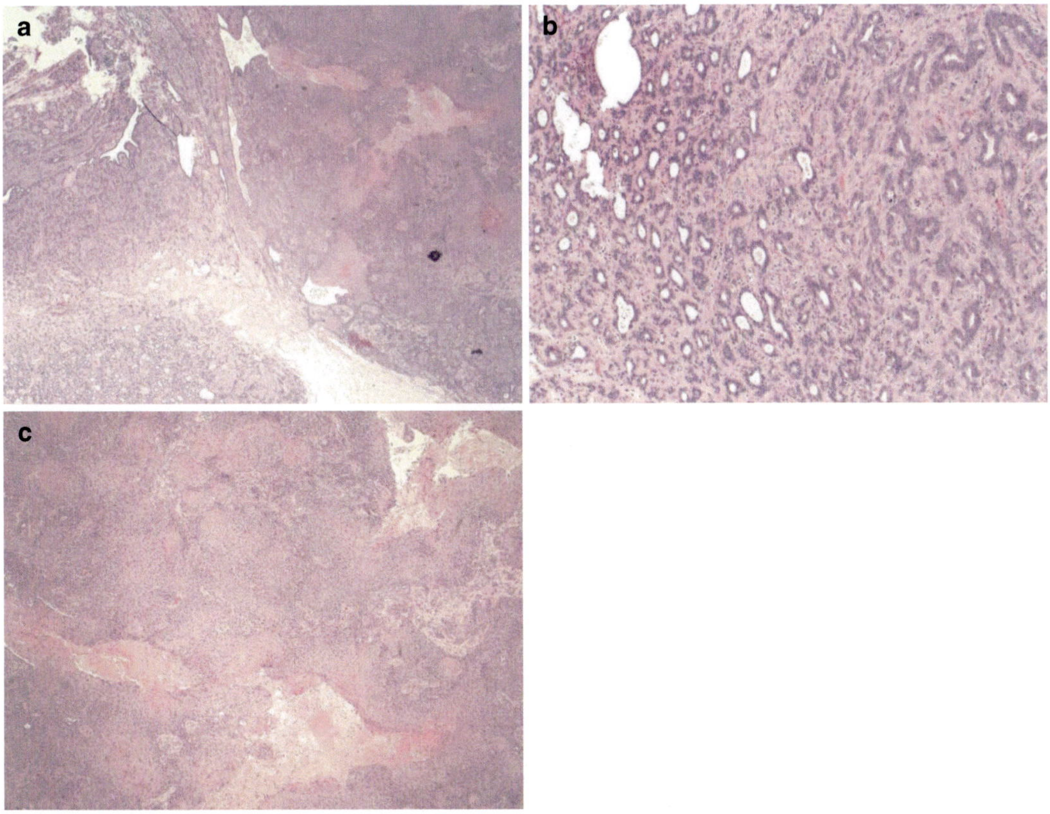

Fig. 3.21 A lumpectomy specimen in a patient with an enlarging left breast mass demonstrating biphasic growth with small glands and intervening spindle-shaped myoepithelial component (**a**, **b**). An area of squamous differentiation was also present (**c**)

Squamous Cell Carcinoma

Squamous Cell Carcinoma: Primary squamous cell carcinoma (SCC) of the breast is a rare entity, representing <0.1% of breast cancers [31]. Therefore, a metastatic lesion from another source should first be considered in the context of the patient's prior oncologic history, as well as comprehensive imaging findings. Because of its rarity, the epidemiologic features are not fully characterized. However, most primary SCCs of the breast are associated with aggressive histologic features and studies comparing triple-negative breast cancer and primary SCC seem to suggest that SCC is more aggressive [44].

The outcomes, etiology, and classification continue to be studied and characterized. In terms of radiologic features, varying presentations have been reported in the literature. While SCC of the breast may form a solid spiculated mass, some studies describe the presence of a partially solid/partially cystic mass on imaging and gross pathology [45].

- **Clinical Presentation**: Squamous cell carcinoma may be screening detected or palpable and tends to affect older women in the 75–79 age group [31]. If SCC is diagnosed in the breast, a CT scan of the chest is recommended to exclude a lung SCC that has metastasized to the breast. Approximately half of patients have positive axillary lymph nodes at the time of diagnosis [31].
- **Imaging Findings**:
  - **Mammography**: Round or oval mass, may be circumscribed (Fig. 3.22).
  - **US**: Oval or round mass, may be complex cystic and solid.

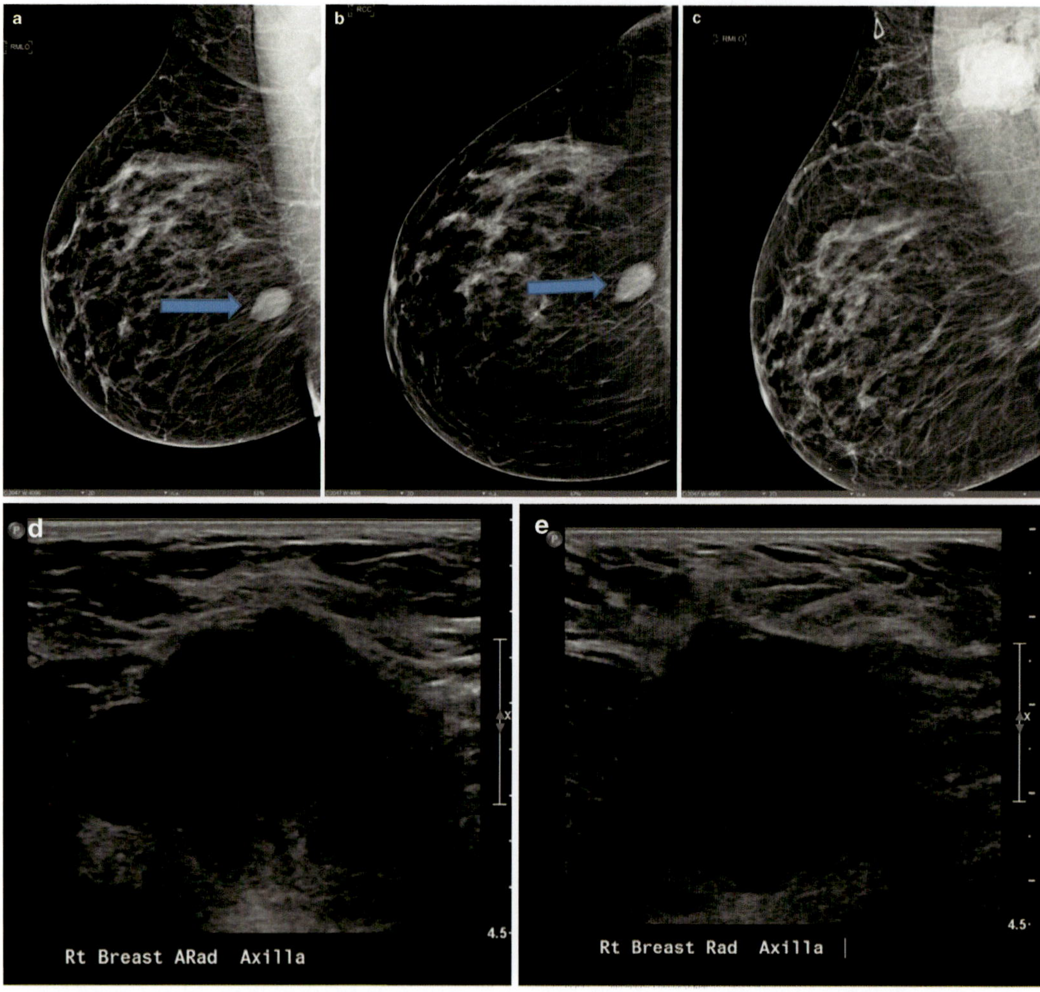

Fig. 3.22 A 48-year-old female presented for screening mammography. Ten years ago, the patient had a palpable mass biopsied at the 6 o'clock position of the right breast, which was shown to be an epidermoid inclusion cyst. Currently mammography shows an oval, circumscribed, hyperdense mass in the location of the previously biopsied epidermoid inclusion cyst (**a**, **b**) and an ultrasound was not performed. The lesion was characterized as BI-RADS: 2, benign, but the mass was noted to have increased slightly since the prior mammogram 10 years ago. The patient underwent a surgical excision of the mass. Follow up 2 years later, the patient palpated a right axillary mass, and diagnostic imaging was obtained. Mammography showed a round, hyperdense right axillary mass with an indistinct margin (**c**) and ultrasound showed a round, microlobulated, complex cystic and solid mass (**d**, **e**). The mass was now considered BI-RADS 4 and an US-guided biopsy was recommended and performed revealing squamous cell carcinoma. A chest CT was performed and yielded no evidence of a lung mass to suggest that this would be a metastatic lesion

- **BI-RADS**: 4, but many findings may overlap with those of probably benign lesions.
- **Differential Diagnosis**: Invasive ductal carcinoma, fibroadenoma, epidermoid cyst, phyllodes.

- **Pathology Findings**:
  - **Microscopic Histology**: The histologic origin of primary SCC of the breast is not clear. Two different etiologies have recently been proposed:

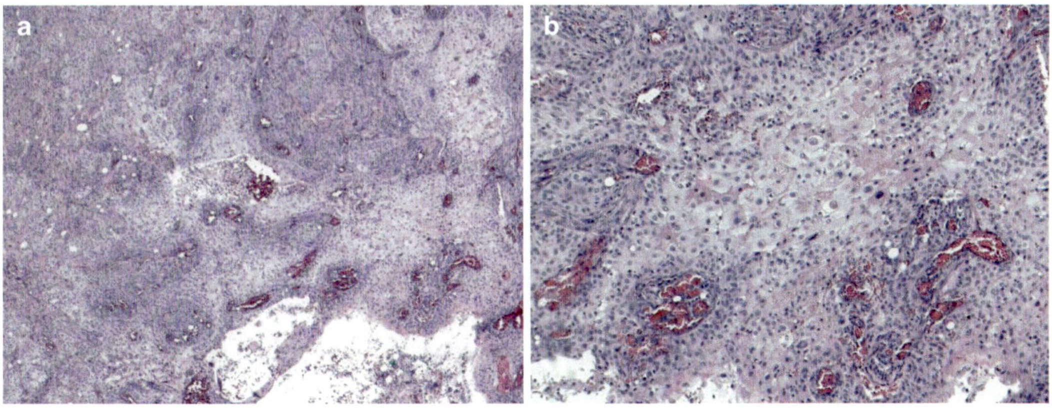

Fig. 3.23 A 56-year-old woman underwent lumpectomy for a round, solid cystic mass seen on ultrasound. On histology there were sheets of squamous epithelium invading the breast, diagnostic of squamous cell carcinoma of the breast (**a**, **b**)

Some authors believe that the precursor lesion is benign squamous metaplasia that occurs in benign breast cysts, fibroepithelial lesions, and hyperplasia (ductal or lobular) [46].

Others suggest that SCC of the breast is derived from extensive squamous metaplasia involving invasive ductal carcinoma [46].

The different proposed origins imply there are two histologic phenotypes, one that is predominantly squamous cell (>90% squamous morphology), and a second that represents a combination of squamous cell carcinoma and adenocarcinoma, what is currently known as metaplastic squamous breast carcinoma [46].

SCC is similar to the "basal-like" breast tumors and is likely to be hormone receptor negative, have aggressive histological features and be associated with a poor outcome (Fig. 3.23).

- **Differential Diagnosis**: Metastatic SCC, metaplastic squamous breast carcinoma, benign processes involved by extensive squamous metaplasia.
- **Management**: Mastectomy or breast conserving surgery followed by radiation, with possible adjuvant chemotherapy [47].

Triple Negative and Basal-Like Breast Cancer

Triple Negative and Basal-Like Breast Cancer: Hormone receptor (estrogen and progesterone) and HER2-negative breast cancers are a heterogeneous group with a spectrum of morphologies. Most of these invasive carcinomas are high grade, poorly differentiated tumors with solid growth, and pushing margins. There are limited treatment options, and these tumors have a significantly poorer prognosis compared to hormone receptor-positive breast cancers, with a mortality rate of 40% within the first 5 years after diagnosis [48, 49]. Approximately 46% have distal metastases at the time of diagnosis [48]. Relapse rates are high, occurring within 5 years of initial treatment [48, 50].

- **Clinical Presentation**: These aggressive tumors frequently present as interval cancers palpated by the patient or clinician and may grow rapidly. They are more frequent in younger women, particularly African American women, with up to 34% of cases occurring in patients with BRCA mutations [51].
- **Imaging Findings**:
  - **Mammography**: Round or oval masses with circumscribed or indistinct margins (Fig. 3.24).
  - **US**: Oval, hypoechoic masses with circumscribed or irregular margins. Often complex cystic and solid, frequently with increased internal vascularity [52].

    These may mimic benign lesions (fibroadenomas).
  - **BI-RADS**: 4 or 5, but may be mistaken for probably benign lesions (fibroadenomas) and given a BI-RADS 3 designation.
  - **Differential Diagnosis**: Papillary lesion, fibroadenoma, phyllodes, abscess, mucinous carcinoma, sarcoma.
- **Pathology Findings**.
  - **Microscopic Histology**: On histology the tumor cells exhibit a high nuclear to cytoplasmic ratio, nuclear pleomorphism, and high mitotic count (Fig. 3.25).

    There often is a central scar and geographic areas of necrosis.

    A significant number of these tumors have associated dense stromal lymphocytic response.

    Core needle biopsy shows poorly differentiated invasive cancer with focal or no associated DCIS.

      In such situations it is prudent to do immunostains for breast-specific markers like GATA3, mammaglobin, and GCDFP-15, to exclude a metastatic carcinoma [53].

      More recently, it has been shown that 20–30% of triple-negative cancers also stain positive for the transcription factor SOX10 [53].

      Immunostains for basal phenotype such as keratin CK5/6 and EGFR are not routinely performed.
  - **Differential Diagnosis**: Metastatic carcinoma.
  - **Management**: Neoadjuvant chemotherapy followed by surgery and radiation therapy is the mainstay of treatment.

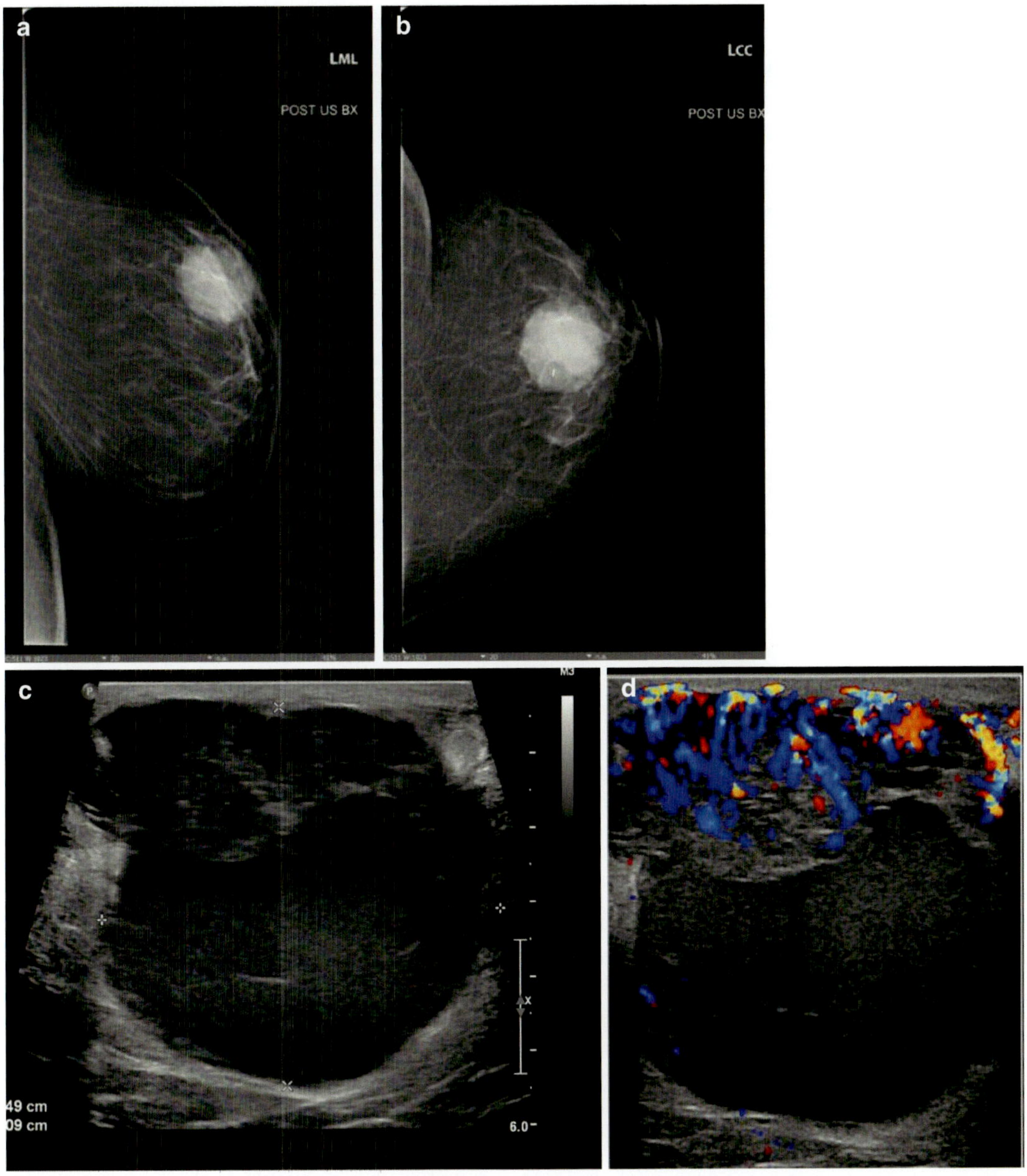

Fig. 3.24 A 35-year-old nulliparous female without significant family history of breast carcinoma presents with a palpable left breast mass. Mammography shows a round, hyperdense 3-cm mass with indistinct margins (**a**, **b**). Ultrasound shows a round, complex cystic and solid, hypervascular mass (**c**, **d**). MRI revealed a round mass with an irregular margin, and heterogeneous rim enhancement (**e**). The mass is considered BI-RADS 4, suspicious. An US-guided biopsy was performed revealing a triple-negative invasive ductal carcinoma. The patient underwent neoadjuvant chemotherapy, but the mass continued to enlarge. The solid component of the mass continuously secreted bloody fluid into the cystic component which caused distention of the component and was painful for the patient. Serial aspirations of the cystic component were performed for symptomatic relief, yielding large amounts of bloody fluid. The patient became anemic due to the intratumoral hemorrhages and required blood transfusions. Repeat MRI showed interval enlargement of the mass, and now edema, skin thickening and enhancement of the left breast (**f**)

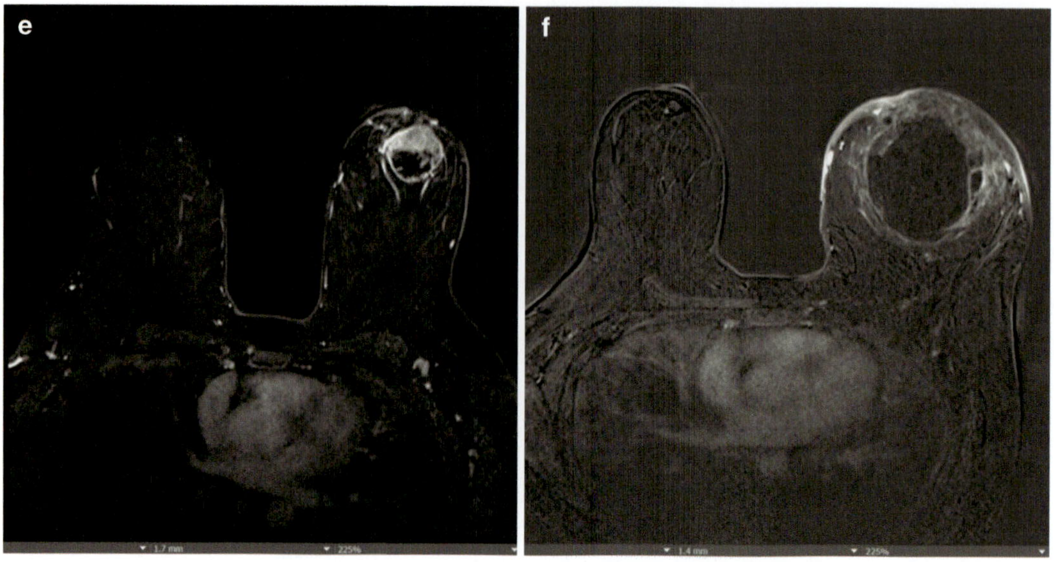

Fig. 3.24 (continued)

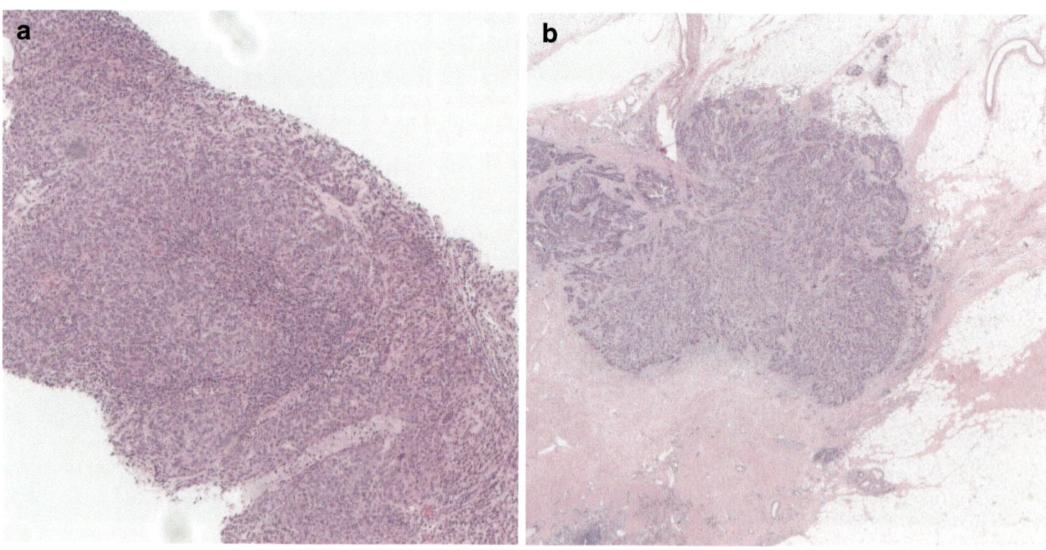

Fig. 3.25 A 42-year-old woman presented with a palpable mass. Mammography showed an irregular hyperdense mass. An US-guided biopsy was performed revealing sheets of poorly differentiated carcinoma with nuclear pleomorphism, and high mitotic rate (**a**). Steroid hormone receptors performed on the biopsy showed the lesion was ER negative, PR negative, and HER2 negative. The patient subsequently underwent left mastectomy and sentinel axillary lymph node sampling after receiving neoadjuvant chemotherapy which showed more foci of poorly differentiated tumor still present (**b, c**)

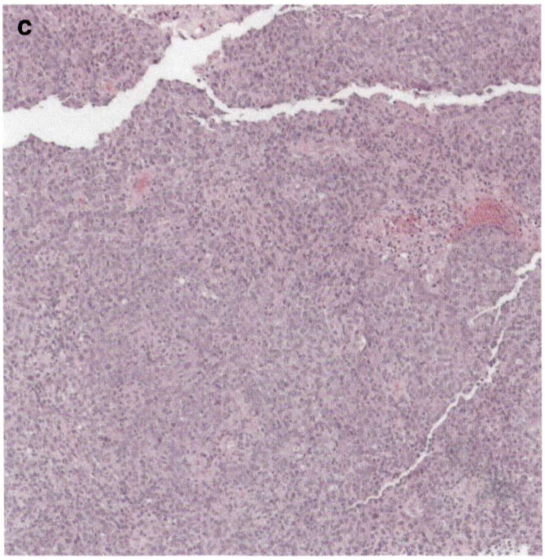

Fig. 3.25 (continued)

Metaplastic Carcinoma

See Chap. 2.

Encapsulated Papillary Carcinoma

Encapsulated Papillary Carcinoma: This is a rare, indolent lesion accounting for less than 2% of all breast cancers and is frequently associated with DCIS and IDC which exists in the periphery of the lesion; it is therefore important to include the cyst wall in the biopsy [31, 54, 55]. The prognosis is excellent, with rare distant metastases [54]. Axillary metastases are infrequent at the time of diagnosis.

- **Clinical Presentation**: May present as a palpable or screening detected mass, and may be associated with suspicious nipple discharge if subareolar in location.
- **Imaging Findings**:
  - **Mammography**: Round or oval mass, may be circumscribed and associated with pleomorphic calcifications (Fig. 3.26).
  - **US**: Round or oval complex cystic and solid mass with possible internal vascularity.
  - **BI-RADS**: 4, but may be mistaken for a probably benign lesion and assigned a BI-RADS 3 designation.
  - **Differential Diagnosis**: Papilloma, papillary lesion, phyllodes tumor, IDC.
- **Pathology Findings**:
  - **Microscopic Histology**: Core needle biopsy of papillary carcinoma is particularly challenging as some are cystic and others are solid.

    The epithelial cells in papillary carcinoma are less orderly than papillomas with loss of polarity in the epithelium, stratification and complex arborizing architecture with cribriform and micropapillary structures (Fig. 3.27).

    There is nuclear hyperchromasia, high nuclear to cytoplasmic ratio and increased mitoses.

    Occasionally, low-grade papillary carcinomas are orderly with delicate fibrovascular cores as well as regular and uniform columnar epithelium.

    Immunostains for myoepithelial markers, cytokeratin CK5/6 (used as a differentiation marker), along with estrogen receptor will help elucidate the malignant nature of the lesion [35].

    The friable nature of the malignant papillary lesion on core needle biopsy may show detached fragments of malignant epithelium without adjacent ducts.

    There may be intracytoplasmic and extracellular mucin formation. In such cases distinguishing between in situ and invasive carcinoma on core biopsy is impossible and therefore the diagnosis of at least in situ carcinoma is generated in the final pathology report.

    On excision, the difficulty between in situ and invasive carcinoma may continue to persist as displaced epithelium from the prior core biopsy may have dislodged clusters of cells into the stroma.

      Immunostains for myoepithelial markers are not helpful as they are lost both around in situ and invasive carcinoma [35, 56, 57].

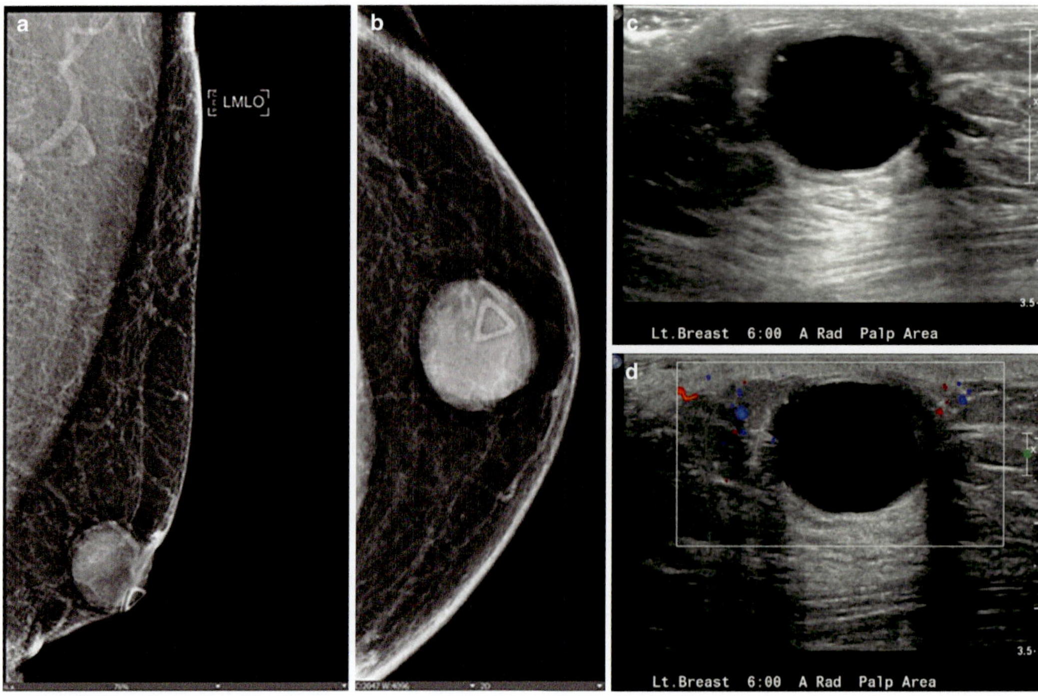

Fig. 3.26 A 69-year-old male experienced pruritus of the left nipple and the development of a small subareolar mass, which subsequently increased in size over the course of a year. On mammography there was a round, circumscribed 2.5-cm hyperdense mass in the left retroareolar region (**a**, **b**). Ultrasound showed a round, circumscribed mass that is complex cystic and solid, with minimal internal vascularity (**c**, **d**). The mass was categorized as BI-RADS 4, suspicious. An US-guided biopsy of the solid component was recommended and performed revealing an encapsulated papillary carcinoma

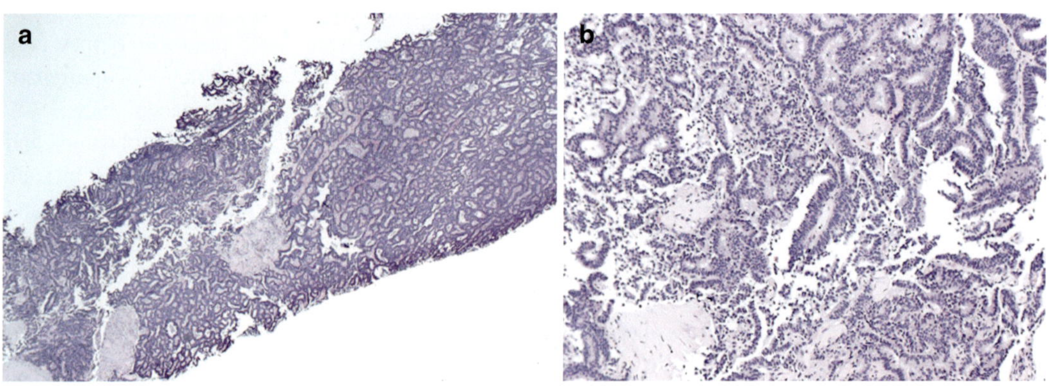

Fig. 3.27 A 59-year-old woman was found to have a 3.8-cm solid cystic mass on ultrasound. An US-guided biopsy of the solid component was performed revealing a well circumscribed, encapsulated papillary lesion (**a**, **b**). Smooth muscle myosin immunohistochemical staining demonstrates a lack of myoepithelial cells in the papillary proliferation (**c**). The patient subsequently underwent a left mastectomy and axillary sentinel node biopsy demonstrating an encapsulated papillary carcinoma (**d**, **e**) with metastasis to the lymph nodes

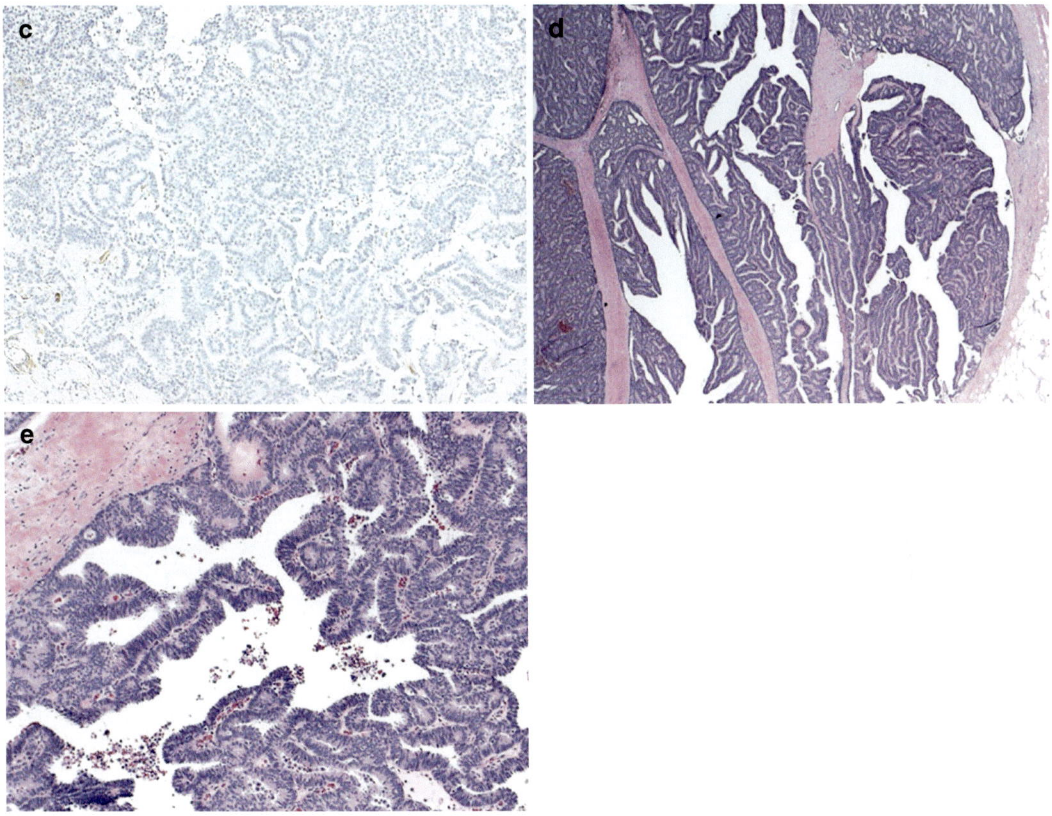

Fig. 3.27 (continued)

Only when there is unequivocal invasion extending beyond the perimeter of the papillary carcinoma is a diagnosis of invasion is rendered.

– **Management**: Wide local excision, with adjuvant hormonal and radiation therapy.

Phyllodes Tumor

See Chap. 2.

Apocrine Carcinoma

See Chap. 13.

Non-Hodgkin Lymphoma

Non-Hodgkin Lymphoma: Involvement of the breast by lymphoma is a rare occurrence. The diagnosis of lymphoma of the breast is classified into either a primary or secondary type, both of which account for <1% of all breast malignancies, though secondary lymphoma is more prevalent [58]. Breast lymphomas are usually B-cell lymphomas (except for implant-associated anaplastic large cell lymphoma discussed below) and the etiology is not completely understood. It has been hypothesized that the breast may act as a mucosal immune site which develops lymphoid tissue in autoimmune disease or other causal events [58]. Lymphomas may also arise in pre-existing mam-

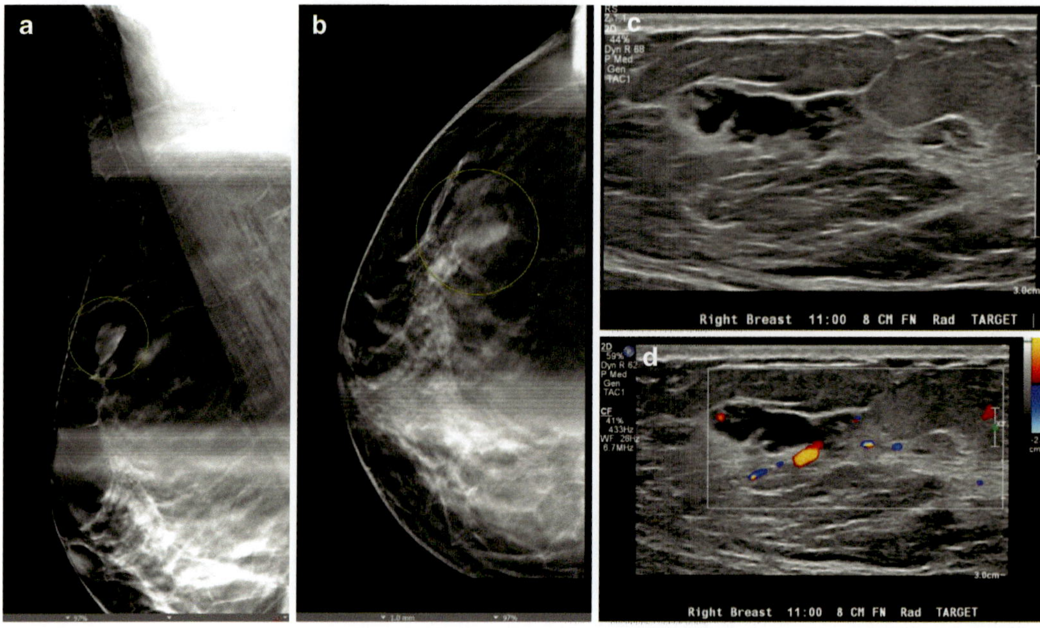

Fig. 3.28 A 42-year-old multiparous woman underwent screening mammography that demonstrated a new mass. On mammography there was an oval, equal density mass with an obscured margin (**a**, **b**). Ultrasound showed an oval, microlobulated hypoechoic complex cystic and solid mass with an echogenic rim and internal vascularity (**c**, **d**). The mass was considered BI-RADS 4, suspicious. An ultrasound-guided biopsy was recommended and performed revealing follicular lymphoma of the breast

mary lymph nodes. Primary breast lymphoma is most frequently diffuse large B-cell lymphoma, whereas the most prevalent type of secondary lymphoma is follicular lymphoma [59, 60]. Primary and secondary forms cannot be distinguished based on radiology or histology, though secondary lymphomas can develop multiple nodules, whereas primary lymphomas generally comprise a single large mass. A recent series of over 40,000 breast biopsies found that 75–80% of breast lymphomas were solid masses radiologically, while 20–25% were described as mixed solid/cystic lesions [61]. Given that up to 30% of breast lymphomas demonstrate necrosis and/or liquefaction histologically, this likely accounts for the nonsolid or cystic component of the lesion [59]. Most lymphomas also show well-defined margins rather than spiculated, poorly defined borders on imaging. Of note, because most lymphomas of the breast present as palpable masses, most receive an ultrasound-guided biopsy, where the appearance is always hypoechoic.

Breast implant-associated anaplastic large cell lymphoma (BIA-ALCL) is a more recently recognized entity of T-cell origin that is associated with breast implant insertion. The most common presentation of BIA-ALCL is generalized swelling of the breast secondary to peri-implant effusion, though mass forming lesions can develop in advanced disease. Ultrasound is often the initial radiologic assessment for swelling in the setting of implants and is highly sensitive for detection of periprosthetic effusions. Ultrasound is also sensitive for detecting mass-forming lesions associated with advanced forms of BIA-ALCL. Masses formed by BIA-ALCL have mostly been described as solid well-defined lesions that lack the hypervascularity of the other B-cell lymphomas seen in the breast. They are not usually complex cystic masses, though it has been reported in rare cases [62].

- **Clinical Presentation**: May present in the breast as a rapidly enlarging, painless, palpable mass. May also present with multiple masses. Occasionally, may be asymptomatic and be screening detected.

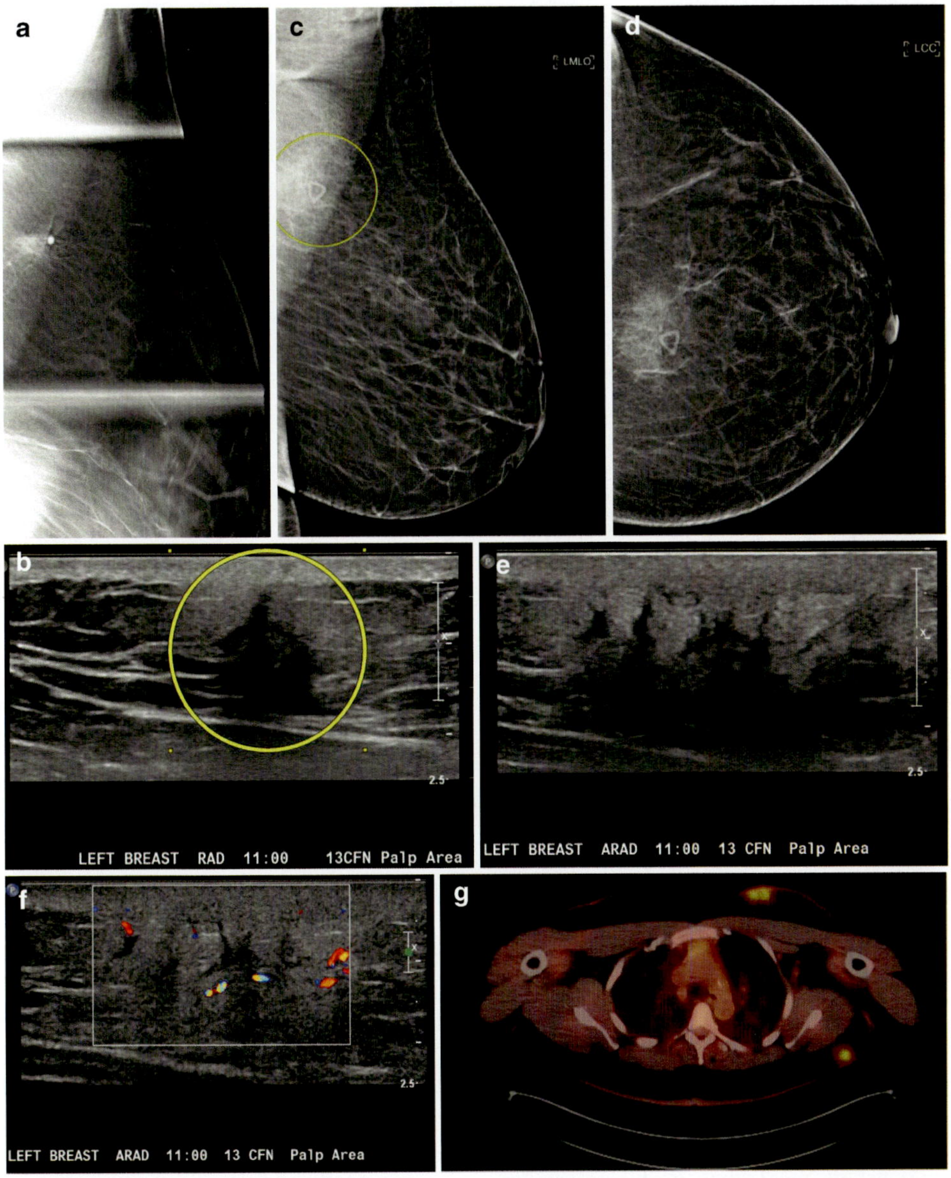

Fig. 3.29 A 32-year-old female presents with a palpable mass in the left breast. She works in a nursing home, frequently helping patients with dementia, and was recently hit in the breast area. She believes that the palpable area occurred after the trauma. Mammogram shows asymmetry seen on the MLO view only that correlates with the palpable area (**a**). On ultrasound there is a heterogeneous lesion with no demonstrable internal vascularity, contiguous with the skin surface (**b**). The lesion is graded BI-RADS 3, probably benign findings. Given history of recent trauma, this finding was thought to likely be fat necrosis, and the patient was instructed to return for a 6-month follow-up ultrasound with a possible mammogram, and to contact her referring clinician immediately if her symptoms worsened in the interim. The patient had a similar finding in the right breast in the prior year that had been imaged and had subsequently resolved. The patient returned at the recommended time for a 6-month follow-up. She reported that the lesion had not changed in size. Mammography at this time revealed that a large focal asymmetry in the left breast corresponding to the palpable area, increased in size since the prior study (**c, d**). Ultrasound showed a large heterogeneous area with internal vascularity (**e, f**). At this time the lesion was called BI-RADS 4, suspicious of malignancy. An US-guided biopsy was recommended and performed, yielding T-cell lymphoma, with features compatible with subcutaneous panniculitis-like T-cell lymphoma. The patient then underwent a PET/CT scan for staging, which demonstrated an intensely hypermetabolic lesion in the left breast, consistent with the biopsied lesion, and a smaller hypermetabolic lesion in the left upper back, also suspicious for T-cell lymphoma (**g**)

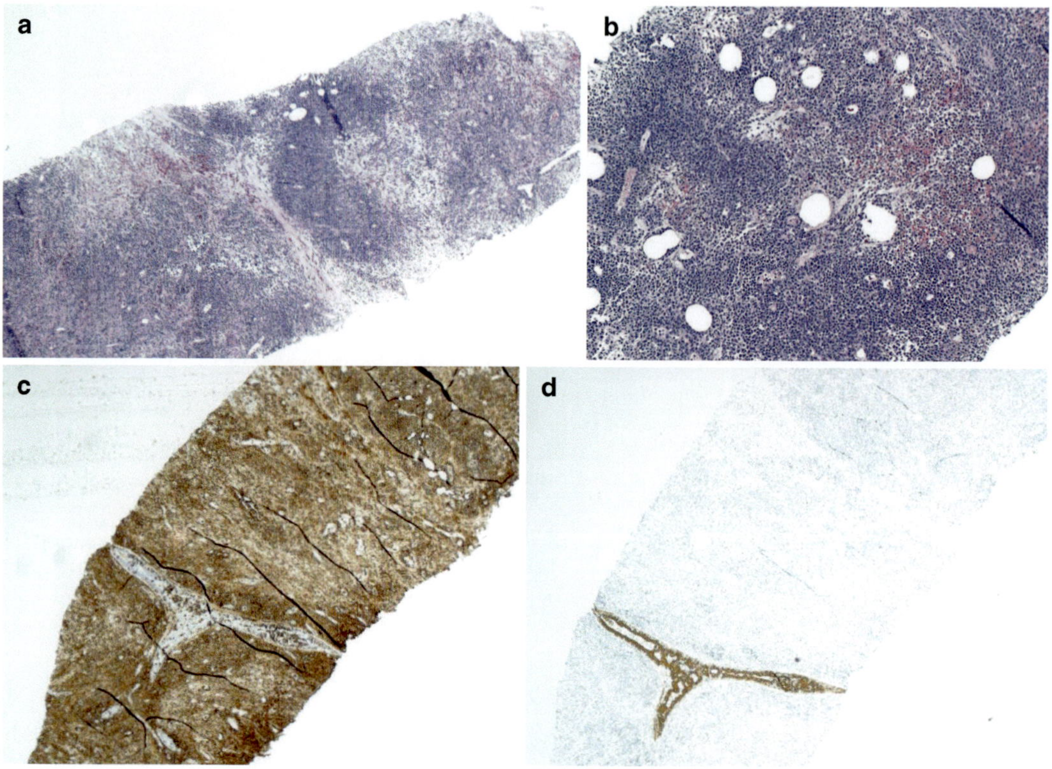

Fig. 3.30 An 83-year-old woman presented with large palpable bilateral breast masses which on imaging were considered BI-RADS 5. Core needle biopsy of the masses revealed diffuse sheets of large, atypical cells (**a**, **b**) with strong diffuse CD20 (**c**) and CD45 staining on immunohistochemistry but were negative for AE1/AE3 (**d**) supporting the diagnosis of diffuse large B-cell lymphoma

- **Imaging Findings**:
  - **Mammography**: Oval mass with circumscribed, microlobulated or indistinct margins, or a focal asymmetry (Figs. 3.28 and 3.29).
    No associated calcifications.
  - **US**: May range from oval to irregular, very hypoechoic mass, may be hypervascular, complex cystic and solid.
  - **BI-RADS**: 4, but may be mistaken for probably benign lesions such as complicated cysts.
  - **Differential Diagnosis**: Complicated cysts, clustered cysts, FA, phyllodes, abscess, IDC, mucinous carcinoma.
- **Pathology Findings**:
  - **Microscopic Histology**:
    Diffuse large B-cell lymphoma shows diffuse infiltration of the breast parenchyma by large atypical lymphoid cells (Fig. 3.30).
    They more commonly show a non-germinal center B-cell (non-GCB) like phenotype.
    Extranodal marginal zone lymphoma show features similar to other marginal zone lymphomas and show a predominantly nodular architecture (Fig. 3.31).
    The atypical lymphocytes are monocytoid, intermediate sized with moderate pale to clear cytoplasm.
    Neoplastic cells with plasmacytic differentiation, plasma cells and reactive follicles may also be identified.
    The neoplastic lymphocytes occasionally colonize the epithelial cells forming lympho-epithelial lesions.
    Follicular lymphoma of the breast, similar to nodal follicular lymphomas demonstrate a back-to-back follicular architecture with prolifera-

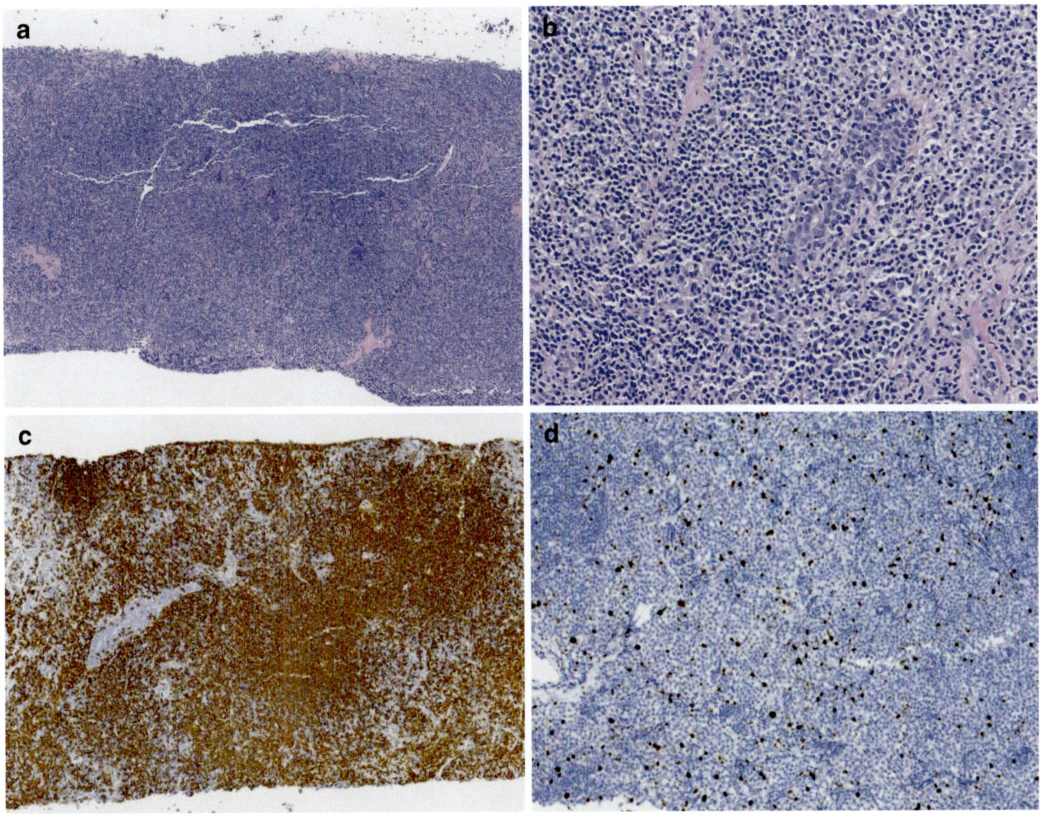

Fig. 3.31 Screening mammography and ultrasound of a 51-year-old woman demonstrated multiple heterogeneous hypoechoic lobulated masses in the bilateral breasts with internal vascularity and was categorized as BI-RADS 4C. A core biopsy from the right breast mass showed effacement of breast tissue by a diffuse and vague nodular lymphoplasmacytic infiltrate (**a**). The atypical lymphocytes are predominantly small-to-medium in size with clear cytoplasm and involve the interspersed ducts forming lymphoepithelial lesions (**b**). On immunohistochemistry these atypical lymphoid cells were positive for CD20 (**c**), BCL2 and CD43, but negative for CD5, CD10, and BCL6. KI67 index was about 5% (**d**). The histological and immunohistochemical features were suggestive of an extra-nodal marginal zone lymphoma

tion of a monotonous population of cells composed of small centrocytes with scattered centroblasts possible (Fig. 3.32).

All grades (grade 1–3) depending on the number of centroblasts have been documented in the breast [63].

Peripheral infiltration of the parenchyma by atypical lymphoid cells can also be seen.

Lymphoepithelial lesions are less common than in marginal zone lymphoma.

Cells may be arranged in cords or a linear pattern mimicking invasive lobular carcinoma.

Associated sclerosis can also lead to a single file pattern.

BIA-ALCL is characterized by proliferation of large anaplastic cells with large horseshoe-shaped nuclei, prominent nucleoli, vesicular chromatin, and abundant cytoplasm (Fig. 3.33).

These cells line the capsular surface or are present in the seroma fluid.

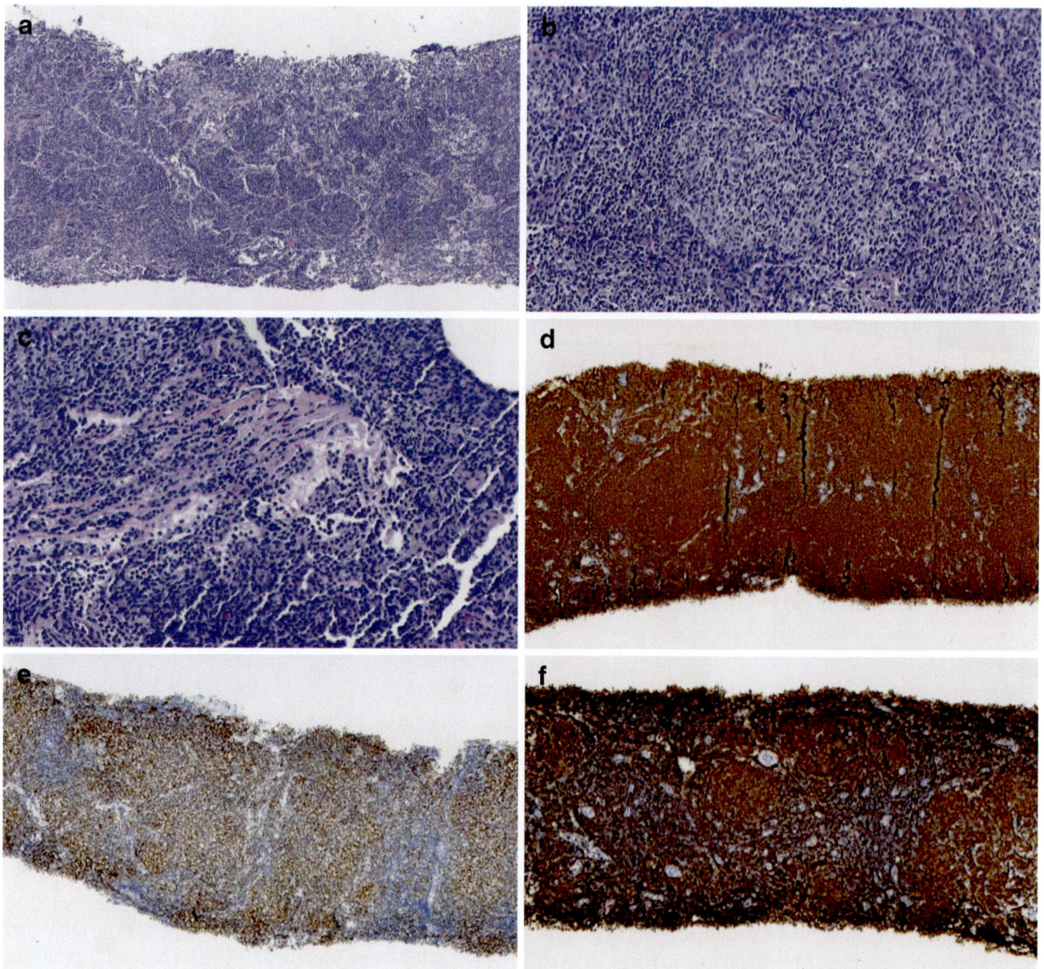

Fig. 3.32 An 87-year-old woman presented with a golf ball-sized lump in her right breast. An ultrasound revealed a 6.0 × 4.0 × 4.3 cm hypoechoic mass and was considered BI-RADS 4. A core biopsy from the mass showed a follicular growth pattern (**a**). The follicles were predominantly composed of atypical small lymphocytes with angulated nuclei, cells with moderate amounts of pale cytoplasm (centrocytes) and occasional interspersed large cells (centroblasts) (**b**). Focal areas with sclerosis showed cells in a single file pattern (**c**). These atypical lymphocytes were positive for CD20 (**d**), BCL6 (**e**), CD10, and BCL2 (**f**) and were negative for CD3, CD5, Cyclin D1, and LEF1. These features were suggestive of a low-grade follicular lymphoma

Extremely rarely they can show trans-capsular invasion and infiltration into the breast parenchyma.

The neoplastic cells are negative for ALK immunostaining.

Immunostains for hormone receptors and lymphoid markers can be used to help differentiate lymphoma from mimickers.

- **Differential Diagnosis**: Invasive lobular carcinoma, poorly differentiated invasive carcinoma with medullary features, chronic inflammation.
- **Management**: Treatment is typically chemotherapy, with surgical therapy not playing a significant role.

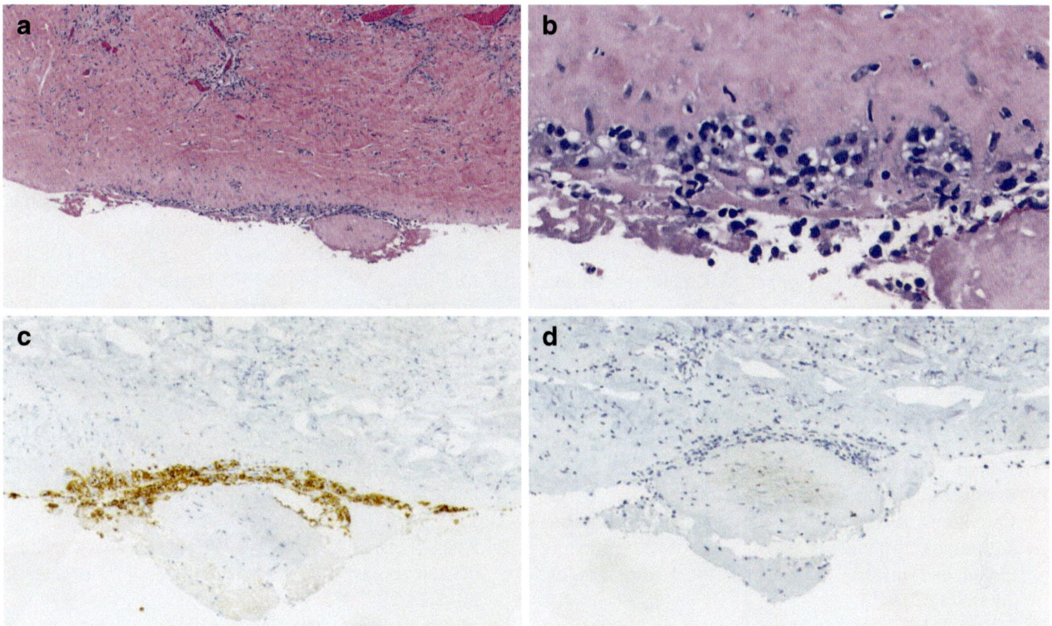

Fig. 3.33 A 50-year-old female presented with right breast swelling for 3 days. She has a history of right breast invasive ductal carcinoma status post-bilateral mastectomy with bilateral saline implant placement. An ultrasound was suggestive of ruptured implant in her right breast and she eventually underwent implant removal and capsulectomy. Sections from the capsule predominantly show dense fibrous tissue with chronic inflammation and fibrin deposition (**a**). On the capsular surface, focal clusters of large cells, some with horseshoe nuclei, prominent nucleoli, and eosinophilic cytoplasm were identified (**b**). These large anaplastic cells were positive for CD30 (**c**), CD3, and CD45, but negative for CD20 and ALK (**d**). These features are diagnostic of ALK-negative breast implant-associated anaplastic large cell lymphoma (BIA-ALCL). A T-cell gene rearrangement study demonstrated clonal gamma T-cell receptor gene rearrangement

References

1. Taboada JL, Stephens TW, Krishnamurthy S, et al. The many faces of fat necrosis. AJR. 2009;192:815–25.
2. Daly CP, Jaeger B, Sill DS. Variable appearances of fat necrosis on breast MRI. AJR. 2008;191:1374–80.
3. Rosen PP, Hoda SA. Breast Pathology: Diagnosis by Needle Core Biopsy. 3rd edition. WoltersKluwer/Lippincott Williams & Wilkins Health. 2015.
4. Schmitt SJ, Collins LC. Biopsy interpretation of the breast. 3rd ed. Wolters Kluwer Health; 2018.
5. Mahoney MC, Ingram AD. Breast emergencies: types, imaging features, and management. AJF. 2014;202:W390–9.
6. Tariq H, Menon PD, Fan H, Vadlamudi KV, Pandeswara SL, Nazarullah AN, Mais DD. Detection of Corynebacterium kroppenstedtii in granulomatous lobular mastitis using real-time polymerase chain reaction and sanger sequencing on formalin-fixed, paraffin-embedded tissues. Arch Pathol Lab Med. 2022;146(6):749–54. https://doi.org/10.5858/arpa.2021-0061-OA.
7. Liang Y, Zhan H, Krishnamurti U, Harigopal M, Sun T. Further characterization of clinicopathologic features of cystic neutrophilic granulomatous mastitis. Am J Clin Pathol. 2022;158(4):488–93. https://doi.org/10.1093/ajcp/aqac074.
8. Berg WA, Yang WT. Diagnostic imaging: Breast. 2nd ed. Philadelphia, PA: Lippincott Williams&Wilkins; 2013.
9. Dixon JM, et al. Periductal mastitis and duct ectasia: different conditions with different etiologies. Br J Surg. 1996;83(6):820–2.
10. Dixon JM, Anderson TJ, Lumsden AB, et al. Mammary duct ectasia. Br J Surg. 1983;70(10):601–3.
11. Haagensen CD. Diseases of the breast. 3rd ed. Philadelphia, PA: WB Saunders; 1986.
12. D'Alonso TM, et al. A review of inflammatory processes of the breast with a focus on diagnosis in core needle biopsy samples. J Pathol Transl Med. 2015;49(4):279–87.
13. Visscher DW, Nassar A, Degnim AC, et al. Sclerosing adenosis and risk of breast cancer. Breast Cancer Res Treat. 2014;144(1):205–12.

14. Jensen RA, Page DL, Dupont WD, et al. Invasive breast cancer risk in women sclerosing adenosis. Cancer. 1989;64(10):1977–83.
15. Carter DJ, Rosen PP. Atypical apocrine metaplasia in sclerosing lesions of the breast: a study of 51 patients. Mod Pathol. 1991;4(1):1–5.
16. Seidman JD, Ashton M, Lefkowitz M. Atypical apocrine adenosis of the breast: a Clinicopathologic study of 37 patients with 8.7-year follow-up. Cancer. 1996;77(12):2529–37.
17. Harmon M, Fuller B, Copper K. Carcinoma arising in microglandular adenosis of the breast. Int J Surg Pathol. 2001;9(4):344.
18. Khalifeh IM, Albarracin C, Diaz LK, et al. Clinical histopathologic, and immunohistochemical features of microglandular adenosis and transition into in situ and invasive carcinoma. Am J Surg Pathol. 2008;32(4):544–52.
19. Koenig C, Dadmanesh F, Bratthauer GL, et al. Carcinoma rising in the microglandular adenosis: an immunohistochemical analysis of 20 intraepithelial and invasive neoplasms. Int J Surg Pathol. 2000;8(4):303–15.
20. Sabate JM, Clotet M, Torrubia S, et al. Radiologic evaluation of breast disorders related to pregnancy and lactation. Radiographics. 2007:S101–24.
21. Vashi R, Hooley R, Butler R, et al. Breast imaging of the pregnant and lactating patient: physiologic changes and common benign entities. AJR. 2013;200:329–36.
22. Ironside JW, Guthrie W. The galactocele: a light- and electron microscopic study. Histopathology. 1985;9(4):457–67.
23. Paliotta A, Sapienza P, D'Ermo G, et al. Epidermal inclusion cyst of the breast: a literature review. Oncol Lett. 2016;11:657–60.
24. Wynne E, Louie A. Epidermoid cyst of the breast: mammography, ultrasound, MRI. Radiol Case Rep. 2011;6(3):431.
25. Crystal P, Shaco-Levy R. Case report: concentric rings within a breast mass on sonography: lamellated keratin in an epidermoid inclusion cyst. AJR. 2005;184:S47–8.
26. Vitug AF, Newman LA. Complications in breast surgery. Surg Clin N Am. 2007;87:431–51.
27. Neal CH, Yilmaz ZN, Noroozian M, et al. Imaging of breast cancer-related changes after surgical therapy. AJR. 2014;202:262–72.
28. Suzuki S, Oura S, Makimoto S. Prolonged large seroma formation after breast-conserving therapy. Case Rep Oncol. 2022;15(1):382–7. https://doi.org/10.1159/000522557. PMID: 35529287; PMCID: PMC9035919
29. Kurumety S, Morris M, Aydi ZB. New-onset axillary lymphangioma: a case report. J Med Case Rep. 2022;16(1):242. https://doi.org/10.1186/s13256-022-03461-0. PMID: 35717390; PMCID: PMC9206747
30. Chung SY, Oh KK, Kim DJ. Mammographic and sonographic findings of a breast cystic lymphangioma. J Ultrasound Med. 2003;22:307–9.
31. WHO Classification of Tumours Editorial Board. Breast tumours. WHO classification of tumour series, 5th ed., vol. 2. Lyon (France): International Agency for Research on Cancer; 2019.
32. Eiada R, Chong J, Kulkarni S, et al. Papillary lesions of the breast: MRI, US, and mammographic appearances. AJR. 2012;198:264–71.
33. Mulligan AM, O'Malley FP. Papillary lesions of the breast: a review. Adv Anat Pathol. 2007;14(2):108–19.
34. Ueng SH, Mezzetti T, Tavassoli FA. Papillary neoplasms of the breast: a review. Arch Pathol Lab Med. 2009;133(6):893–907.
35. Raju UB, Lee MW, Zarbo RJ, et al. Papillary neoplasia of the breast: immunohistochemically defined myoepithelial cells in the diagnosis of benign and malignant papillary breast neoplasms. Mod Pathol. 1989;2(6):569–76.
36. Khan S, Diaz A, Archer KJ, et al. Papillary lesions of the breast: to excise or observe? Breast J. 2018;24:227–452.
37. Moynihan A, Quinn EM, Smith CS. Benign breast papilloma: is surgical excision necessary? Breast J. 2020;26:705–10.
38. Newstead GM, Baute PM, Toth HK. Invasive lobular and ductal carcinoma: mammographic findings and stage of diagnosis. 1992;184:593–888.
39. Hayes MM. Adenomyoepithelioma of the breast: a review stressing its propensity for malignant transformation. J Clin Pathol. 2011;64(6):477–84.
40. Moro K, Sakata ER, Nakahara A, et al. Malignant Adenomyoepithlioma of the breast. Surg Case Rep. 2020:106–18.
41. Zhang Z, Wang Y, Xie X. Malignant epithelioma of the breast. Medicine. 2021:100–5.
42. Hicks, David G., and Susan Carole Lester. Diagnostic Pathology: Breast. Elsevier, 2021.
43. Rosen PP. Adenomyoepithelioma of the breast. Hum Pathol. 1987;18(12):1232–7.
44. Yadav S, Yadav D, Zakalik D. Squamous cell carcinoma of the breast in the United States: incidence, demographics, tumor characteristics, and survival. Breast Cancer Res Treat. 2017;164:201–8.
45. Candelaria RP, Krishnamurthy S, Huang ML, Santiago L, Adrada BE. Imaging and pathological findings in a case of invasive squamous cell carcinoma of the breast. Breast J. 2018;24(2):203–4.
46. Pirot F, et al. Squamous cell carcinoma of the breast, are there two entities with distinct prognosis? A series of 39 patients. Breast Cancer Res Treat. 2020;180:87–95.
47. Nayak A, Wu Y, Gilcrease MZ. Primary squamous cell carcinoma of the breast: predictors of locoregional recurrence and overall survival. Am J Surg Pathol. 2013;37(6):867–73.

48. Alluri P, Newman P. Basal-like and triple negative breast cancers: searching for positives among many negatives. Surg Oncol Clin N Am. 2014;23(3):567–77.
49. Li Y, Duan JJ, Bian XW, Yu SC. Triple-negative breast cancer molecular subtyping and treatment progress. Breast Cancer Res. 2020;22:61.
50. Bianchini G, De Angelis C, Licata L, Gianni L. Treatment landscape of triple-negative breast cancer—expanded options, evolving needs. Nat Rev Clin Oncol. 2022;19(2):91–113.
51. Howard FM, Olopade OI. Epidemiology of triple-negative breast cancer: a review. Cancer J. 2021;27(1):8–16.
52. Krizmanich-Conniff KM, Paramagul C, Patterson SK, et al. Triple receptor-negative breast cancer: imaging and clinical characteristics. AJR. 2012;198:458–64.
53. Kumar P, Aggarwal R. An overview of triple-negative breast cancer. Arch Gynecol Obstet. 2016;293(2):247–69.
54. Rakha EA, Gandhi N, Climent F, et al. Encapsulated papillary carcinoma of the breast: and invasive tumor with excellent prognosis. Am J Surg Pathol. 2011;35(8):1093–103.
55. Nassar H, Qureshi H, Volkanadsay N, et al. Clinicopathologic analysis of solid papillary carcinoma of the breast and associated invasive carcinomas. Am J Surg Pathol. 2006;30(4):501–7.
56. Hill CB, Yeh IT. Myoepithelial cell staining patterns of papillary breast lesions: from intra intraductal papillomas to invasive papillary carcinomas. Am J Clin Pathol. 2005;123(1):36–44.
57. Rakha EA, Tun M, Junainah E, et al. Encapsulated papillary carcinoma of the breast: a study of invasion associated markers. J Clin Pathol. 2012;65(8):710–4.
58. Picasso R, Tagliafico A, Calabrese M, et al. Primary and secondary breast lymphoma: focus on epidemiology and imaging features. Pathol Oncol Res. 2020;26:1483–8.
59. Raj SD, Shurafa M, Shah Z, Raj KM, Fishman MDC, Dialani VM. Primary and secondary breast lymphoma: clinical, pathologic, and multimodality imaging review. Radiographics. 2019;39(3):610–25.
60. Gholam D, Bibeau F, El Weshi A, et al. Primary breast lymphoma. Leuk Lymphoma. 2003;44(7):1173–8.
61. Nicholson B, Bhatti R, Glassman L. Extranodal lymphoma of the breast. Radiol Clin North Am. 2016;54:711–26.
62. Sharma B, Jurgenson-Rauch A, Pace E, et al. Breast implant-associated anaplastic large cell lymphoma: review and multiparametric imaging paradigms. Radiographics. 2020;40:609–28.
63. James ER, Miranda RN, Turner SD. Primary Lymphomas of the Breast: A Review. JPRAS Open. 2022;32:127–43. https://doi.org/10.1016/j.jpra.2022.01.004. PMID: 35402679; PMCID: PMC8987598.

Masses with Indistinct Margins

4

Kamaljeet Singh, James Lee, Malini Harigopal, and Liva Andrejeva

Fat Necrosis

Fat Necrosis: Fat necrosis is a common, benign lesion formed as an inflammatory reaction to local trauma, both accidental and iatrogenic trauma, such as breast surgery. Depending on its acuity, fat necrosis may demonstrate a wide range of morphological features, including as a mass with an indistinct margin [1]

- **Clinical Presentation**: Clinically, it may present as a painful, palpable mass accompanied by skin bruising after trauma, or it may be asymptomatic and detected on a screening exam [2, 3].

K. Singh (✉)
Department of Pathology and Laboratory Medicine, Brown University and Women and Infants Hospital of RI, Providence, RI, USA
e-mail: kamaljeet_singh@brown.edu

J. Lee
Department of Radiology and Biomedical Imaging, Yale University, New Haven, CT, USA
e-mail: james.lee@yale.edu

M. Harigopal
Department of Pathology, Yale University, New Haven, CT, USA
e-mail: malini.harigopal@yale.edu

L. Andrejeva
Department of Radiology and Biomedical Imaging, Yale School of Medicine, New Haven, CT, USA
e-mail: liva.andrejeva@yale.edu

- **Imaging Findings**:
  - **Mammogram**: The mammographic appearance of fat necrosis depends on the acuity of the lesion. In the early stages, it may mimic malignancy, presenting as a mass with a spiculated or indistinct margin. It may evolve into a circumscribed oil cyst in the late stage, occasionally with peripheral curvilinear or rim calcification [4, 5].
  - **US**: The sonographic appearance of fat necrosis is widely variable and depends on the degree of fibrosis. It may appear as an oval or irregular mass with an indistinct or spiculated margin and variable echogenicity or a complex cystic and solid mass.
  - **MRI**: The MRI findings of fat necrosis are varied and nonspecific. A fat intensity signal (hyperintense signal on T1 and T2 sequences and hypointense signal on fat suppression) is often detected. However, ancillary findings such as necrotic fat (low intensity on T1) may also be seen. Fat necrosis also demonstrates a wide array of enhancement patterns with IV contrast, ranging from washout to gradual enhancement. These features of fat necrosis render them difficult to distinguish from malignant lesions on MRI.
  - **BIRADS**: Variable; 2–5 depending on appearance.
  - **Differential Diagnosis**: Benign: abscess, cyst; Malignant: breast cancer [6, 7].

M. Harigopal et al. (eds.), *Radiology Pathology Correlations of Breast Lesions*,
https://doi.org/10.1007/978-3-031-65711-5_4

- **Pathology Findings**: The gross and microscopic appearance of the fat necrosis depends on the duration of the lesion.
  - **Gross**: Early lesions can appear hemorrhagic. After a few weeks, the lesion often becomes indurated and more well-defined with a tan-yellow cut surface. Pseudocystic change with oil and necrotic consistency may be present. Fibrosis and dystrophic calcification are present in older lesions.
  - **Microscopic Findings**: The histological findings mirror the aforementioned gross appearance of the lesion, which depends on the age/duration. Early lesions consist of disruption of adipocytes with accompanying histiocytic and lymphoplasmacytic infiltrate. Multinucleated histiocytes can be present. This leads to a peripheral rim of fibrosis with variable cellularity; a central pseudocystic space can form. Older lesions show dense fibrosis and calcification. Liquified degenerated fat can persist in the center of the lesion. Post-radiation therapy, adjacent breast lobules show atrophy and radiation-related cytologic atypia.
  - **Differential Diagnosis**: Reactive histiocytic proliferation/pseudotumors and carcinoma recurrence at radiation/surgery site. A radiological, pathological correlation is required when histological findings show fat necrosis without any carcinoma.
- **Management**: Fat necrosis is a benign lesion that does not require urgent or invasive intervention in cases whose appearance overlaps that of malignant lesions; a radiology pathology correlation and a close follow-up are required.

Case 1

Clinical History: A 69-year-old female presented with a palpable lump in the right breast for 1 month. There was no history of trauma to the breast (Figs. 4.1 and 4.2).

BI-RADS: 4.

An ultrasound-guided biopsy was recommended (Fig. 4.3).

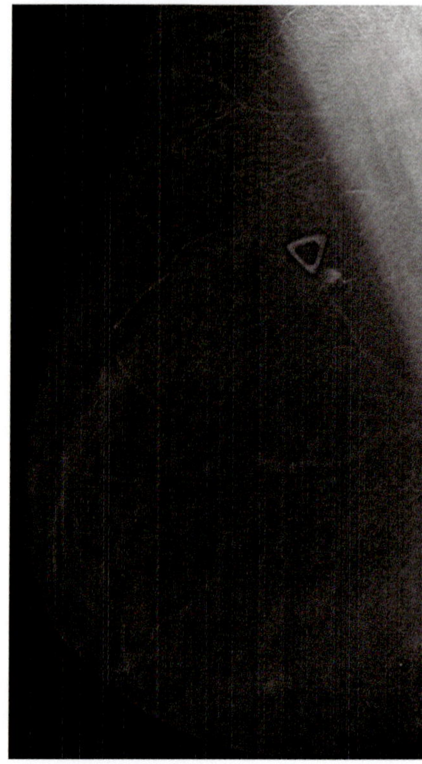

Fig. 4.1 Mammographic findings: Irregular mass with an indistinct margin in the right breast

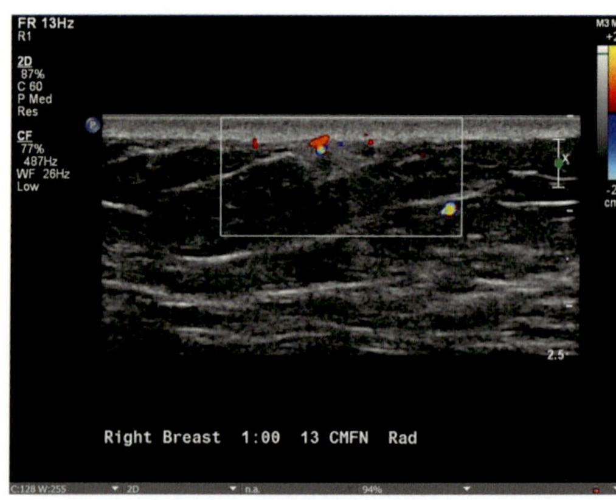

Fig. 4.2 Ultrasound findings: Hypoechoic irregular mass with echogenic halo and peripheral vascularity

Case 2

Clinical History: A 53-year-old female with a history of left breast cancer status post-bilateral mastectomy and implant reconstruction (Figs. 4.4, 4.5 and 4.6).

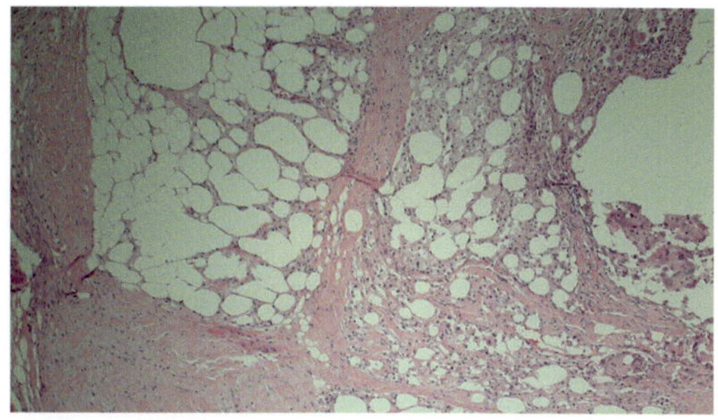

Fig. 4.3 Fat necrosis (H&E, 10×): The adipocytes show loss of nuclei and distorted cell shapes, accompanying histiocytic infiltrate and giant cells. A pseudocystic space is present near the right border of the image

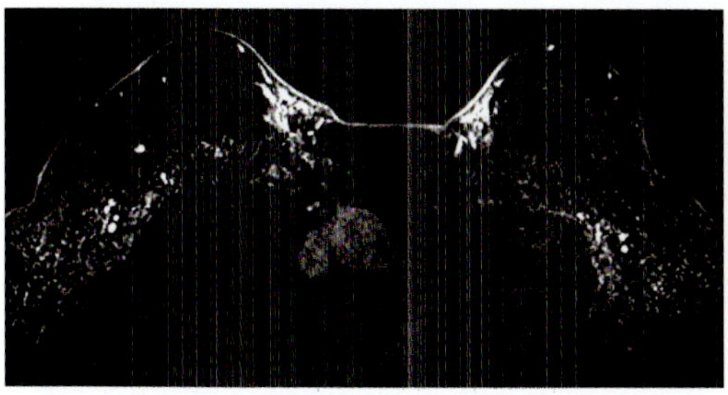

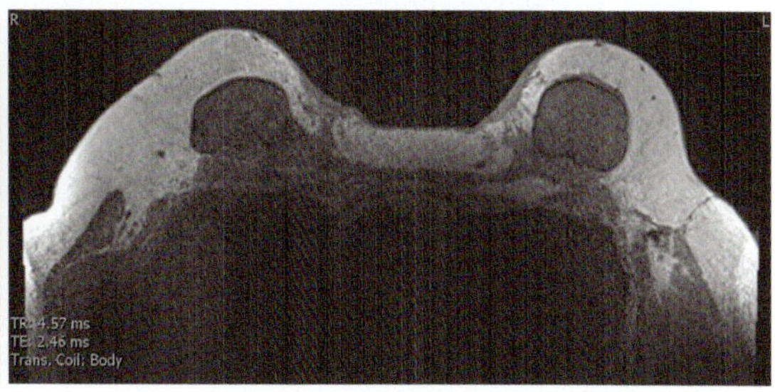

Figs. 4.4 and 4.5 **MRI findings**: Regional areas of non-mass enhancement with mixed enhancement kinetics in the upper, inner aspect of the reconstructed breasts

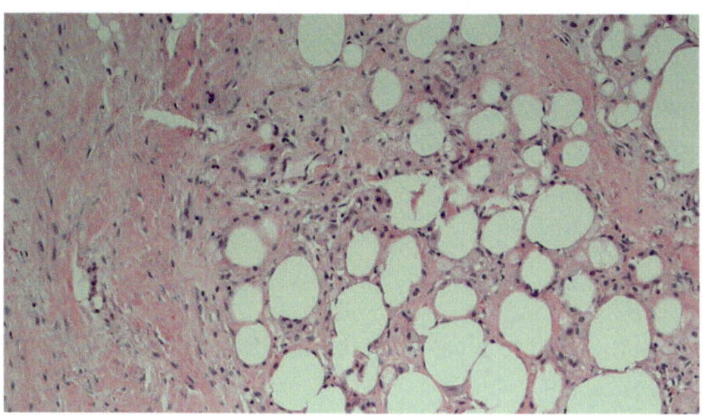

Fig. 4.6 (H&E, 20×): Fat necrosis consisting of disrupted adipocytes, fibrosis, and histiocytic infiltrate

Case 3

Clinical History: A 55-year-old female with possible minor trauma to the right breast. Recall from screening (Figs. 4.7, 4.8, 4.9 and 4.10).

BI-RADS: 3.

A 6-month follow-up was recommended. The follow-up ultrasound demonstrated the resolution of the previously seen mass (Fig. 4.11).

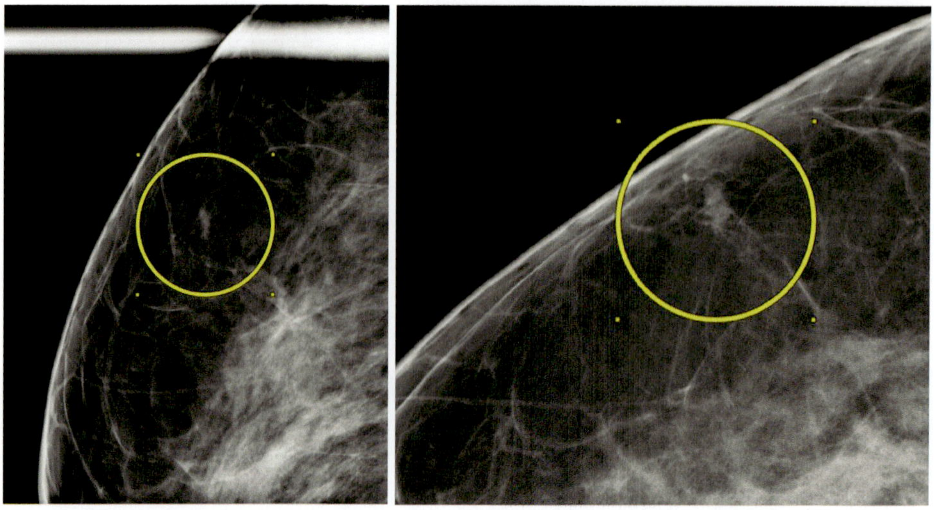

Figs. 4.7 and 4.8 **Mammographic findings**: 0.9 cm mass with an indistinct margin in the right breast

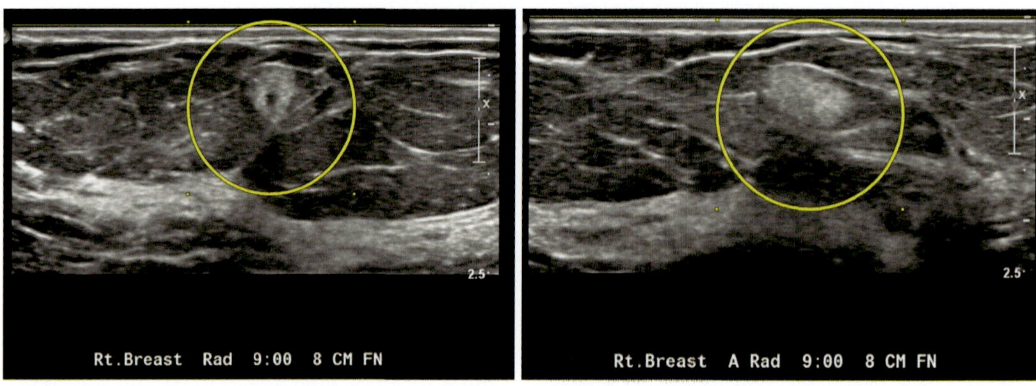

Figs. 4.9 and 4.10 **Ultrasound findings**: Oval, predominantly hyperechoic mass with indistinct margin in the right breast

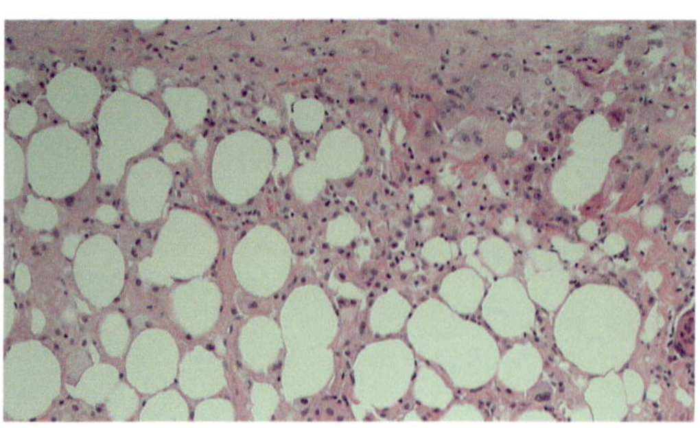

Fig. 4.11 Fat necrosis (H&E, 20×): Fibrosis, disrupted adipocytes, and histiocytic infiltrate

Abscess

Abscess: A breast abscess is categorized as puerperal (lactational) or nonpuerperal type, with lactation as the leading cause of abscess formation. It is commonly subareolar and caused by *Staphylococcus aureus* bacteria entering via a nipple fissure [8, 9].

- **Clinical Presentation**: Clinical presentations of breast abscess include a palpable, fluctuant, tender mass with associated systemic symptoms such as fever and body aches. However, breast abscesses may also occur in smokers, following recreational nipple/breast piercing or without a clear predisposing cause.
- **Imaging Findings**:
  - **Mammogram**: Due to pain and edema, patients with abscesses frequently find it difficult to undergo mammography. An oval or irregular mass with an indistinct margin may be observed. There are commonly associated findings, such as skin thickening and adjacent soft tissue edema.
  - **US**: A breast abscess commonly presents as a complex solid and cystic mass with increased peripheral vascularity. Debris related to infection, such as accumulated WBCs, may appear as hyperechoic foci within the mass.
  - **MRI**: A breast abscess may appear as a round or irregular mass with peripheral rim enhancement, demonstrating washout within the rim. The center of the mass is usually T2 hyperintense. Surrounding edema is usually present [10].
  - **BIRADS**: 2, 3, or 4.
  - **Differential Diagnosis**: Benign: galactocele (in the setting of recent pregnancy/lactation), hematoma, seroma. Malignant: necrotic malignancy, inflammatory breast CA [11–13].
- **Pathology Findings**: The pathology findings depend upon the etiologic agent and the clinical setting.
  - **Gross**: There are no specific gross findings for abscess. The breast skin may show signs of infection/inflammation—"red breast". The location of the abscess depends on the clinical setting. The lactation mastitis-related abscess involves peripheral breast parenchyma. The squamous metaplasia of lactiferous ducts leads to abscess formation in periareolar tissue.
  - **Microscopic Findings**: There is acute and chronic inflammatory infiltrate involving breast lobules. Abscess is characterized by a pseudocyst space line by granulation tissue and associated acute and chronic inflammatory infiltrate. The inflammatory cell population varies depending on the etiology of the abscess. Granulomas, eosinophils, and giant cells can be seen lining the abscess.
  - **Differential Diagnosis**: Cytsic neutrophilic granulomatous mastitis, inflammatory breast cancer, radiation effects, Paget disease, squamous metaplasia of lactiferous ducts.
- **Management**: Antibiotic therapy combined with needle aspiration is the mainstay of abscess treatment. Needle aspiration allows for obtaining microbiology samples for cultures and antibiotic sensitivity. It also serves as a therapeutic intervention with a greater success rate if the abscess is sufficiently small (<3 cm). If the abscess recurs or persists after multiple rounds of aspiration and antibiotic therapy, surgical incision and drainage or indwelling catheter placement could be considered as a more definitive measure. Additionally, if signs and symptoms persist after appropriate care and treatment, the mass should be biopsied to exclude malignancy [14].

Case 1

Clinical History: A 37-year-old male presenting with a lump in his right breast that is tender to palpation. No axillary lymphadenopathy or nipple discharge is present (Figs. 4.12, 4.13, 4.14 and 4.15).

BI-RADS: 2.

A follow-up ultrasound in 1 month was recommended to monitor response to treatment (Figs. 4.16–4.19).

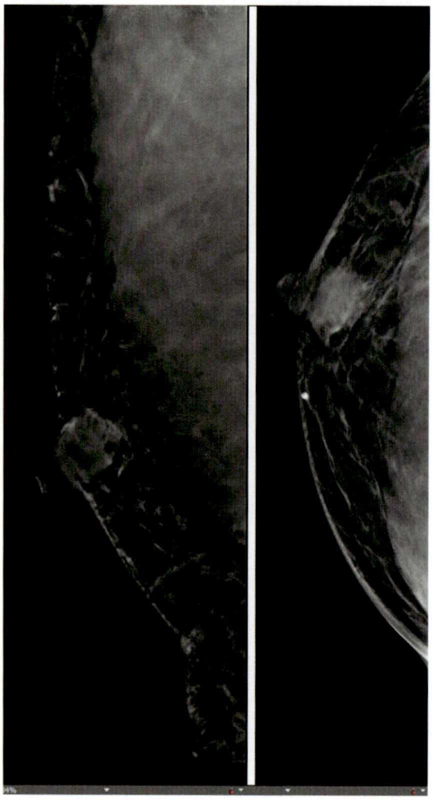

Figs. 4.12 and 4.13 Mammographic findings: Irregular retroareolar mass with an indistinct margin in the right breast

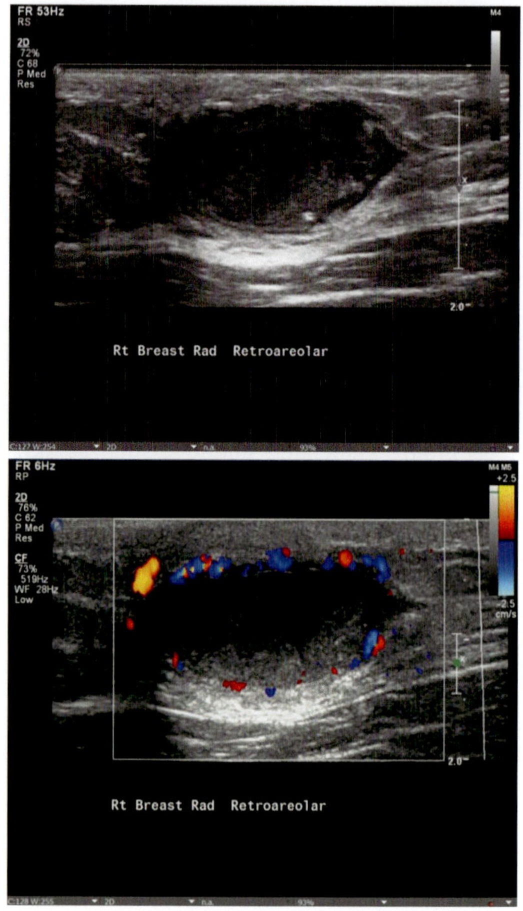

Figs. 4.14 and 4.15 Ultrasound findings: Hypoechoic oval mass with complex internal echoes and posterior acoustic enhancement. Increased vascularity is present in the surrounding tissue

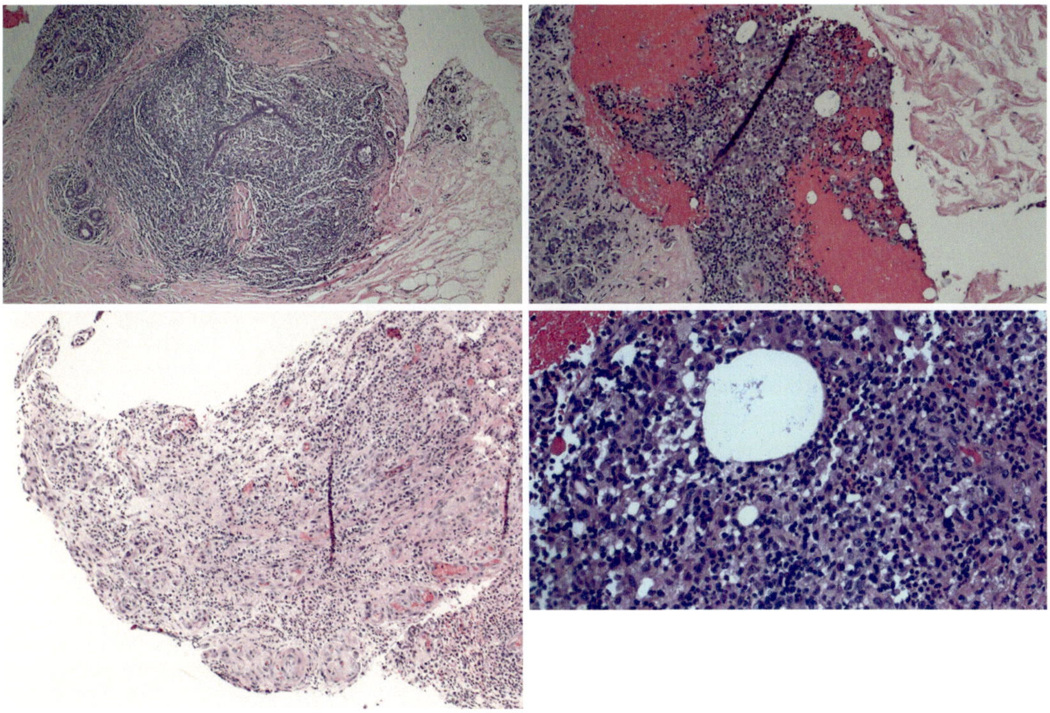

Figs. 4.16–4.19 Breast abscess (H&E, 4×, two 10×, and 20×). The breast tissue shows acute and chronic inflammatory infiltrate surrounding lobules and ducts. There is pseudocystic space (abscess lining) lined by granulation tissue and acute inflammatory cells. The empty rounded space shows profiles of the bacterial organisms

Pseudoangiomatous Stromal Hyperplasia (PASH)

Pseudoangiomatous Stromal Hyperplasia: Pseudoangiomatous stromal hyperplasia (PASH) is an uncommon, benign disease of the breast with unclear etiology and no association with malignancy. The proposed pathophysiology of PASH is the response of myofibroblasts to hormonal stimuli, linking its increased prevalence in premenopausal women or postmenopausal women to hormonal therapy [15].

Clinical Presentation: PASH may present as a suspicious mass with an indistinct margin, which prompts a biopsy and eventual excision. Patients may report a palpable mass, but asymptomatic presentation is also common.

- **Imaging Findings**:
  - **Mammogram**: A classic mammographic presentation of PASH is a mass with a circumscribed or indistinct margin. It may also present as a focal asymmetry. Associated punctate calcifications may be present.
  - **US**: A typical sonographic appearance of PASH is round or oval, hypoechoic mass with a circumscribed margin.
  - **MRI**: PASH on MRI exhibits nonspecific features, most commonly appearing as a circumscribed oval or round, persistently enhancing mass with internal areas of increased T2 signal or clumped non-mass enhancement with persistent kinetics.
  - **BIRADS**: Variable, may range from 3 to 5.
  - **Differential Diagnosis**: Benign: fibroadenoma, adenosis, fibrocystic changes, phyllodes tumor; Malignant: breast cancer, low-grade angiosarcoma [16–18].
- **Pathology Findings**: PASH can present as a well-formed mass called nodular PASH. More commonly, PASH is associated with other

proliferative and cystic changes involving the breast tissue.

- **Gross**: The nodular PASH can form a circumscribed solid tan-white mass with a gelatinous cut surface.
- **Microscopic Findings**: PASH comprises the proliferation of benign myofibroblastic stromal cells that mimic thin-walled vessels. The stromal cells are separated by collagenous fibrous tissue, which can be edematous, especially surrounding the epithelial line duct. PASH can contain hypercellular areas with fascicular patterns. A range of mesenchymal metaplastic changes have been described involving PASH. PASH can involve intralobular as well as interlobular breast tissue. The epithelium of adjacent breast lobules often shows gynecomastia-type usual ductal hyperplasia.
- **Differential Diagnosis**: The histological differential diagnoses include benign and malignant spindle cell lesions of the breast. PASH also needs to be differentiated from the breast's combined epithelial and stromal lesions. Distinction of fibroadenoma with PASH-like stroma from nodular PASH can be extremely difficult, especially in small needle biopsies. Since both are benign lesions, this distinction is redundant. PASH-like stroma can also be seen in phyllodes tumor [19].

• **Management**: Although PASH demonstrates no association with malignancy, its imaging appearance may mimic malignant lesions; a biopsy is frequently necessary for confirmation. Although most lesions remain stable, some may exhibit growth or be symptomatic; these lesions are usually excised.

Case 1

Clinical History: A 40-year-old female with a history of bilateral breast reduction mammoplasty presents with a new palpable lump in the left breast (Figs. 4.20 and 4.21).

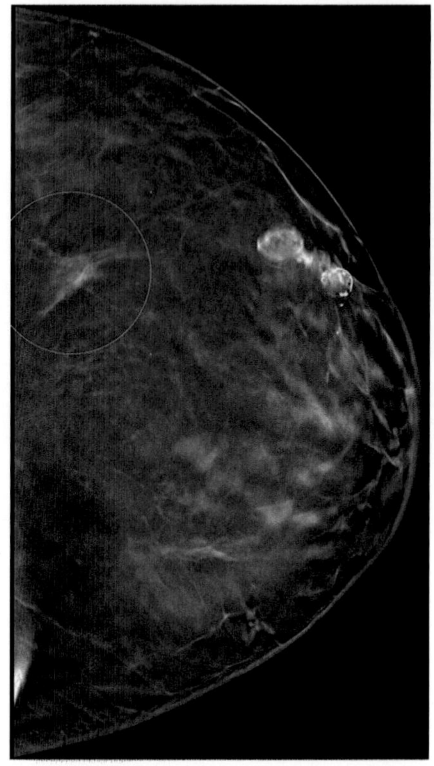

Fig. 4.20 **Mammographic findings**: Focal asymmetry with an indistinct margin in the left breast

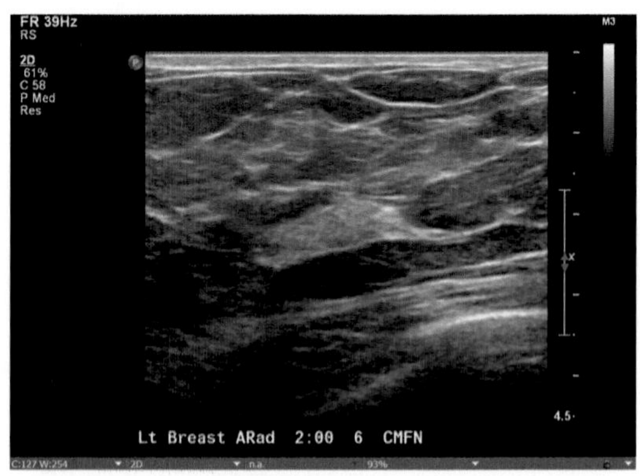

Fig. 4.21 **Ultrasound findings**: Hyperechoic, avascular mass with indistinct margin

BI-RADS: 4.

A tomosynthesis-guided biopsy was recommended (Figs. 4.22 and 4.23).

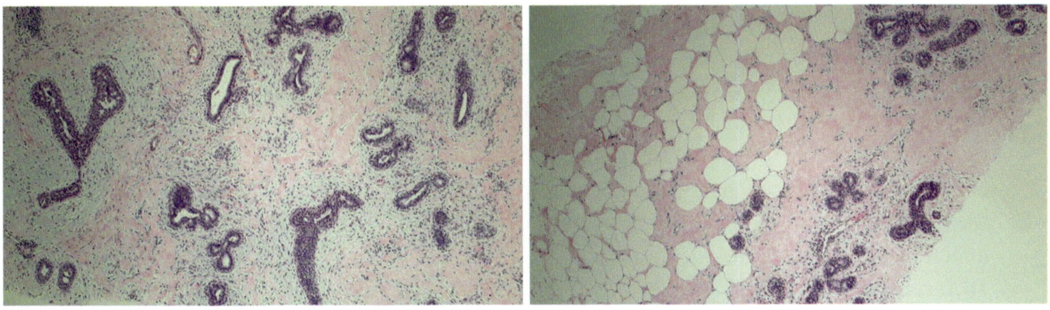

Figs. 4.22 and 4.23 PASH (H&E, 10×): Stromal expansion by PASH involving periductal stroma. PASH extends into the interlobular adipose tissue

Invasive Breast Cancer

Invasive Breast Cancer: The presence of an irregular mass with indistinct margins must first raise suspicion of malignancy.

Clinical Presentation: Invasive ductal carcinoma manifests as an irregular mass with indistinct margins more frequently than its pure mucinous counterpart. Interestingly, DCIS is often found in the vicinity of or surrounding invasive ductal carcinoma, regarded as field cancerization, due to the accumulation of genetic or molecular aberrations in the same area of the breast. Invasive lobular carcinoma has a very variable manifestation but may also present as an irregular mass with indistinct margins [20–27].

- **Imaging Findings**:
  - **Mammogram**: Invasive ductal carcinoma is classically described as an irregular, high-density mass with an indistinct or spiculated margin, often accompanied by pleomorphic calcifications. In contrast, invasive lobular carcinoma may present as a mass or a focal developing asymmetry and usually lacks microcalcifications. Associated architectural distortion and axillary adenopathy can also be observed [24, 25, 27].
  - **US**: Sonographic findings of invasive carcinoma are varied. A common representation is an irregular, nonparallel hypoechoic mass with a spiculated or indistinct margin with posterior acoustic shadowing. Microcalcifications and internal vascularity may also be detected. An echogenic rim or halo around the margin may be present [22].
  - **MRI**: Characteristic MRI features of invasive carcinoma include a mass with a spiculated or indistinct margin. It is T1 and T2 hypointense and avidly enhances with either plateau or washout kinetics. MRI may demonstrate mammographically occult multifocal or multicentric disease [23].
  - **BIRADS**: 4 to 5.
  - **Differential Diagnosis**: Benign: fat necrosis, PASH, nodular adenosis, complex sclerosing lesions; Malignant: sarcoma, lymphoma.
- **Pathology Findings**: The pathology findings depend on the presence of in situ and or invasive disease. Mass-forming lesions can also be formed by a benign breast lesion-like a papilloma, sclerosing lesion, or a fibroadenoma that is involved by carcinoma.
  - **Gross**: The macroscopic appearance can change with the histological tumor type. The ductal carcinoma is often a tan, white firm mass with irregular infiltrative borders. The cut surface can be mucinous in mucinous carcinoma or cystic in the papillary lesion. The hemorrhagic tan, red surface has been described with invasive carcinomas with osteoclast-like giant cells.
  - **Microscopic Findings**: The invasive carcinomas comprise infiltrating malignant epithelial cells accompanied by variable amounts of desmoplastic, fibroblastic, and inflammatory cells. The invasive carci-

noma epithelial clusters show an absent myoepithelial layer and lack of basement membrane. In DCIS, involving a mass-forming lesion (fibroadenoma, papilloma, or sclerosing lesion), the benign epithelial component is replaced by malignant epithelial proliferation limited to the intraductal compartment.
  - **Differential Diagnosis**: Invasive ductal carcinoma, no special type, and special histologic subtypes of carcinoma-like mucinous carcinoma, invasive micropapillary carcinoma, and carcinoma with medullary features. Benign proliferative lesions-papilloma with sclerosis, radial and complex sclerosing lesion.
- **Management**: Surgery remains the mainstay of therapy, with neoadjuvant treatment frequently recommended for large tumors prior to surgery and radiation therapy following resection.

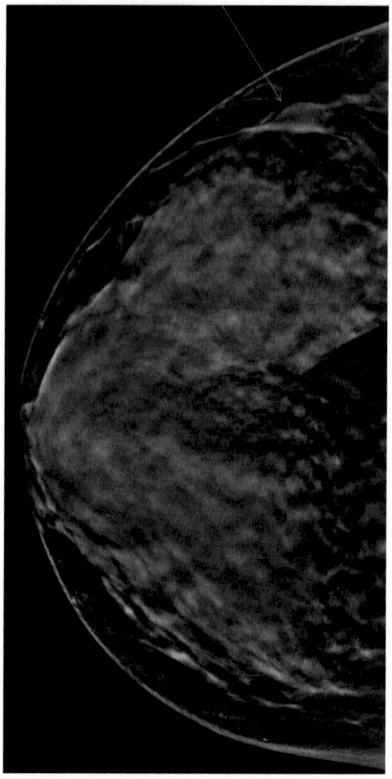

Fig. 4.24 **Mammographic findings**: Oval mass with an indistinct margin

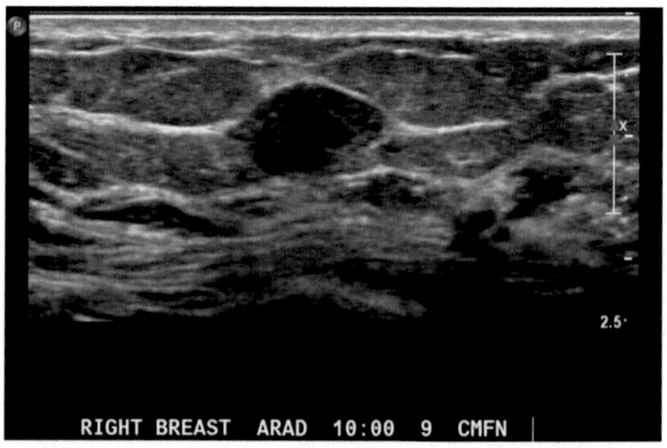

Fig. 4.25 **Ultrasound findings**: Hypoechoic oval mass with indistinct margin and internal vascularity

Case 1

Clinical History: A 67-year-old female's screening mammogram detected a mass in the right breast (Figs. 4.24 and 4.25).

BI-RADS: 4C, suspicious of malignancy.

An US-guided biopsy was performed (Figs. 4.26 and 4.27).

Case 2

Clinical History: A 27-year-old female presenting with left breast pain, soreness, tightness, and firmness. No history of nipple discharge or skin changes at the time of evaluation (Figs. 4.28, 4.29, 4.30, 4.31 and 4.32).

BI-RADS: 4A, suspected of malignancy.

An US-guided biopsy was performed (Figs. 4.33 and 4.34).

Case 3

Clinical History: A 75-year-old female was recalled from screening for a new mass in the right breast (Figs. 4.35, 4.36 and 4.37).

BI-RADS: 4A, low suspicion for malignancy. A biopsy was recommended (Figs. 4.38–4.41).

Case 4

Clinical History: A 76-year-old female recalled from screening for a mass seen in a screening exam (Figs. 4.42, 4.43 and 4.44).

BI-RADS: 4. An US-guided biopsy was recommended (Figs. 4.45 and 4.46).

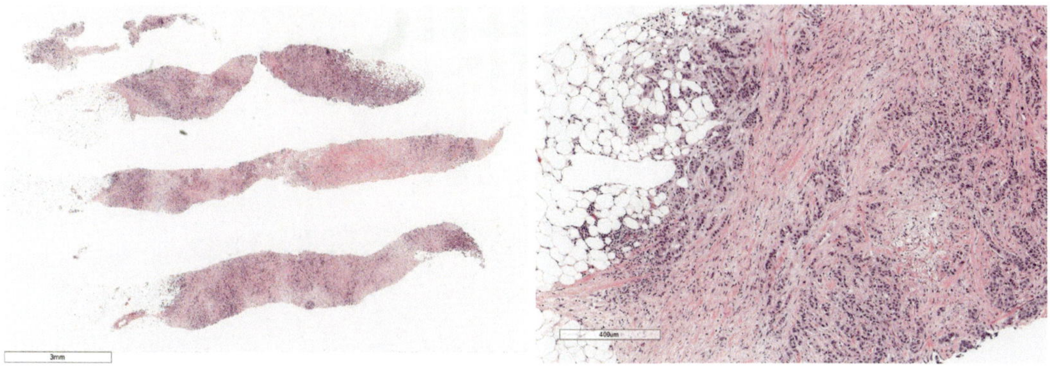

Figs. 4.26 and 4.27 Invasive ductal carcinoma (H&E, low power and 2×): The core needle biopsy shows a histologic grade 2 invasive ductal carcinoma (no special type). The tumor forms a fibrous mass, and tumor cells infiltrate adjacent adipose tissue

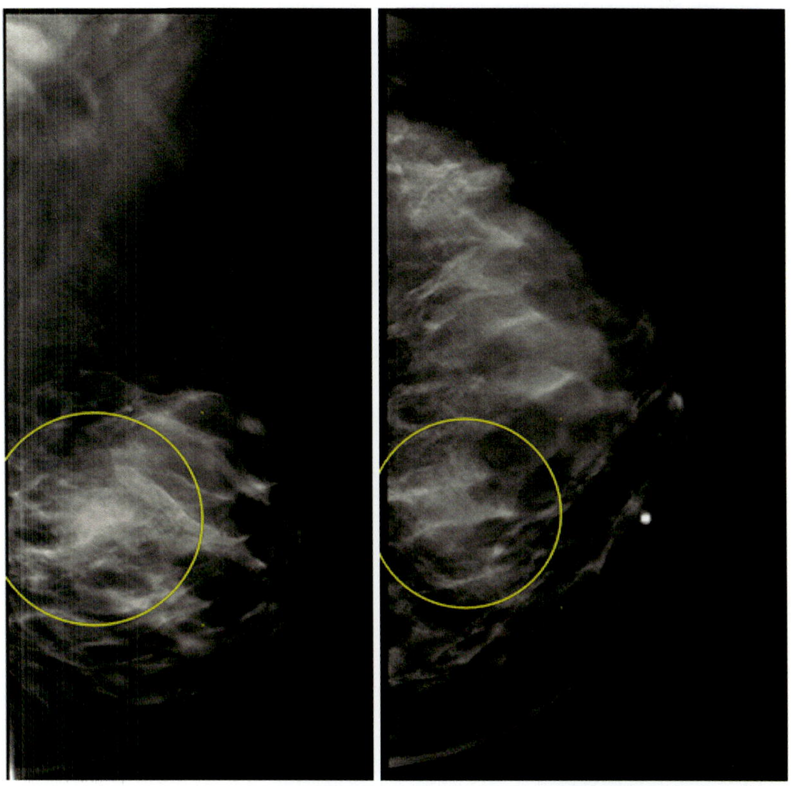

Figs. 4.28 and 4.29 Mammographic findings: Irregular mass with an indistinct margin in the left breast with a prominent lymph node

Case 5

Clinical History: A 78-year-old female. Recall from screening (Figs. 4.47, 4.48 and 4.49).

BI-RADS: 4. Biopsy was recommended.

Pathology: Initial US-guided biopsy demonstrated focal minimal atypical ductal hyperplasia, discordant with the imaging findings. An excisional biopsy was performed, which was concordant with invasive ductal carcinoma (Figs. 4.50, 4.51, 4.52 and 4.53).

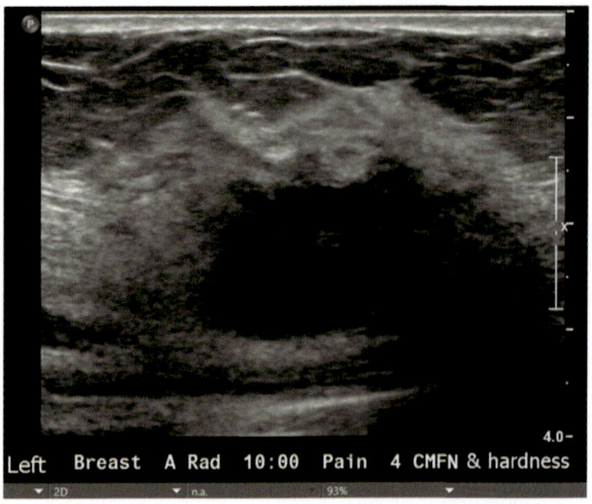

Fig. 4.30 **Ultrasound findings**: Hypoechoic mass with an indistinct margin and with adjacent vascularity

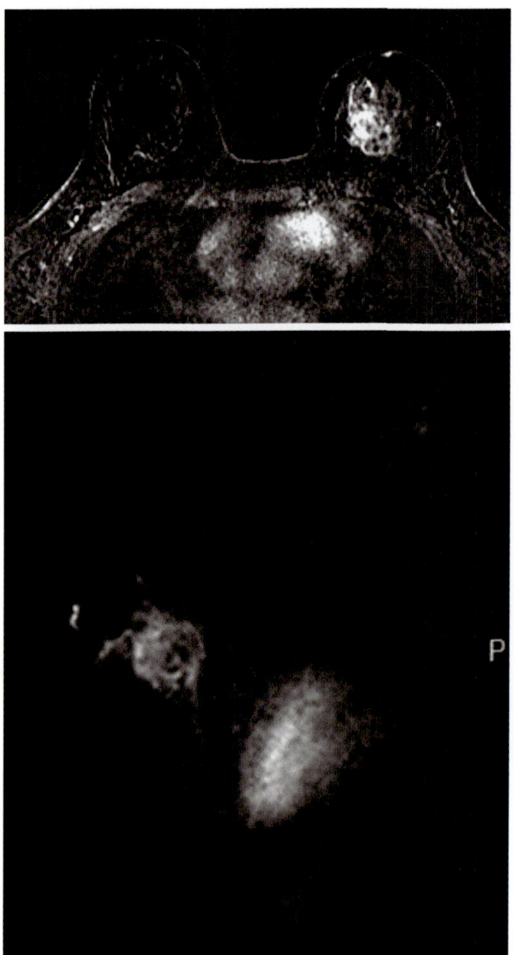

Figs. 4.31 and 4.32 **MRI findings**: Irregular mass with heterogeneous enhancement, peripheral persistent kinetics, and central plateau and washout kinetics

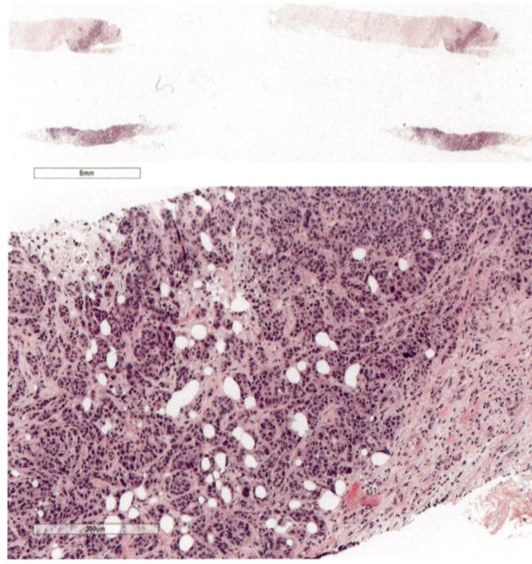

Figs. 4.33 and 4.34 Invasive ductal carcinoma histologic grade 3 (H&E, low power and 10×): Core needle biopsy shows a poorly differentiated ductal carcinoma with sheets of tumor cells with high-grade nuclei and prominent mitotic activity

Case 6

Clinical History: A 57-year-old female presented with a new right breast mass on a screening mammogram (Figs. 4.54, 4.55 and 4.56).

BI-RADS: 4C, suspected of malignancy. An US-guided biopsy was performed.

Pathology: Invasive ductal carcinoma with mucinous features and focal ductal carcinoma in situ, moderately differentiated (Figs. 4.57 and 4.58).

Case 7

Clinical History: A 61-year-old female, asymmetry on screening mammogram (Figs. 4.59 and 4.60).

Ultrasound findings: No correlate mass was seen on ultrasound.

BI-RADS: 4. Biopsy was recommended.

Pathology: Invasive mucinous carcinoma with multifocal mucinous ductal carcinoma in situ (Figs. 4.61, 4.62 and 4.63).

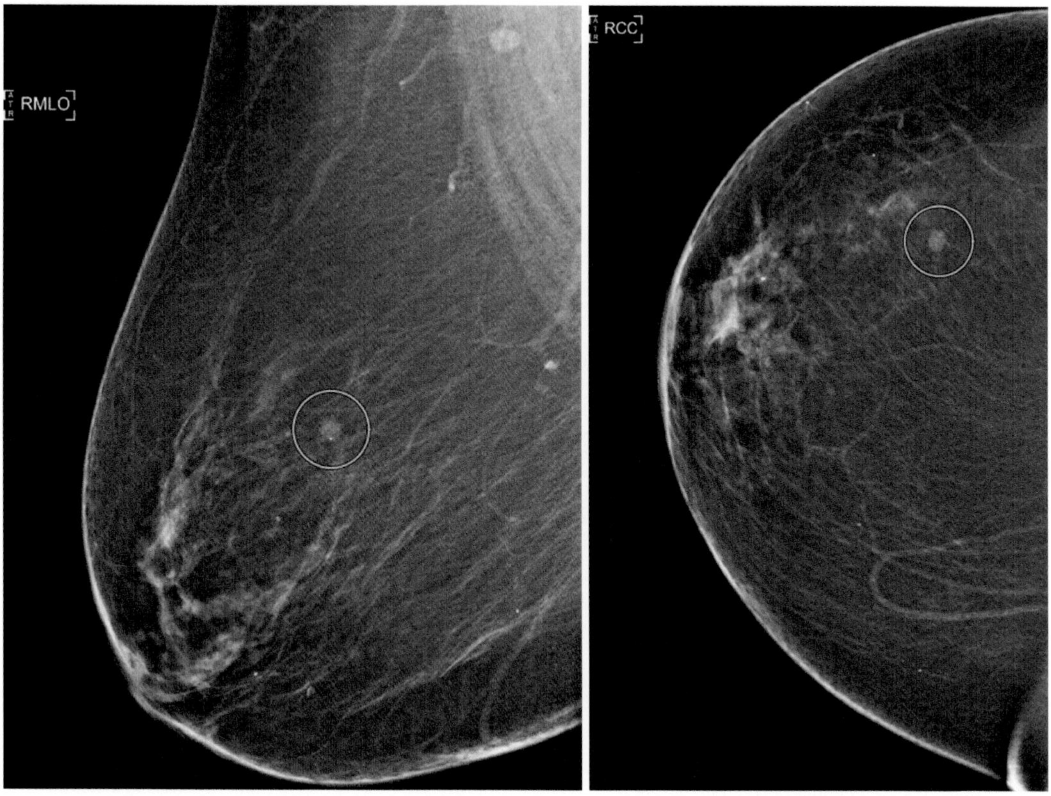

Figs. 4.35 and 4.36 Mammographic findings: Oval mass with an indistinct margin in the right breast

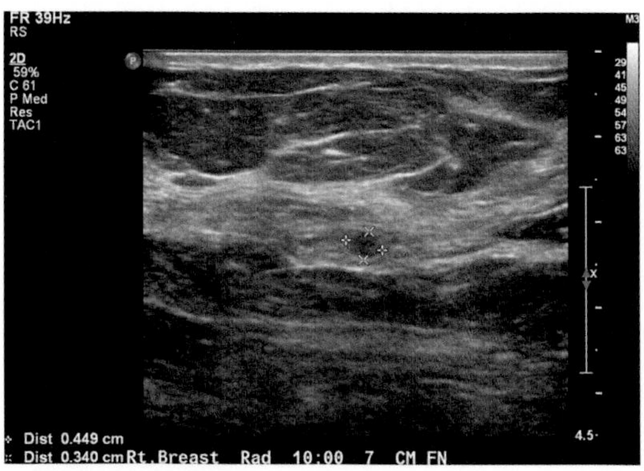

Fig. 4.37 Ultrasound findings: Hypoechoic, oval mass with an indistinct margin

Case 8

Clinical History: A 46-year-old female with left breast focal asymmetry was seen on a screening mammogram and recalled for additional evaluation (Figs. 4.64, 4.65, 4.66 and 4.67).

BI-RADS: 4B, suspicious for malignancy. Biopsy was recommended.

Pathology: Invasive lobular carcinoma with axillary lymph node metastasis (Figs. 4.68, 4.69, 4.70 and 4.71).

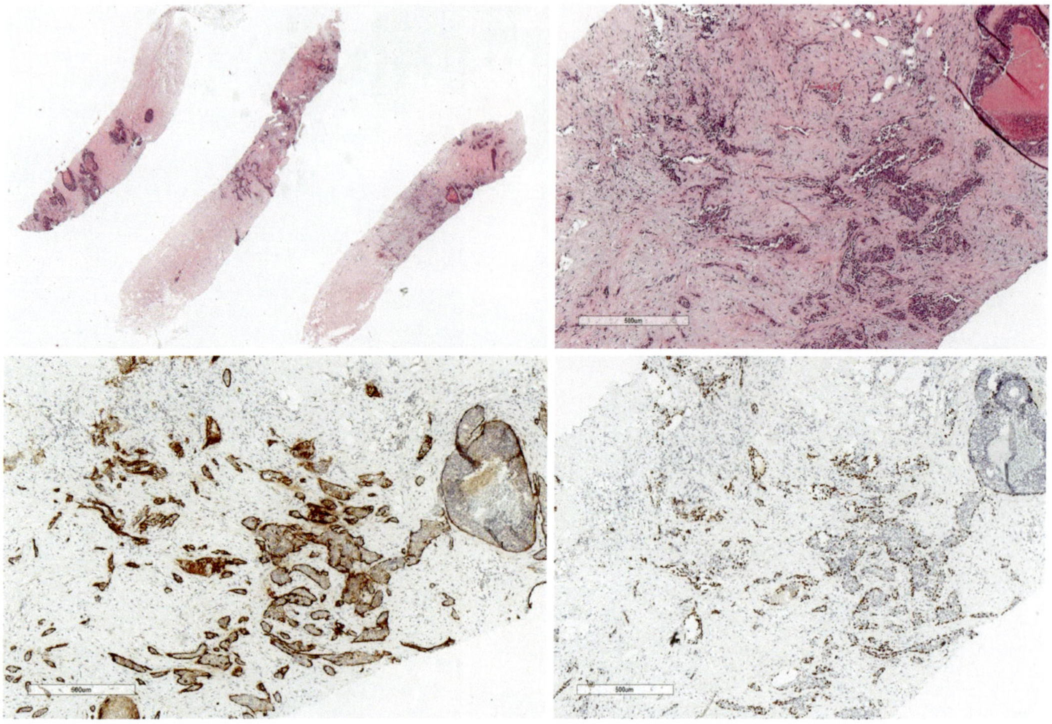

Figs. 4.38–4.41 DCIS (H&E, low power and 10× and smooth muscle myosin and p63 IHC) involving a sclerosing lesion. Prominent fibrous stroma forms part of the mass. The myoepithelial cell IHC confirms the intact myoepithelial layer and the in-situ nature of the carcinoma

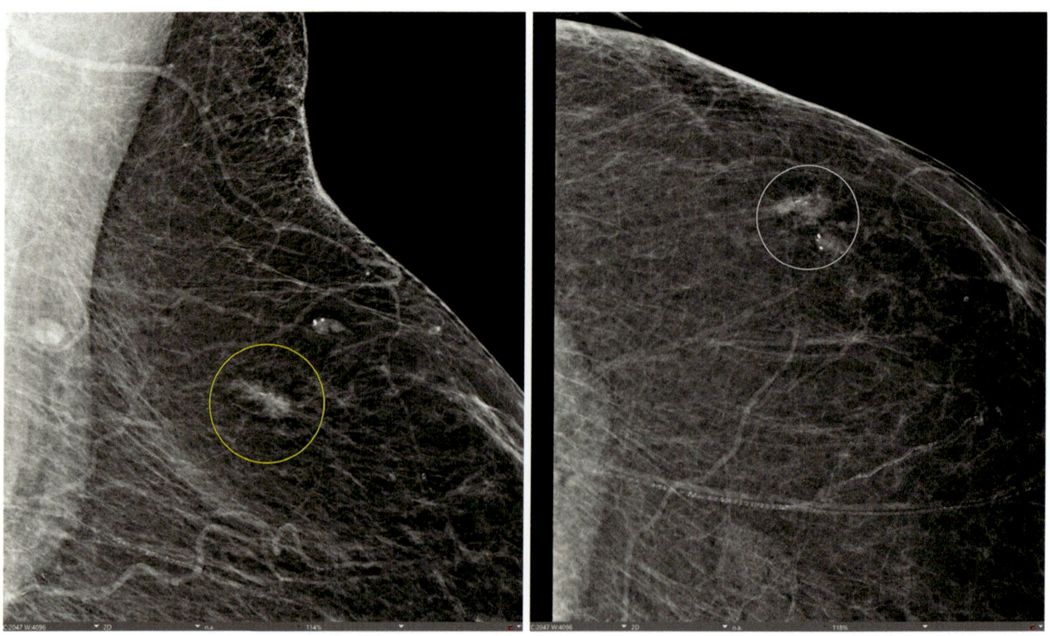

Figs. 4.42 and 4.43 Mammographic findings: Irregular mass with an indistinct margin and with heterogeneous calcifications

Fig. 4.44 **Ultrasound findings**: Irregular, hypoechoic mass with an indistinct margin and hyperechoic halo

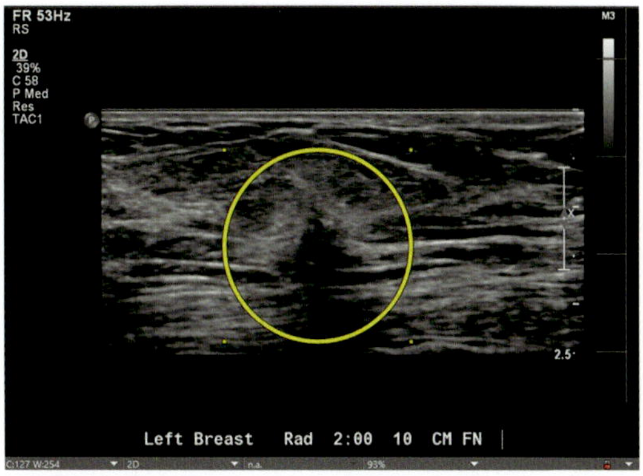

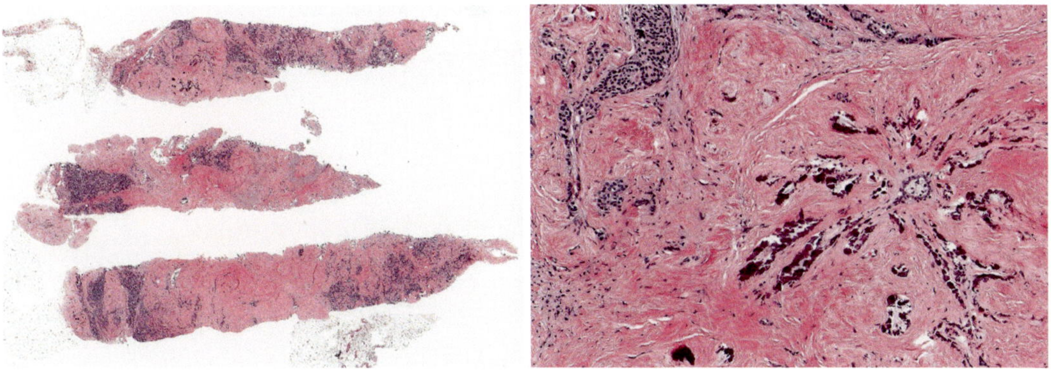

Figs. 4.45 and 4.46 Core needle biopsy with histologic grade 2 invasive ductal carcinoma (H&E, low power) and intermediate nuclear grade DCIS (H&E, 10×) with associated calcifications

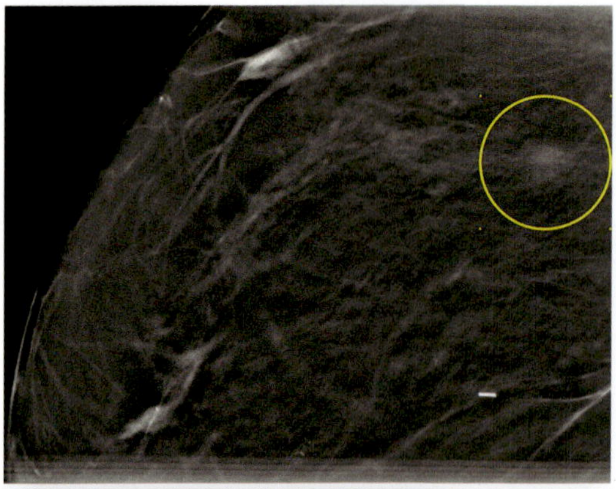

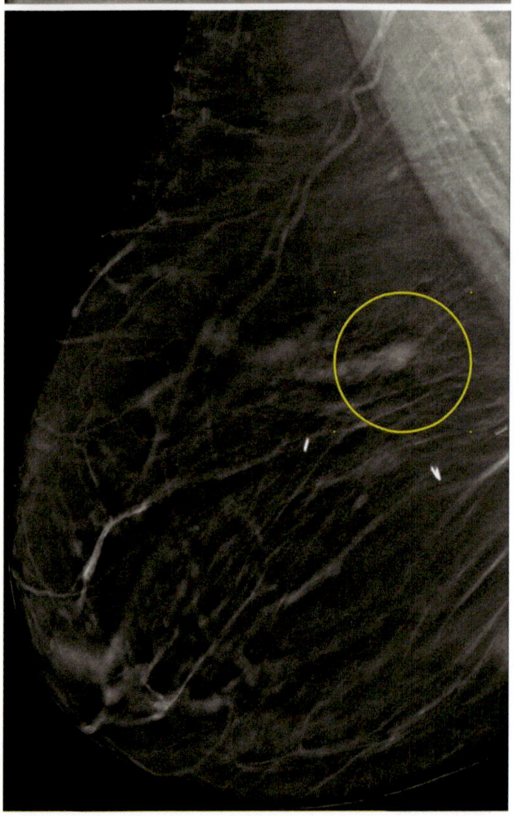

Figs. 4.47 and 4.48 Mammographic findings: Oval mass with an indistinct margin

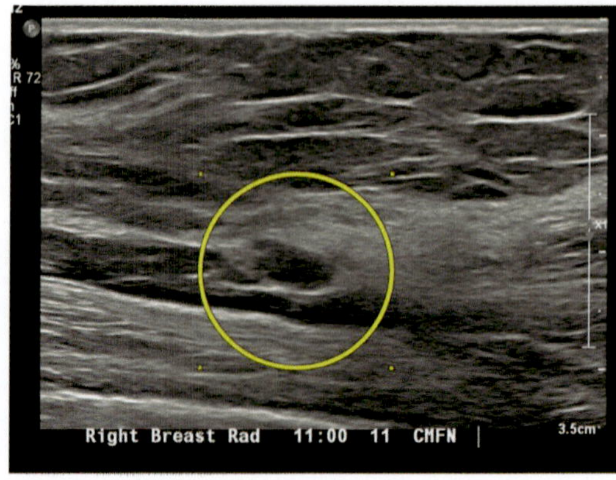

Fig. 4.49 Ultrasound findings: Hypoechoic oval mass with a circumscribed margin parallel to the nipple. No vascularity was detected

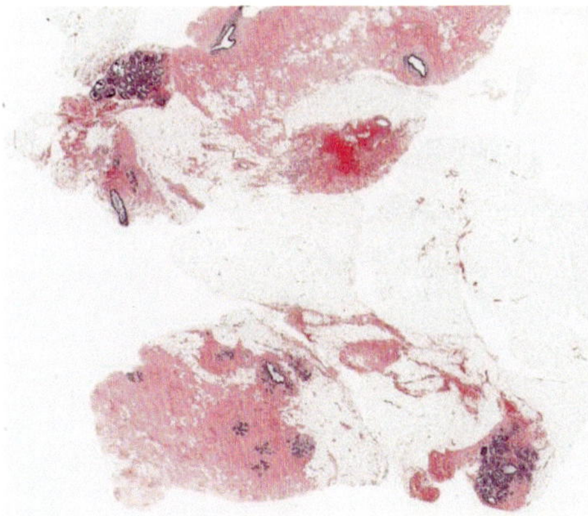
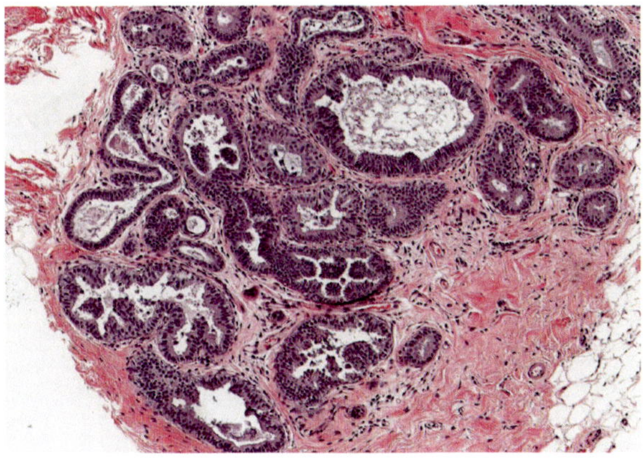

Figs. 4.50 and 4.51 Core needle biopsy (H&E low power and 10×) shows atypical ductal hyperplasia focus with micropapillary pattern and associated calcifications. Histological findings do not explain mass-forming lesion, and therefore, pathology is discordant with radiological findings

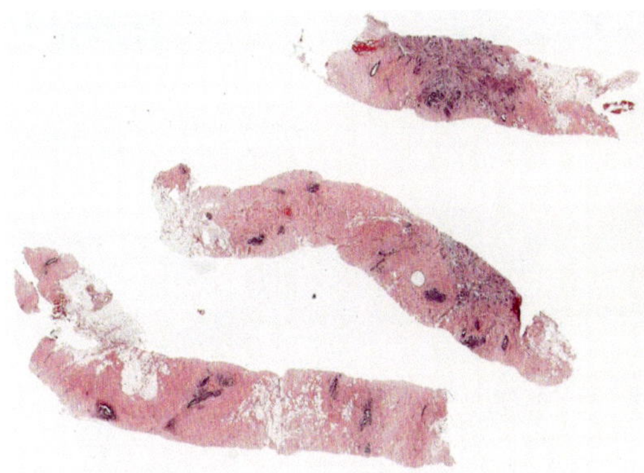
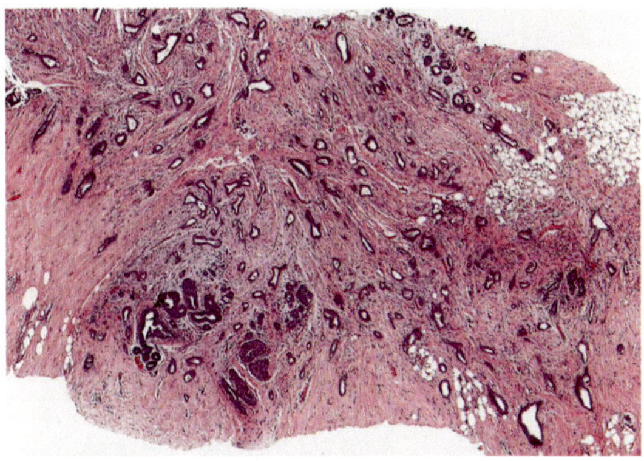

Figs. 4.52 and 4.53 Tubular carcinoma (H&E, low power, and 4×) represented the mass lesion. More than 90% of carcinoma is comprised of well-formed tubules with low nuclear grade and absent to minimal mitotic activity

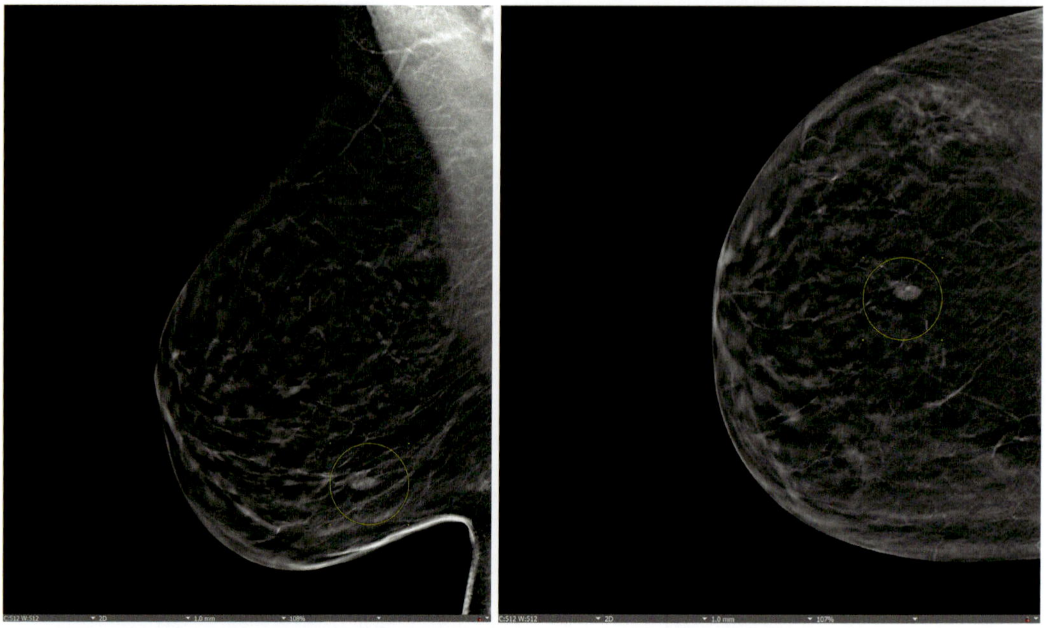

Figs. 4.54 and 4.55 Mammographic findings: Irregular mass with an indistinct margin

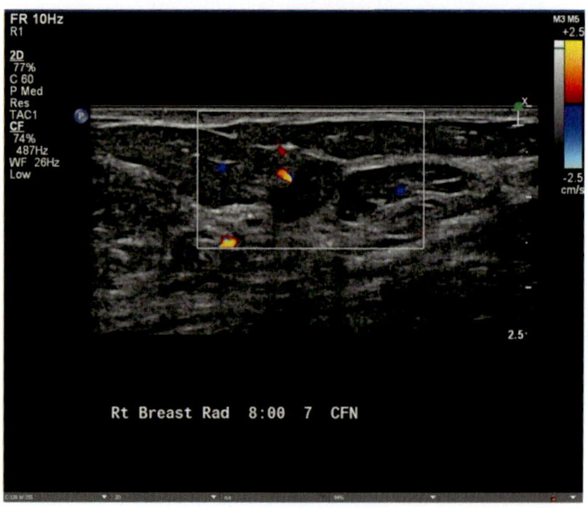

Fig. 4.56 Ultrasound findings: Irregular, hypoechoic mass with increased adjacent vascularity

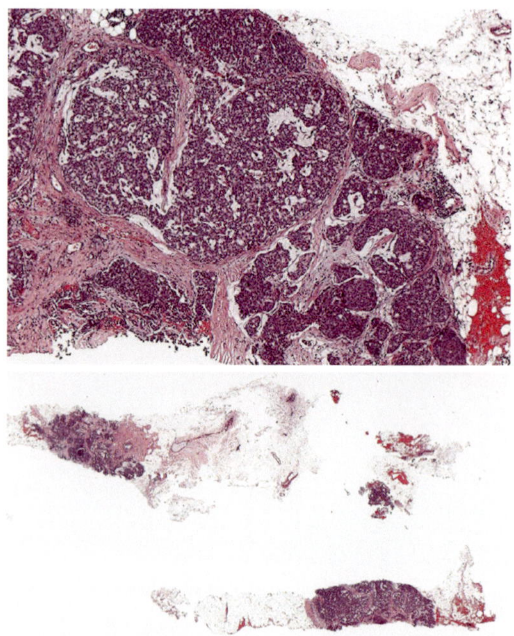

Figs. 4.57 and 4.58 Invasive carcinoma with mucinous features (H&E, low power and 2×). The mass is formed of infiltrative malignant epithelial cells with duct formation and pools of extracellular mucin

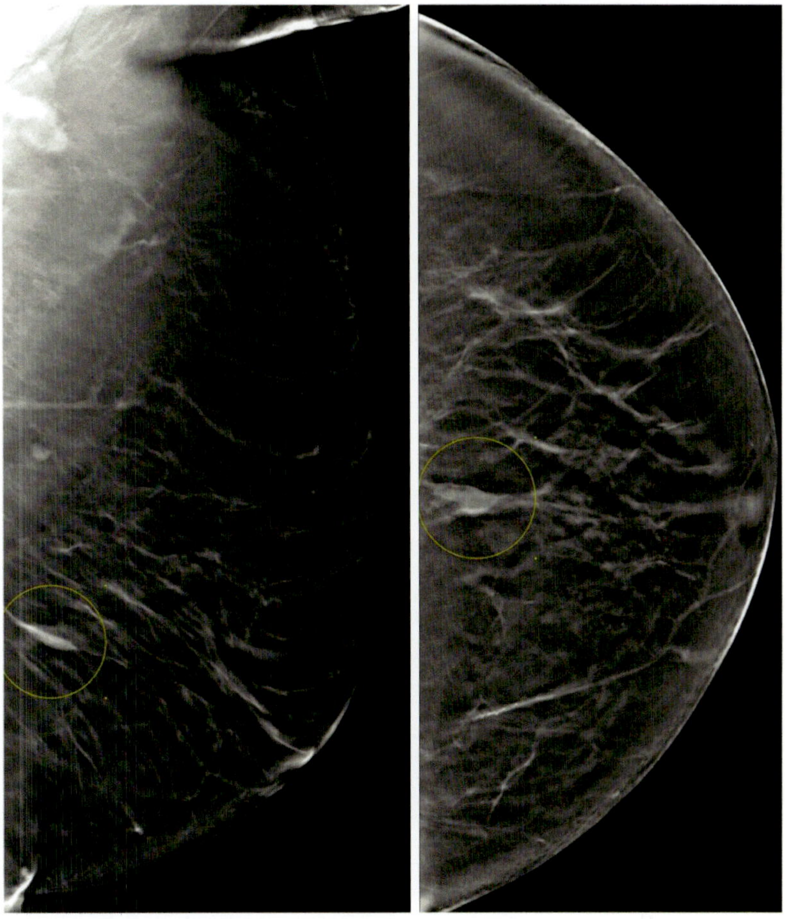

Figs. 4.59 and 4.60 Mammographic findings: Equal density focal asymmetry

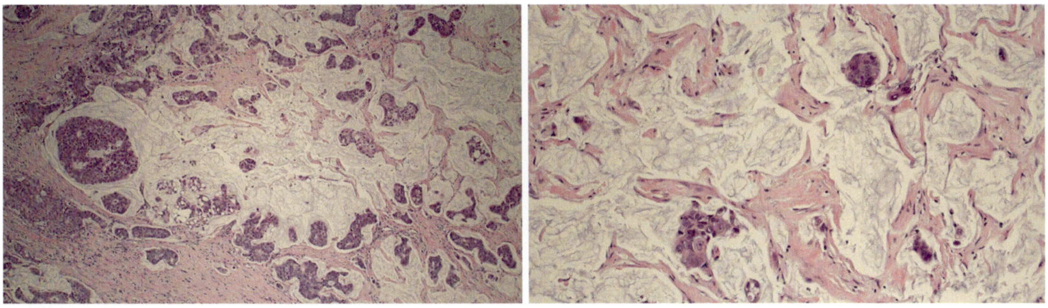

Figs. 4.61 and 4.62 Mucinous carcinoma (H&E, 4× and 20×) Mass is formed by invasive mucinous carcinoma histologic grade 2 comprising of malignant epithelial cells floating in the stromal mucin pools

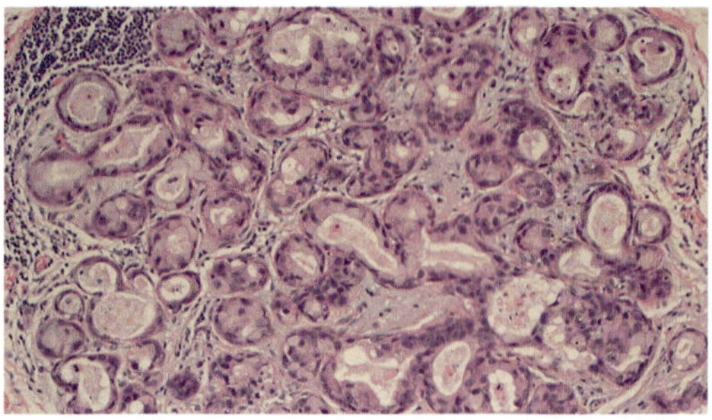

Fig. 4.63 Ductal carcinoma in situ (H&E, 10×) with mucinous features involving lobules

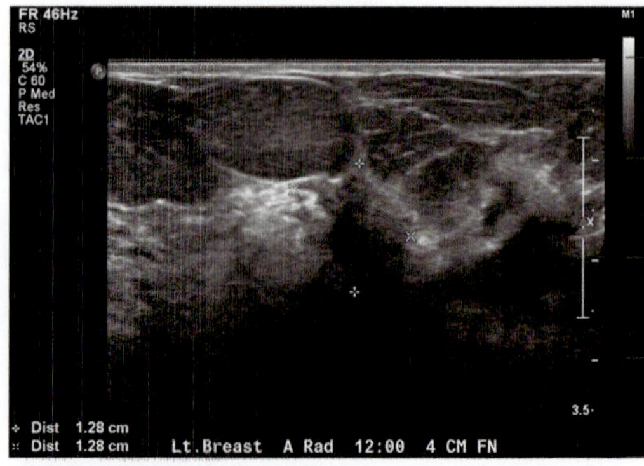

Fig. 4.66 Ultrasound findings: Hypoechoic irregular area, which corresponds to a palpable lump. Additionally, A few lymph nodes with cortical thickening and asymmetry in the left axilla

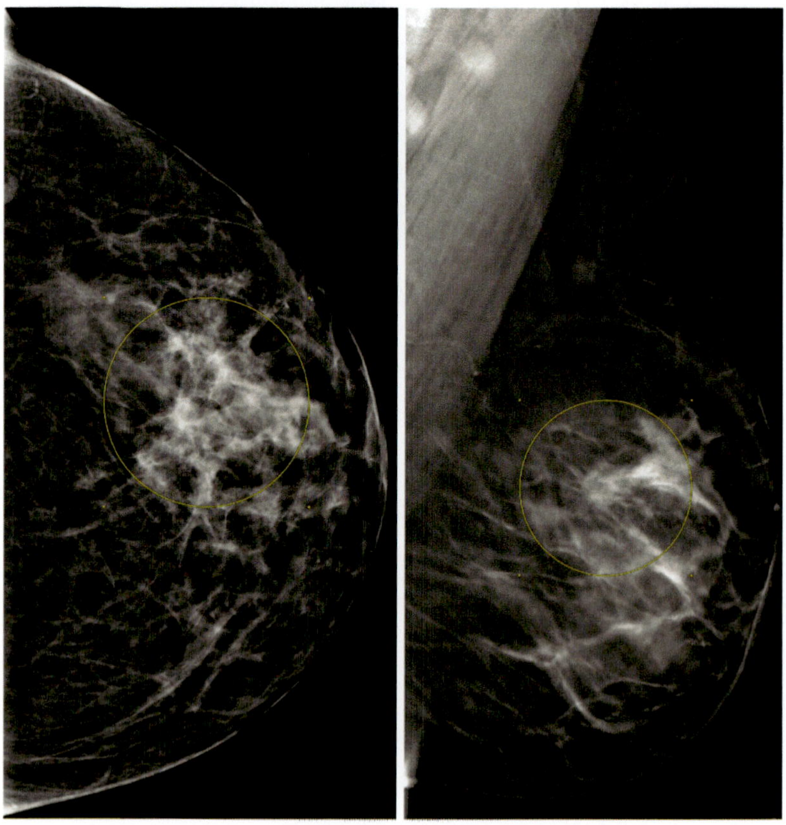

Figs. 4.64 and 4.65 Mammographic findings: Irregular, focal asymmetry with architectural distortion

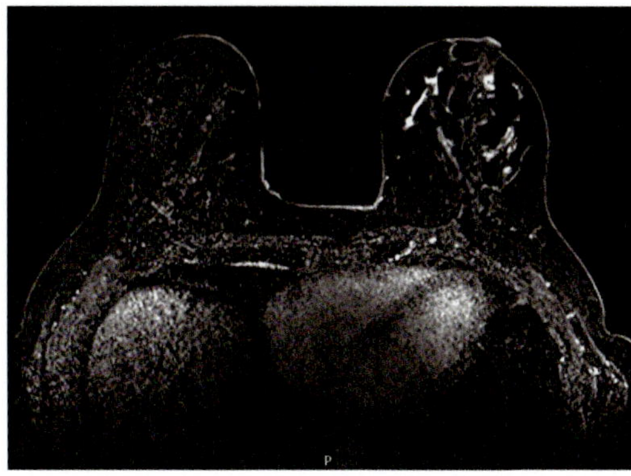

Fig. 4.67 **MRI findings**: Multiple areas of non-mass enhancement in the left breast

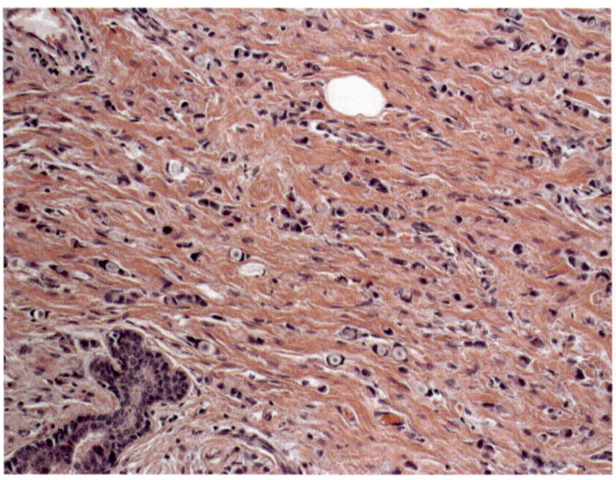

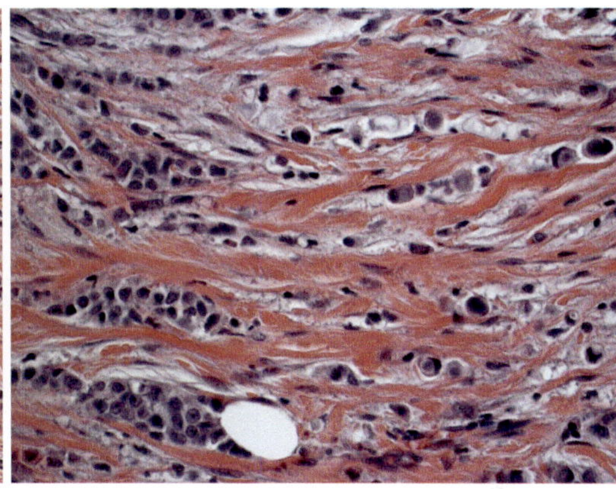

Figs. 4.68 and 4.69 Invasive lobular carcinoma (H&E, 10×, and 20×) histologic grade 2 showing dyshesive tumor cells with linear single file arrangement, intracytoplasmic mucin vacuoles, and signet-ring cell morphology

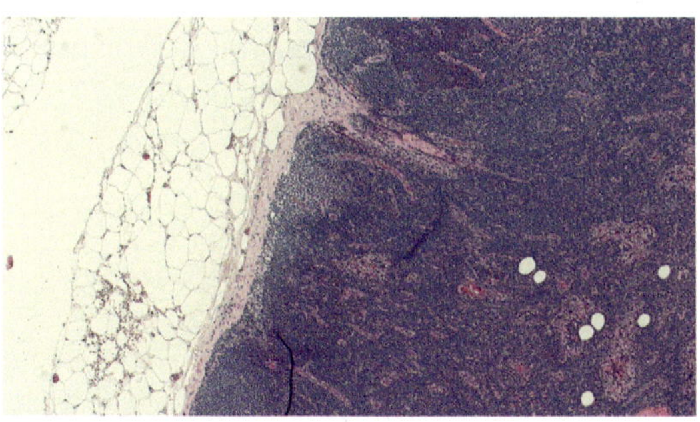

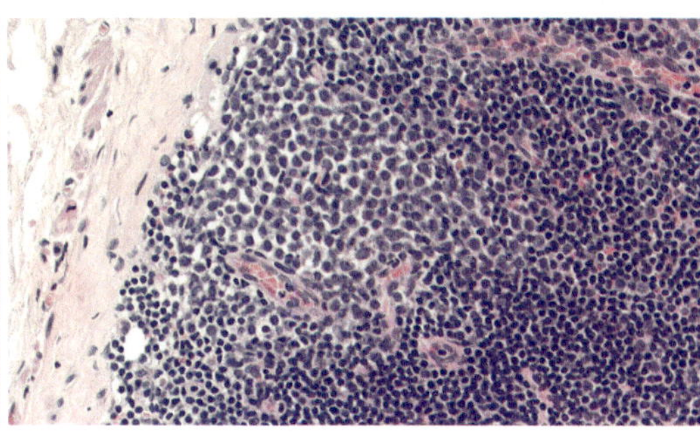

Figs. 4.70 and 4.71 Metastatic lobular carcinoma (H&E, 4× and 20×) involving the subcapsular area of the axillary lymph node. The tumor cells form loose clusters and are slightly larger than lymphoid cells

Invasive Micropapillary Carcinoma

Invasive Micropapillary Carcinoma: Invasive micropapillary carcinoma is a distinct histologic subtype of invasive breast cancer. The tumor cells form morular clusters and tubules suspended in empty clear spaces on hematoxylin and eosin-stained sections. The individual tumor cells show so-called reversed polarity: the luminal apical surface of the tumor cells faces the stromal tissue [28].

- **Clinical Presentation:** Although usually indistinguishable on imaging from IDC, this is an aggressive cancer. It often presents as a high-stage tumor with a palpable mass and axillary adenopathy. The IMC has a poorer prognosis than the IDC, no special type.
- **Imaging Findings:**
  - **Mammogram:** The most common presentation is an irregular, high-density mass with indistinct or spiculated margins and microcalcification (fine pleomorphic, clustered, or segmental). Axillary lymphadenopathy is frequently associated [29–31].
  - **US:** Irregular, hypoechoic mass with indistinct or spiculated margin. Enlarged axillary lymph nodes may also be observed.
  - **MRI:** Although nonspecific, this tumor may manifest as an irregular, spiculated mass or, less frequently, as non-mass-like enhancement (diffuse, clumped, or segmental), with either plateau or washout enhancement kinetics.
  - **BIRADS:** 4 or 5.
  - **Differential Diagnosis:** Benign: fat necrosis, diabetic mastopathy; Malignant: IDC or ILC.
- **Pathology Findings:**
  - **Gross:** The IMC is often a large high-stage tumor and forms a firm tan, white solid mass.
  - **Microscopic Findings:** The tumor comprises morula and tubules populated by reverse polarized cells. The carcinoma is often very cellular and intermediate to high histologic grade. The tumor is often positive for estrogen receptor and frequently positive for HER2 (up to 50%). Lymphovascular invasion is frequently identified, and local lymph nodes are positive in up to two-thirds of cases [32, 33].
  - **Differential Diagnosis:** Metastasis from non-breast primary. Adenocarcinomas in many other organs, including the gynecological tract, lung, and bladder, can show micropapillary architecture. Metastasis from non-breast primary needs to be considered and excluded.
- **Management:** Similar to that for IDC NST.

Case 1

Clinical History: A 51-year-old female with a palpable left breast lump (Figs. 4.72, 4.73, 4.74, 4.75 and 4.76).

BI-RADS: 5, highly suggestive of malignancy. Biopsy was recommended.

Pathology: Invasive ductal carcinoma with micropapillary features, poorly differentiated, with lymphovascular invasion (Figs. 4.77 and 4.78).

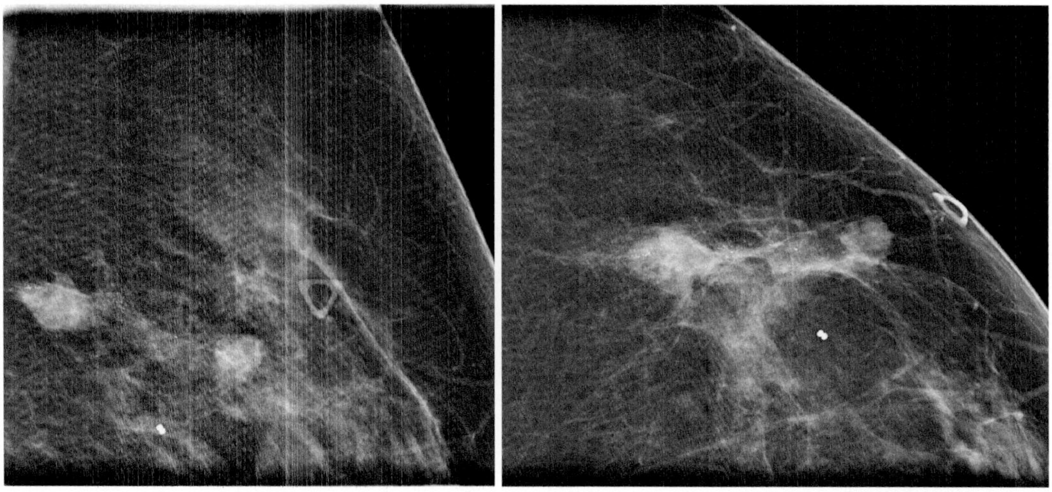

Figs. 4.72 and 4.73 **Mammographic findings**: Irregular masses with linear pleomorphic calcifications and round axillary lymph nodes

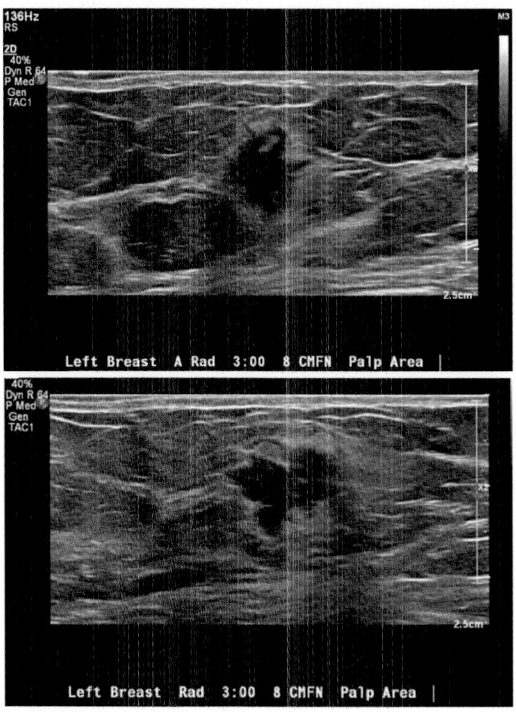

Figs. 4.74 and 4.75 **Ultrasound findings**: Hypoechoic, irregular masses with angular margins

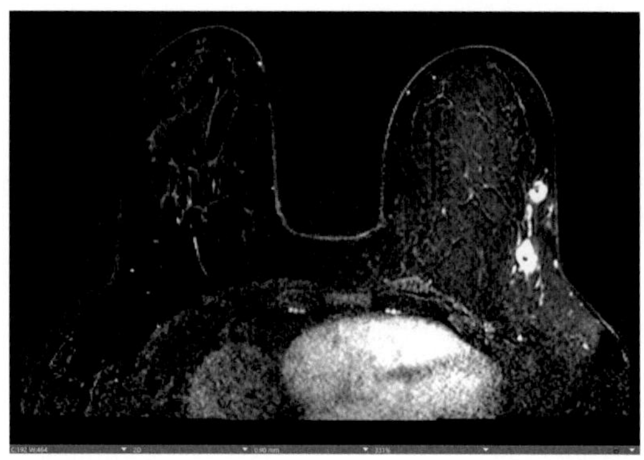

Fig. 4.76 **MRI findings**: Irregular enhancing masses without washout, delayed phase kinetics, associated linear non-mass enhancement, and suspicious calcifications

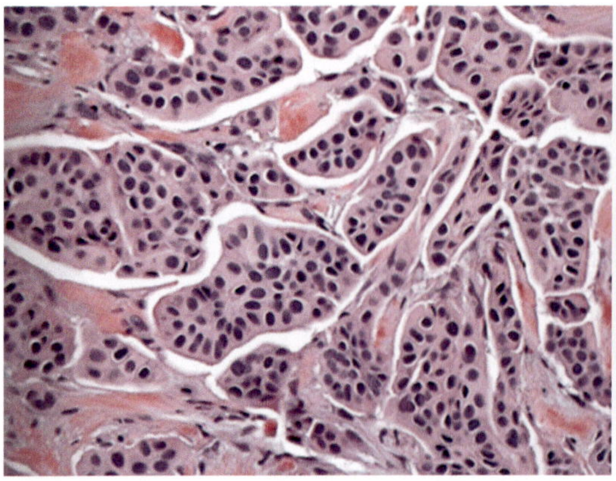

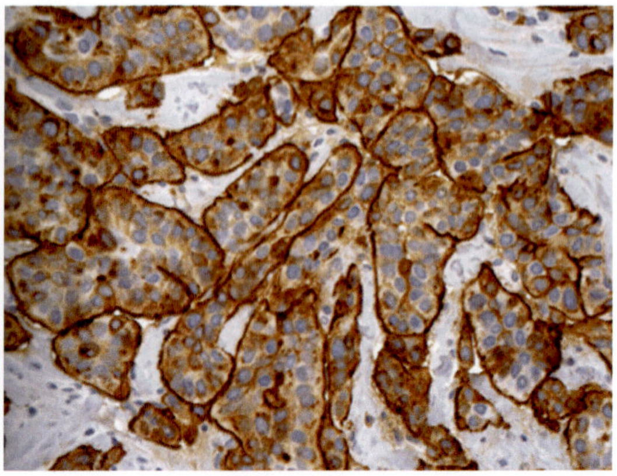

Figs. 4.77 and 4.78 IMC (H&E 20× and EMA IHC) comprises of micropapillary fronds, tubules and morulae of tumor cells floating in empty spaces. The epithelial membrane antigen IHC highlights the outward-facing luminal border of the tumor cells confirming the reverse polarity

Other Cases

Several other disease entities can present with indistinct margins. This section provides examples of metastasis, granulomatous mastitis, and myofibroblastoma with indistinct margins.

Metastasis to Breast

Clinical History: A 71-year-old female with a history of high-grade serous carcinoma (Figs. 4.79, 4.80, 4.81 and 4.82).

BI-RADS: 5. Biopsy was recommended.

Pathology: Metastatic high-grade serous carcinoma (Figs. 4.83 and 4.84).

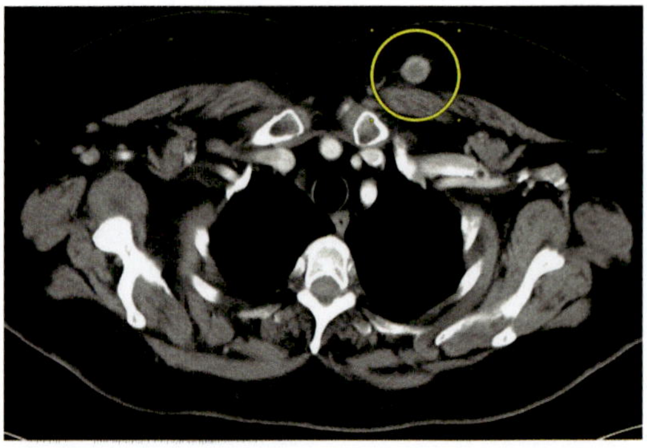

Fig. 4.79 Left upper breast lesion on surveillance CT

Granulomatous Mastitis

Clinical History: A 42-year-old female presents with a painful palpable left breast mass for 1 week (Figs. 4.85, 4.86, 4.87 and 4.88).

BI-RADS: 5, suspected of malignancy. Biopsy was recommended.

Pathology: Granulomatous lobular mastitis (Figs. 4.89, 4.90 and 4.91).

Myofibroblastoma

Clinical History: A 56-year-old female was recalled from screening (Figs. 4.92, 4.93, 4.94, 4.95 and 4.96).

Ultrasound findings: The mass was not seen on targeted ultrasound.

BI-RADS: 4. Biopsy was recommended.

Pathology: Myofibroblastoma.

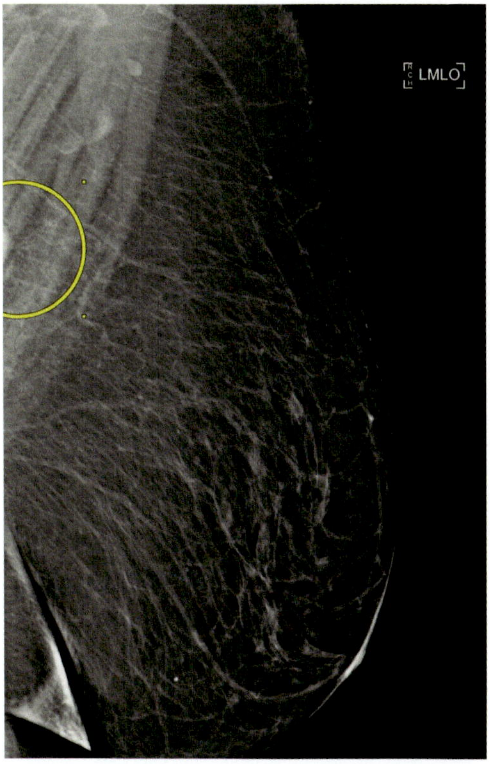

Fig. 4.80 **Mammographic findings**: Not well visualized on mammography as the mass is far too medial and superior

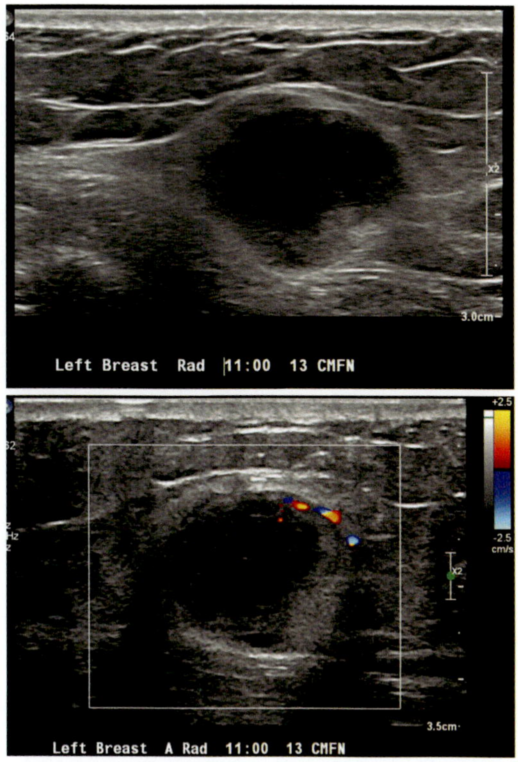

Figs. 4.81 and 4.82 **Ultrasound findings**: Hypoechoic irregular mass with an indistinct margin and echogenic boundaries

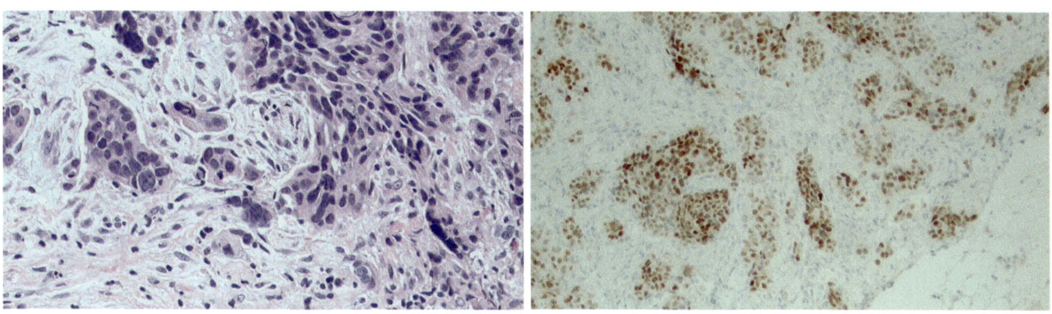

Figs. 4.83 and 4.84 Adenocarcinoma (H&E, 20× and PAX8 IHC) with micropapillary clusters of high-grade carcinoma cells. By immunohistochemistry, the tumor cells are positive for the Mullerian marker PAX8

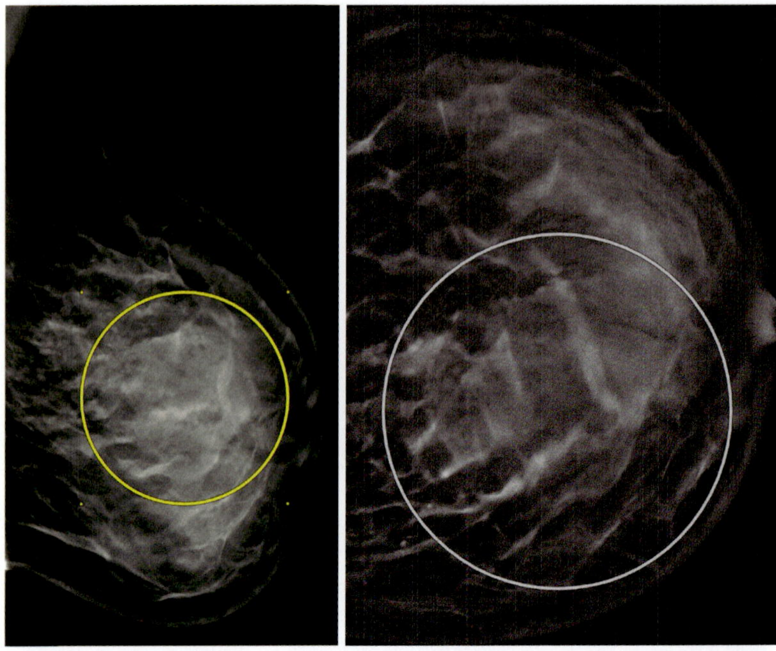

Figs. 4.85 and 4.86 Mammographic findings: New asymmetry in the left breast

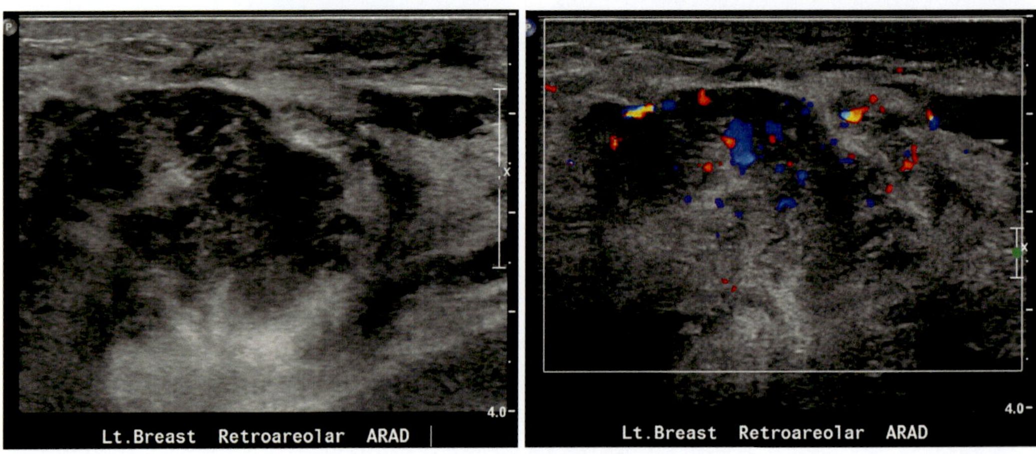

Figs. 4.87 and 4.88 Ultrasound findings: Irregular mass with mixed echogenicity correlates with the palpable lump

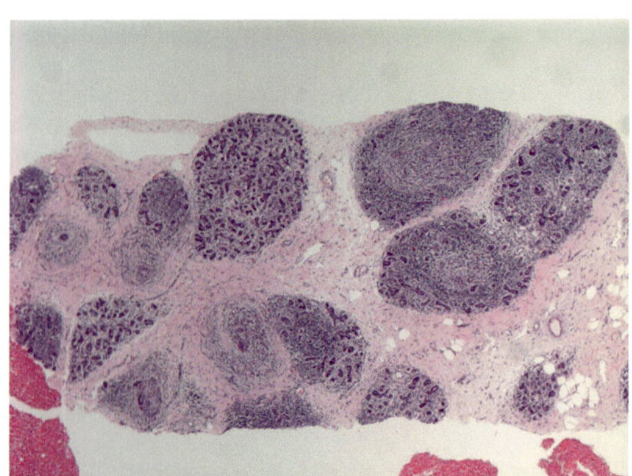

Fig. 4.89 (H&E, 4×) Cystic neutrophilic granulomatous mastitis (CNGM). There is lobulocentric acute and chronic inflammation. Non-necrotizing granulomas are present. Round empty spaces with a ring of neutrophils are present. These features have been described in mastitis associated with *Corynebacterium* species, and histological features are labeled as cystic neutrophilic granulomatous mastitis (CNGM)

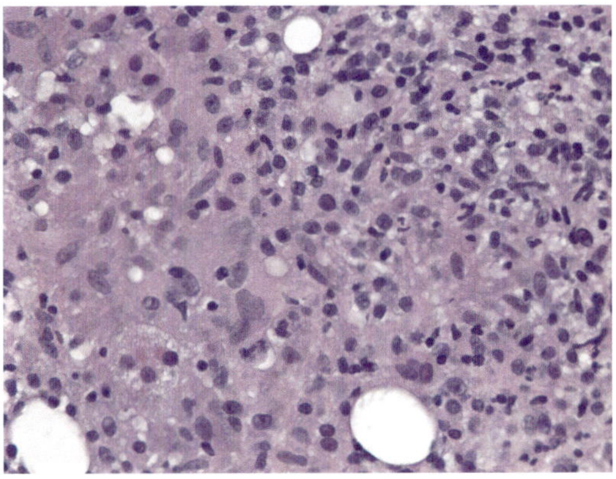

Fig. 4.90 (H&E, 40×)

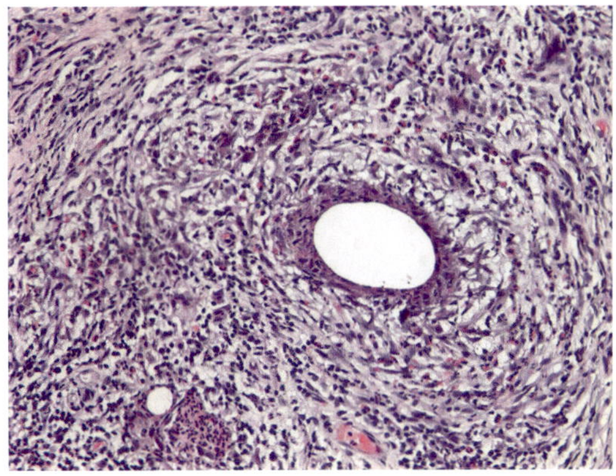

Fig. 4.91 (H&E, 20×)

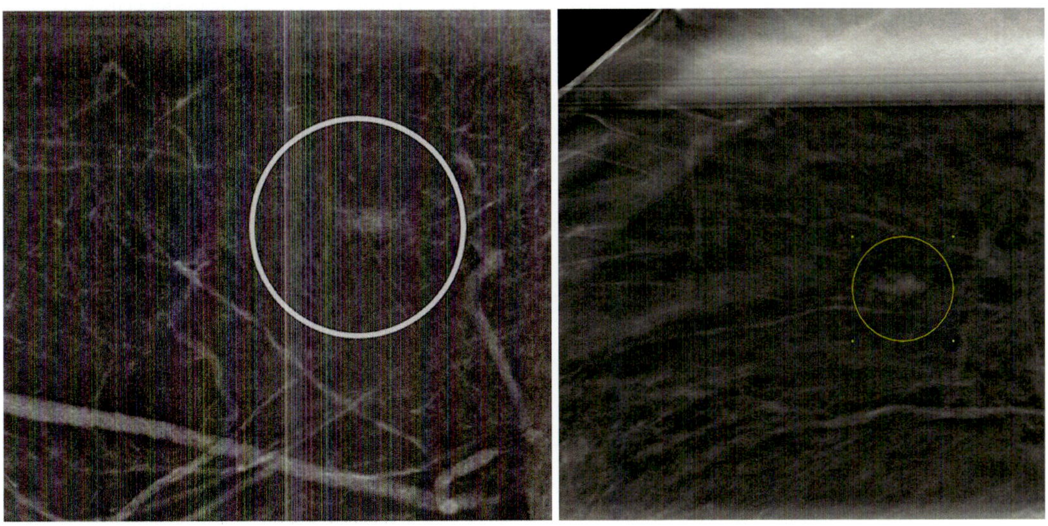

Figs. 4.92 and 4.93 **Mammographic findings**: Irregular focal asymmetry seen on multiple views

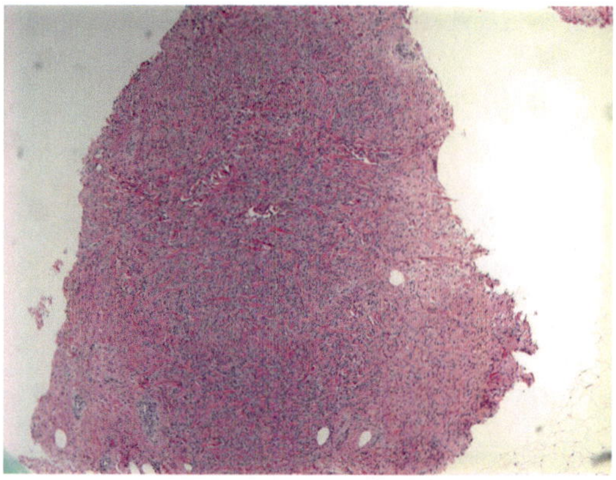

Fig. 4.94 (H&E, 4×) Myofibroblastoma. The tumor comprises bland-appearing myofibroblastic spindle cells separated by fibrous tissue

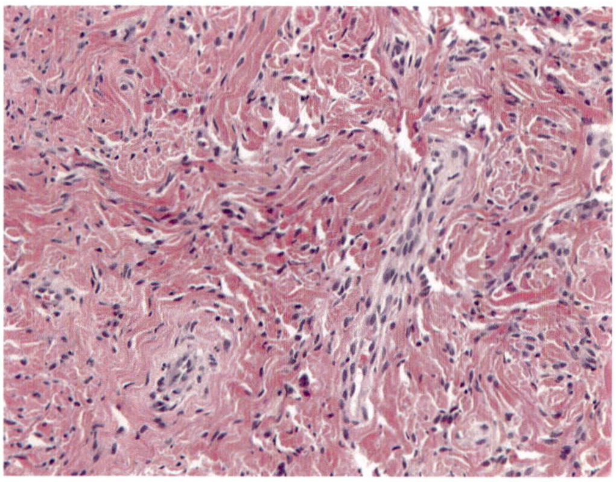

Fig. 4.95 (H&E, 20×) Myofibroblastoma. The tumor comprises of homogenous moderately cellular spindle cell lesion. The lesional cells show oval to elongated nuclei, seperated by dense fibrous tissue

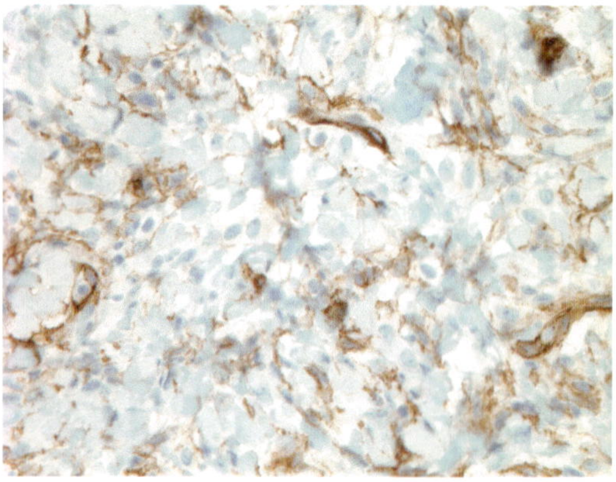

Fig. 4.96 (CD34 IHC 20×) Myofibroblastoma. Most mammary myofibroblastoma are CD34 positive by immunohistochemistry

References

1. Tan PH, Lai LM, Carrington EV, Opaluwa AS, Ravikumar KH, Chetty N, Kaplan V, Kelley CJ, Babu ED. Fat necrosis of the breast—a review. Breast. 2006;15(3):313–8. https://doi.org/10.1016/j.breast.2005.07.003. Epub 2005 Sep 29

Fat Necrosis

2. Miyake KK, Ikeda DM. Mammographic and ultrasound analysis of breast masses. In: Ikeda DM, Miyake KK, editors. Breast imaging: the requisites. 3rd ed. St. Louis, Missouri: Elsevier; 2016. p. 122–70.
3. Raza S, Goldkamp AL, Chikarmane SA, Birdwell RL, et al. US of breast masses categorized as BI-RADS 3, 4, and 5: pictorial review of factors influencing clinical management. Radiographics. 2010;30(5):1199–213. https://doi.org/10.1148/rg.305095144.
4. Mario J, Venkataraman S, Dialani V, Slanetz P. Benign breast lesions that mimic cancer: determining radiologic-pathologic concordance. Appl Radiol. 2015;44(9):28–32.
5. Vasei N, Shishegar A, Ghalkhani F, Darvishi M. Fat necrosis in the breast: a systematic review of clinical. Lipids Health Dis. 2019;18:139. https://doi.org/10.1186/s12944-019-1078-4.
6. Lee J, Park HY, Kim WW, et al. Natural course of fat necrosis after breast reconstruction: a 10-year follow-up study. BMC Cancer. 2021;21:166. https://doi.org/10.1186/s12885-021-07881-x.
7. Taboada JL, Stephens TW, Krishnamurthy S, Brandt KR, Whitman GJ. The many faces of fat necrosis in the breast. AJR. 2009;192(3):815–25. https://doi.org/10.2214/AJR.08.1250.

Abscess

8. Kasales CJ, et al. Nonpuerperal mastitis and subareolar abscess of the breast. AJR. 2014;202(2):W133–9. https://doi.org/10.2214/AJR.13.10551.
9. Adrada B, Wu Y, Yang W. Hyperechoic lesions of the breast: radiologic-histopathologic correlation. AJR. 2013;200(5):W518–30. https://doi.org/10.2214/AJR.12.9263.
10. Fu P, et al. High-resolution MRI in detecting subareolar breast abscess. AJR. 2007;188(6):1568–72. https://doi.org/10.2214/AJR.06.0099.
11. Mahoney MC, Ingram AD. Breast emergencies: types, imaging features, and management. AJR. 2014;202(4):W390–9. https://doi.org/10.2214/AJR.13.11758.
12. Kaneda HJ, Mack J, Kasales CJ, Schetter S. Pediatric and adolescent breast masses: a review of pathophysiology, imaging, diagnosis, and treatment. AJR.

2013;200(2):W204–12. https://doi.org/10.2214/AJR.12.9560.
13. Toomey A, Le JK. Breast abscess. [updated 2021 Dec 16]. In: StatPearls [internet]. Treasure Island (FL): StatPearls Publishing; 2022. Available from: https://www.ncbi.nlm.nih.gov/books/NBK459122/.
14. Snider HC. Management of Mastitis, abscess, and fistula. Surg Clin North Am. 2022;102(6):1103–16. https://doi.org/10.1016/j.suc.2022.06.007.

PASH

15. Speer ME, Yoon EC, Berg WA, Chang Sen LQ. Pseudoangiomatous stromal hyperplasia: radiologic-pathologic correlation. J Breast Imaging. 2022;5(1):67–72. https://doi.org/10.1093/jbi/wbac051. PMID: 36778653; PMCID: PMC9901424
16. Jones KN, Glazebrook KN, Reynolds C. Pseudoangiomatous stromal hyperplasia: imaging findings with pathologic and clinical correlation. AJR. 2010;195(4):1036–42. https://doi.org/10.2214/AJR.09.3284.
17. Polger MR, Denison CM, Lester S, Meyer JE. Pseudoangiomatous stromal hyperplasia: mammographic and sonographic appearances. AJR. 1996;166(2):349–52. https://doi.org/10.2214/ajr.166.2.8553945.
18. Raza R, Fatima K, Tariq MU. Breast imaging chameleon: Pseudoangiomatous stromal hyperplasia presenting as breast malignancy. Cureus. 2020;12(5):e8359. https://doi.org/10.7759/cureus.8359.
19. Taliaferro AS, et al. Imaging features of spindle cell breast lesions. AJR. 2017;209(2):454–64. https://doi.org/10.2214/AJR.16.17610.

Breast Cancer

20. Heaphy CM, Griffith JK, Bisoffi M. Mammary field cancerization: molecular evidence and clinical importance. Breast Cancer Res Treat. 2009;118:229–39. https://doi.org/10.1007/s10549-009-0504-0.
21. Lam WWM, Chu WCW, Tse GM, Ma TK. Sonographic appearance of mucinous carcinoma of the breast. AJR. 2004;182(4):1069–74. https://doi.org/10.2214/ajr.182.4.1821069.
22. Kawashima M, et al. MR imaging of mucinous carcinoma of the breast. AJR. 2002;179(1):179–83. https://doi.org/10.2214/ajr.179.1.1790179.
23. Wison TE, Helvie MA, Oberman HA, Joynt LK. Pure and mixed mucinous carcinoma of the breast: pathologic basis for differences in mammographic appearance. AJR. 1995;165(2):285–9. https://doi.org/10.2214/ajr.165.2.7618541.
24. Matsuda M, Yoshimoto M, Iwase T, et al. Mammographic and clinicopathological features of mucinous carcinoma of the breast. Breast Cancer. 2000;2000(7):65–70. https://doi.org/10.1007/BF02967190.
25. Reed AEM, et al. Invasive lobular carcinoma of the breast: morphology, biomarkers and 'omics. Breast Cancer Res. 2015;17:12. https://doi.org/10.1186/s13058-015-0519-x.
26. van Bommel RMG, et al. Incidence and tumour characteristics of bilateral and unilateral interval breast cancers at screening mammography. Breast. 2018;38:101–6. https://doi.org/10.1016/j.breast.2017.12.018.
27. Winston CB, et al. Metastatic lobular carcinoma of the breast. AJR. 2000;175(3):795–800. https://doi.org/10.2214/ajr.175.3.1750795.

Papillary/Micropapillary

28. Yang YL, Liu BB, Zhang X, Fu L. Invasive micropapillary carcinoma of the breast: an update. Arch Pathol Lab Med. 2016;140(8):799–805. https://doi.org/10.5858/arpa.2016-0040-RA.
29. Adrada B, Arribas E, Gilcrease M, Yang WT. Invasive micropapillary carcinoma of the breast: mammographic, sonographic, and MRI features. AJR. 2009;193(1):W58–63. https://doi.org/10.2214/AJR.08.1537.
30. Yun SE, et al. Imaging findings of invasive micropapillary carcinoma of the breast. J Breast Cancer. 2012;15(1):57–64. https://doi.org/10.4048/jbc.2012.15.1.57.
31. Rhee SJ, Han BK, Ko EY, Shin JH. Invasive micropapillary carcinoma of the breast: mammographic, sonographic and MR imaging findings. JKSMRM. 2012;16(3):205–16.
32. Hao S, Zhao YY, Peng JJ, et al. Invasive micropapillary carcinoma of the breast had no difference in prognosis compared with invasive ductal carcinoma: a propensity-matched analysis. Sci Rep. 2019;9:286. https://doi.org/10.1038/s41598-018-36362-8.
33. Lewis GD, Xing Y, Haque W, et al. Prognosis of lymphotropic invasive micropapillary breast carcinoma analyzed by using data from the National Cancer Database. Cancer Commun. 2019;39:60. https://doi.org/10.1186/s40880-019-0406-4.

5 Spiculated Masses

Malini Harigopal, Liva Andrejeva, Sonali Lanjewar, and Peter Podany

Benign

Radial Scar

See Chap. 7.

Postsurgical Scar

See Chap. 7.

Infection (Abscess)

See Chap. 2.

Fat Necrosis

Fat Necrosis: Fat necrosis develops in response to breast tissue injury related to either prior trauma or surgery. Because of its protean manifestations, it has sometimes been described as "the great mimicker" [3].

- **Clinical Presentation**: The patient may present for diagnostic mammography and/or ultrasound with a palpable mass and may recall an episode of trauma to the breast. When a clinical history of trauma in the region of suspected fat necrosis is available, the imaging findings can often be safely monitored with short-term follow-up studies. However, when imaging findings are highly suspicious or in the absence of supporting clinical history, biopsy may be required.
- **Imaging Findings**:
  - **Mammography**: The typical mammographic appearance of fat necrosis is a lucent mass with dystrophic or rim calcifications. This finding may be associated with architectural distortion in the surrounding tissue (Figs. 5.1).

    When such pathognomonic findings are seen in conjunction with a clinical history of surgery or trauma, routine follow-up can be resumed.

    The appearance of fat necrosis is variable and may overlap with malignancy

M. Harigopal · P. Podany
Department of Pathology, Yale University, New Haven, CT, USA
e-mail: malini.harigopal@yale.edu; peter.podany@yale.edu

L. Andrejeva (✉)
Department of Radiology and Biomedical Imaging, Yale School of Medicine, New Haven, CT, USA
e-mail: liva.andrejeva@yale.edu

S. Lanjewar
Department of Pathology, University of Chicago, Chicago, IL, USA

M. Harigopal et al. (eds.), *Radiology Pathology Correlations of Breast Lesions*,
https://doi.org/10.1007/978-3-031-65711-5_5

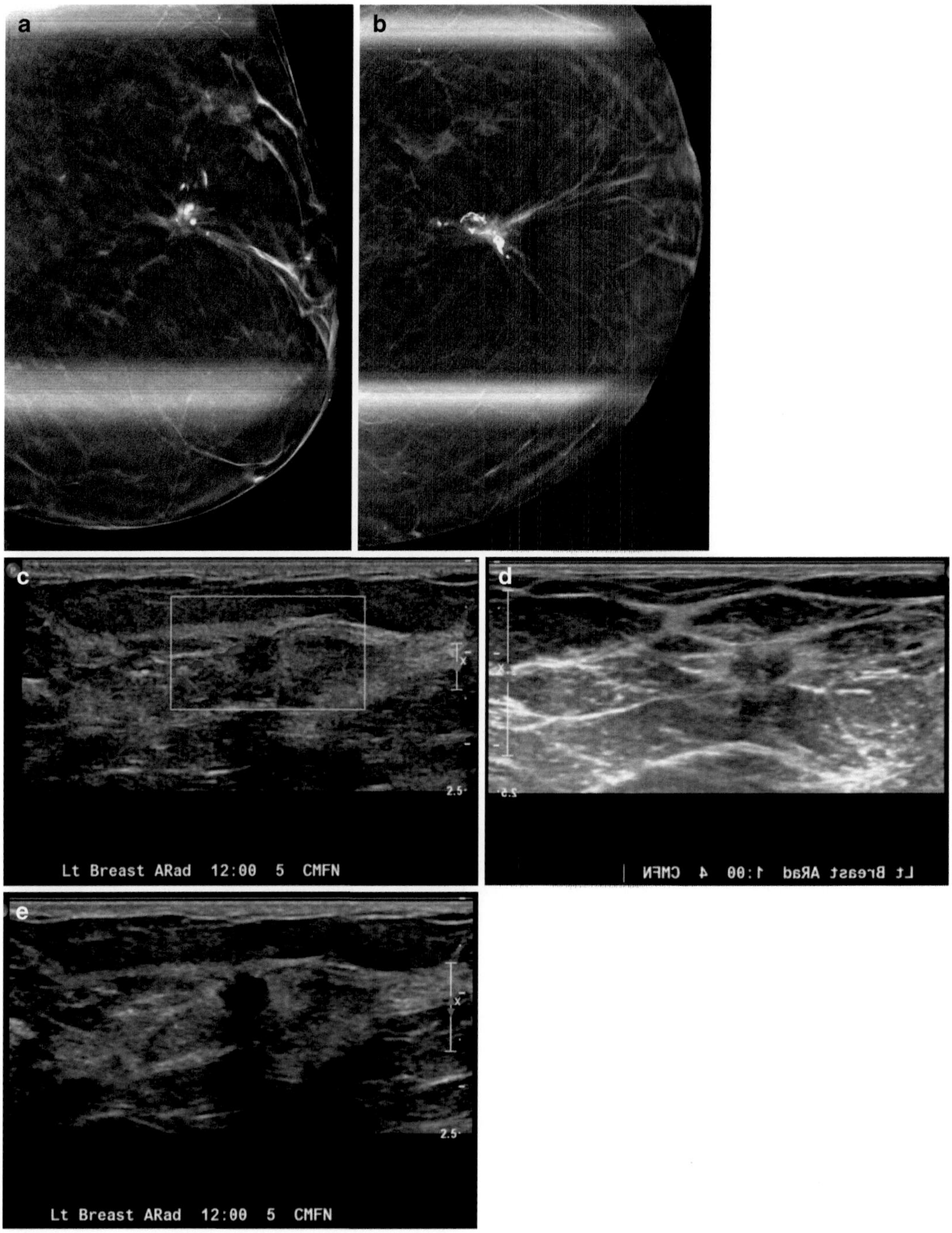

Fig. 5.1 A 46-year-old female with history of left breast cancer, status post lumpectomy and radiation 12 years ago presents for follow up. She was found to have two new spiculated masses in her left breast, near the lumpectomy site. On mammogram (**a**, **b**) there are two isodense, spiculated masses in the upper outer quadrant, near the lumpectomy site. Ultrasound (**c**, **d**, **e**) shows two adjacent, hypoechoic irregular masses with spiculated margins, one with adjacent vascularity which corresponds to the mammographic findings. The findings were considered BI-RADS 4, suspicious findings. An US-guided biopsy of the more suspicious of the two lesions (the one with adjacent vascularity) was recommended. This yielded fat necrosis

and biopsy may be required to confirm the diagnosis.

- **US**: The most common sonographic appearance of fat necrosis is a heterogeneous mass, often containing both hyperechoic and cystic components.

  In cases of fat necrosis presenting only with architectural distortion on mammography, ultrasound may show an area of shadowing without a definable mass.
- **MRI**: As with mammography and ultrasound, the MRI appearance of fat necrosis is variable and includes both mass and non-mass enhancement.

  A pre-contrast, nonfat suppressed T1-weighted sequence may be helpful in confirming signal intensity consistent with fat within the lesion of interest.
- **BI-RADS**: 2, 3, 4, or 5, depending on clinical history and imaging features.
- **Differential Diagnosis**: Invasive ductal carcinoma, invasive lobular carcinoma, radial scar/complex sclerosing lesion.

- **Pathology Findings**:
  - **Microscopic Histology**: Needle core biopsy shows infarction of fat cells and hemorrhage initially followed by histiocytes along with foreign body material and multinucleated giant cells depending on the etiology, along with a variable infiltrate of plasma cells, lymphocytes, and eosinophils [4] (Figs. 5.2).

    As the lesion evolves with cavitation of fat, fibrosis is evident around the focus of fat necrosis with scar formation and calcifications [4].

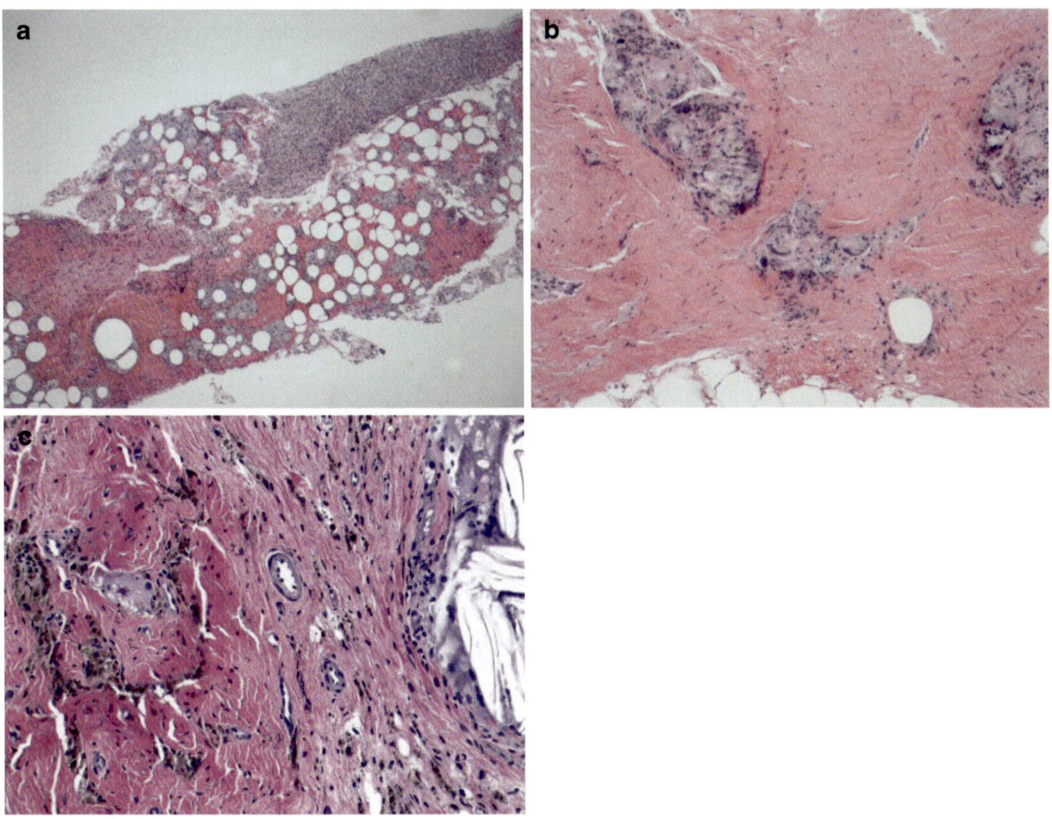

Fig. 5.2 A 1.1-cm hypoechoic right breast mass in a 64-year-old female with a question of fat necrosis. Ultrasound was performed, and the lesion was called probably benign/BIRADS 3. Five cores were collected from the right breast 12 o'clock position demonstrating fat necrosis (**a**, **b**). On higher power we can see hemosiderin laden macrophages and cholesterol clefts associated with the fat necrosis (**c**)

Surrounding ducts and lobules may develop squamous metaplasia [4].

Even in older lesions, a few histiocytes persist and may be highlighted by CD68.

Additional deeper H&E levels may be useful for definitive diagnosis in clinically and mammographically concerning lesions.

- **Differential Diagnosis**: Cystically dilated ducts, duct ectasia, granulomatous inflammation.
- **Management**: Fat necrosis can be managed by observation when concordant with imaging findings. Due to the relatively rapid evolution of fat necrosis, the patient may be asked to return in as little as 6 weeks for repeat imaging to confirm that the area is changing as would be expected for fat necrosis.

  Smaller areas of fat necrosis may resolve completely.

  Larger areas will gradually become more cystic and assume the typical oil cyst appearance on mammography.

  At times, fat necrosis may be indistinguishable from malignant lesions, such as breast cancers, particularly in patients who have been treated for breast cancer in the past. In such cases, a needle biopsy may be necessary and can be virtually diagnostic of fat necrosis.

  Excision is usually not indicated and may result in additional fat necrosis.

Diabetic Mastopathy

Diabetic Mastopathy: Diabetic mastopathy is a mass forming fibrous proliferation of breast characteristically occurring in patients with diabetes mellitus, autoimmune, and endocrine disorders. Long standing diabetic mellitus results in glycosylation of collagen, accumulation of advanced glycosylation products and incites a B-cell autoimmune lymphocytic response, cytokine release and matrix expansion giving the characteristic histologic appearance [5–7]. Changes of diabetic mastopathy can occasionally be found in patients with no evidence of autoimmune disorder or diabetes mellitus [6, 8]. Radiographic examination may show variable appearances raising concern of malignancy in some cases.

- **Clinical Presentation**: Diabetic mastopathy refers to tumor forming stromal proliferations occurring in patients with insulin-dependent diabetes, type 2 diabetes, and other autoimmune thyroid diseases [9]. Diabetic mastopathy typically occurs in women from the second to fourth decade of life and rarely can be seen in men [5–8]. Patients present with a non-painful palpable mass, which could be unifocal, multifocal, or may present with diffuse nodularity. It can affect unilateral or bilateral breasts [10]. On imaging, diabetic mastopathy is difficult to distinguish from a malignancy, and even though history of diabetes may suggest this diagnosis, a biopsy is usually needed to confirm benignity. This process is caused by perivascular lymphocytic infiltrates surrounding lobules, ducts, and vascular structures. On imaging diabetic mastitis can mimic carcinoma. The stromal changes are thought to occur as a result of increased resistance to normal degradation [6].
- **Imaging Findings**:
  - **Mammography**: Mammographically can present as a hyperdense spiculated mass or can be obscured by dense tissue (Fig. 5.3).
  - **US**: On US it can be seen as an irregular hypoechoic mass with posterior shadowing [11].

    A coexistent carcinoma may be obscured which can be detected by MRI.
  - **BI-RADS**: 4 or 5; biopsy is usually warranted as cannot be distinguished from malignancy.
  - **Differential Diagnosis**: Benign: stromal fibrosis, fibromatosis, PASH; Malignant: IDC, ILC.
- **Pathology Findings**:
  - **Gross**: Dense white mass with circumscribed or ill-defined margins [12].
  - **Microscopic Histology**: Diabetic mastopathy is characterized by stromal fibrosis, periductular, peri-lobular and perivascular

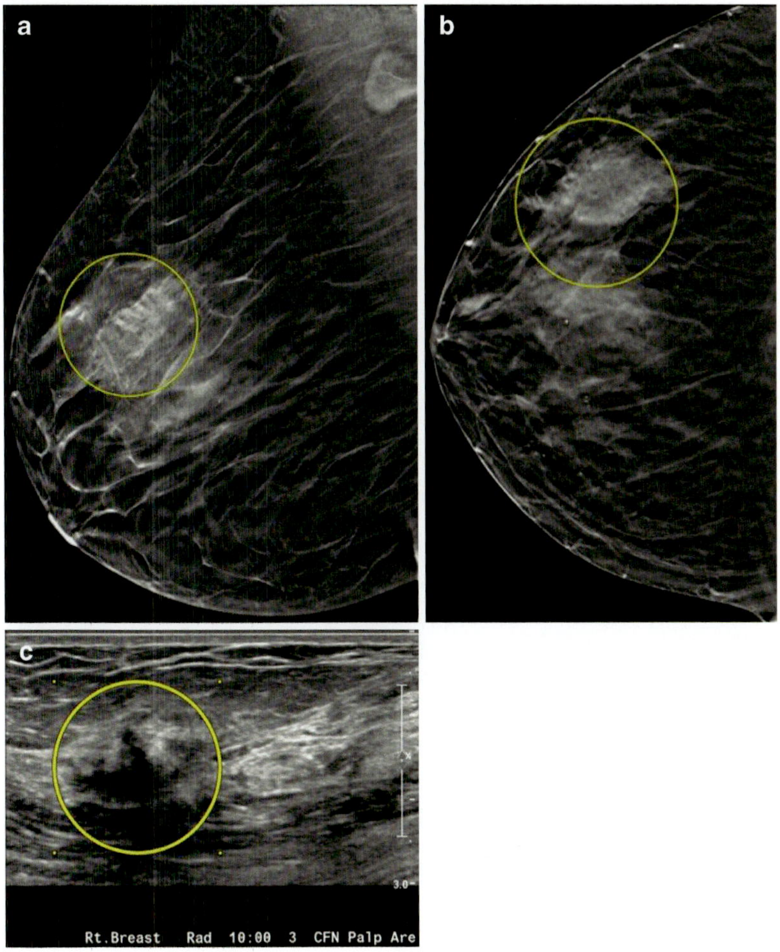

Fig. 5.3 A 59-year-old female, status post left breast lumpectomy many years ago, with long standing IDDM, presents with a palpable mass in the right breast. On mammography (**a**, **b**) there was an irregular focal asymmetry in the upper outer quadrant of the right breast. Ultrasound (**c**) showed an irregular, spiculated hypoechoic mass that correlates as palpated to the mammographic asymmetry. The mass was considered BI-RADS 4, suspicious finding. An ultrasound-guided biopsy was recommended and performed, revealing diabetic mastopathy. On follow-up the biopsy result was deemed concordant, and a 6-month follow-up right diagnostic mammogram and US were recommended. However, the patient did not return until 2 years later, when she experienced pain in her right breast. At this time, a diagnostic mammogram and US were again performed. Mammogram now showed an irregular, spiculated mass in the right breast, 9 o'clock position (**d**, **e**), and an irregular focal asymmetry is demonstrated in the right breast, 12 o'clock position (**g**, **h**). In addition, a markedly enlarged lymph node is demonstrated in the right axilla. On ultrasound there was an irregular, hypoechoic mass with an angular to spiculated margin at the 9 o'clock position (**f**), and an irregular, hypoechoic mass with an angular to spiculated margin at the 12 o'clock position (**i**). A markedly enlarged right axillary lymph node is also seen on US. At this time the mass was still considered BI-RADS 4, suspicious of malignancy. An US-guided biopsy was recommended and performed for both findings. The 12 o'clock mass yielded diabetic mastopathy, and the 9 o'clock mass yielded a poorly differentiated IDC. The right axillary lymph node biopsy revealed metastatic carcinoma similar to the breast primary. The patient was treated with neoadjuvant chemotherapy and underwent a modified radical mastectomy and axillary lymph node dissection, yielding multifocal residual poorly differentiated IDC and 6 out of 11 axillary lymph nodes positive for metastatic breast cancer

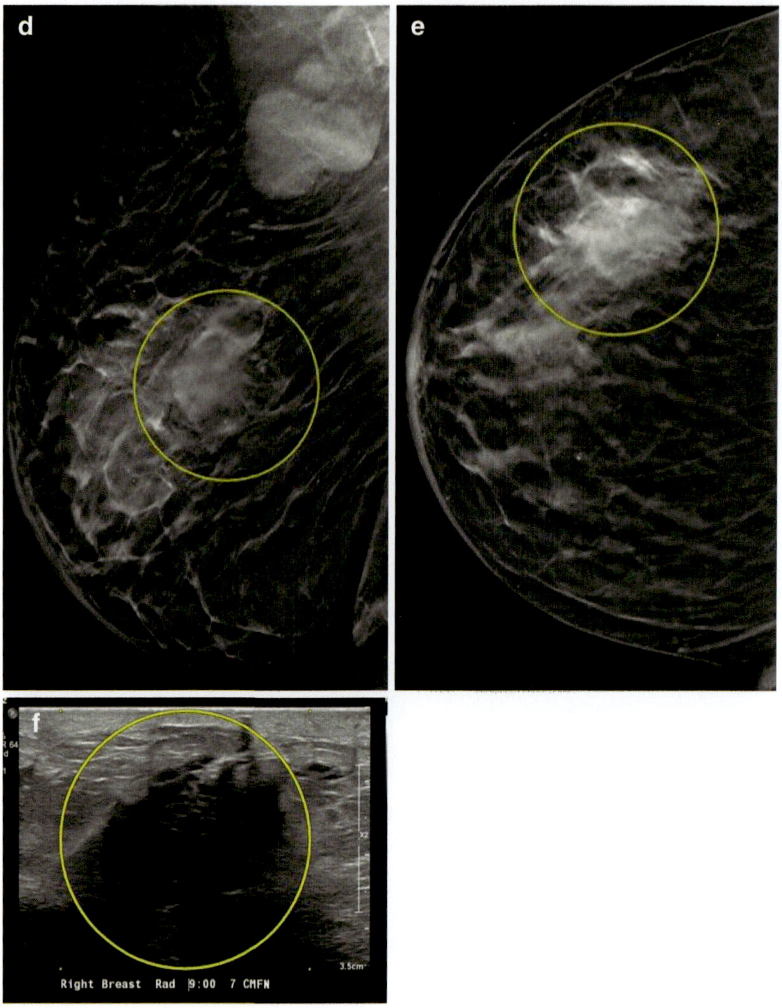

Fig. 5.3 (continued)

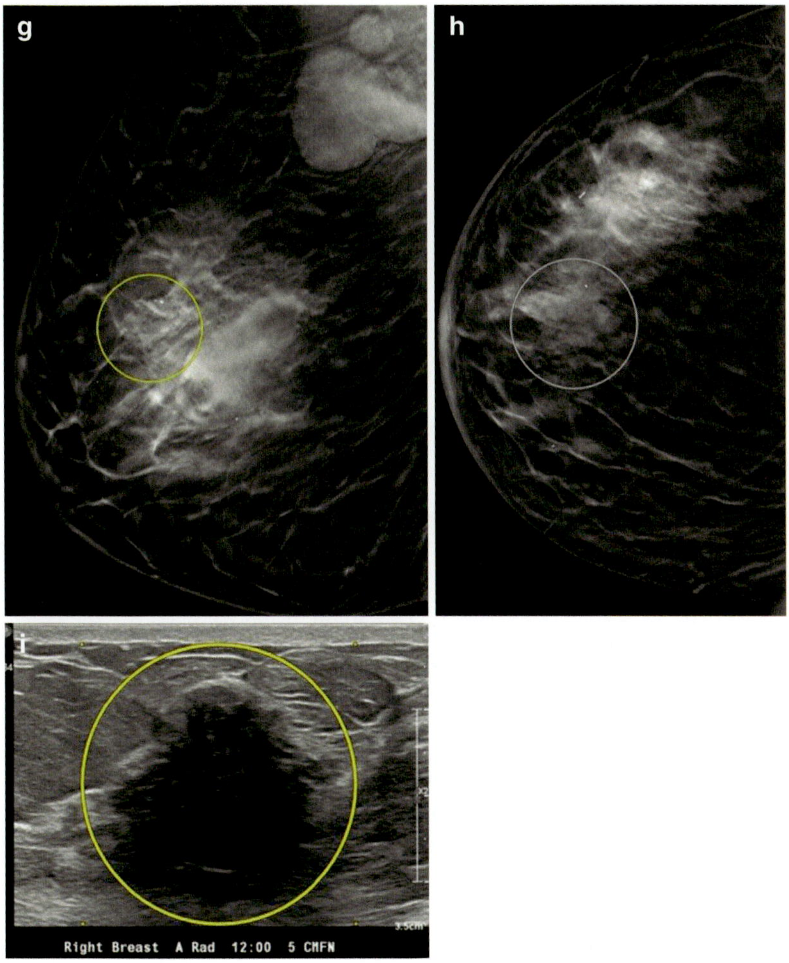

Fig. 5.3 (continued)

lymphocytic infiltrates, lobular atrophy, and epithelioid stromal fibroblasts (Fig. 5.4).

The fibrous stroma is dense keloidal and has a glassy appearance. The epithelioid stromal fibroblasts are plump with round to ovoid vesicular nuclei and abundant eosinophilic cytoplasm.

Lymphoid aggregates are composed mostly of mature B lymphocytes and are prominent around ducts, lobules, and vessels. Germinal centers are usually not present [10, 13].

– **Differential Diagnosis**: Invasive carcinoma, granular cell tumor, lymphoma, IgG4-related sclerosing mastitis, T-cell lymphocytic lobulitis, fibrous nodules.

Invasive Carcinoma: The palpable nature of the lesion and presence of epithelioid fibroblasts can mimic an invasive carcinoma. Keratin immunostaining can be performed to rule out a malignant process.

Granular Cell Tumor: Due to abundant eosinophilic cytoplasm in epithelioid stromal fibroblasts, these cells can be confused with granular cell tumors and immunostaining for S100 and CD68 can help to rule out granular cell tumor.

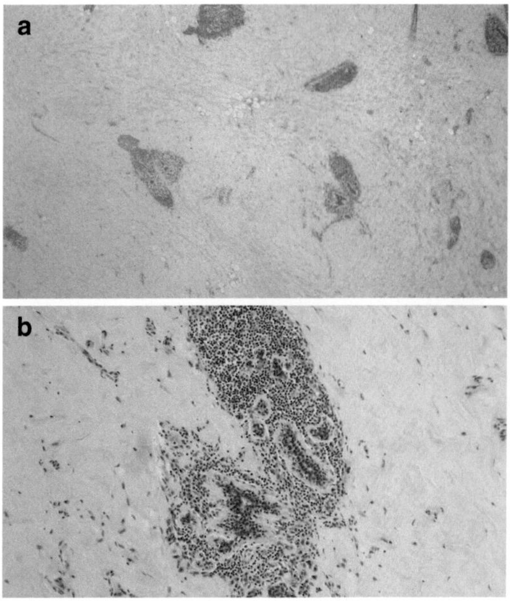

Fig. 5.4 Surgical resection specimen demonstrating diabetic mastopathy with a perilobular lymphocytic infiltration (**a**, **b**)

Lymphoma: Lymphoid infiltrate may raise suspicion for lymphoma. Neoplastic lymphoma cells may surround glands and vessels but characteristically show diffuse involvement of glands and stroma. Their monoclonality can be established by immunostaining and molecular studies. The stroma is usually of normal appearance.

IgG4-Related Sclerosing Mastitis: These present with multiple, bilateral masses composed of dense lymphoplasmacytic infiltrate with prominent germinal centers. Plasma cells are predominantly IgG4+. They have sclerotic stroma with the presence of ducts and lobules in the periphery.

T-Cell Lymphocytic Lobulitis: Represents a non-mass forming lesion, showing aggregates of lymphocytes surrounding normal appearing lobules. Seen incidentally in prophylactic mastectomies in high-risk women.

Fibrous Nodules: Comprised of a proliferation of interlobular fibroblasts, lacks lymphocytic infiltrates, and plump epithelioid fibroblasts.

- **Management**: Diabetic mastopathy is a benign disease with no increased risk of carcinoma and/or lymphoma [7, 13, 14]. Unless there is a clinical suspicion of malignancy, surgical excision is not recommended.

Granular Cell Tumor

Granular Cell Tumor: Accounts for about 5% of tumors that originate in the breast [15]. Granular cell tumors (GCTs) are rare, usually benign, and arise from peripheral nerve schwann cells in patients ranging from 17 to 75 years old [15]. GCTs are somewhat more common in African American patients and 10% of the patients diagnosed are male. It is associated with Bannyan-Ruvalcaba-Riley, NF type 1, and LEOPARD syndromes [15]. GCT mimics breast cancer as it presents as a firm, painless mass with focal skin or nipple retraction, may involve the underlying pectoralis, and is more common in the upper inner quadrant of the breast. GCT

- **Clinical Presentation**: Patients present with a palpable, solitary, firm or hard, painless mass which is usually located in the upper and medial quadrants of the breast [15]. Prognosis is good except in the rare malignant cases which can metastasize to distant sites [15].
- **Imaging Findings**:
  - **Mammography**: Difficult to distinguish from carcinoma as they form a stellate mass without calcifications [15] (Fig. 5.5).

    They can also present as circumscribed lobulated masses.

    Multiple tumors may be present.

    Calcifications are generally not present [15, 16].

    Occasionally may have focal skin retraction.

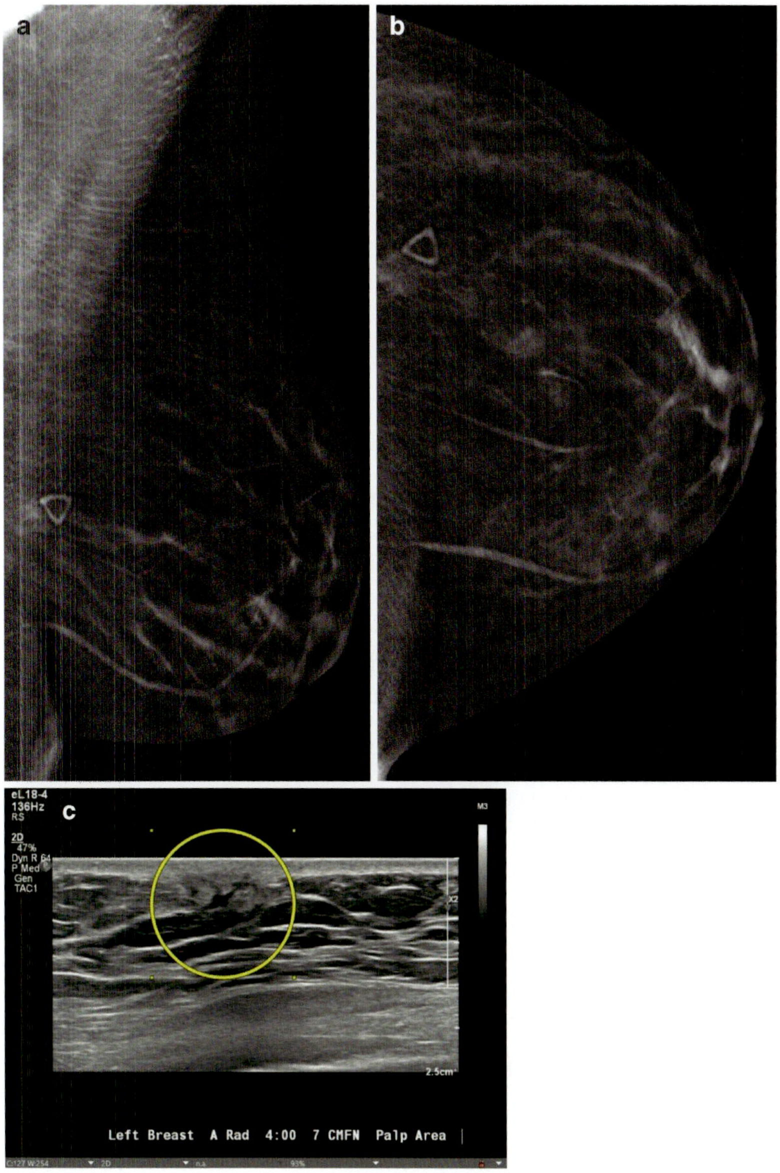

Fig. 5.5 A 46-year-old white female presented with a small, superficial palpable mass in the lower outer aspect of the left breast, near the inframammary fold. Mammography (**a**, **b**) revealed an irregular, spiculated mass in the lower outer quadrant of the left breast. Ultrasound (**c**) showed a heterogeneous, irregular mass with an indistinct margin without demonstrable vascularity involving the skin. The mass was graded as BI-RADS 4, suspicious of malignancy. An ultrasound-guided biopsy was recommended and performed, yielding a granular cell tumor. A subsequent surgical excision also demonstrated a granular cell tumor

  - **US**: Irregular, hypoechoic mass with a spiculated margin.
  - **BI-RADS**: 4 or 5, as GCT is indistinguishable from breast cancer.
  - **Differential Diagnosis**: Fibromatosis, tubular carcinoma, IDC, ILC.
- **Pathology Findings**:
  - **Microscopic Histology**: On microscopic examination the tumor is composed of sheets and nests of round to polygonal or spindle-shaped tumor cells in collagenous breast stroma [17] (Fig. 5.6).
    - Infiltration into adjacent fat and stroma gives the tumor a spiculated margin.
    - The tumor cells are characterized by abundant granular eosinophilic cytoplasm.
      - The granules stain positive for PAS (periodic acid-Schiff) and are diastase resistant [17].

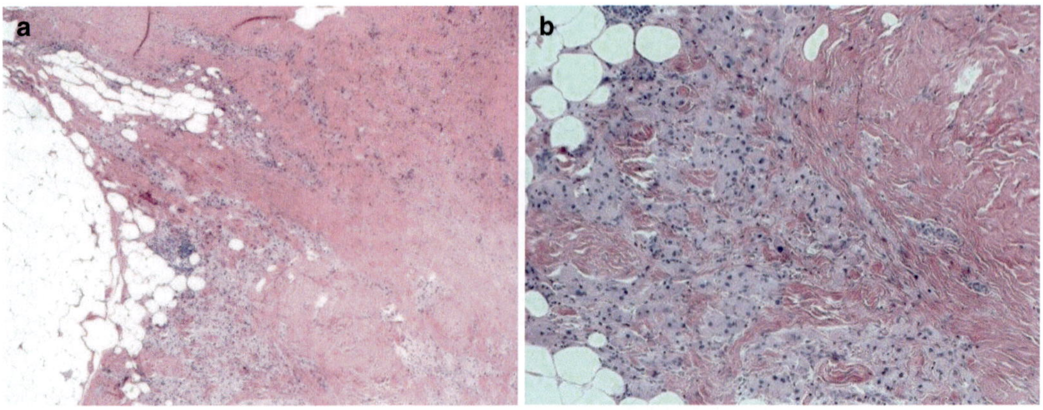

Fig. 5.6 A partial mastectomy specimen from a 56-year-old woman demonstrating a 0.6-cm granular cell tumor (**a**, **b**) composed of nests of polygonal to spindle shaped tumor cells with abundant granular cytoplasm and uniform round to oval nuclei infiltrating through the breast stroma and fat

The nuclei are uniform, and round to oval with prominent or inconspicuous nucleoli.

They can be benign or malignant. The majority are benign with rare malignant examples.

Criteria used to distinguish malignant from benign lesions are large tumor size >5 cm, the presence of necrosis, nuclear pleomorphism, conspicuous nucleoli, increased mitotic activity, and local recurrence [17, 18].

– **Differential Diagnosis**: Includes benign proliferations with abundant histiocytes and malignant tumors like apocrine carcinoma and carcinomas with histiocytic appearance.

Granular cell tumors are strongly and diffusely positive for S-100 protein, supporting neuronal origin.

Granular cell tumors are negative for epithelial markers like cytokeratin in all cases.

Calretinin and CD 68 (also used as a marker of histiocytes) can be positive in most of these tumors [17].

Hormone receptors (ER and PR) are negative and muscle markers (SMA) are negative.

S100 positivity can also be seen in metastatic melanoma to the breast but granular cell tumors are negative for other markers of melanocytic differentiation such as HMB45.

Metastatic renal cell carcinoma to the breast has abundant granular cytoplasm and can therefore mimic granular cell tumors. However, these tumors are cytokeratin positive.

Management: These lesions may be missed on core needle biopsy due to limited sampling or mistaking them for histiocytic proliferation. When diagnosed on core needle biopsy an excision is recommended. Local excision is recommended as the risk of local recurrence is minimum even with positive margins. Malignant tumors can recur if incompletely excised. may also be screening-detected.

Sclerosing Adenosis

Sclerosing Adenosis: Sclerosing adenosis is characterized by an increased number of glands in the terminal duct lobular units and coexistent stromal sclerosis resulting in compression and distortion of normal tissue. The sclerosis and compressed glands mimic invasive carcinoma.

Rarely sclerosing adenosis can infiltrate surrounding parenchyma and fat and can be difficult to differentiate from invasive carcinoma on needle core biopsies [19].

- **Clinical Presentation**: Sclerosing adenosis is commonly found in women of reproductive age in their third and fourth decade [19]. It is found incidentally in benign biopsies. When it forms an adenosis tumor, it can form a clinically detectable mass. Sclerosing adenosis is a common incidental finding that infrequently produces mammographic architectural distortion. When it is considered as the primary diagnosis, careful imaging-pathology correlation is essential to ensure that the process is exuberant enough to explain the mammographic findings.

- **Imaging Findings**:
  - **Mammography**: The most common mammographic manifestation of sclerosing adenosis is scattered regional or diffuse punctate calcifications [20].

    When the associated sclerosis is profuse, it may create architectural distortion and overlap in appearance with malignancy (Fig. 5.7).

    Nodular sclerosing adenosis may appear as a high-density mass with circumscribed or indistinct margins (Fig. 5.8).

    Adequate histologic sampling at core needle biopsy and communication with the interpreting pathologist are advisable to confirm the diagnosis.
  - **US**: Sclerosing adenosis is typically sonographically occult.
    - Exuberant sclerosing adenosis associated with mammographic distortion may produce areas of shadowing on ultrasound without a discrete mass (Fig. 5.9).
  - **MRI**: The appearance of sclerosing adenosis on MRI ranges from no abnormal enhancement to areas of non-mass enhancement in a stellate pattern that mirrors the architectural distortion seen mammographically. Mass enhancement is uncommon (Fig. 5.10).
  - **BI-RADS**: 2, 3, 4, depending on imaging appearance and clinical history.
  - **Differential Diagnosis**: Radial scar/complex sclerosing lesion; invasive ductal carcinoma, especially tubular carcinoma; invasive lobular carcinoma.**Pathology Findings**:
  - **Gross**: Gross appearance of sclerosing adenosis varies based on its histologic pattern.

    Nodular adenosis, appears as a circumscribed mass with a firm consistency and grey, white to pale tan cut surface.

    When sclerosing adenosis forms multiple nodules, it tends to have more irregular borders.

    When involved by calcifications it tends to have a gritty texture.

    Scattered lobules when involved by sclerosing adenosis are usually inapparent on gross examination [10].
  - **Microscopic Histology**: Sclerosing adenosis (SA) is characterized by glandular proliferation, stromal sclerosis, and lobular atrophy all arranged in a lobulocentric fashion (Figs. 5.11 and 5.12).

    It can be focal, diffuse or form tumor-like lesions and could be sclerotic or florid.

    Myoepithelial cells are always retained.

    Sclerosis is often accentuated in the center. Areas of less sclerosis contain round glands with open lumens and elongated glands with compressed lumens.

    Eosinophilic secretions may be present within the open lumens.

    The luminal epithelium has bland cytomorphologic features.

    In extremely sclerotic lesions, the glands appear as small nests or cords of epithelioid or spindled myoepithelial cells. The glands are surrounded by a thick basement membrane and variably

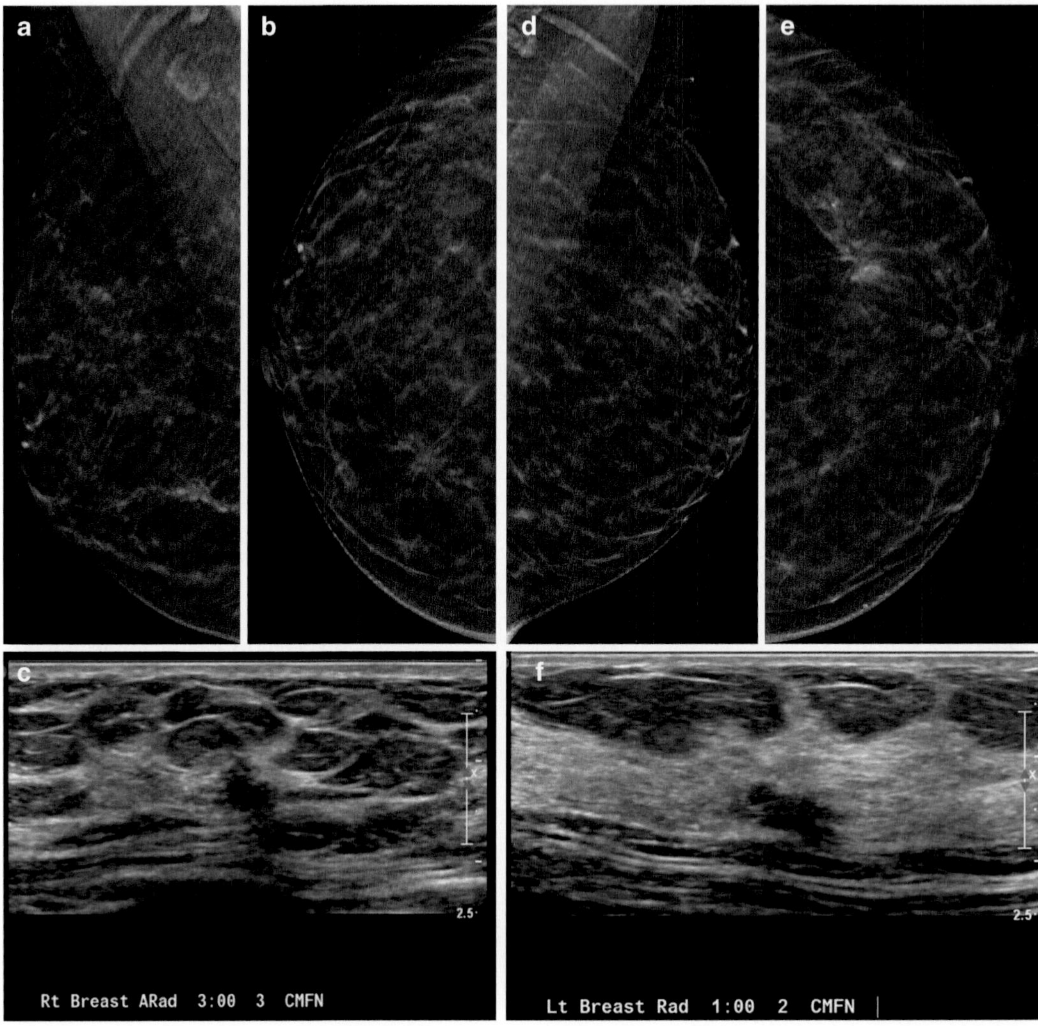

Fig. 5.7 A 46-year-old female presents for annual screening mammography which showed an isodense spiculated mass in the right breast, 3 o'clock position (**a**, **b**) and an isodense spiculated mass in the left breast, 1 o'clock position (**d**, **e**). Ultrasound revealed an irregular mass with a spiculated margin in the right breast, 3 o'clock position (**c**) and an irregular mass with a spiculated margin was noted in the left breast, 1 o'clock position (**f**). The findings were considered BI-RADS 4, suspicious findings. A bilateral US-guided biopsy was recommended and performed. The right breast mass was found to be nodular sclerosing adenosis, and the left breast mass was found to be sclerosing adenosis

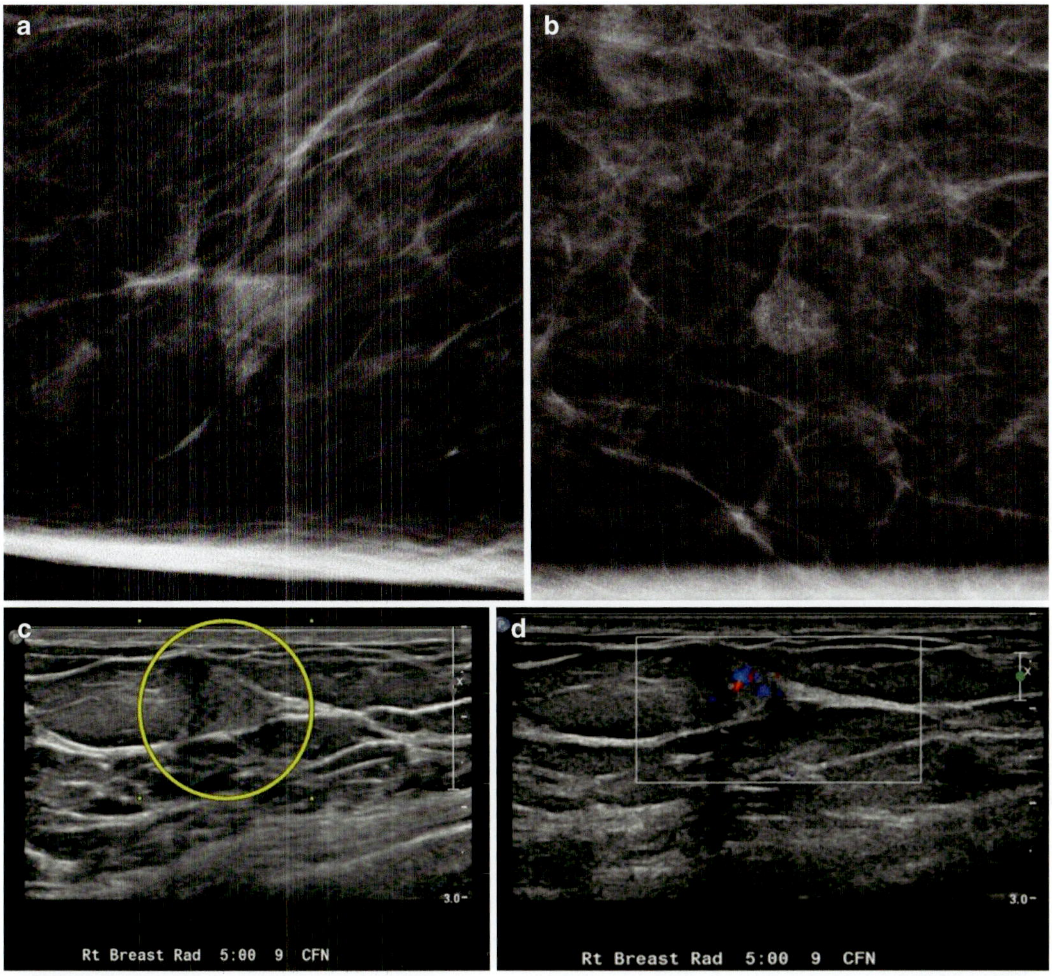

Fig. 5.8 A 46-year-old female presents for mammography (**a**, **b**) which reveals an 8-mm oval mass with a spiculated margin and calcifications at 5:00. On ultrasound (**c**, **d**) there is an oval, isoechoic mass with a circumscribed margin with internal vascularity. The mass is graded BI-RADS 4, suspicious: an ultrasound-guided biopsy was recommended and performed, which showed sclerosing adenosis involved by atypical lobular hyperplasia

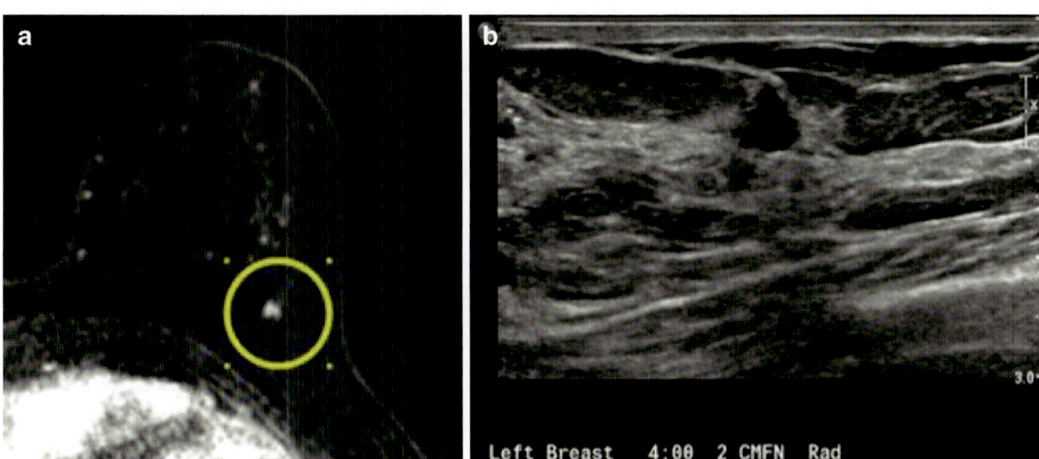

Fig. 5.9 A 47-year-old female presenting with a new left breast mass. On MRI (**a**) and US (**b**) there is a 9-mm oval mass with an irregular margin at 4 o'clock. The lesion was subsequently biopsied revealing sclerosing adenosis

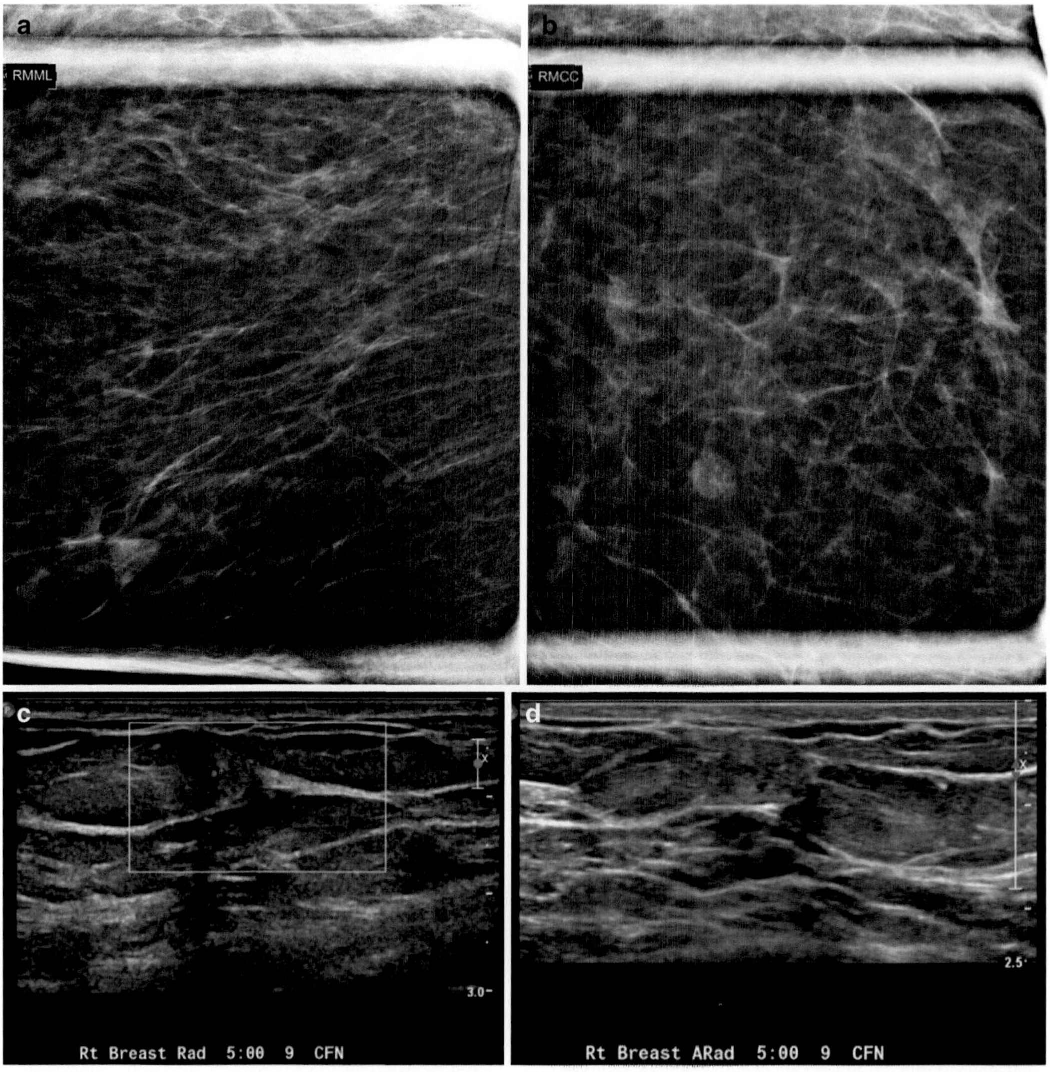

Fig. 5.10 A 46-year-old female with strong family history of breast carcinoma underwent a screening breast MRI (**a**, **b**) which showed a 6-mm irregular mass with a spiculated margin in the left breast. On mammogram there was no corresponding mammographic finding. Ultrasound (**c**, **d**) showed a 6-mm irregular mass with a spiculated margin that appears to correspond to the MRI finding. The lesion was graded as BI-RADS 4, suspicious: an ultrasound-guided core needle biopsy was recommended and performed, which yielded nodular adenosis

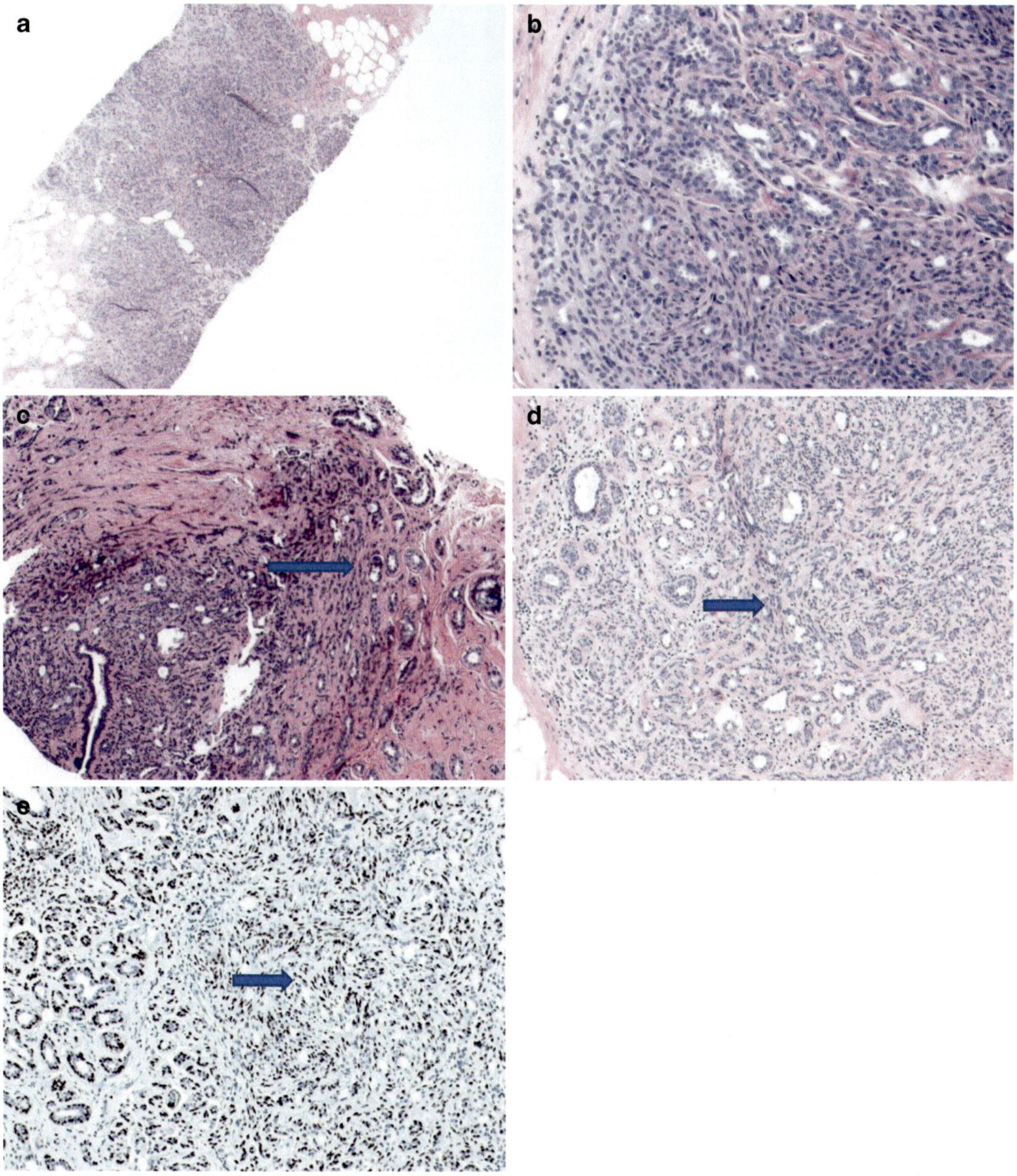

Fig. 5.11 A 38-year-old female presenting with a 7-mm oval mass with an irregular margin on imaging underwent biopsy which revealed adenosis glands of varying sizes with circumscribed margins (**a**). High magnification shows a dense proliferation of epithelial and myoepithelial cells (**b**) and adenosis glands with associated microcalcifications (**c**). Later excision of the lesion shows dense proliferation of epithelial and myoepithelial cells and low power shows myoepithelial hyperplasia (**d**). P63 immunostain highlights myoepithelial hyperplasia (nuclear stain) around adenosis glands (**e**)

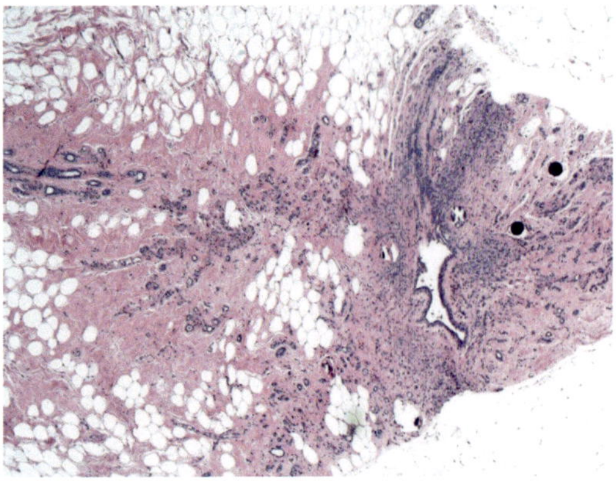

Fig. 5.12 Sclerosing adenosis with associated calcifications

expanded dense fibrotic or hyalinized stroma.

Sclerosing adenosis can be commonly seen in association with fibrocystic changes, atypical proliferation and in situ carcinoma [21–24] (Figs. 5.13 and 5.14).

Florid adenosis consists of enlarged or coalescent lobules of densely packed ductules and glands.

These mass forming confluent areas are commonly referred to as nodular adenosis.

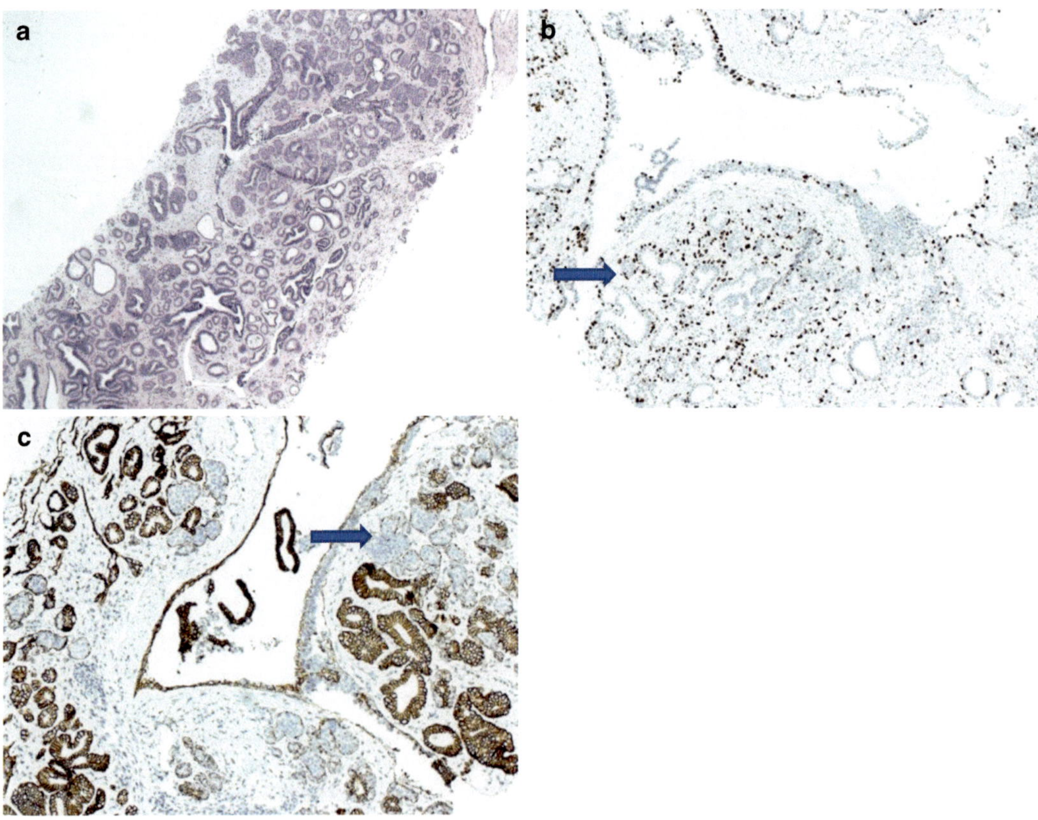

Fig. 5.13 A 52-year-old female underwent biopsy after mammography revealed a 6-mm round mass with spiculated margins. On biopsy there is sclerosing adenosis with expansion of some glands with atypical epithelial proliferation and loss of cohesion (**a**). An immunostain for p63 highlights myoepithelial cells around glands involved by LCIS, confirming absence of invasion (**b**). An immunostain for E-cadherin shows absence of staining in the epithelial proliferation, confirming LCIS (**c**)

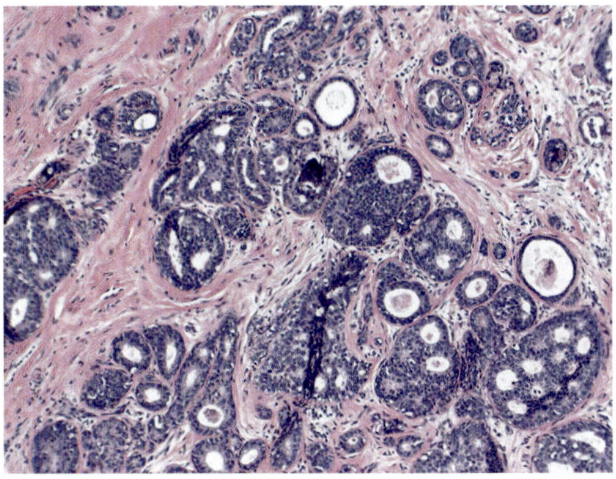

Fig. 5.14 Surgical resection demonstrating sclerosing adenosis involved by DCIS

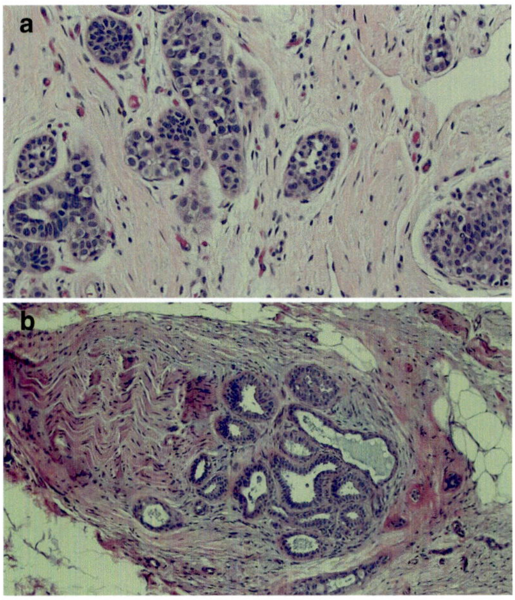

Fig. 5.15 Surgical resection demonstrating sclerosing adenosis involved by LCIS (**a**) and sclerosing adenosis mimicking perineural invasion (**b**)

Rarely one can find perineural invasion, and infiltration of blood vessel walls by benign glands [25, 26] (Fig. 5.15).

Core biopsy findings: On core biopsy, presence of a well-demarcated border is helpful in determining the benign nature of florid cases. In cases with extreme sclerosis and extension of glands in the stroma and fat, immunostaining with myoepithelial cells can support the diagnosis of sclerosing adenosis.

Immunohistochemistry to demonstrate myoepithelial cells may be useful in distinguishing sclerosing adenosis from invasive carcinoma using myoepithelial markers such as p63 and calponin [27].

– **Differential Diagnoses**: Tubular carcinoma, invasive lobular carcinoma, sclerosing adenosis involved by LCIS or DCIS, atypical apocrine adenosis.

Tubular Carcinoma: Sclerosing adenosis with less sclerosis and extending into adipose tissue or with perineural invasion is a well-known mimic of tubular carcinoma.

Tubular carcinoma shows haphazard proliferation of well-formed glands with sharp angulated contours, tapering ends, and open lumens with bland cytology. The tumor cells are columnar and have little to no attenuation. The stroma is desmoplastic rather than hyalinized or fibrotic as seen in sclerosing adenosis.

The glands in sclerosing adenosis are compressed and show the presence of myoepithelial cells on immunohistochemical study.

Invasive Lobular Carcinoma: Sclerosing adenosis with marked sclerosis and glandular atrophy closely mimics lobular carcinoma.

Invasive lobular carcinoma is cellular, shows infiltration of tumor cells with epithelioid morphology and lacks myoepithelial cells.

Sclerosing Adenosis Involved by LCIS or DCIS: Important to distinguish from invasive carcinoma.

Myoepithelial markers, at least two to three (p63, calponin, and SMM) are helpful as they are lost in invasive carcinoma but present around adenosis glands [24].

DCIS involving sclerosing adenosis would show an intact myoepithelial layer, but the atypical epithelial proliferation will be negative for CK5/6 (an epithelial differentiation marker) and diffusely positive for ER with a membranous staining pattern with E-cadherin [24].

Similarly, LCIS involving sclerosing adenosis would show preserved myoepithelial cells but will show absence of staining with E-cadherin.

Atypical Apocrine Adenosis: Defined as nodular sclerosing adenosis involved by apocrine atypia.

Rare (0.4% of cases) [24].

Apocrine cells show threefold variation in nuclear size and prominent nucleoli.

Distinction from apocrine DCIS is not clear cut.

Limited data on management, surgical excision.

Management: When radiologic findings are concordant with the biopsy diagnosis of sclerosing adenosis, it can be managed by observation [26]. Sclerosing adenosis in spiculated masses is best managed by excision to rule out other possible radiologic differentials which include radial sclerosing lesions and invasive carcinoma [28].

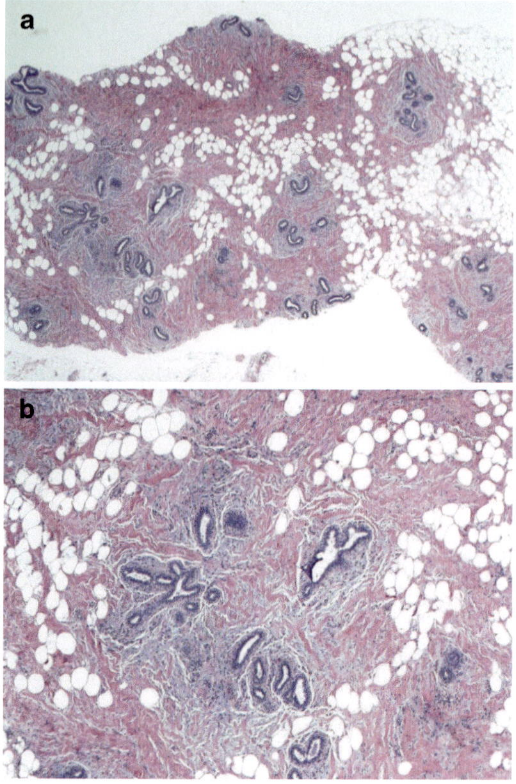

Fig. 5.16 PASH with characteristic slit like empty spaces mimicking vascular channels (**a**, **b**)

Pseudoangiomatous Stromal Hyperplasia (PASH)

See Chap. 7 for text (Fig. 5.16).

Fibromatosis

See Chap. 7 for pathology text and additional information.

Fibromatosis: Fibromatosis in the breast is a rare, benign lesion occurring in women of reproductive age that presents as a spiculated mass, mimics malignancies, and is caused by a proliferation of fibroblasts and myofibroblasts that infiltrate the surrounding tissue but have no metastatic potential [2] (Fig. 5.17). Its etiology is not clearly established, although prior trauma to the breast, both iatrogenic and accidental, has been implicated, and this lesion may be more common in patients with adenomatous polyposis coli (APC) gene mutations [29–31]. Although these lesions may spontaneously regress, excision is usually performed after diagnosis. After excision, this lesion has a relatively high recurrence rate of 20–30% within 3 years [2, 32].

- **Clinical Presentation**: Fibromatosis may manifest as a palpable, painful mass in the posterior aspect of the breast, frequently attached to the pectoralis muscle.

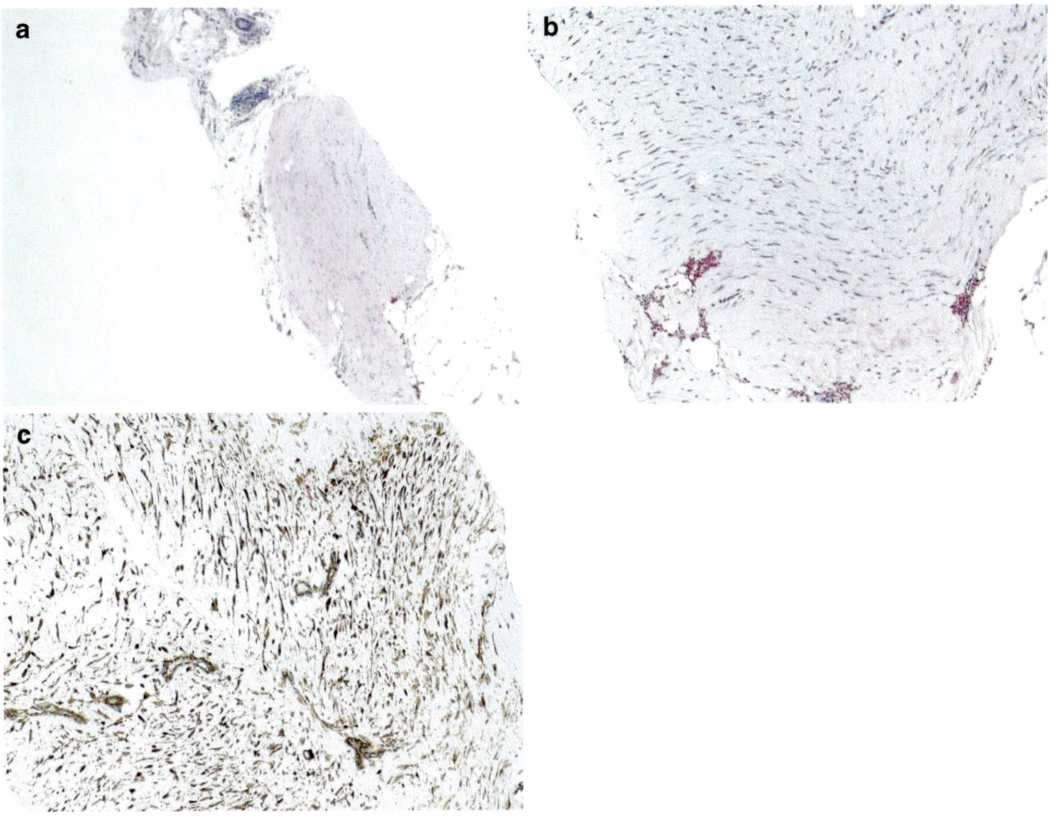

Fig. 5.17 A 57-year-old female status post bilateral mastectomy for invasive ductal carcinoma was incidentally found to have a mass in her reconstructed right mass. On core needle biopsy there are areas with cellular stroma extending into adipose tissue and dense collagenous tissue with lymphoid aggregate at the periphery (**a**). On high magnification the tumor cells are arranged in broad sheets and interlacing bundles with oval and spindled nuclei with no pleomorphism or mitosis (**b**). An immunostain for beta catenin shows nuclear staining in the stromal cells which helps confirm the diagnosis (**c**)

- **Imaging Findings**:
  - **Mammography**: Irregular, spiculated high density mass in the posterior aspect of the breast that may appear to arise from the pectoralis muscle (Fig. 5.18).

    Associated calcifications are uncommon.

    When large and occupying a large portion of the breast, breast skin thickening, nipple retraction, and overall breast shrinkage may occur.

    Axillary adenopathy is absent.
  - **US**: Hypoechoic, irregular mass with angular or speculated margins. An echogenic rim may be present.
  - **CT**: Soft tissue density mass within the posterior breast, attached to the chest wall musculature (Fig. 5.19).
  - **BI-RADS**: 4 or 5, these lesions are usually indistinguishable from malignancy and a core biopsy is recommended.
  - **Differential Diagnosis**: Benign: postoperative scar, fat necrosis, diabetic mastopathy; Malignant: IDC, ILC, sarcoma.
  - **Management**: Wide local excision is typically performed. However, the lesion recurs in 20–30% of patients within 3 years [2, 32]. If surgical excision is not possible due to potential significant morbidity, observation may be considered, as up to 50% of

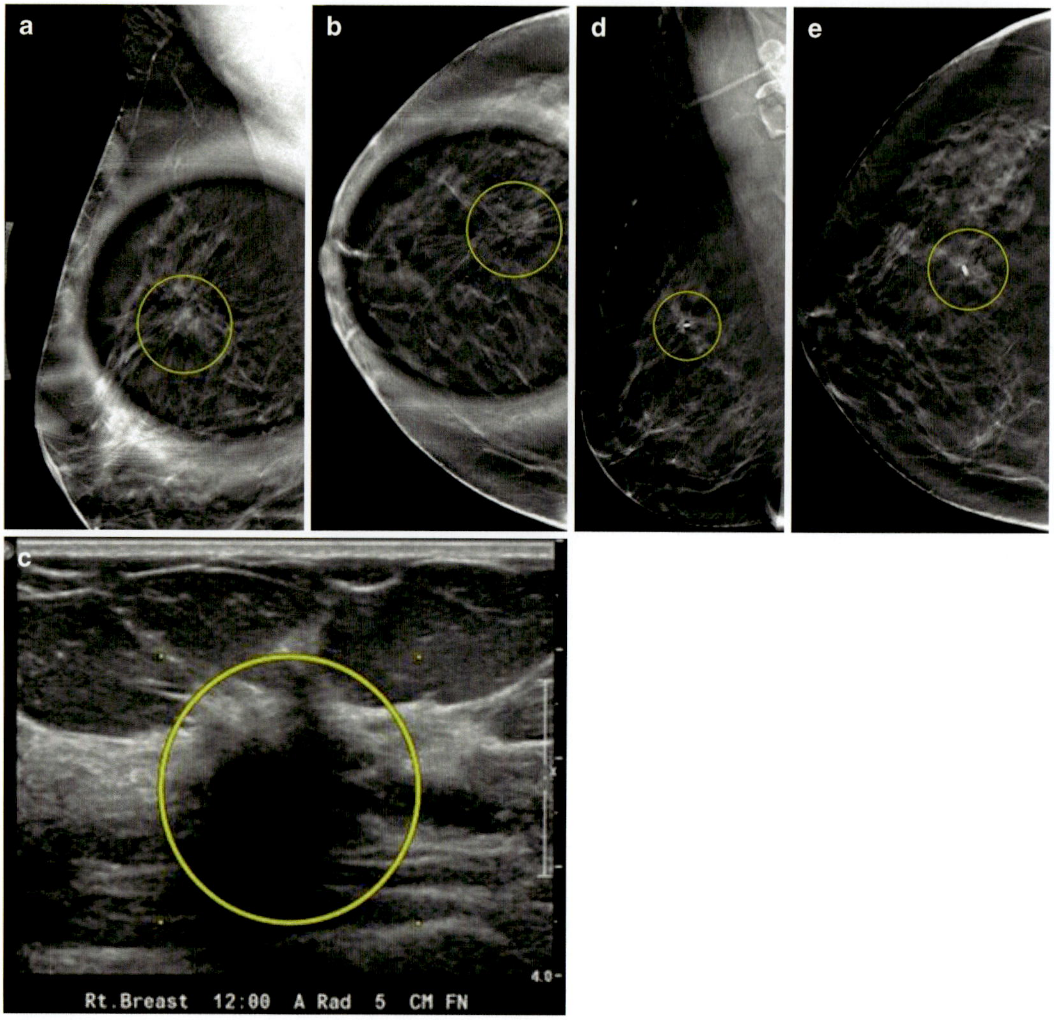

Fig. 5.18 A 55-year-old female was recalled from screening mammography due to an area of architectural distortion in the upper outer aspect of the right breast. The mammography showed focal irregular asymmetry, better seen on the MLO spot view, with associated architectural distortion (**a**, **b**). On ultrasound there was an irregular, hypoechoic, spiculated mass with posterior acoustic shadowing and no demonstrable vascularity (**c**). The lesion was graded as BI-RADS 4, suspicious finding. An US-guided biopsy was recommended and performed, yielding portions of hyalinized, involuting fibromatosis. Since this diagnosis was deemed concordant, short-term follow-up was recommended, and the finding remained stable. Three years after the biopsy, the finding remains mammographically stable (**d**, **e**)

extra-abdominal desmoid tumors may regress spontaneously [32] however, about 50% will progress [32]. Newer therapies, including cryoablation and high intensity focused US, are being investigated as potential means to treat fibromatosis. Radiation and medical therapy are not clearly indicated [30].

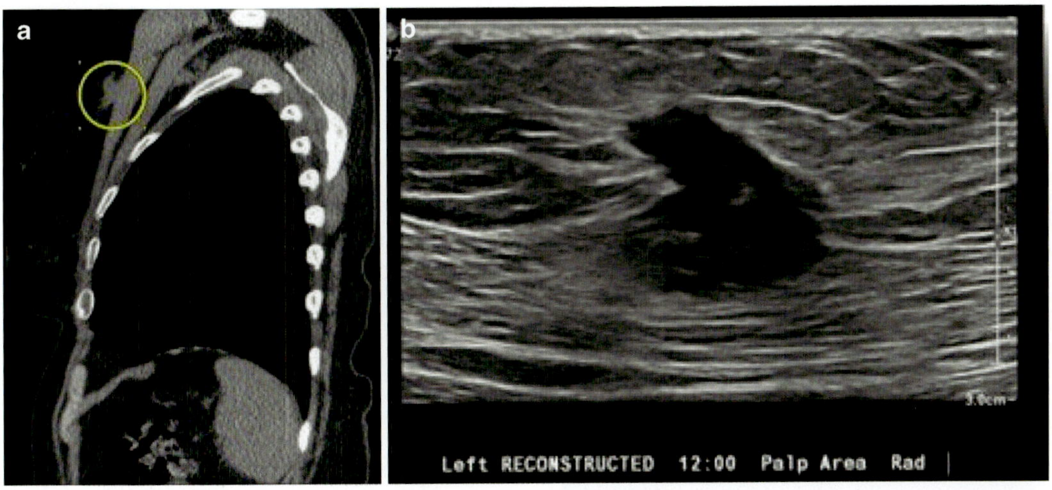

Fig. 5.19 A 68-year-old female status post right mastectomy for extensive DCIS and prophylactic left mastectomy underwent annual non-contrast CT screening of her lungs due to a history of non-small cell lung carcinoma. Incidentally noted was a lesion in the reconstructed left upper breast. On CT a soft tissue density irregular mass in the upper aspect of the left autologous breast reconstruction, tethered to the left pectoralis major muscle was seen (**a**). Targeted US reveals a hypoechoic, irregular, spiculated mass with no demonstrable internal vascularity and no posterior acoustic features (**b**). The lesion was graded as BI-RADS 4, suspicious of malignancy; an US-guided biopsy was recommended and performed revealing fibromatosis

Malignant

Mucinous Carcinoma

See Chap. 2.

Tubular Carcinoma

Tubular Carcinoma: Considered a special type of invasive carcinoma with excellent prognosis [33–35]. The incidence in screened populations is higher than in unscreened populations as they rarely form palpable masses and measure <1 cm [35]. It accounts for about 2% of breast cancers, and it is usually detected on screening mammography in women aged 50 and over as a small, spiculated mass that frequently contains pleomorphic calcifications [33, 34]. Lymph node metastases at presentation are very rare [35]. Tubular carcinomas generally have favorable prognoses, with a 10-year breast cancer-specific survival of up to 98% [36, 37].

- **Clinical Presentation**: Tubular carcinoma presents mammographically as a stellate mass with irregular spicules on mammogram or as architectural distortion and overlaps with radial sclerosing lesions [33].
- **Imaging Findings**:
  - **Mammography**: Although tubular carcinoma classically presents as a small, slow growing spiculated mass, it may also manifest as an asymmetry or an architectural distortion. In about 50% of cases, associated pleomorphic calcifications are present (Fig. 5.20).
  - **US**: Irregular, spiculated mass with posterior acoustic shadowing.
  - **MRI**: Irregular, spiculated mass with rapid initial enhancement and washout kinetics.
  - **BIRADS**: 4, 5.
  - **Differential Diagnosis**: Postsurgical scar, fat necrosis, radial scar/CSL, granular cell tumor, IDC not otherwise specified, ILC, DCIS.

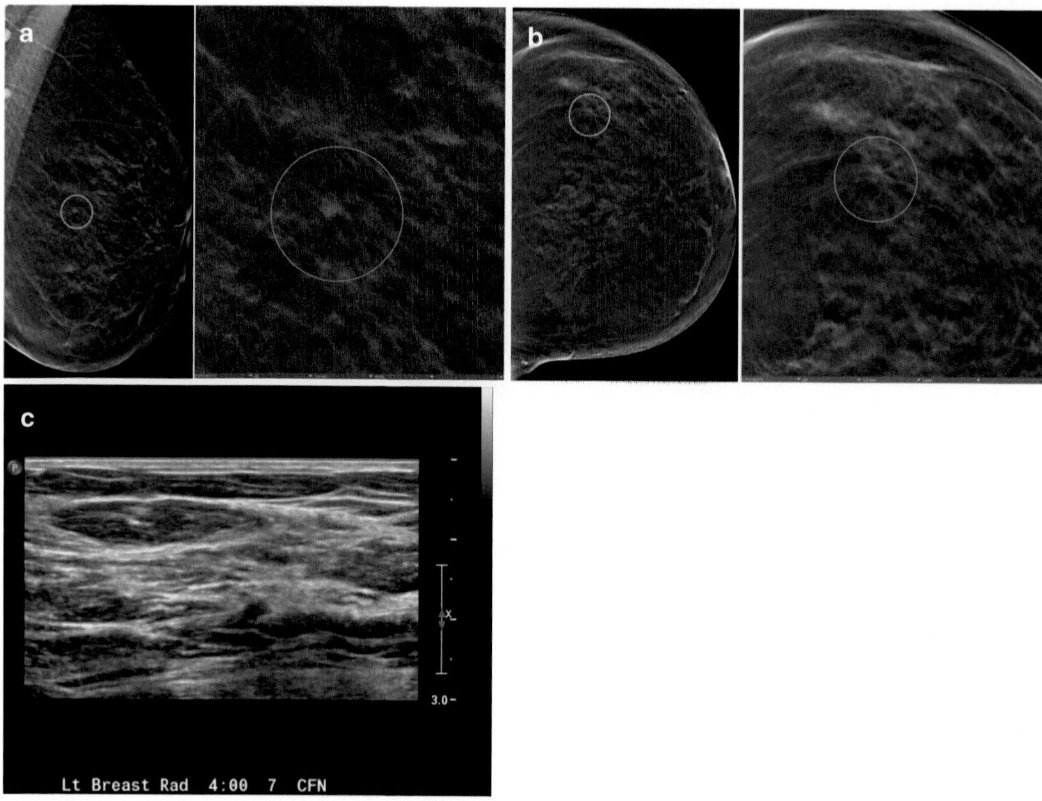

Fig. 5.20 A 51-year-old perimenopausal female with history of breast reduction surgery presents for screening mammography (**a**, **b**) which reveals a small, irregular spiculated mass in the left breast within the area of the post-reduction scar. On ultrasound (**c**) there is a small, irregular spiculated mass with posterior acoustic shadowing. The mass is graded as BI-RADS 4, suspicious. An ultrasound-guided core biopsy was recommended and performed, yielding tubular carcinoma. The patient subsequently underwent a double mastectomy

- **Pathology Findings**:
  - **Microscopic Histology**: Invasive tubular carcinomas are comprised of glands with open lumina distributed haphazardly in a desmoplastic stroma (Fig. 5.21).

    The tubules are lined by a single layer of epithelial cells and lack an outer layer of myoepithelial cells. The glands are angulated with low-grade nuclei, small uniform nucleoli, and apical cytoplasmic snouts [34].

    Mitoses are relatively rare.

    Greater than 90% of the tumor should be comprised of classic tubular morphology to be regarded as the special type, tubular carcinoma [2, 34]. The well-formed glands are often seen infiltrating into and around normal breast ducts and lobules.

    Tubular carcinoma may be associated with flat epithelial atypia, columnar cell changes, atypical lobular and ductal hyperplasia, lobular carcinoma in situ and DCIS in the adjacent breast [34].

    Tubular carcinomas are strongly positive for ER and PR, and negative for HER2. Immunohistochemistry for myoepithelial markers (p63, calponin, and SMM) are helpful in differentiating these glands from entrapped glands in radial sclerosing lesions and small glandular proliferations such as adenosis glands seen in sclerosing adenosis.

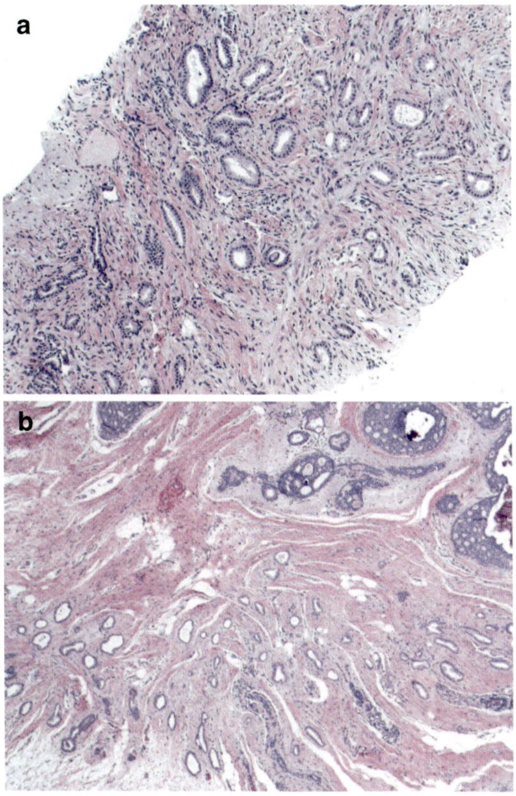

Fig. 5.21 A breast biopsy (**a**) showing the oval and angular glands of tubular carcinoma in a cellular stroma. A surgical excision (**b**) with well-formed tubules characteristic of well differentiated tubular carcinoma seen adjacent to a low to intermediate grade DCIS with cribriform architecture and necrosis

- **Differential Diagnosis**: Radial sclerosing lesions, sclerosing adenosis, microglandular adenosis, low-grade adenosquamous carcinoma, syringomatous adenoma, well-differentiated invasive ductal carcinoma [38].
- **Management**: Diagnosis on core needle biopsy may be challenging on limited samples. An unequivocal diagnosis of tubular carcinoma on core needle biopsy warrants a complete surgical excision with lymph node sampling.

Invasive Ductal Carcinoma

See Chap. 7 for additional information and pathology text.

Invasive Ductal Carcinoma: Invasive ductal carcinoma accounts for nearly 80% of all invasive breast cancers [39, 40]. Of these, invasive ductal carcinoma, no special type (IDC NST), which represents about 60% of all breast cancers, is the most common [39] (Fig. 5.22). Often, IDC is associated with a DCIS component that manifests as linear and/or pleomorphic calcifications in the vicinity of the mass.

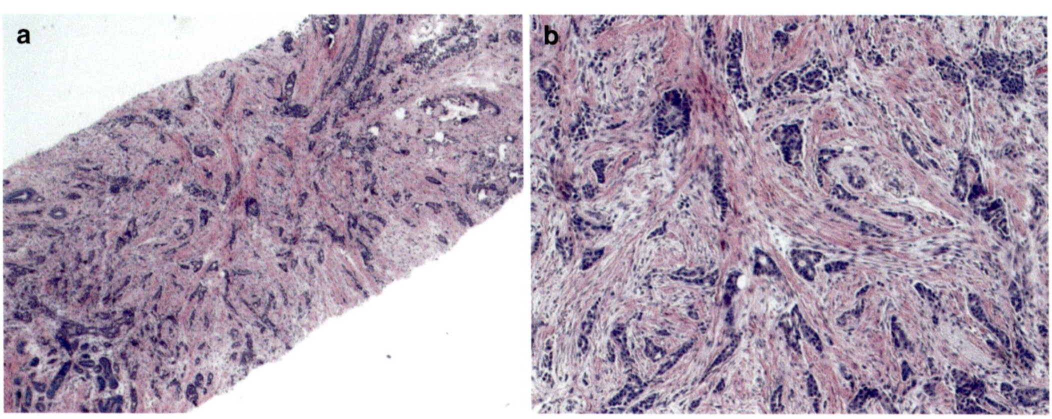

Fig. 5.22 Invasive ductal carcinoma with angulated, irregular gland formation in a haphazard pattern seen on core needle biopsy (**a**, **b**)

- **Clinical Presentation**: In the era of digital mammography and digital breast tomosynthesis, IDC NST is frequently screening detected. However, it may also present as a palpable mass, and may be associated with nipple or skin retraction and axillary or internal mammary adenopathy [41, 42].

- **Imaging Findings**:
  - **Mammography**: About 66% of IDCs NST present as spiculated masses and are frequently seen on both screening views, particularly when DBT is performed [39, 47, 50] (Figs. 5.23 and 5.24).

    May also present as a one-view only finding, particularly when occurring in dense breast tissue or a posterior location.

    It is frequently associated with architectural distortion due to tethering of Cooper ligaments.

    Pleomorphic and/or linear calcifications are frequently present within and in the vicinity of the spiculated mass.
  - **US**: Irregular, spiculated mass, anti-parallel in orientation, hypoechoic or heterogeneous, with or without associated vascularity.

    Frequently with posterior shadowing and a hyperechoic rim.

    Ultrasound is frequently helpful in assessing the axilla for adenopathy.

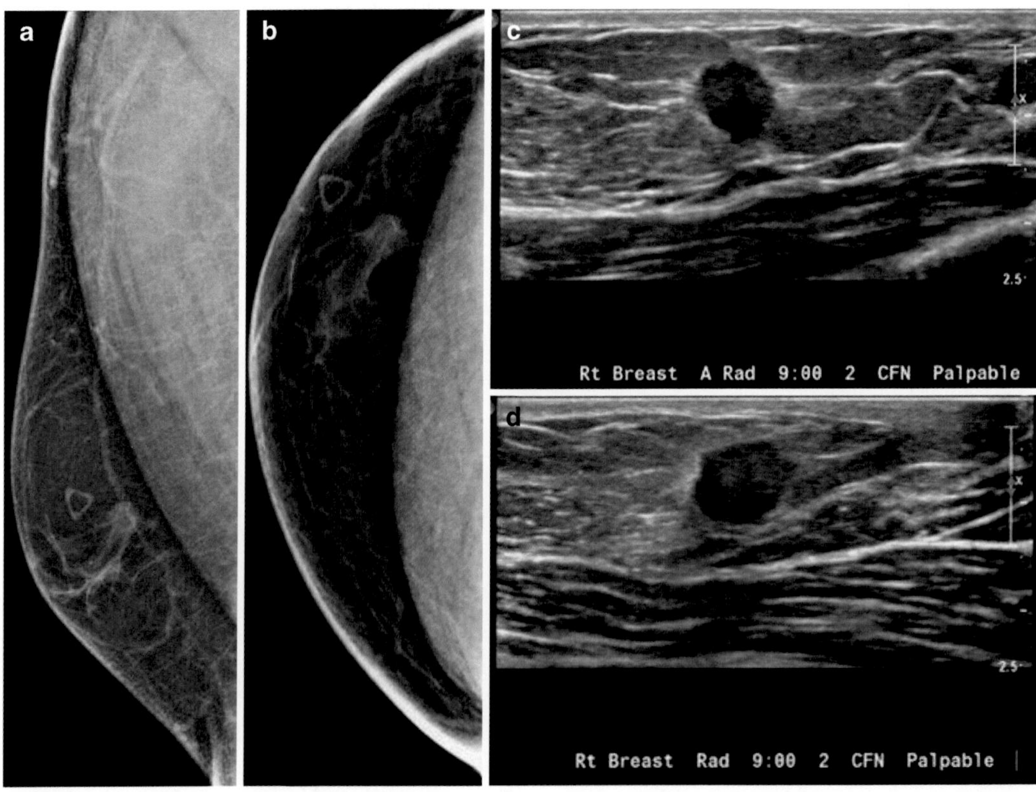

Fig. 5.23 A 95-year-old female, recalled from screening mammography (**a**, **b**) due to a subtle, incompletely visualized mass in the medial and posterior aspect of the right breast, seen on the CC view only. Based on this appearance, the mass may mimic an atypical appearance of the sternalis muscle; however, this was a new finding and was correctly interpreted as a potential abnormality. Mammography was incompletely visualized. There was a high-density irregular mass with a spiculated margin in the medial posterior aspect of the right breast. A medially exaggerated CC view of the right breast reveals an irregular, spiculated mass with associated pleomorphic calcifications. On ultrasound (**c**, **d**) there was a mixed hypoechoic and hyperechoic irregular mass with an indistinct margin, with internal and rim vascularity. The mass was graded as BI-RADS 5, highly suspicious of malignancy. An US-guided biopsy was recommended and performed yielding IDC, moderately differentiated. The patient subsequently underwent a lumpectomy, which confirmed moderately differentiated IDC

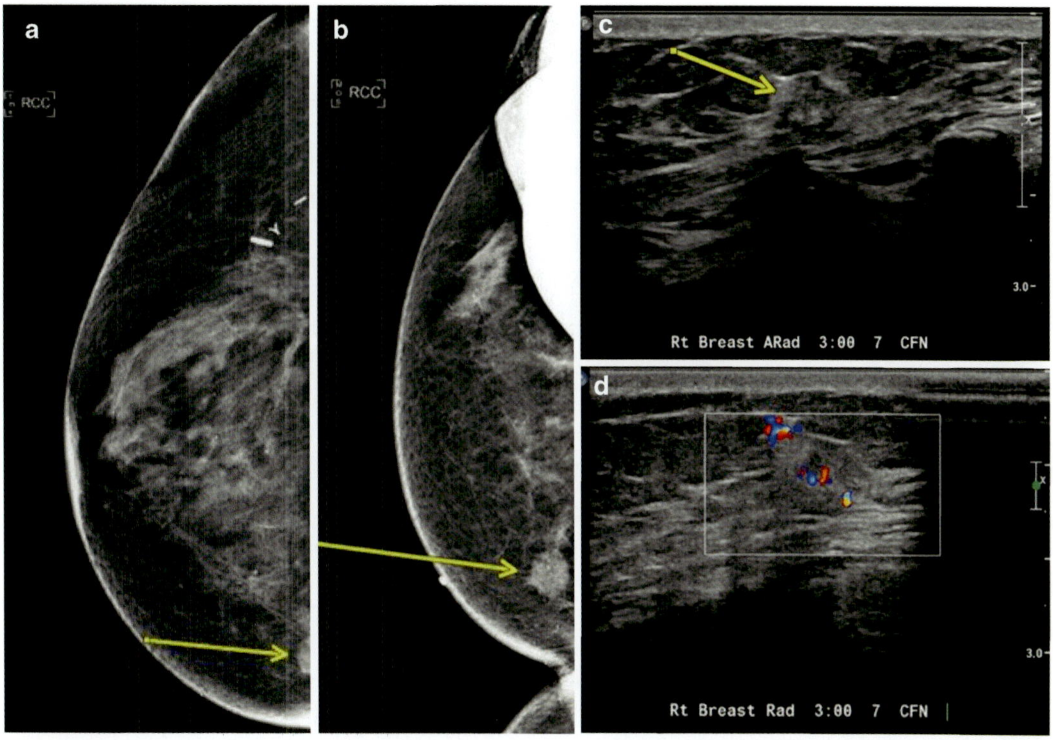

Fig. 5.24 An example of mammography (**a, b**) and ultrasound (**c**, **d**) demonstrating IDC with a medial location mimicking sternal muscle s

- **MRI**: Irregular spiculated mass that is hypointense on T1WI (Fig. 5.25).
  Variable intensity on T2WI.
  Fat may be entrapped within the mass.
  Although classically described as having washout kinetics following contrast administration, plateau and persistent enhancement are not uncommon.
  Rim enhancement can occur when central necrosis is present.
- **BIRADS**: 4 or 5. A biopsy is indicated.
- **Differential Diagnosis**: Benign: postsurgical scar, fat necrosis, radial scar, sclerosing adenosis, granular cell tumor, fibromatosis, granulomatous mastitis, diabetic mastopathy. Malignant: tubular carcinoma, ILC.
- **Management**: Surgery remains the mainstay of treatment of IDC. If breast conservation is performed, radiation therapy is recommended in most cases, as well as endocrine therapy and/or chemotherapy, depending on the grade and stage of the tumor.

Invasive Lobular Carcinoma

Invasive Lobular Carcinoma, Classic and Variants: Invasive lobular carcinoma is a special histologic type of breast cancer that constitutes 10–15% of all breast cancers [43]. Although ILC is less common, on imaging it is more frequently present as architectural distortion [43]. Pathologically, ILC may be associated with lobular carcinoma in situ (LCIS). LCIS can be further subdivided into classic, pleomorphic, or florid subtypes. Reported upgrade rates of pleomorphic and florid LCIS at surgical excision after core

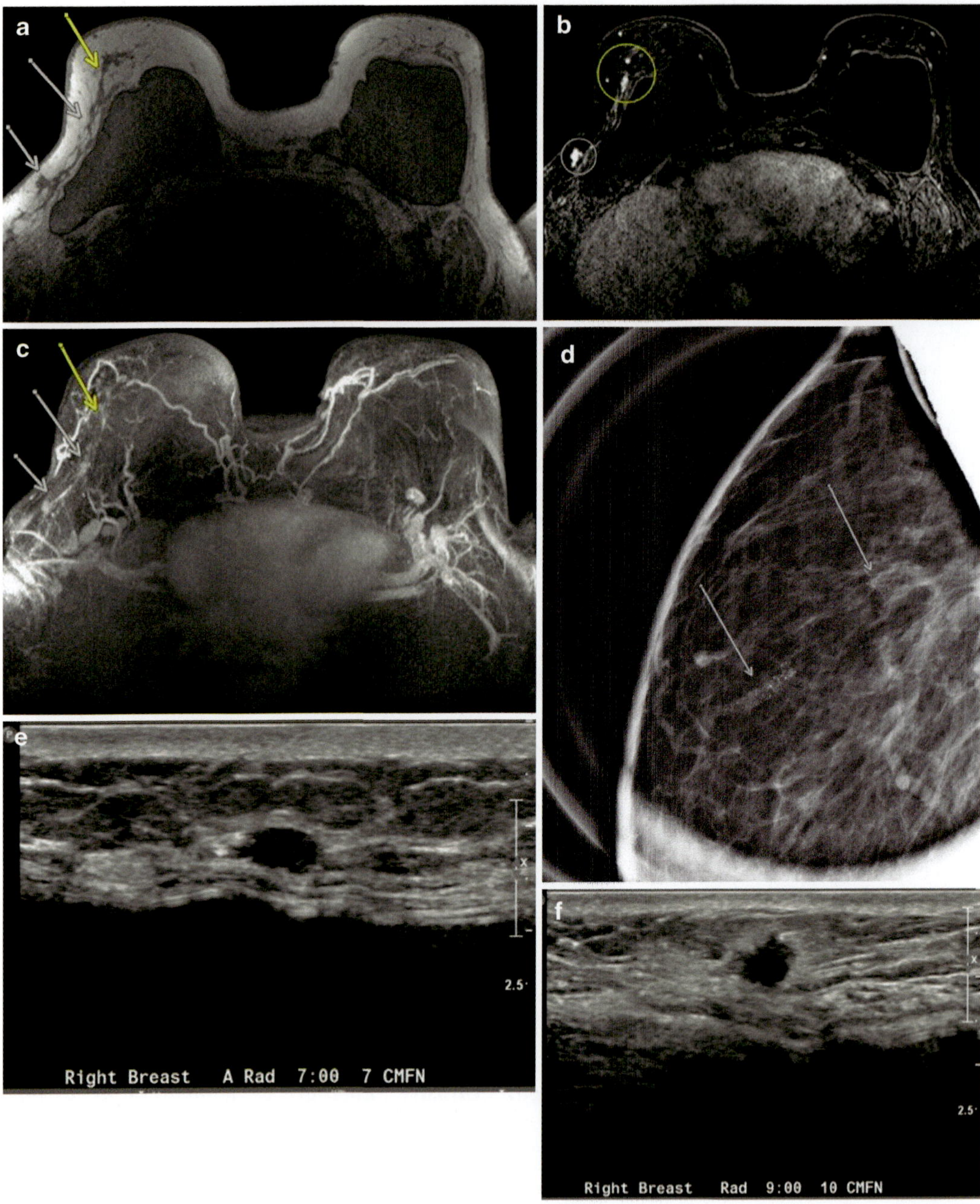

Fig. 5.25 A 53-year-old female palpated a mass in the outer aspect of her reconstructed right breast. She has a history of grade 3 DCIS of the right breast upper outer quadrant 5 years ago, status post bilateral mastectomy with silicone implant reconstruction. The clinician ordered an MRI to evaluate (**a**–**c**). On MRI there was an irregular, spiculated mass with persistent enhancement, and areas of linear non-mass enhancement in a segmental distribution located anterior to the mass, all located within retained axillary tail breast tissue. A diagnostic mammogram (**d**) and a second look US (**e, f**) were recommended and performed. The mammogram showed linear, pleomorphic calcifications within residual breast tissues, corresponding to the areas of non-mass enhancement seen on MRI. The spiculated mass was not definitively seen on mammography due to its posterior location and implant presence. On ultrasound there was a hypoechoic, irregular, spiculated mass corresponding to the MRI-detected finding. The findings were considered BI-RADS 5, highly suggestive of malignancy. An US-guided biopsy of the mass was performed, yielding IDC, moderately differentiated. The patient subsequently underwent a lumpectomy, which revealed IDC and recurrent/residual grade 3 DCIS

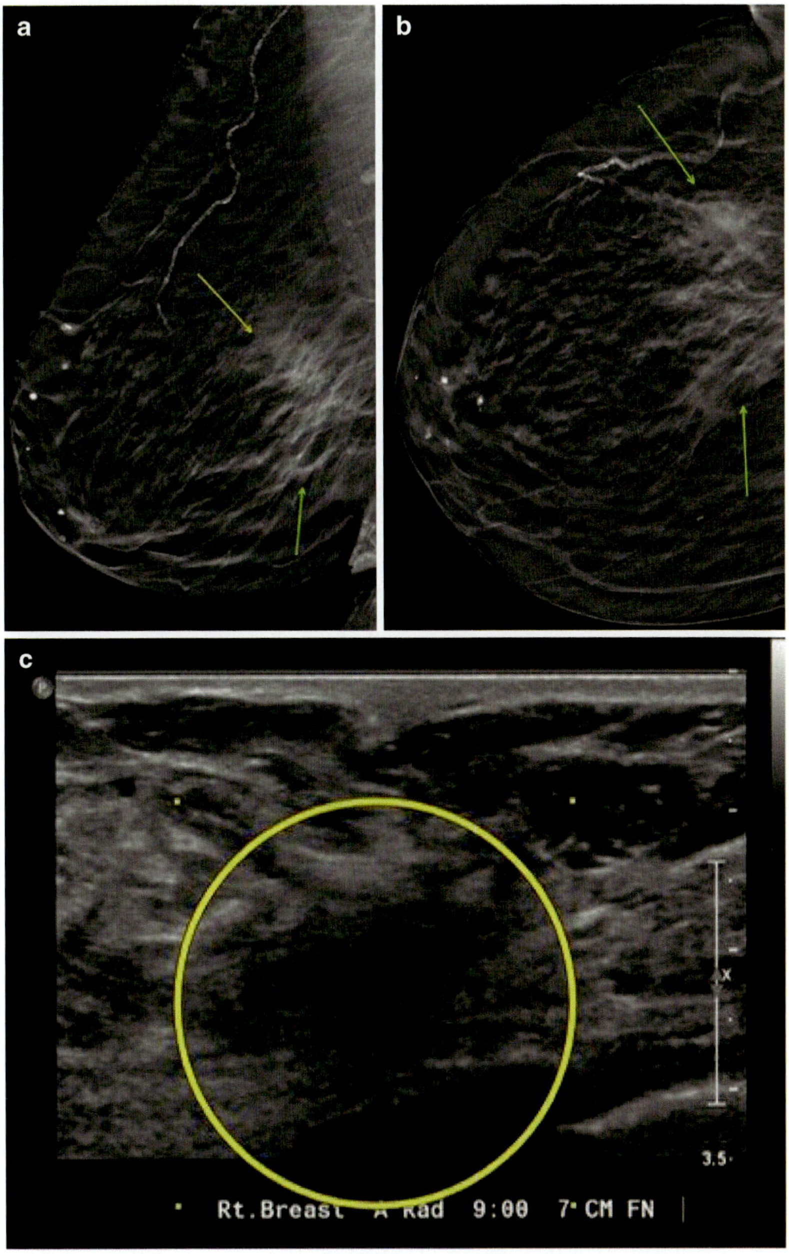

Fig. 5.26 An 83-year-old female, recalled from screening mammography due to a spiculated mass surrounded by architectural distortion and focal asymmetry in the right breast, posterior aspect. Mammography (**a**, **b**) showed a high-density irregular spiculated mass in the upper outer quadrant of the right breast, surrounded by focal asymmetry and architectural distortion. On ultrasound (**c**) there was an irregular mass with an indistinct/spiculated margin, posterior acoustic shadowing, and no detectable internal vascularity. The mass was considered BI-RADS 5, highly suggestive of malignancy. An US-guided biopsy was recommended and performed, yielding ILC, classic type. Due to multiple comorbidities, the patient is not a surgical candidate, and her disease is managed by endocrine therapy

needle biopsy average ~40%, with a range of 25–80% [1, 44, 45]. As such, routine excision following core needle biopsy of pleomorphic or florid LCIS is warranted [46].

- **Clinical Presentation**: Though typically asymptomatic, presentations may include a palpable lump, shrinking breast, or nipple retraction.
- **Imaging Findings**:
  - **Mammography**: Most common appearance is a spiculated mass (Fig. 5.26).

    May also manifest as a developing asymmetry, occasionally seen on one view only, as well as architectural distortion [36].

    ILC is also more likely to be multifocal and multicentric.

If the ILC is diffuse, the breast may appear shrunken and retracted, and skin thickening, and axillary adenopathy may be present.

Calcifications are infrequent [47].

- **US**: Irregular, hypoechoic mass, with indistinct or spiculated margins and posterior acoustic shadowing.

  It may also appear as a vague area of shadowing and may be mistaken for dense fibroglandular breast tissue.
- **MRI**: Most commonly, ILC appears as an irregular, spiculated mass with heterogeneous enhancement.

  Frequently surrounded by smaller masses or foci that represent extent of disease, which may not be visible on mammography or sonography.
- **BIRADS**: 4 or 5. A biopsy is recommended. However, a BI-RADS 3 or even a 2 designation may be erroneously assigned when ILC mimics benign processes.
- **Differential Diagnosis**: Benign: dense benign fibroglandular breast tissue, fibrosis, postoperative scar, radial scar, diabetic mastopathy. Malignant: IDC, tubular carcinoma.

• **Pathology Findings**:

Microscopic Histology: The defining feature of this type of cancer is the lack normal cell adhesion due to loss of the E-cadherin gene and other catenin genes due to germline mutations [43, 48, 49]. This results in the dispersed pattern of growth with discohesive tumor cells in single files in fibrous stroma around normal ducts (Fig. 5.27). The diffuse growth of these tumors makes them hard to be detected by macroscopic or microscopic examination and even on imaging.

The most common variant of invasive lobular carcinoma is the classic type.

There are other architectural and cytologic variants such as solid, alveolar, tubulolobular, pleomorphic, apocrine pleomorphic, and histiocytoid variants [32, 43, 48]. These variant forms are important to recognize in order to avoid misclassification with other types of breast cancer and because the lobular histologic type is frequently associated with distant systemic metastases to serosal surfaces such as the gyn and GI tracts, leptomeninges and bone [43].

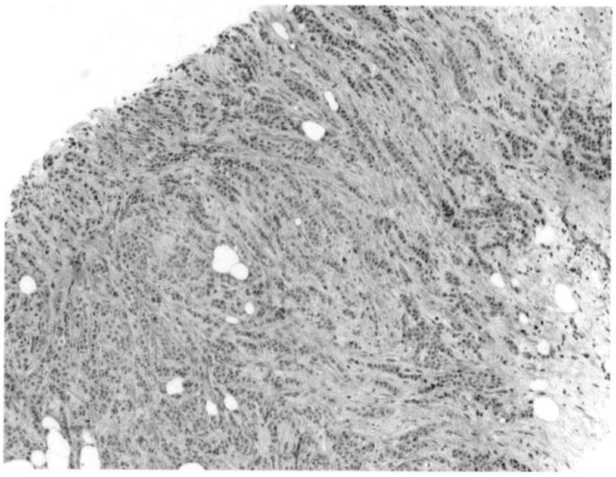

Fig. 5.27 Single filing invasive lobular carcinoma in a 40-year-old female with an irregular mass on imaging

Greater than 90% of ILC show complete loss of E-cadherin with approximately 10–15% expressing membranous E-cadherin that is nonfunctional [43, 49]. Aberrant cytoplasmic diffuse and dot-like expressions of e-cadherin are also described [2, 43]. These cases should be classified as ILC and not ductal based on the growth pattern [50].

The majority of ILCs are hormone receptor (ER and PR) positive and HER2 negative. High-grade ILC and variant forms may be ER negative and HER2 positive [43, 48].

Differential Diagnosis: IDC, lymphomas, metastatic melanoma to breast.

Management: Surgical therapy followed by radiation with endocrine therapy and/or chemotherapy depending on stage of disease.

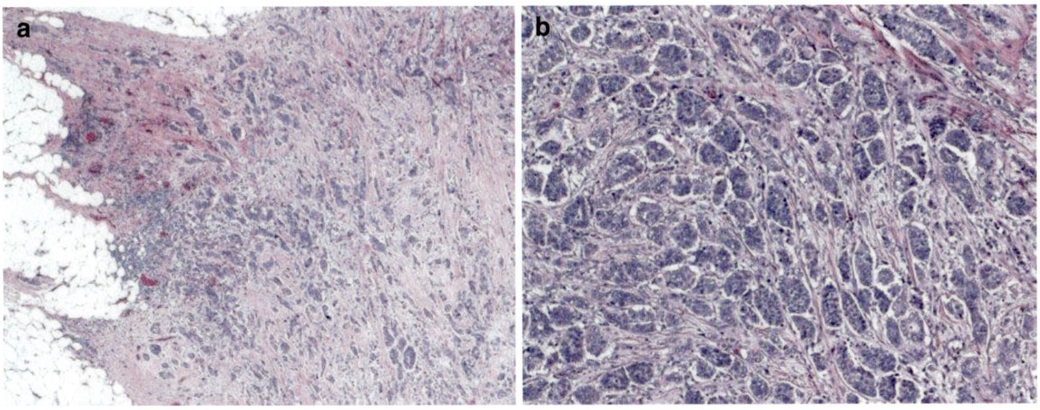

Fig. 5.28 A 69-year-old female undergoes lumpectomy after biopsy of her left breast for a spiculated mass seen on mammography reveals carcinoma. The excisional specimen shows the irregular spiculated outline of the tumor with small nests of tumor cells (**a**). Higher magnification of the tumor demonstrates the inside-out pattern with solid clusters of tumor with the apical portion of the tumor cells towards the empty spaces characteristic of invasive micropapillary carcinoma (**b**)

Invasive Micropapillary Carcinoma

See Chap. 4 for additional information.

Invasive Micropapillary Carcinoma: Invasive micropapillary carcinoma is a rare, aggressive form of IDC, accounting for fewer than 2% of breast cancers [51] (Fig. 5.28).

- **Clinical Presentation**: It frequently presents as a palpable mass in women aged 50–62 commonly with axillary nodal metastases [51].
- **Imaging Findings**:
  - **Mammography**: Irregular mass with a spiculated margin, frequently associated with pleomorphic calcifications (Fig. 5.29).

    Axillary adenopathy may be present.
  - **US**: Irregular mass with indistinct or spiculated margins.

    Frequently associated with axillary adenopathy at the time of diagnosis.
  - **BI-RADS**: 4 or 5.
  - **Differential Diagnosis**: Fat necrosis, fibromatosis, granular cell tumor, diabetic mastopathy, IDC NOS, ILC, metastasis.
  - **Management**: Invasive micropapillary carcinoma is managed in a manner similar to IDC NOS.

Ductal Carcinoma In Situ

See Chaps. 7 and 8.

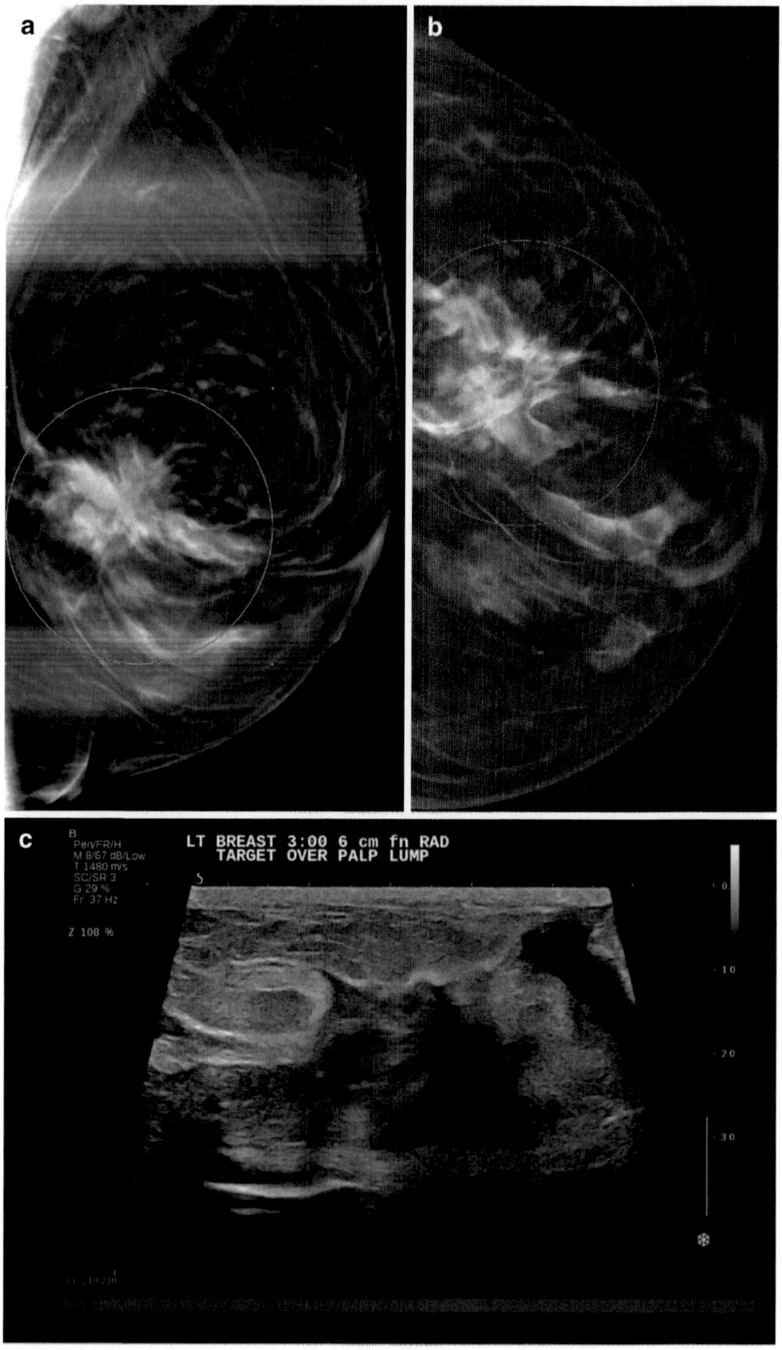

Fig. 5.29 A 78-year-old female with history of breast reduction surgery presents with a palpable mass in the left breast. On mammography there is a conglomerate of several irregular, hyperdense masses with spiculated margins in the left breast within the reduction scar (**a**, **b**). Enlarged left axillary lymph nodes are also demonstrated. On ultrasound several irregular masses with spiculated margins in the left breast are seen (**c**). Enlarged left axillary lymph nodes are confirmed. The lesion is graded as BI-RADS 4, suspicious findings. The excisional specimen reveals invasive micropapillary carcinoma

References

1. Kuba M, et al. Morphologic subtypes of lobular carcinoma in situ diagnosed on core needle biopsy: clinicopathologic features and findings at follow up excision. Mod Pathol. 2021; published online
2. WHO Classification of Tumors Editorial Board. Breast tumours. WHO classification of tumors. 5th ed. Lyon: IARC; 2019.
3. Taboada JL, Stephens TW, Krishnamurthy S, Brandt KR, Whitman GJ. The many faces of fat necrosis in the breast. AJR Am J Roentgenol. 2009;192(3): 815–25.

4. Rosen PP, Hoda SA. Breast Pathology: Diagnosis by needle core biopsy. 3rd edition. Lippincott Williams&Wilkins, 2015.
5. Tomaszewski JE, Brooks JS, Hicks D, Livolsi VA. Diabetic mastopathy: a report of 5 cases and a review of literature. Arch Surg. 2000;135(10):1190–3.
6. Soler NG, Khardori R. Fibrous disease of the breast, thyroiditis and cheiroarthropathy in type 1 diabetes mellitus. Lancet. 1984;1(8370):193–5.
7. Logan WW, Hoffman NY. Diabetic fibrous breast disease. Radiology. 1989;172(3):667–70.
8. Ely KA, Tse G, Simpson JF, Clarfeld R, Page DL. Diabetic mastopathy: a diagnostic challenge in breast sonography. J Clin Ultrasound. 2015;43(2):113–7.
9. Accurso A, et al. Unusual breast lesion mimicking cancer. Diabetic mastopathy. Int J Surg. 2014;12(Suppl1):S79–82.
10. Shin SJ. A comprehensive guide to core needle biopsies of the breast. Springer International Publishing Switzerland; 2016.
11. Moschetta M, Telegrafo M, Triggiani V, et al. Diabetic mastopathy: a diagnostic challenge in breast sonography. J Clin Ultrasound. 2015;43(2):113–7.
12. Schmitt SJ, Collins LC. Biopsy interpretation of the breast. 3rd ed. Wolters Kluwer Health; 2018.
13. Valdez R, Thorson J, Finn WG, Schnitzer B, Kleer CG. Lymphocytic mastitis and diabetic mastopathy: a molecular, immunophenotypic, and clinicopathologic evaluation of 11 cases. Mod Pathol. 2003;16(3):223–8.
14. Kudva YC, Reynolds C, O'Brien T, Powell C, Oberg AL, Crotty TB. Diabetic mastopathy or sclerosing lymphocytic lobulitis, is strongly associated with type 1 diabetes mellitus. Diabetes Care. 2002;25(1):121–6.
15. Gavriilidis P, Michalopoulou I, Baliaka A, et alGranular cell breast tumour mimicking infiltrating carcinoma Case Reports. 2013;2013:bcr2012008178.
16. Chen J, et al. Malignant granular cell tumor with breast metastases. A case report and review of the literature. Oncol Lett. 2012;4(1):63–6.
17. WHO Classification of Tumors Editorial Board. Breast tumours. WHO classification of tumors. 5th ed. Lyon, France: IARC; 2019.
18. Lack EE, Worsham GF, Callihan MD, et al. Granular cell tumor: a clinicopathologic study of 110 patients. J Surg Oncol. 1980;13(4):301–16.
19. Hoda SA, Rosen PP, Brogi E, Koerner F, Rosen PP. Rosen's breast pathology. Lippincott Williams & Wilkins; 2020.
20. Tan H, Zhang H, Lei Z, Fu F, Wang M. Radiological and clinical findings in sclerosing adenosis of the breast. Medicine (Baltimore). 2019;98(39):e17061.
21. Chan JK, Ng WF. Sclerosing adenosis cancerized by intraductal carcinoma. Pathology. 1987;19(4):425–8.
22. Fechner RE. Lobular carcinoma in situ in sclerosing adenosis. A potential source of confusion with invasive carcinoma. Am J Surg Pathol. 1981;5(3):223–9.
23. Fechner RE. Carcinoma in situ involving sclerosing adenosis. Histopathology. 1996;28(6):570.
24. Oberman HA, Markey BA. Noninvasive carcinoma of the breast presenting in adenosis. Mod Pathol. 1991;4(1):31–5.
25. Davies JD. Neural invasion in benign mammary dysplasia. J Pathol. 1973;109(3):225–31.
26. Eusebi V, Azzopardi JG. Vascular infiltration in benign breast disease. J Pathol. 1976;118(1):9–16.
27. Palvaskis K, et al. Myoepithelial cell cocktail (p63 +SMA) for the evaluation of sclerosing breast lesions. Breast. 2006;15(6):705–12.
28. Franquet T, et al. Spiculated lesions of the breast: mammographic-pathologic correlation. Radiographics. 1993;1394:841–52.
29. McMenamin ME, DeSchryver K, Fletcher CD. Fibrous lesions of the breast: a review. Int J Surg Pathol. 2008;8(2):99–108.
30. Wargotz ES, Norris HJ, Austin RM, et al. Fibromatosis of the breast. A clinical and pathological study of 28 cases. Am J Surg Pathol. 1987;11(1):38–45.
31. Rosen PP, Ernsberger D, Mammary fibromatosis. A benign spindle-cell tumor with significant risk for local recurrence. Cancer. 1989;63(7):1363–9.
32. Schnitt SJ, Collins LC. Biopsy interpretation of the breast. 3rd ed. Wolter Kluwer Health; 2018.
33. Rajakariar R, Walker RA. Pathological and biological features of mammographically detected invasive breast carcinomas. Br J Cancer. 1995;71(1):150–4.
34. Romano AM, Wages N, Smolkin M, et al. Tubular carcinoma of the breast: institutional and SEER database analysis supporting a unique classification. Breast Dis. 2015;35(2):103–11.
35. Rakha EA, Lee AH, Evans AJ, et al. Tubular carcinoma of the breast: further evidence to support its excellent prognosis. J Clin Oncol. 2010;28(1):99–104.
36. Harvey J, March. *Making the diagnosis*: a practical guided to breast imaging. Philadelphia, PA: Elsevier; 2013.
37. Sun J, Zhou J, Zhang W, et al. Tubular carcinomas of the breast: an epidemiologic study. Future Oncol. 2018;14(20):3037–47.
38. Rosen PP, Ernsberger D. Low-grade Adenosquamous carcinoma. A variant of metaplastic carcinoma. Am J Surg Pathol. 1987;11(5):351–8.
39. Ellis I, Collins L, Ichhara S, et al. Invasive carcinoma of no special type (NST). In: Lakhani S, Ellis IO, Schnitt SJ, et al, eds. WHO classification of tumors of the breast. 4th Lyon, France: IARC Press;2012.
40. Weigelt B, Horlings HM, Kreike B, et al. Refinement of breast cancer classification by molecular characterization of histological special types. J Pathol. 2008;216(2):141–50.
41. Cady B, Stone MD, Schuler JG, et al. The new era in breast cancer: invasion, size and nodal involvement

dramatically decreaing as a result of mammographic screening. Arch Surg. 1996;131(3):301–8.
42. Haakinson DJ, et al. A significant number of women present with palpable breast cancer even with normal mammogram within 1 year. Am J Surg. 2010;20(6):712–7.
43. Lakhani S, Rakha E, Simpson PT. Invasive lobular carcinoma. In: Lakhani S, Ellis IO, Schnitt SJ, et al., editors. WHO classification of tumors of the breast. Lyon, France: IARC Press; 2012.
44. Schnitt SJ, et al. American registry of pathology expert opinions: the spectrum of lobular carcinoma in situ: diagnostic features and clinical implications. Ann Diagn Pathol. 2020;45:151481.
45. Nakhlis F, et al. Evaluating the rate of upgrade to invasive breast cancer and/or DCIS following a core biopsy diagnosis of non-classic LCIS. Ann Surg Oncol. 2019;26:55–61.
46. American Society of Breast Surgeons Consensus Guidelines, copyright 2018.
47. Durand MA, Wang S, Hooley RJ, et al. Tomosynthesis-detected architectural distortion: management algorithm with radiologic-pathologic correlation. Radiographics. 2016;36(2):311–21.
48. Hicks, David G., and Susan Carole Lester. Diagnostic Pathology: Breast. Elsevier, 2021.
49. Da Silva L, Parry S, Reid L, et al. Aberrant expression of E-cadherin in lobular carcinomas of the breast. Am J Surg Pathol. 2008;32(5):773–83.
50. Zengel B, et al. Comparison of the clinicopathological features of invasive ductal, invasive lobular and mixed (invasive ductal +invasive lobular) carcinoma of the breast. Breast Cancer. 2013;22(4):374–81.
51. Leung JWT, Yang WT. 'Invasive Micropapillary Carcinoma'. In: Berg WA, Leung JWT, editors. Diagnostic Imaging: Breast. Philadelphia: Elsevier. 2019;720–23.

Focal and Developing Asymmetries

6

Steffanie Charlyne Tamayo, Liva Andrejeva, and Kamaljeet Singh

Pseudoangiomatous Stromal Hyperplasia (PASH)

Pseudoangiomatous Stromal Hyperplasia (PASH): PASH is a benign myofibroblastic proliferation involving breast fibrous stroma. PASH has possible hormonal etiology and it typically affects women in the reproductive age group. Male breasts can show PASH changes in a setting of gynecomastia. Often PASH is an incidental histological finding in breast biopsies performed for other lesions. Rarely PASH can present as a firm painless circumscribed mass, which has been called nodular PASH.

- **Clinical Presentation**: PASH occurs mainly in premenopausal women or postmenopausal women taking HRT and is thought to be hormonally induced. It is also commonly detected as an incidental histological finding alongside other entities, including breast cancer; therefore, careful clinical, imaging, and pathologic correlation is necessary. PASH forms the stromal component of the gynecomastia. Nodular PASH presents as a slow-growing breast mass that can clinically mimic fibroadenoma. PASH can involve axillary breast tissue.
- **Imaging Findings**: PASH can have a variable presentation: it may be palpable or screening detected or appear as a mass, architectural distortion, calcifications, or a focal or developing asymmetry [1, 2]. If imaging findings are highly suspicious (spiculated mass, highly suspicious architectural distortion, pleomorphic calcifications), then excision should be considered.
  - **Mammogram**: Variable appearance: focal or developing asymmetry is a common presentation [3].
  - **US**: May be sonographically occult. When a sonographic correlate is present, its appearance varies, ranging from circumscribed to irregular mass(es) to vague hypoechoic areas.
  - **MRI**: Areas of non-mass enhancement are most frequent, followed by enhancing masses and foci. Kinetics are most often persistent, with washout and plateau kinetics less common.
- **BIRADS**: Variable [2–4]
- **Differential Diagnosis**: Benign: fibrocystic change, fibrosis. Malignant: ILC.

S. C. Tamayo
Department of Pathology and Laboratory Medicine, Women and Infants Hospital of Rhode Island, Providence, RI, USA
e-mail: scatamayo1031@gmail.com

L. Andrejeva
Department of Radiology and Biomedical Imaging, Yale School of Medicine, New Haven, CT, USA
e-mail: liva.andrejeva@yale.edu

K. Singh (✉)
Department of Pathology and Laboratory Medicine, Brown University and Women and Infants Hospital of RI, Providence, RI, USA
e-mail: kamaljeet_singh@brown.edu

M. Harigopal et al. (eds.), *Radiology Pathology Correlations of Breast Lesions*,
https://doi.org/10.1007/978-3-031-65711-5_6

- **Pathology Findings**:
  - **Gross**: Nodular PASH size can range from 0.6 to 12 cm. Grossly, the mass is solid, tan-white, well-circumscribed, and firm.
  - **Microscopic Findings**: A typical PASH lesion is composed of dense fibrous stroma with slit-like spaces lined by benign myofibroblastic cells. The spaces in the fibrous tissue mimic thin-walled vessels, hence the name "pseudoangiomatous". The spindle cells have myofibroblastic phenotype, and the lining cells immunostain with CD34, vimentin, and smooth muscle actin. The lesion can involve intralobular as well as interlobular tissue. Adjacent lobules can show variable degrees of usual ductal hyperplasia, and overall changes are reminiscent of gynecomastoid hyperplasia. PASH can be composed of cellular stroma with a fascicular pattern. PASH can show unusual and alarming histological changes, including nuclear atypia, multinucleation, and metaplastic stromal differentiation [4].
- **Differential Diagnosis**: Myofibroblastoma, fibroadenoma, mammary hamartoma, angiosarcoma, and lobular carcinoma.
  - Myofibroblastoma is a benign myofibroblastic proliferation that often presents a well-circumscribed mass in postmenopausal females or males. No entrapped lobules or epithelial components are identified.
  - Nodular PASH can mimic fibroadenoma. The stroma of fibroadenoma can show PASH-like changes and therefore be confused with nodular PASH.
  - Epithelioid morphology of the stromal cells can raise a differential diagnosis of infiltrative epithelial lesion, especially invasive lobular carcinoma.
  - Angiosarcoma can be excluded by lack of specific vascular markers (ERG).
- **Management**: PASH is a benign lesion. The treatment depends upon clinical presentation. Nodular PASH can be managed by conservative excision. No treatment is required for incidental PASH that is not a target lesion.

Case 1

Clinical History: A 43-year-old female presented with palpable left breast nodularity (Figs. 6.1 and 6.2).

A surgical biopsy was recommended and performed as a stereotactic biopsy was deemed to be too difficult (Figs. 6.3, 6.4, 6.5, 6.6 and 6.7).

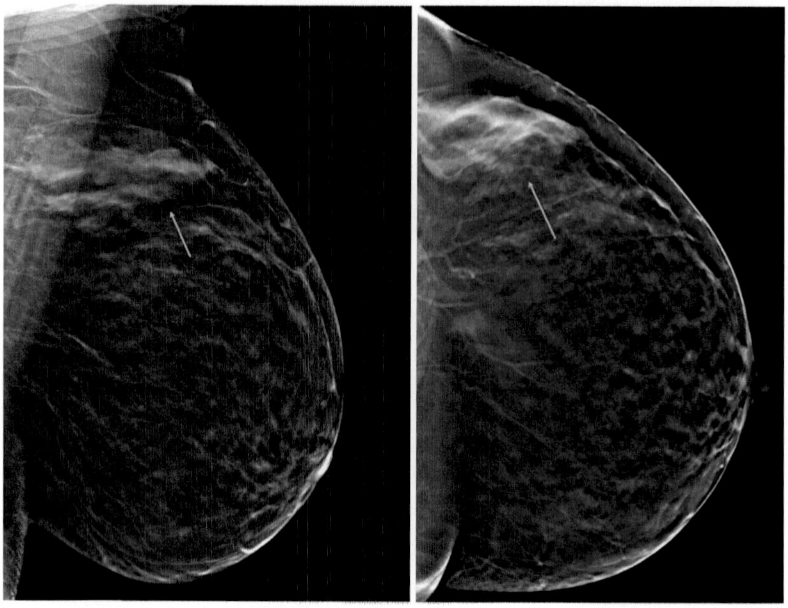

Figs. 6.1 and 6.2 Diagnostic mammogram images were evaluated and initially deemed probably benign, but the lesion became more palpable and more prominent on mammography

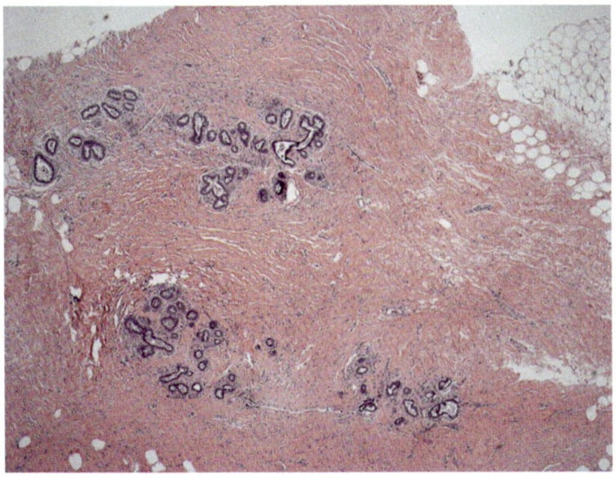

Fig. 6.3 (H&E, 2×) Benign breast tissue with lobules and fibrous stroma. The stroma is cellular and spindle cells form pseudovascular spaces. Pseudoangiomatous stromal hyperplasia (PASH)

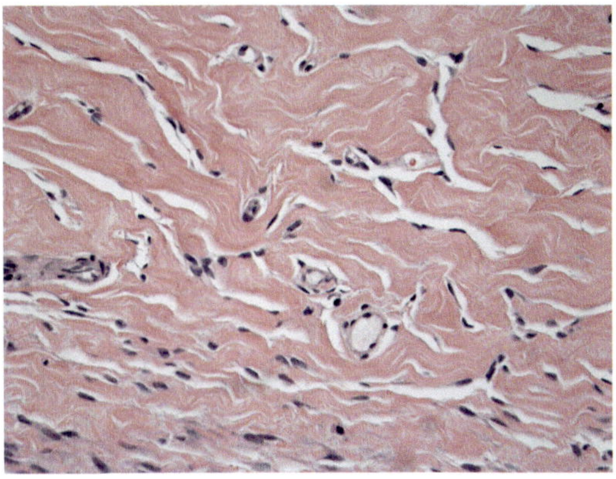

Fig. 6.5 (H&E, 20×) Benign breast tissue with pseudo-angiomatous stromal hyperplasia (PASH). Stromal spindle cells form pseudovascular spaces

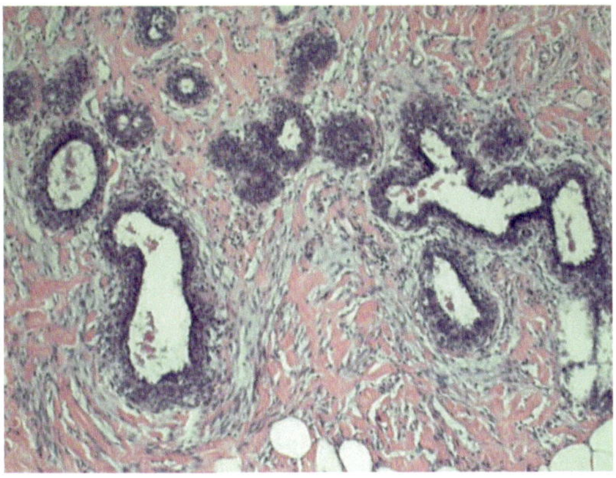

Fig. 6.4 (H&E, 10×) Benign breast tissue with pseudo-angiomatous stromal hyperplasia (PASH). The fibrous stroma is populated by spindle cells forming pseudovascular spaces and fascicular architecture

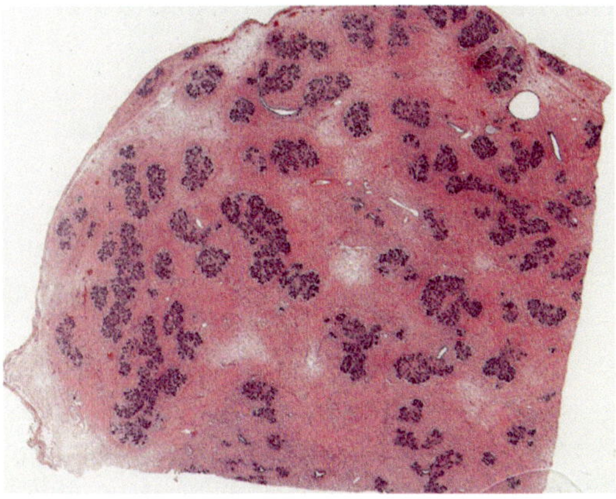

Fig. 6.6 (H&E low power) Nodular pseudoangiomatous stromal hyperplasia (PASH). The circumscribed nodule comprises benign lobules embedded in fibrous stroma diffusely involved by PASH

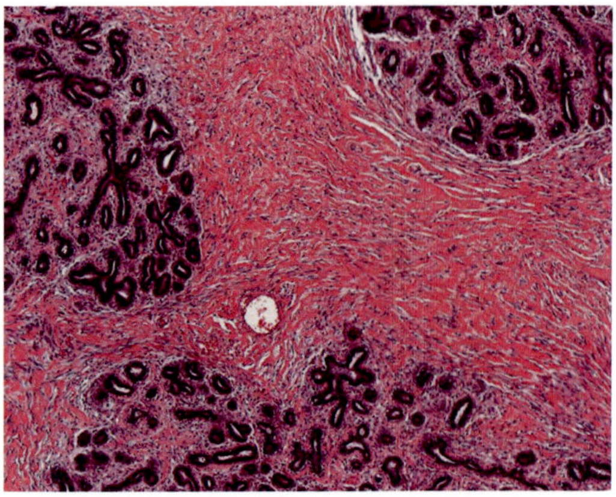

Fig. 6.7 (H&E, 10×) Nodular pseudoangiomatous stromal hyperplasia (PASH)

Normal Asymmetric Fibroglandular Tissue

Normal Asymmetric Fibroglandular Tissue:

- **Clinical Presentation**:
  Normal asymmetric fibroglandular tissue presents as an incidentally detected finding of focal or developing asymmetry.
- **Imaging Findings**: Islands of fibroglandular tissue are frequent causes of focal asymmetries. When these areas are dense than the remainder of the fibroglandular tissue and/or are positioned in an extreme posterior or medial position within the breast, where predominantly fatty tissue is usually found, the patient may be called back from screening for further evaluation. Weight loss can accentuate such islands of breast tissue as the interspersed fat diminishes. In premenopausal women, hormonal fluctuations may result in focal asymmetries due to fibroglandular breast tissue varying in prominence.
  - **Mammogram**: Round or oval focal asymmetries with internal fat, concave outward borders, similar in density to fibroglandular tissue elsewhere in the breast.
  - **US**: Negative, but can sometimes identify an island of breast tissue within surrounding fatty tissue.
  - **MRI**: Demonstrates background enhancement similar to fibroglandular tissue elsewhere in the breast, and has a T1 and T2 correlate.
  - **BIRADS**: 1, 2, or 3; occasionally, a 4 if features are atypical and cannot differentiate from a suspicious lesion.
  - **Differential Diagnosis**:
    Benign: Fibrocystic changes, fibroadenomatoid changes, fibrosis, fat necrosis, PASH.
    Malignant: ILC.
- **Pathology Findings**:
  - **Gross**: There are no distinct gross findings.
  - **Microscopic Findings**: The biopsy material shows benign breast tissue, including terminal duct lobular units and larger ducts embedded in fibrous stroma. A variable amount of adipose tissue is also present. However, many of these samples contain prominent fibrous stroma. Other stromal changes like pseudoangiomatous stromal hyperplasia can be present focally. The breast epithelial tissue may show variable minimal proliferative changes like mild usual ductal hyperplasia, columnar cell change, and small cysts. These epithelial and stromal changes are focal and do not account for any specific lesion.
  - **Differential Diagnosis**: Fibroadenoma, nodular PASH, radial scar. Focal PASH-like changes may raise a question of etiological association with the radiological findings. Nodular fibrous stroma may histologically mimic a fibroadenoma. However, there is no well-defined border to this change, and often, the nodular fibrous stroma merges with adjacent benign fibrous breast tissue indicating just nodular fibrous stroma rather than a fibroadenoma. The absence of fibroelastotic stroma would exclude radial scar.
- **Management**: A radiologic-pathologic correlation is needed to ensure the target lesion is sampled.

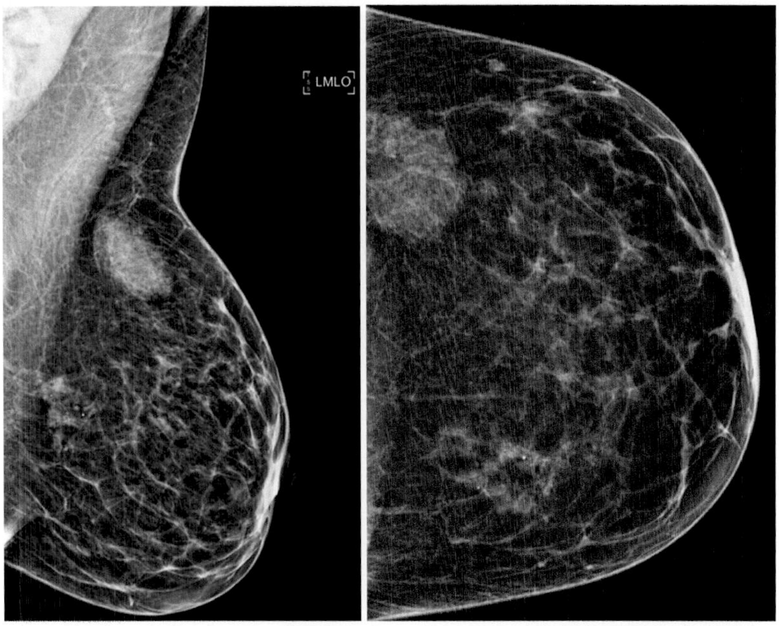

Figs. 6.8 and 6.9 Current mammogram

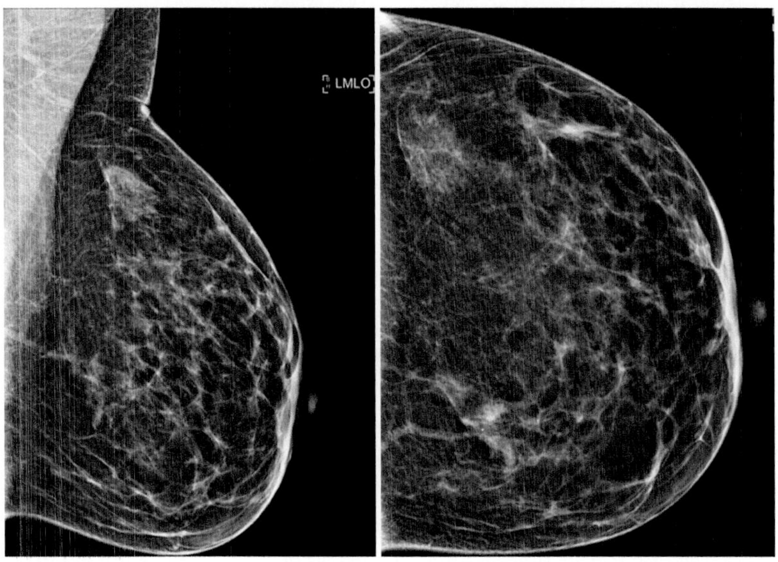

Figs. 6.10 and 6.11 MMG 3 years ago

Case 1

Clinical History: A 43-year-old female showed a developing asymmetry on a screening mammogram (Figs. 6.8, 6.9, 6.10, 6.11, 6.12 and 6.13).

Granulomatous Mastitis

Granulomatous Mastitis: Granulomatous mastitis (GM) is a benign inflammatory condition of the breast characterized by non-caseating granu-

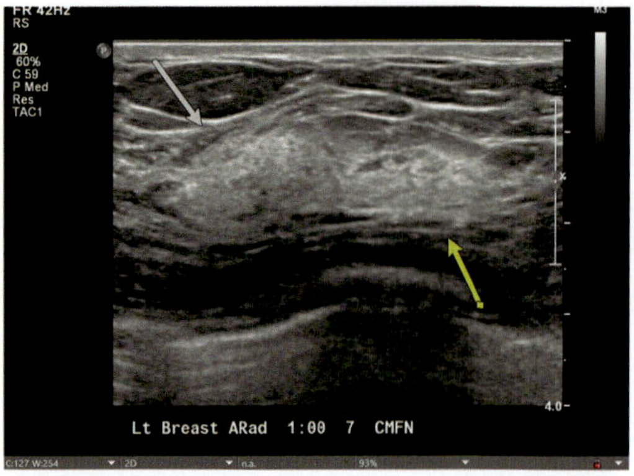

Fig. 6.12 Ultrasound shows a vague poorly defined mass-like area with variable echogenicity

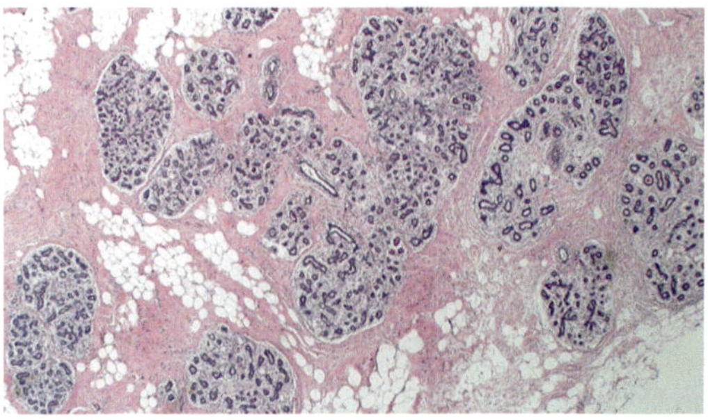

Fig. 6.13 Benign breast tissue (H&E, 4×). The core needle biopsy showed breast tissue with benign terminal duct lobular units. No histologic correlation was present for asymmetry

lomas accompanied by acute and chronic inflammatory infiltrate involving breast lobules and ducts. Most cases occur in women of reproductive age, rare cases are reported in male breast. The GM has a predilection for Hispanic women. Granulomatous mastitis is linked to rheumatic autoimmune diseases, high prolactin levels, and *corynebacteria* infection. Cystic neutrophilic granulomatous mastitis (CNGM), a subtype of granulomatous mastitis, shows distinct histological features, and it is recently linked to *Croynebacterium* species. The CNGM presents as a single or multiple symptomatic masses in a multiparous breastfeeding women. The GM can present with abscesses and periareolar skin fistulas. Relapse and chronic course are seen in a significant minority of GM patients [5, 6].

- **Clinical Presentation**:
  Granulomatous mastitis has nonspecific clinical features, often presenting as a painful palpable lump in a woman of reproductive age with or without associated nipple retraction or discharge and axillary lymphadenopathy. Other inflammatory features such as erythema, skin thickening, and sinus tract formation can also be seen, thereby mimicking inflammatory breast carcinoma [7]. Delay in diagnosis is common.
- **Imaging Findings**: Non-puerperal mastitis can occur in women of all ages and may be bacterial or nonbacterial, the latter including plasma cell and granulomatous mastitis. The exact etiology of this disorder is not known. The patients may present with breast mass(es), pain, breast edema and erythema, and occasionally nipple discharge.
  - **Mammogram**: Findings are variable, a focal asymmetry being the most common. An US-guided biopsy may frequently be necessary to establish the diagnosis, as the patients, even when demonstrating signs and symptoms of mastitis, may not respond to antibiotic treatment. Associated axillary adenopathy may be present. However, with diffuse involvement of the breast, the mammographic findings may mimic those of inflammatory breast cancer, with diffuse skin and trabecular thickening present.
  - **US**: Hypoechoic masses or coalescent hypoechoic serpiginous areas in ductal distribution may be seen. Hypervascularity may be demonstrated in the surrounding tissue.
  - **MRI**: Although MRI is not indicated for the evaluation or follow-up of mastitis and does not aid in distinguishing mastitis from malignancy, it is still occasionally performed due to suspicious clinical signs and symptoms. The MRI findings can also be variable, with non-mass enhancement in regional distribution, with T2 bright correlates being most common.
  - **BIRADS**: 4A-4C.
  - **Differential Diagnosis**: Benign: diabetic mastopathy. Malignant: inflammatory breast CA, ILC, noncalcified DCIS.

- **Pathology Findings**:
  - **Gross**: There are no specific gross findings of granulomatous mastitis. Most histological diagnoses are rendered on core needle biopsies with no specific findings. The excised tissue can show firm, ill-defined gray tan mass with ill-defined margins. Chronic and persistent disease can present with skin fistula.
  - **Microscopic Findings**: The histological findings depend on the duration of the disease. In the early stages, the core needle biopsy specimen shows a variable amount of lobule-centric acute and chronic inflammation accompanied by non-necrotizing granulomas. Microscopic empty spaces rimmed with neutrophils are often seen adjacent to the granulomas. Histiocytic giant cells can be present. Inflammation involves surrounding ducts and interlobular fibrous tissue. In later stages, abscess formation, pseudocystic change with granulation tissue, and fibrosis can be seen. Bacterial microorganisms can be identified in the empty spaces.
  - **Differential Diagnosis**: Carcinoma, ruptured cyst, duct ectasia, mastitis. Mastitis can mimic carcinoma. Therefore the goal of tissue sampling is to exclude carcinoma and discern the etiology of mastitis. Microbiology studies like culture can help to pin down the etiology of mastitis and guide medical management. Tubercular mastitis needs to be excluded. Unlike tuberculosis, granulomas in CNGM are non-necrotizing.
- **Management**: Because of unclear and variable etiology, managing granulomatous mastitis is controversial. Treatment options include surveillance, systemic antibiotics, oral corticosteroids, limited or wide surgical excision and mastectomies [8–10].

Case 1

Clinical History: A 32-year-old female presented with a painful palpable area in the left breast (Figs. 6.14, 6.15, 6.16 and 6.17–6.19).

BI-RADS: 4a, low suspicion of malignancy.

An US-guided biopsy was performed (Figs. 6.20, 6.21 and 6.22).

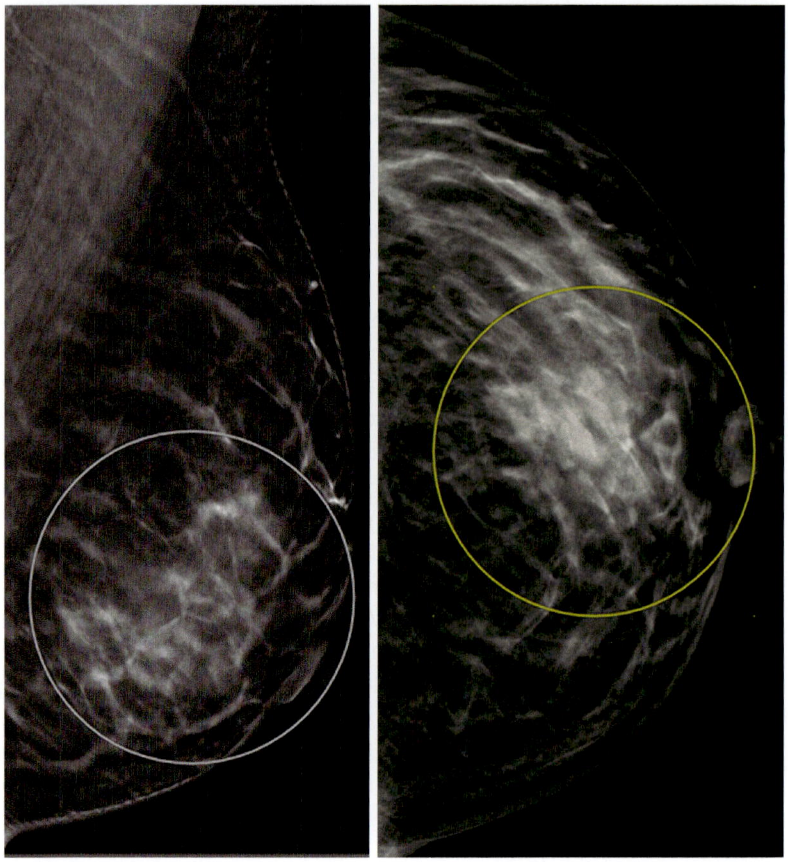

Figs. 6.14 and 6.15 MG: Mammogram demonstrates a relatively hyperdense focal asymmetry in the central aspect of the breast

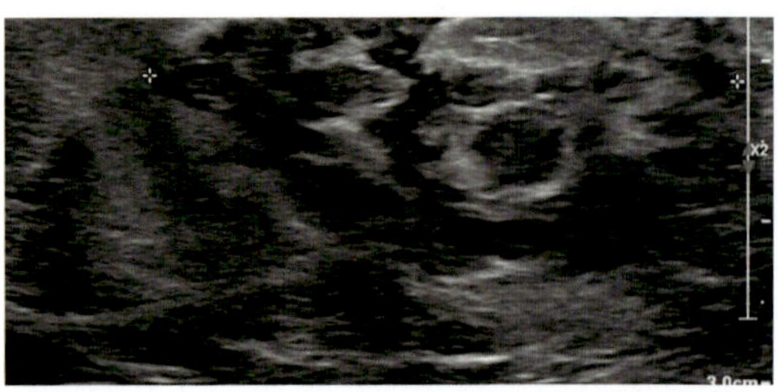

Fig. 6.16 US: Hypoechoic serpiginous areas in ductal distribution

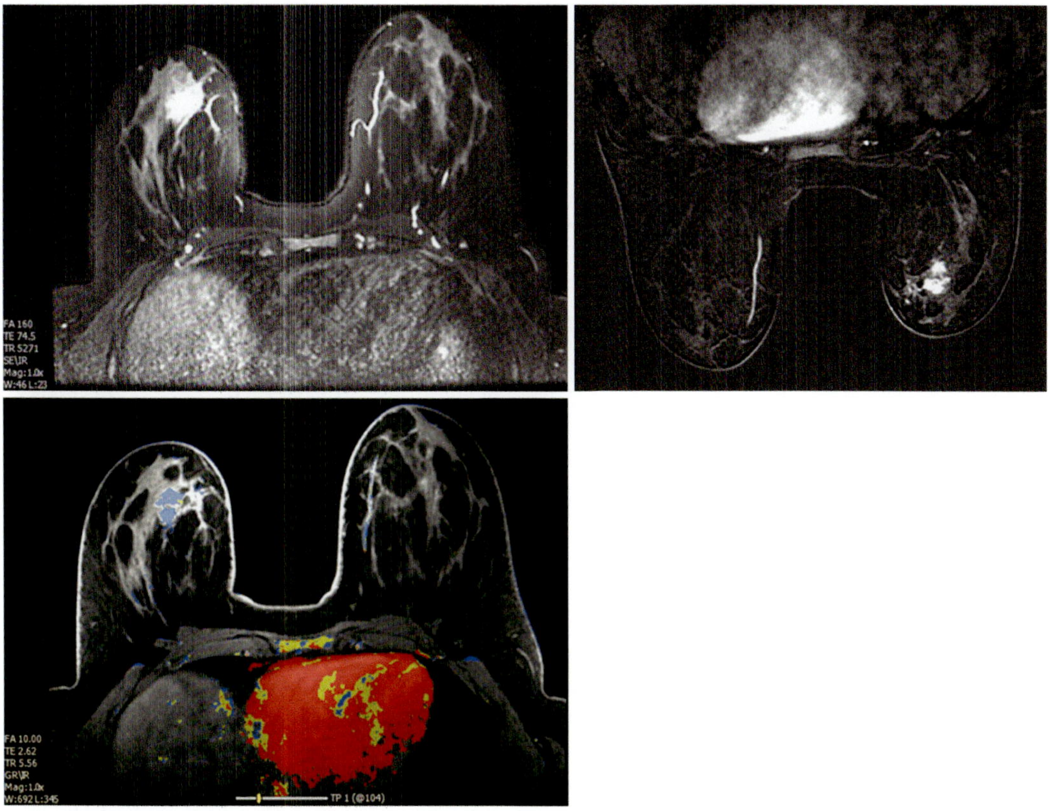

Figs. 6.17–6.19 MRI showed an irregular mass with an irregular margin, persistently and homogeneously enhancing. This is a somewhat atypical presentation

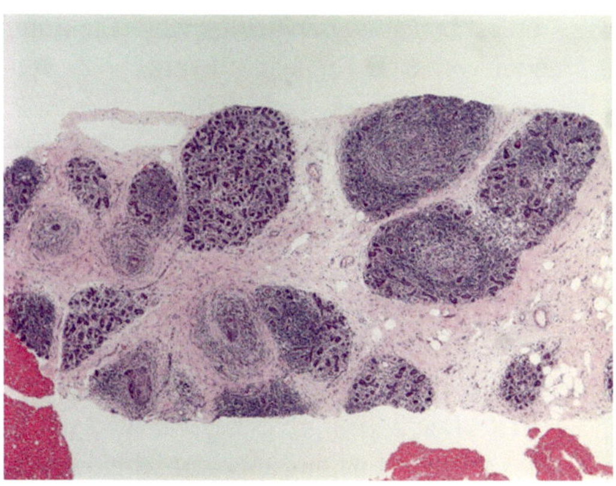

Fig. 6.20 Granulomatous mastitis (H&E, 4×). Benign breast tissue with inflammatory infiltrate involving the lobules and ducts

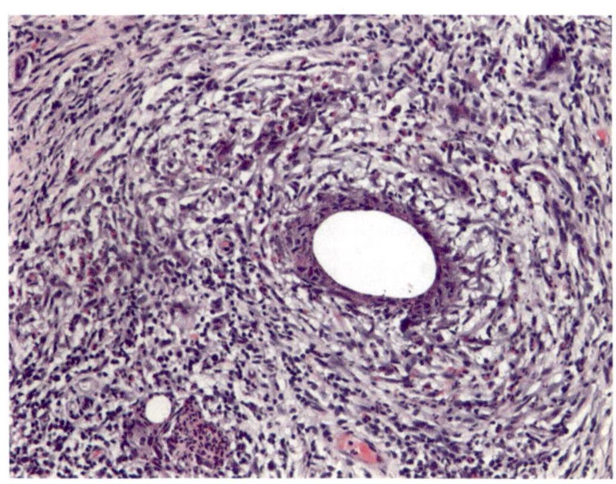

Fig. 6.21 Granulomatous mastitis (H&E, 20×). The inflammatory infiltrate comprises epithelioid histiocytes, lymphocytes, plasma cells, eosinophils, and some neutrophils. Round spaces in the center of inflammation are distinct histological changes of cystic neutrophilic granulomatous mastitis (CNGM)

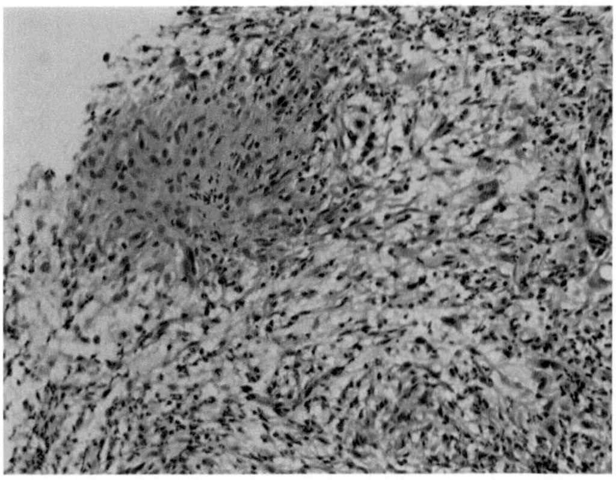

Fig. 6.22 Granulomatous mastitis (H&E, 40×). A granuloma composed of a nodular collection of epithelioid histiocytes is surrounded by lymphocytes, plasma cells, eosinophils, and neutrophils

Gynecomastia

Gynecomastia: Gynecomastia is a non-neoplastic enlargement of the male breast, presenting as a painful, palpable, firm, mobile mass in newborns, adolescents, and older individuals. It has been associated with physiologic fluctuations in estrogen levels and with pathologic states such as androgen deficiency, obesity, certain medication intake, and liver and kidney disease. Physiologic gynecomastia is seen in almost 25% of cases [11].

- **Clinical Presentation**: Gynecomastia occurs as a result of physiologic and pathologic imbalances of androgen and estrogen levels in males, which may be idiopathic or due to various medical conditions (hepatic dysfunction, hypogonadism, testicular malignancy, and others) or due to use of different prescription and nonprescription drugs. Gynecomastia may occur in the newborn period, during puberty, and after the age of 60. It is usually bilateral but may be unilateral.
- **Imaging Findings**: Frequently suspected clinically, men are referred for mammography to evaluate a retroareolar lump, which is frequently tender, or breast enlargement. Regardless of its etiology, the imaging appearance is similar. The three types of gynecomastia are: nodular, dendritic, and diffuse, which correlate with mammographic appearance. Ultrasound is a helpful adjunct tool to evaluate gynecomastia presenting with dense fibroglandular tissue, which can obscure an associated breast cancer.
  - **Mammogram**: Findings vary depending on the phase. Nodular gynecomastia, the acute phase, may present with a dense, nearly spherical, or oval focal area of fibroglandular tissue in the retroareolar region, sometimes extending into the upper outer quadrant. This type of gynecomastia may recede if the precipitating cause is resolved. However, if the underlying cause persists, gynecomastia may progress into a transitional phase, when progressive deposition of dense fibrous tissue occurs that obliterates the proliferated ducts, which leads to the dendritic phase, where flame-like fibroglandular retroareolar tissue is seen, which resembles a female breast with a scattered fibroglandular tissue density. If there is prolonged exposure to estrogen, diffuse gynecomastia may occur, which has an appearance similar to a heterogeneously dense female breast [12].
  - **US**: Nodular gynecomastia resembles a breast bud sonographically, while dendritic gynecomastia appears hypoechoic retroareolar tissue with fingerlike hypoechoic areas extending posteriorly. Diffuse gynecomastia mimics the sonographic appearance of dense breast tissue in a female.
  - **MRI**: Gynecomastia appears similar to normal fibroglandular breast tissue on all sequences.
  - **BIRADS**: 2, benign; gynecomastia usually has a typical imaging appearance. However, beware of associated breast cancer, which is rare, but the index of suspicion should be raised if additional symptoms, such as nipple discharge, nipple changes, enlarged axillary lymph node(s), or a lump that is not directly retroareolar, are present.
  - **Differential Diagnosis**: Carcinoma, PASH, myofibroblastoma, hamartoma.

- **Pathology Findings**:
  - **Gross**: There are no specific gross findings, and often, breast tissue consists of an ill-defined fibrous breast tissue. The breast tissue is usually fibrous and poorly defined mass-forming tissue, often containing some adipose tissue. The cut surface may be slightly myxoid or shiny without any well-defined mass.
  - **Microscopic Findings**: The breast tissue shows ducts and fibrous stroma with variable extent of proliferative changes. The ductal epithelium often shows mild to moderate usual ductal hyperplasia characterized by loose papillary projections, which can mimic micropapillary ADH or DCIS. The ducts with UDH are often accompanied by variably cellular myxoid or fibrous/hyalinized stroma with pseudoangiomatous stromal hyperplasia (PASH).
  - **Differential Diagnosis**: Pseudogynecomastia (prominence of subareolar adipose tissue), myofibroblastoma, and breast carcinoma.
- **Management**: Symptomatic and supportive treatment for physiologic causes; removal of offending medication; management of co-morbidities; anti-estrogen therapy; surgical excision for symptomatic and persistent lesions.

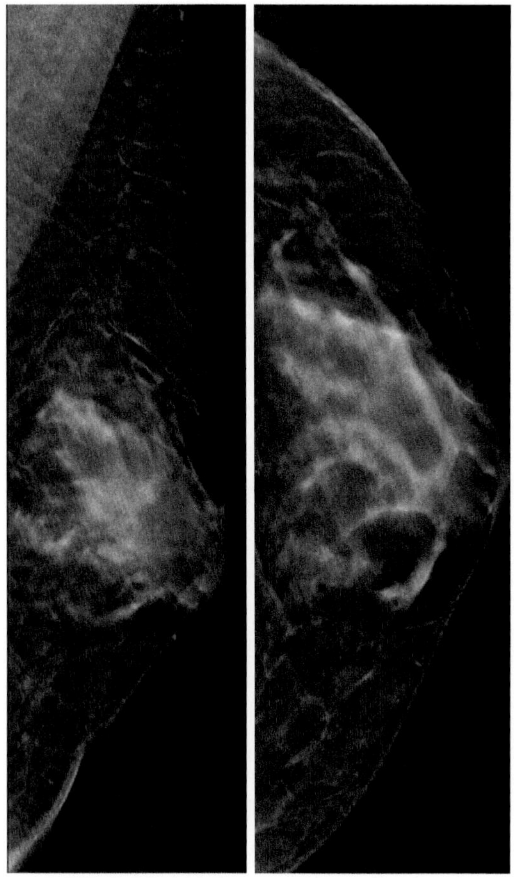

Figs. 6.23 and 6.24 **MG**: Dense retroareaolar fibroglandular tissue which extends into the upper outer quadrant in a pattern resembling nodular gynecomastia

Case 1

Clinical History: A 63-year-old male with a palpable, tender left retroareolar mass (Figs. 6.23, 6.24 and 6.25).

BI-RADS: 2, benign findings. Clinical follow-up was recommended (Fig. 6.26).

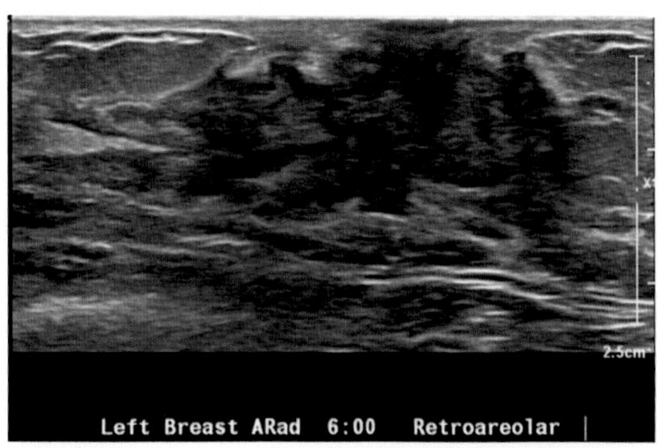

Fig. 6.25 **US**: Dense retroareolar tissue resembles a breast bud. No other abnormalities are demonstrated

Case 2

Clinical History: A 50-year-old male presented with a palpable mass just above the level of the nipple (Figs. 6.27, 6.28, 6.29 and 6.30).

BI-RADS: 4, suspicious findings.

An US-guided biopsy of the mass was recommended and performed, yielding IDC, NOS.

Follow-up: The patient subsequently underwent a mastectomy and axillary lymph node biopsy, which yielded one lymph node positive for metastasis (Figs. 6.31 and 6.32).

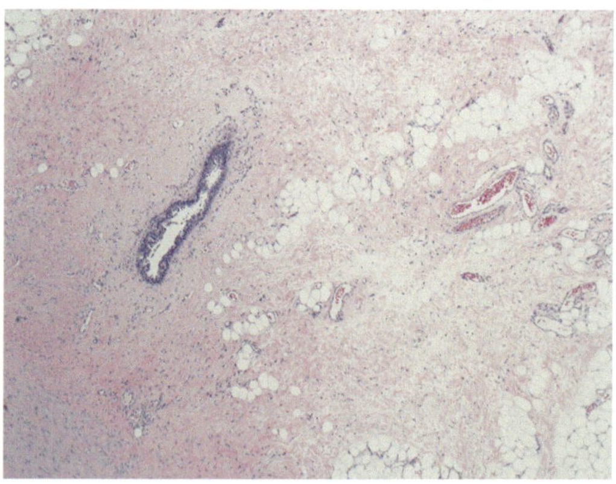

Fig. 6.26 (H&E, 10×) Male breast tissue comprising of duct with usual ductal hyperplasia and prominent fibrous tissue

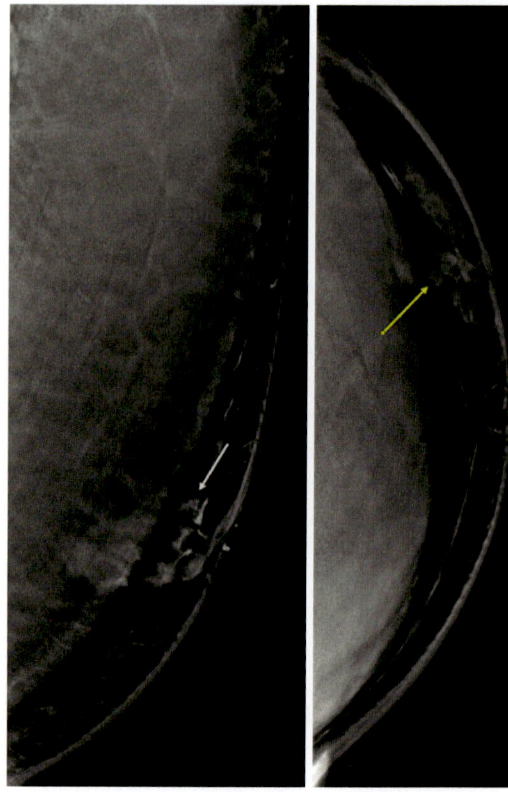

Figs. 6.27 and 6.28 Mammogram findings: Dense retroareolar fibroglandular tissue that extends into the upper outer quadrant, in a pattern resembling nodular gynecomastia, but at the area of palpable nodularity, there is a subtle oval mass with a partially circumscribed, partially obscured margin

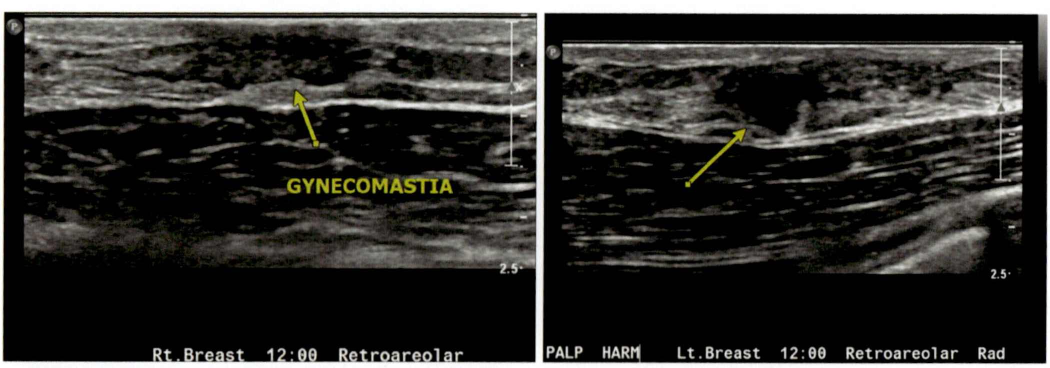

Figs. 6.29 and 6.30 Ultrasound findings: Corresponding to the palpable mass, there is a round, hypoechoic mass with an indistinct margin that is located at the edge of the area of retroareolar gynecomastia. The axillary lymph nodes appeared normal

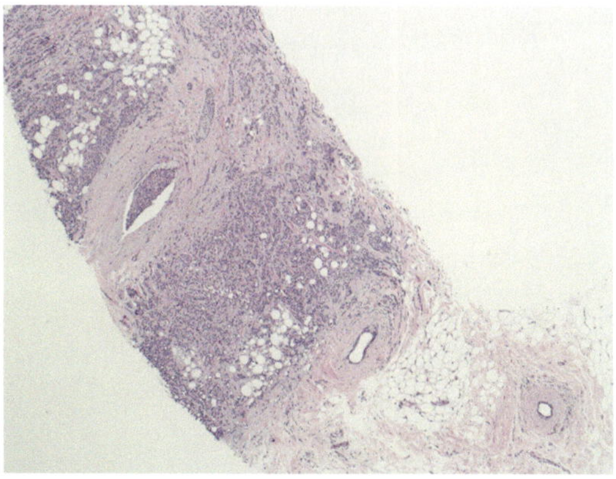

Fig. 6.31 (H&E, 4×) Invasive carcinoma arising in a background of gynecomastia. Male breast tissue consists of ducts and fibrous stroma (lower portion). Invasive breast carcinoma and associated ductal carcinoma in situ (top portion)

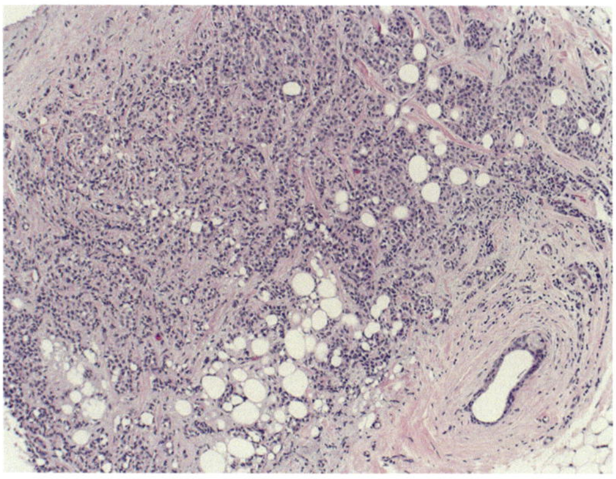

Fig. 6.32 (H&E, 20×) Invasive carcinoma arising in a background of gynecomastia. Male breast tissue involved by an invasive breast carcinoma

Fat Necrosis

Fat Necrosis: Fat necrosis is characterized by infarction of the adipose tissue, which is accompanied by fibrosis and reparative changes. The etiology includes trauma, therapy, and idiopathic. The fat necrosis can clinically and radiologically mimic carcinoma. Therefore correlation with history of trauma or recent intervention is important. Fat necrosis can eventually undergo fibrosis and dystrophic calcification.

- **Clinical Presentation**: Fat necrosis can be an incidental finding or present as a palpable painless lump(s) that may be smooth, round, firm, or irregular. The most common location is in the subareolar and periareolar areas and superficial breast tissue. Associated signs and symptoms include erythema, ecchymosis, skin and nipple retraction, and axillary lymphadenopathy. More than half of palpable cases are adherent to the skin [13], and the overall clinical picture simulates that of carcinoma. History of trauma is not always present, and it is more commonly seen because of surgery or radiotherapy.
- **Imaging Findings**: **(discussed elsewhere)**.
- **Pathology Findings**:
  - **Gross**: Yellow-gray mass that is poorly defined. Hemorrhage, calcification, and cystic degeneration may be seen.
  - **Microscopic Findings**: In the early stage, histopathologic examination reveals disruption of adipose tissue by hemorrhage and an inflammatory infiltrate composed predominantly of histiocytes, hemosiderin-laden macrophages, lymphocytes, and plasma cells. Eosinophils may be present. Fibrosis eventually develops, and late-stage lesions are replaced by fibrous tissue, which may ossify.
- **Differential Diagnosis**: Granular cell tumor, ruptured cyst, radiation/surgery-related changes, amyloidosis involving breast, and breast carcinoma. Fat necrosis due to trauma or any intervention needs clinical correlation. Fat necrosis is part of the spectrum of the histological changes secondary to radiation and surgery, mandating a clinical correlation with the histological findings. Reparative changes following a ruptured cyst can have a component of fat necrosis. Amyloidosis can contain a component of fat necrosis and lymphoplasmacytic infiltrate. Granular cell tumor cells can mimic the histiocytic component of the fat necrosis.
- **Management**: Symptomatic treatment and short-term clinical and radiologic follow-up; surgical excision for suspicious masses.

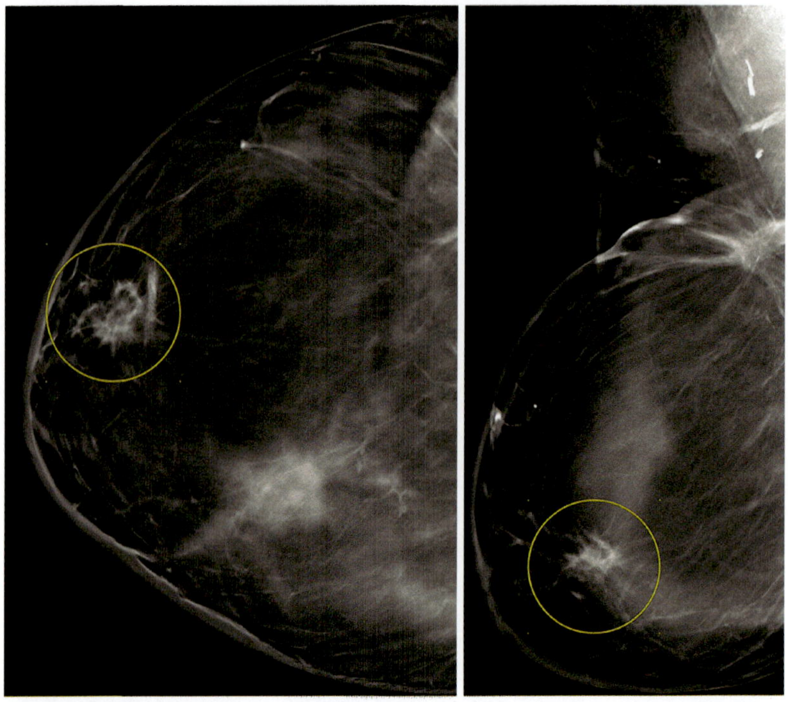

Figs. 6.33 and 6.34 Mammogram findings: Focal developing, fat-containing asymmetry in the lower outer aspect of the right breast

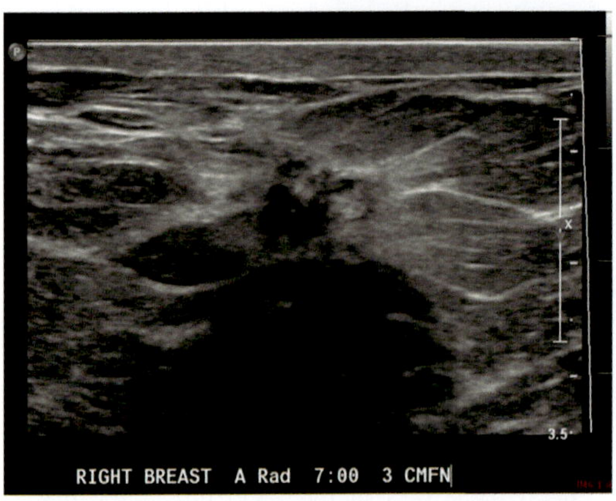

Fig. 6.35 Ultrasound findings: Irregular, largely hypoechoic mass

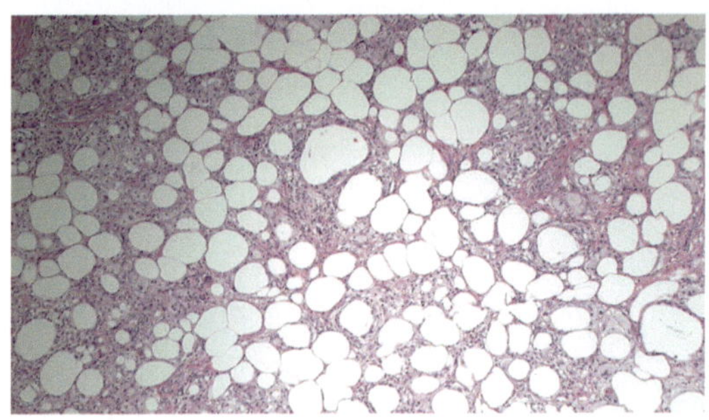

Fig. 6.36 Fat necrosis (H&E, 4×). Adipose tissue is surrounded by histiocytes, multinucleated giant cells, lymphocytes, and neutrophils

Case 1

Clinical History: A 67-year-old female with a history of a right well-differentiated IDC 10 years ago, now with a developing focal asymmetry demonstrated on screening mammography in a site remote from her lumpectomy scar (Figs. 6.33, 6.34 and 6.35).

BI-RADS: 4, suspicious findings.

An US-guided biopsy was performed and demonstrated fat necrosis (Fig. 6.36).

Stromal Fibrosis

Stromal Fibrosis: Stromal fibrosis is a poorly defined entity. Fibrosis is the end result of any tissue injury; therefore, any ischemic, inflammatory event or trauma involving the breast can lead to stromal fibrosis. In many breast biopsies, normal breast tissue can show prominent fibrous stroma, which may be labeled as stromal fibrosis. History of previous surgical intervention, radiation, or trauma may explain the finding of reparative changes and fibrosis. Clinical correlation is required, and radiology pathology correlation is imperative to ascertain that the target lesion is sampled [14].

- **Imaging Findings**: Stromal fibrosis may result in the perimenopausal period from proliferation of fibrous stroma and atrophy of ducts and lobules or as a result of chronic mastitis, diabetic mastopathy, or due to radiation treatment for breast cancer. It may be an incidental finding on screening mammography or present as a firm, painless, palpable area.
  - **Mammography**: Stromal fibrosis may present a focal, developing asymmetry in the axillary tail of the breast. Less frequently, it may appear as a mass or an architectural distortion. Calcifications are infrequent.
  - **Ultrasound**: Most frequently presents as a hypoechoic mass with circumscribed to indistinct margins that may exhibit posterior shadowing.
  - **MRI**: May be difficult to distinguish from breast cancer; may appear as linear non-mass enhancement or, less commonly, an irregular mass, usually with persistent kinetics.
  - **Differential Diagnosis**: Benign: normal dense tissue, PASH, degenerated FA, diabetic mastopathy, sclerosing adenosis. Malignant: IDC, ILC.
- **Pathology Findings**: The histological findings range from benign breast tissue with hypocellular nodular fibrous stroma to a fibrous scar comprising variably cellular fibrous connective tissue populated with reactive myofibroblastic cells and connective tissue.
  - **Gross Findings**: There are no specific gross findings.
  - **Microscopic Findings**:

    Nodular Fibrous Stroma in Benign Breast Tissue: The microscopic examination shows benign breast tissue comprising terminal duct lobules and ducts separated by hypocellular dense collagenous stroma. The stromal cells have benign spindle nuclei without any atypia. The fibrous stroma can form a circumscribed interface with adjacent fatty breast tissue.

    Fibrous Scar: Histological examination reveals fibrosis involving the breast parenchyma comprising reactive myofibroblasts and collagen deposition. Hemosideirn deposits, small congested vessels, and mild chronic inflammation can be evident. Older lesions show a reduction in cellularity and an increase in collagenous tissue. Multinucleated giant may be present. Dystrophic calcifications can be present in stromal fibrosis, especially following radiation treatment.
- **Differential Diagnoses**: Diabetic/lymphocytic mastopathy, benign and malignant spindle cell lesions of the breast: PASH, fibroadenoma, neurofibroma, fibromatosis, and metaplastic carcinoma. The nodular fibrous stroma can mimic nodular PASH. The absence of cleft-like pseudovascular spaces favors nodular fibrous stroma. Fibromatosis and low-grade fibromatosis-like metaplastic carcinoma are infiltrative lesions. The tumor cells have myofibroblastic phenotype, but both of these lesions are characterized by infiltration of breast parenchyma and fatty tissue.
- **Management**: Radiology-pathology correlation is needed to ensure that the target lesion is sampled. In a concordant setting, no excision is warranted.

Case 1

Clinical History: A 39-year-old female complained of a palpable mass in the right axillary tail region (Figs. 6.37 and 6.38 and 6.39).

BI-RADS: 4, suspicious findings.

US-guided biopsy was recommended and performed, yielding stromal fibrosis and perilobular chronic inflammation consistent with diabetic mastopathy (Fig. 6.40 and 6.41).

Case 2

Clinical History: A 58-year-old female with a history of ADH presents for a screening MRI (Figs. 6.42, 6.43, 6.44, 6.45 and 6.46).

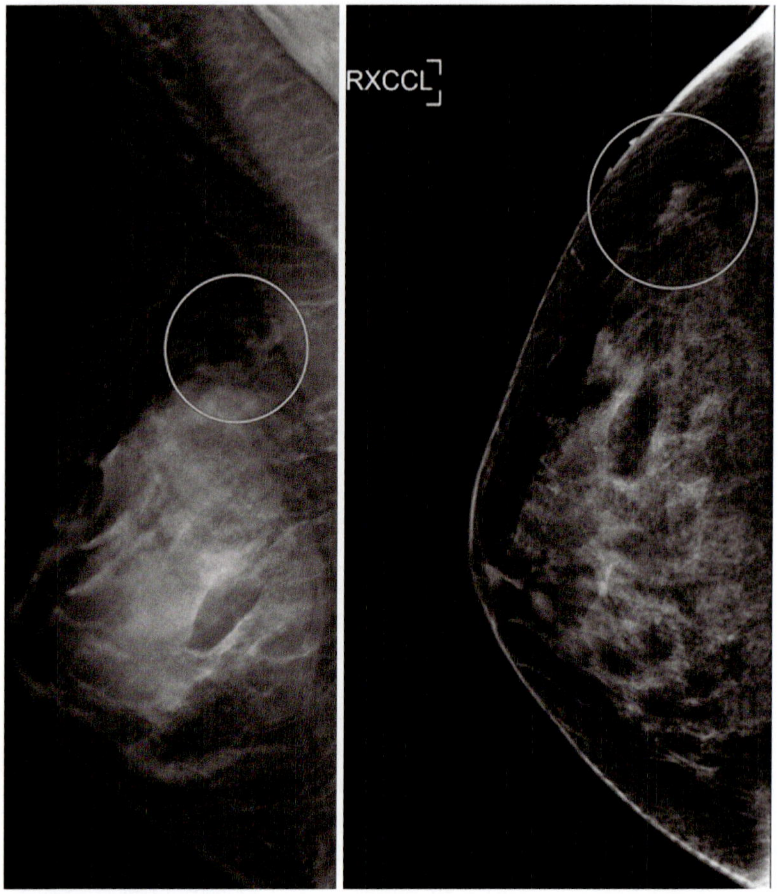

Figs. 6.37 and 6.38 Mammogram findings: A focal, irregular, fat-containing asymmetry correlates as palpated

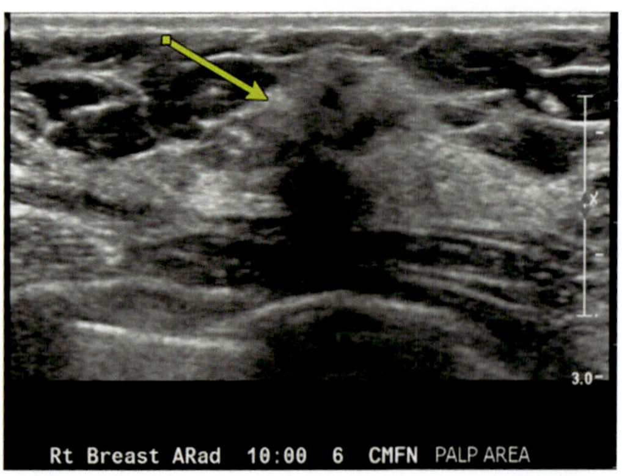

Fig. 6.39 Ultrasound findings: Mixed echogenic and hypoechoic irregular mass with an indistinct margin

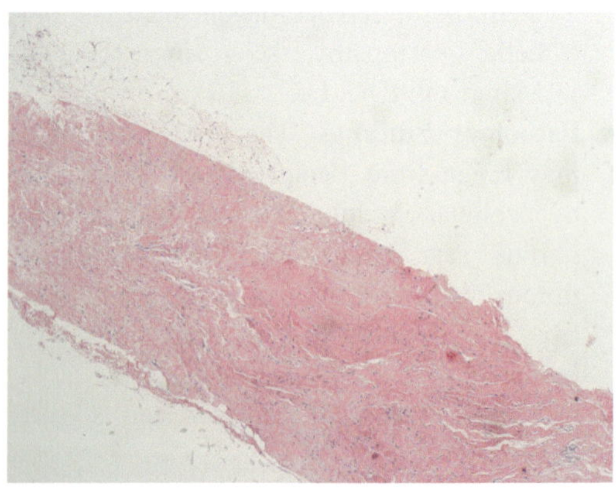

Fig. 6.40 (H&E, 4×) Keloidal collagenous tissue with reactive epithelioid myofibroblasts

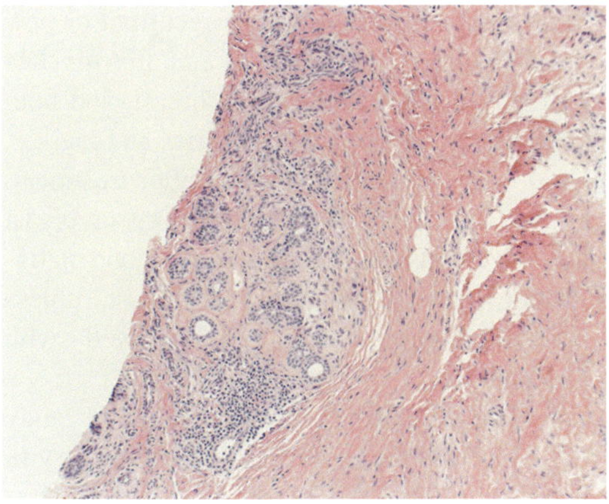

Fig. 6.41 (H&E, 10×) Terminal duct lobule and interlobular stroma with chronic inflammation

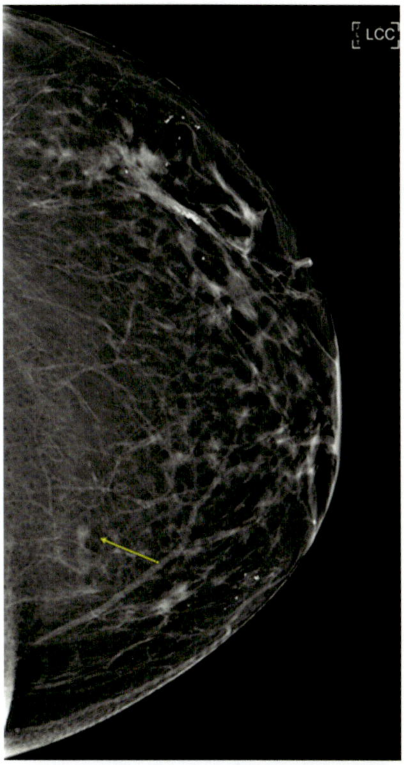

Fig. 6.42 The most recent mammogram was normal

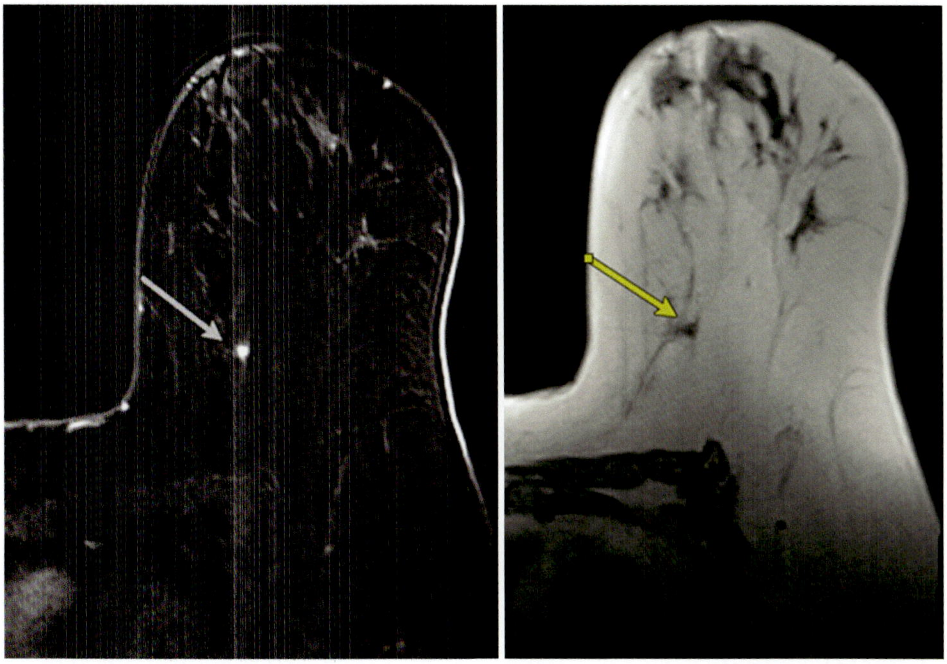

Figs. 6.43 and 6.44 MRI: A small, irregular, persistently enhancing mass in the upper inner left breast has a T1 hypointense correlate. A second look US was negative, and the mammogram showed a possible asymmetry on the CC view only that may correlate with the MRI finding. The MRI finding was subsequently biopsied with MRI guidance, yielding benign breast tissue with stromal fibrosis

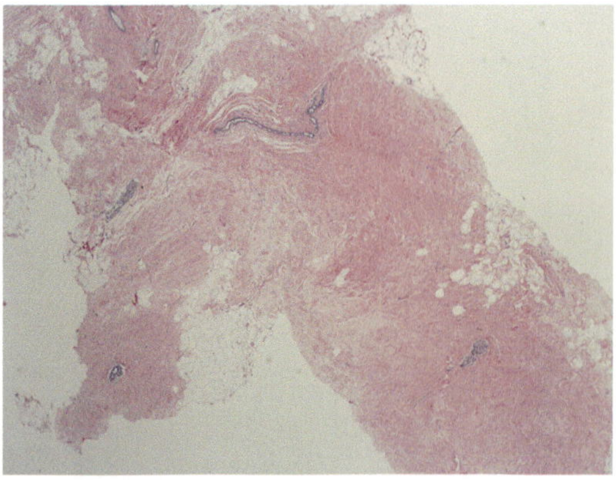

Fig. 6.45 (H&E, 2×) Benign breast tissue with nodular collagenous fibrous stroma

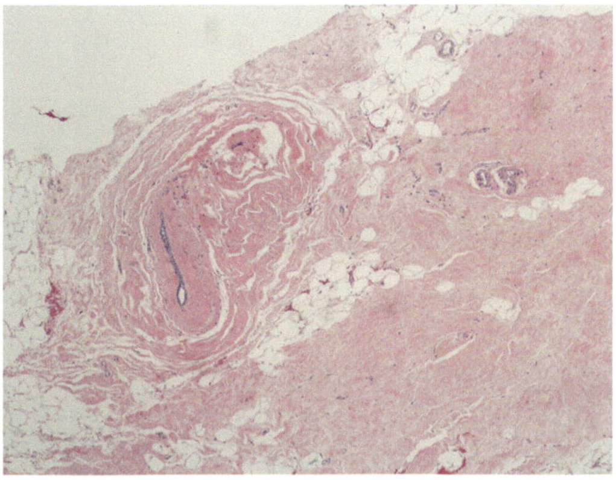

Fig. 6.46 (H&E, 4×) Benign breast tissue with nodular collagenous fibrous stroma

Postsurgical/Radiation Scar

Postsurgical/Radiation Scar:

- **Clinical Presentation**:
  May be an incidental imaging finding during routine follow-up or present clinically as a palpable lump, skin thickening, or skin retraction after biopsy, surgery, or radiation therapy. Symptoms may occur years after a surgical procedure [15, 16].
- **Imaging Findings**: Breast conservation therapy followed by radiation can produce significant changes within the breast, which may be difficult to distinguish from recurrent or new malignancies. Fat necrosis and fibrosis frequently occur in the treated breast, and both can present as focal asymmetries and masses, and both can occur for years after treatment. Given that patients with a history of breast cancer are at increased risk for a second malignancy, new findings in the breast, unless clearly benign, are to be viewed with suspicion.
  - **Mammogram**: Stromal fibrosis may present a focal, developing asymmetry in the axillary tail of the breast. Less frequently, it may appear as a mass or an architectural distortion. Calcifications are infrequent.
  - **US**: Most frequently presents as a hypoechoic mass circumscribed to indistinct margins that may exhibit posterior shadowing.
  - **MRI**: May be difficult to distinguish from breast cancer; may appear as linear non-mass enhancement or, less commonly, an irregular mass, usually with persistent kinetics.
  - **BIRADS**: 2, 3, or 4, depending on appearance and clinical history.
  - **Differential Diagnosis**:
    Benign: normal dense tissue, PASH, degenerated FA, diabetic mastopathy, sclerosing adenosis.
    Malignant: IDC, ILC.
- **Pathology Findings**:
  - **Gross**: Irregular or spiculated, firm, yellow-white mass, which may be 1–3 cm in size.
  - **Microscopic Findings**: Benign breast tissue with dense fibrous stroma. Post-procedural changes such as hemorrhage, clusters of hemosiderin-laden macrophages, necrosis, and squamous metaplasia may also be present.
  - **Differential Diagnosis**: Radial scar/complex sclerosing lesion, tubular carcinoma, low-grade adenosquamous carcinoma.
- **Management**: Observation with close clinical and radiologic follow-up.

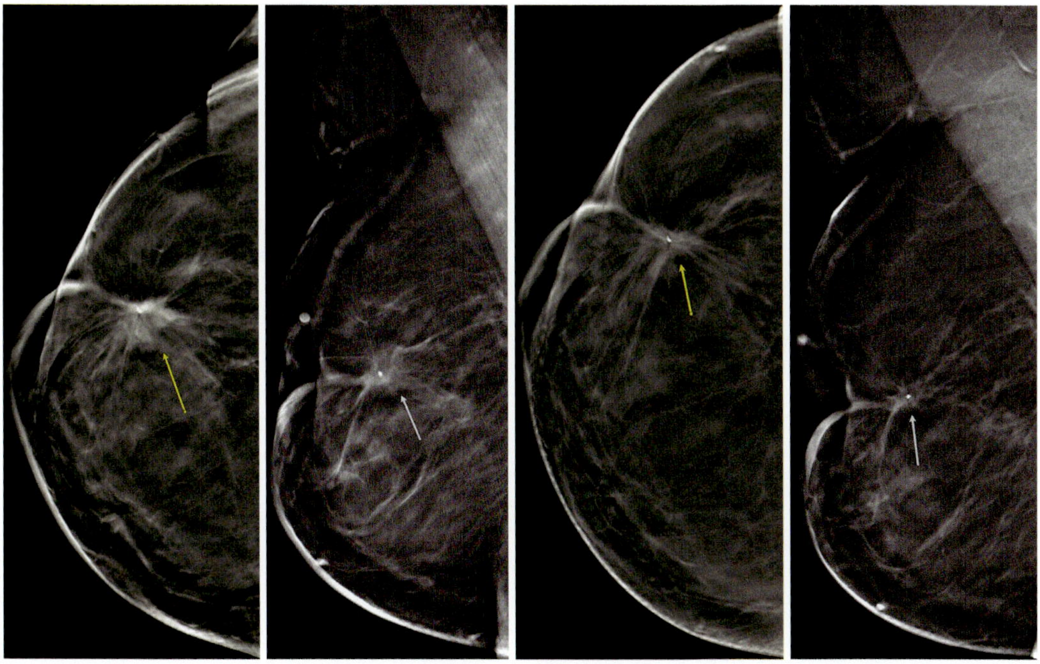

Figs. 6.47–6.50 **Mammogram findings**: Focal developing, fat-containing asymmetry in the lower outer aspect of the right breast

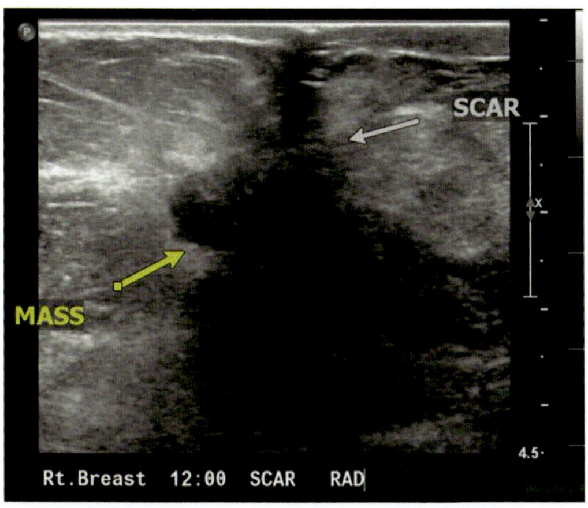

Fig. 6.51 **Ultrasound findings**: Irregular, largely hypoechoic mass

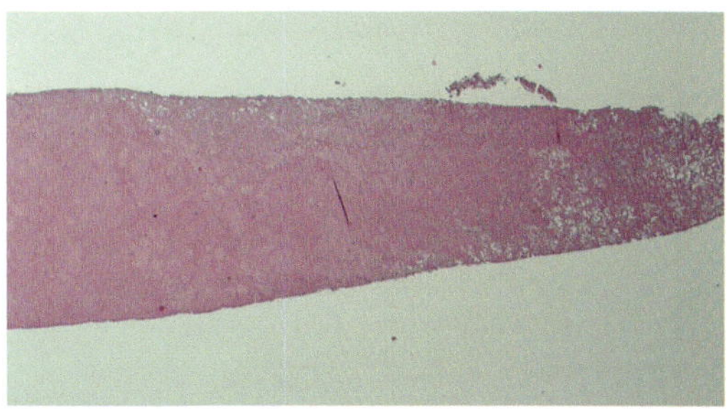

Fig. 6.52 Fibrous scar (H&E, 4×). This core biopsy consists of a hyalinized stroma. No viable tissue is present

Case 1

Clinical History: A 67-year-old female with a history of a right well-differentiated IDC 10 years ago, now with a developing focal asymmetry demonstrated on screening mammography in a site remote from her lumpectomy scar (Figs. 6.47–6.50 and 6.51).

BI-RADS: 4, suspicious findings.

An US-guided biopsy was performed and demonstrated fat necrosis (Fig. 6.52, 6.53 and 6.54).

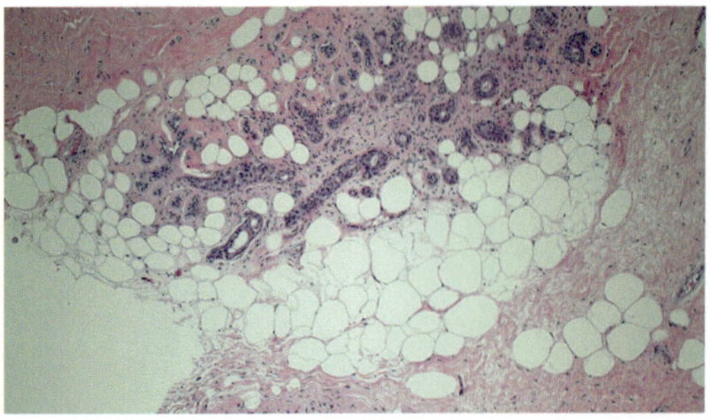

Fig. 6.53 Postradiation change (H&E, 4×) may be seen as nuclear enlargement in the ductal epithelial cells. The nuclear: cytoplasmic ratio is preserved. Stromal fibrosis and hyalinization of the basement membrane can also be appreciated

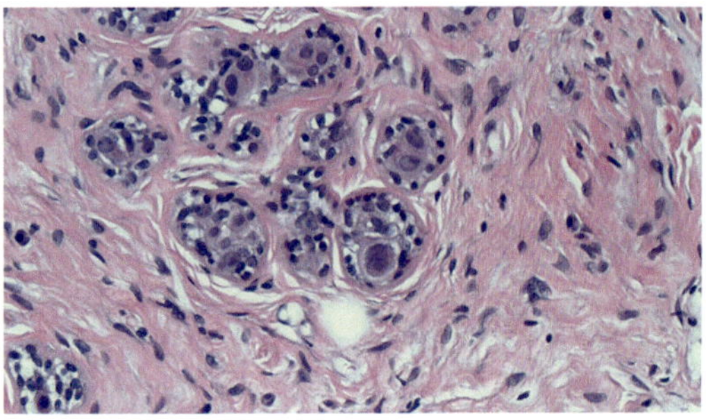

Fig. 6.54 Postradiation change (H&E, 20×). Nuclear enlargement is better appreciated at this magnification. The nuclei are round to ovoid, with smudgy chromatin

Case 2

Clinical History: A 59-year-old female with history of a moderately differentiated, ER/PR+, HER2-, left breast cancer, treated with lumpectomy and radiation, presents with a developing asymmetry in the lumpectomy site detected on screening mammography.

The ultrasound was negative.

BI-RADS: 4, suspicious findings (Figs. 6.55 and 6.56).

A tomosynthesis-guided biopsy yielded focal minimal ADH in the background of radiation-related changes and stromal fibrosis. This was felt to be concordant, and given that the ADH was focal and minimal, surgical excision was deemed unnecessary at the time, and a 6-month follow-up mammogram was recommended.

Below are the radiologic images at the time of the 6-month follow-up (Figs. 6.57, 6.58, 6.59, 6.60 and 6.61):.

BI-RADS: 4, suspicious.

An US-guided biopsy was recommended and demonstrated a poorly differentiated TNBC (Fig. 6.62).

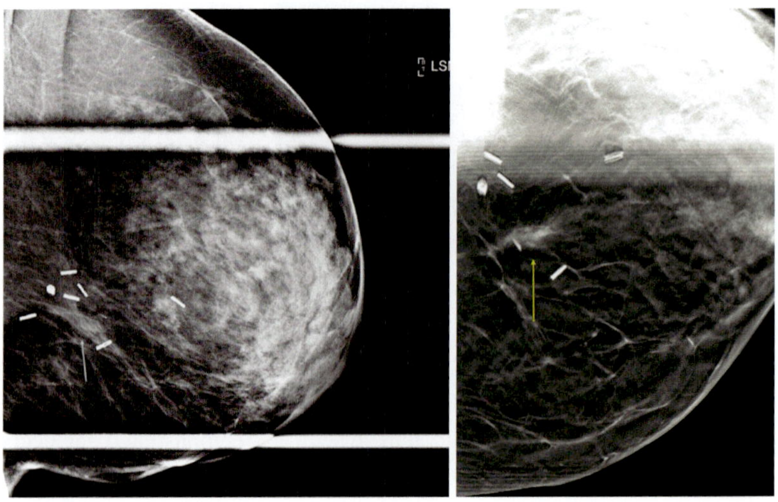

Figs. 6.55 and 6.56 Mammogram findings: Focal developing, fat-containing asymmetry in the lumpectomy site

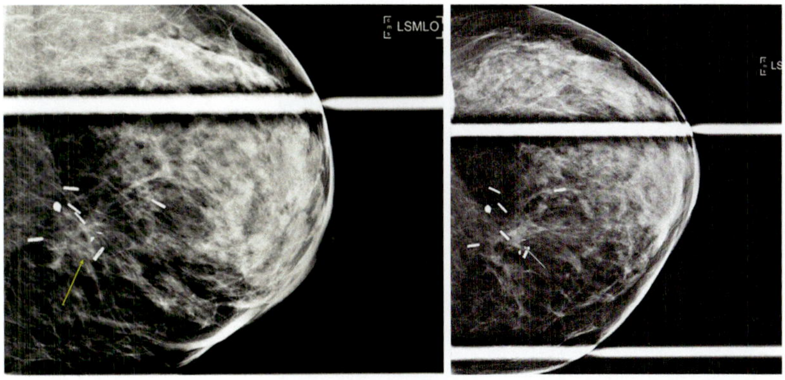

Figs. 6.57 and 6.58 Mammogram findings: The focal asymmetry is larger

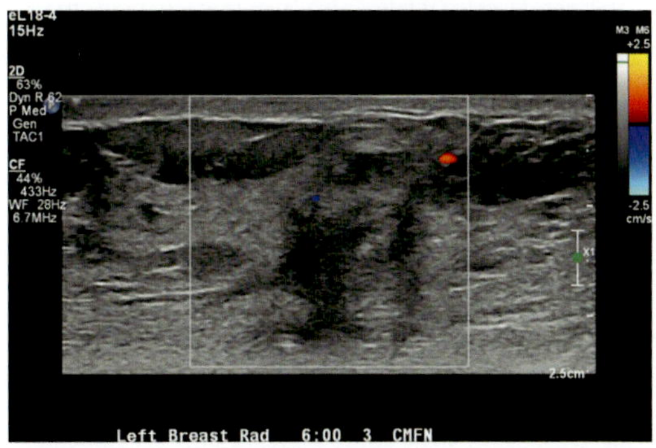

Fig. 6.59 Ultrasound findings: An irregular, hypoechoic mass is now seen, corresponding to the focal asymmetry

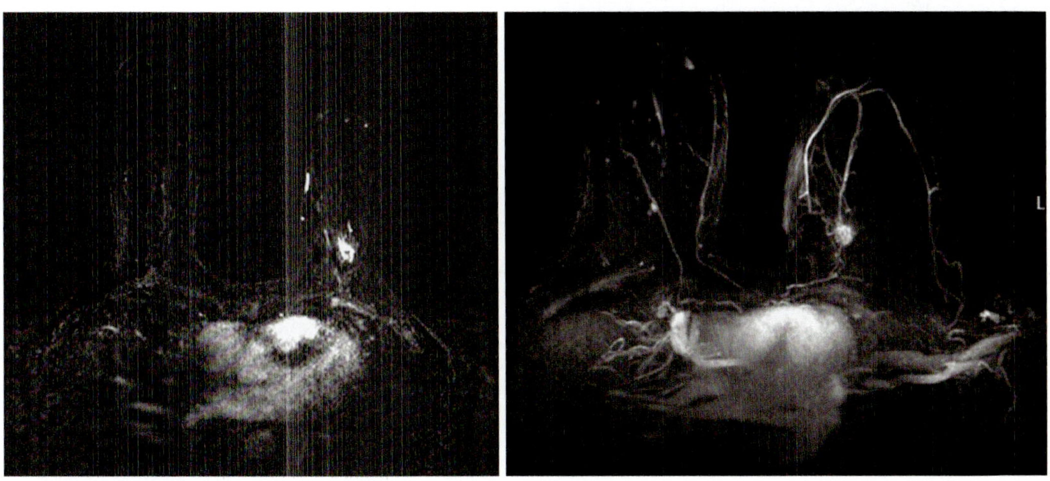

Figs. 6.60 and 6.61 MRI: A bilateral breast MRI showed a suspicious irregular mass, corresponding with the US and mammogram findings

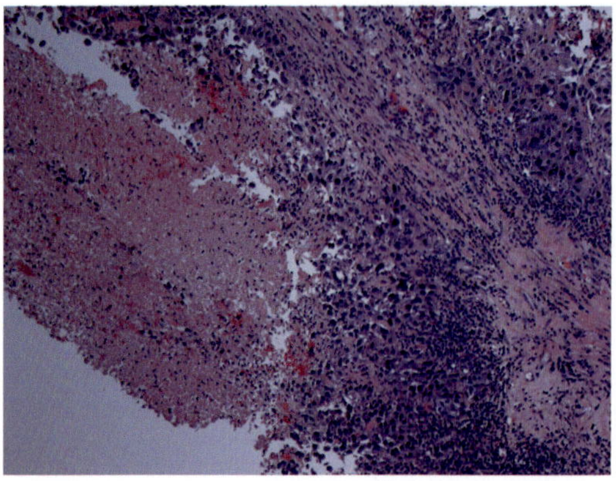

Fig. 6.62 Triple-negative histologic grade 3 invasive ductal carcinoma (H&E, 20×). On the left side, tumor necrosis is present

Invasive Lobular Carcinoma

Invasive Lobular Carcinoma:

- **Clinical Presentation**.
  Invasive lobular carcinoma often presents as a palpable or radiographically detected ill-defined mass. Skin retraction or fixation may be seen in larger tumors. Paget disease of the nipple is uncommon. The relative risk of contralateral carcinoma compared to ductal carcinoma or breast carcinoma in general ranges from 1.6 to 2 [17, 18].
- **Imaging Findings**:
  - The common imaging features of ILC have been described elsewhere within the book. ILC may present as a developing asymmetry and mimic fibroglandular breast tissue.
- **Pathology Findings**:
  - **Gross**: Invasive lobular carcinoma may have subtle gross findings, such as fine, hard nodules that feel like grains of sand or tiny pebbles [17]. Typically, however, it forms a gray to white, firm-to-hard mass with irregular borders which may blend imperceptibly with the surrounding breast parenchyma. Cystic change, hemorrhage, necrosis, or gross calcifications are uncommon [17].
  - **Microscopic Findings**:

The classic form of invasive lobular carcinoma is that of slender strands of discohesive cells with small round nuclei and scant cytoplasm. Tumor cells may also be arranged around ducts and lobules in a concentric or "targetoid" pattern. Variant forms include altered cytology in the form of pleomorphic/apocrine, plasmacytoid, signet ring cell, or histiocytoid cell types characterized by larger nuclei and/or abundant cytoplasm. Variations in growth pattern and architecture include solid (sheet-like growth), alveolar (groups composed of at least 20 cells), trabecular (strands more than 2 cells in width), and tubulolobular.

  - **Differential Diagnosis**: Inflammatory cell infiltrates, invasive ductal carcinoma, lymphoma, melanoma, metastatic (gastric) carcinoma.
- **Management**: Surgical resection, chemotherapy, radiotherapy.

Case 1

Clinical History: A 73-year-old female with a developing focal asymmetry, demonstrated in the lower outer aspect of the left breast on screening mammography (Figs. 6.63–6.66, 6.67, 6.68 and 6.69).

BI-RADS: 4, suspicious.

An US-guided biopsy revealed a moderately differentiated ILC (Fig. 6.70).

Follow-up: The patient underwent a lumpectomy.

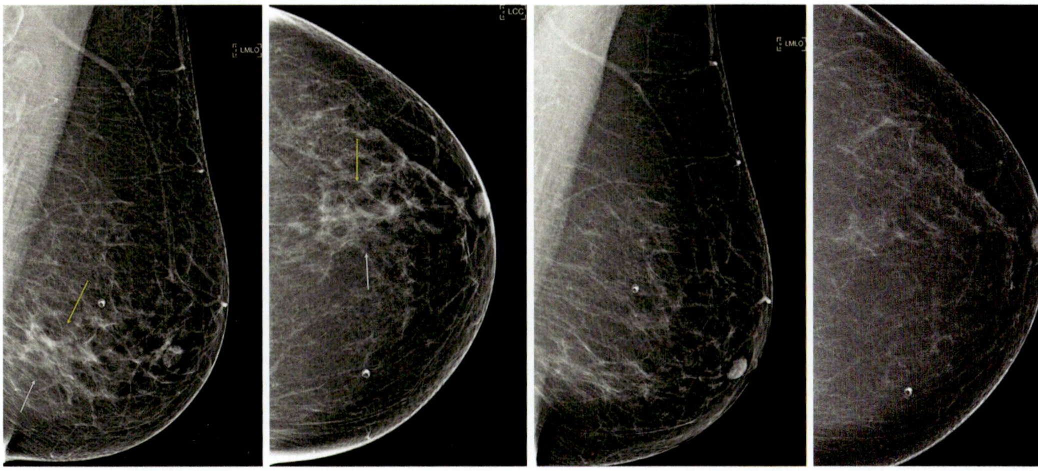

Figs. 6.63–6.66 **Mammogram Findings**: A developing focal asymmetry within a segment of the lower outer aspect, the left breast

Fig. 6.67 **Ultrasound findings**: A vague shadowing area within the lower outer quadrant

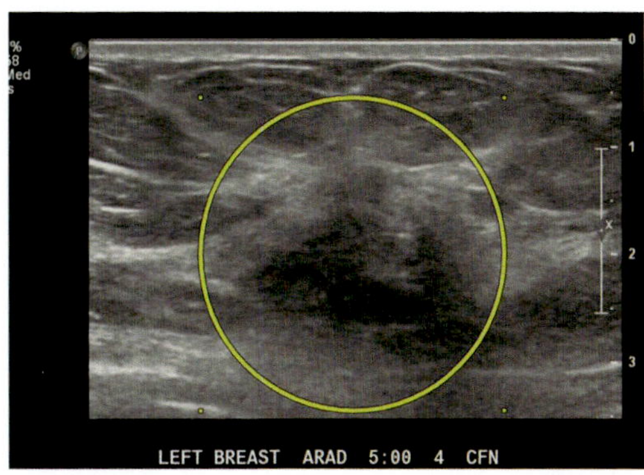

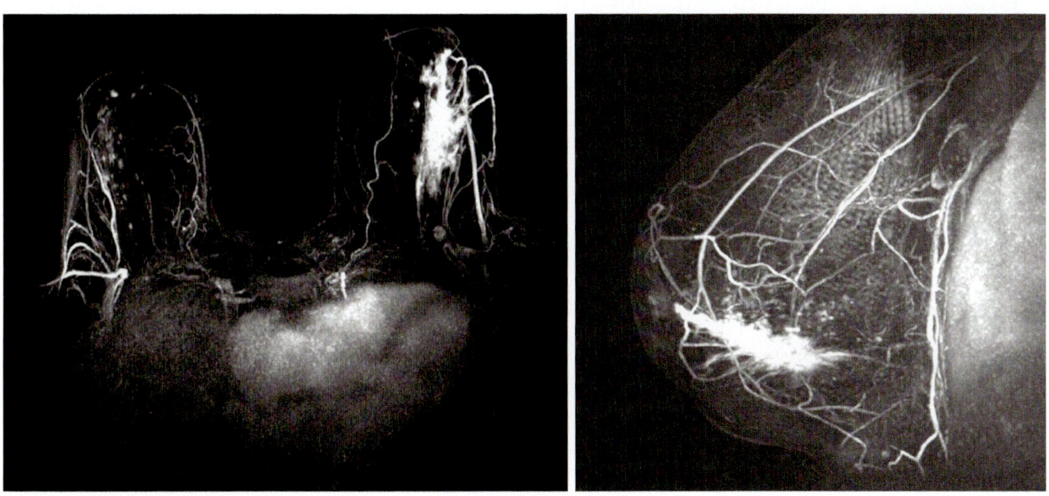

Figs. 6.68 and 6.69 **MRI**: Non-mass enhancement in a segmental distribution

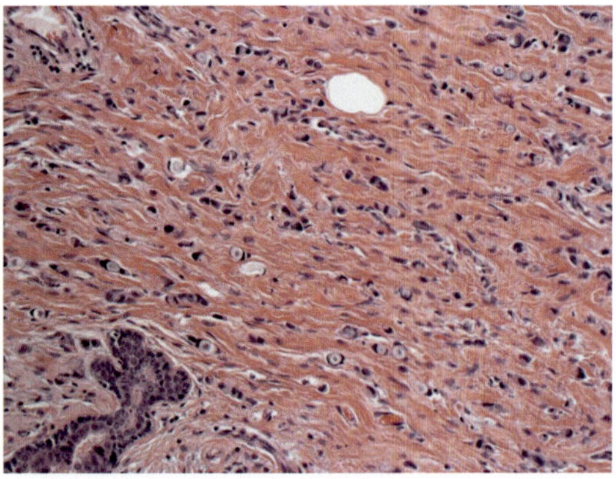

Fig. 6.70 Invasive lobular carcinoma (H&E, 10×). Tumor cells infiltrate in cords, composed of cells with round to ovoid, hyperchromatic nuclei, and ample cytoplasm. Signet ring cells are also seen

Invasive Ductal Carcinoma

Invasive Ductal Carcinoma:

- **Clinical Presentation**:
  Invasive ductal carcinoma presents as a palpable or radiographically detected mass with or without associated skin and nipple changes, nipple discharge, and breast asymmetry.
- **Imaging Findings**: The common imaging features of IDC have been described elsewhere within the book. Although classically presenting as a spiculated mass, IDC may manifest as a focal asymmetry.
- **Pathology Findings**:
  - **Gross**: Invasive ductal carcinoma is grossly visualized as a stellate or nodular mass with irregular borders or palpated as a firm to hard irregular mass that, when associated with calcifications, can have a gritty feel on sectioning. Hemorrhage and necrosis can also be seen.
  - **Microscopic Findings**: Microscopic examination reveals tumor cells of ductal phenotype permeating the surrounding stroma and fat and disrupting the terminal duct-lobular unit. Architecturally, these cells may invade as solid sheets, thin cords (thereby mimicking invasive lobular carcinoma), wider trabeculae, and round nests. Cytology and mitotic activity are variable, with increasing nuclear pleomorphism associated with brisk mitosis. Single-cell or comedo-type necrosis may be identified [18].
  - **Differential Diagnosis**: Radial scar, sclerosing adenosis, ductal carcinoma in-situ, metastatic carcinoma.
- **Management**: Surgical resection, chemotherapy, radiotherapy.

Case 1

Clinical History: A 67-year-old female presented for diagnostic imaging due to a palpable left retroareolar nodule with overlying skin retraction (Figs. 6.71, 6.72, 6.73).

BI-RADS: 4, suspicious findings.

An US-guided biopsy revealed a moderately differentiated IDC (Fig. 6.74).

Follow-up: The patient underwent a central lumpectomy.

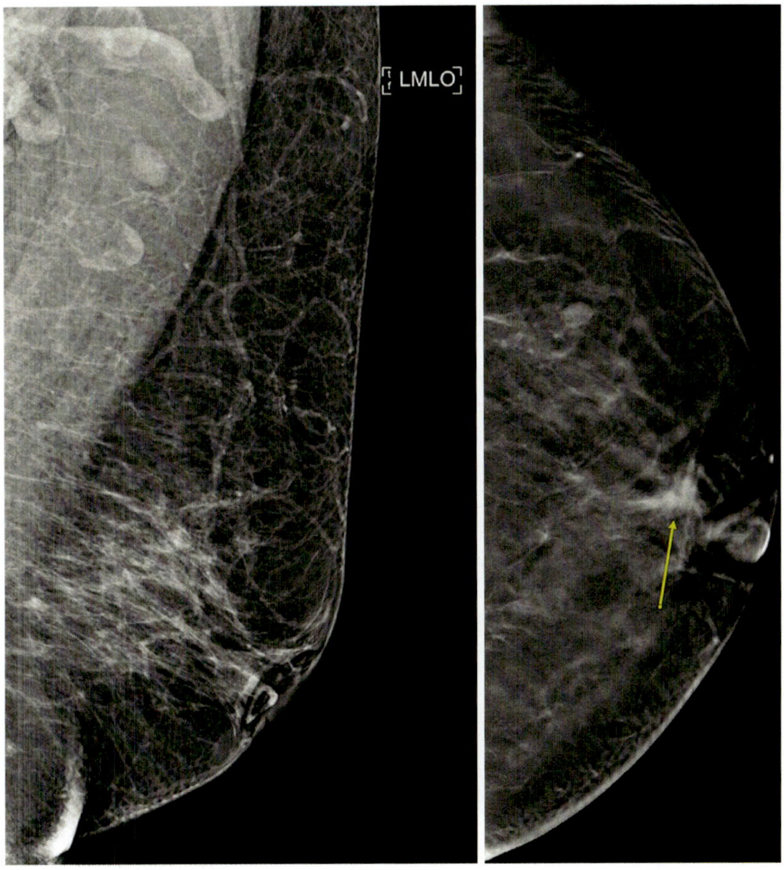

Figs. 6.71 and 6.72 Mammogram findings: A focal asymmetry is seen that corresponds to the palpable nodule, with skin retraction and nipple deviation demonstrated

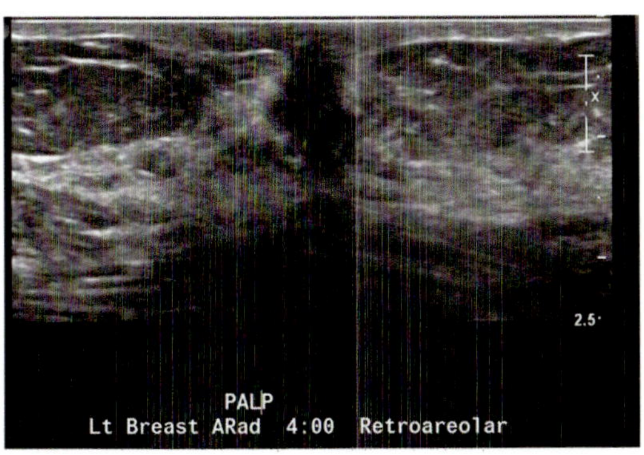

Fig. 6.73 Ultrasound findings: An irregular, hypoechoic mass tethered to the skin, with focal skin thickening

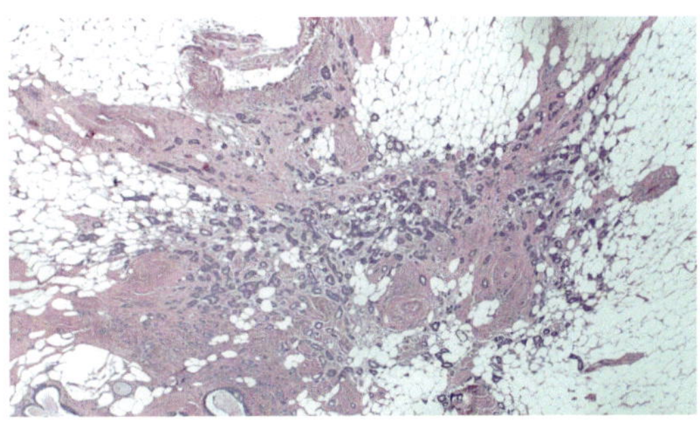

Fig. 6.74 Invasive ductal carcinoma (H&E, 4×). Invasive tumor cells are seen infiltrating into adipose tissue, accompanied by desmoplastic (fibrous) stroma

References

1. Chesebro AL, Winkler NS, Birdwell RL, Giess CS. Developing asymmetries at mammography: a multimodality approach to assessment and management. Radiographics. 2016;36:322–34.
2. Sickles EA. The spectrum of breast asymmetries: imaging features, work-up, management. Radiol Clin North Am. 2007;45(5):765–71.
3. Speer ME, Yoon EC, Berg WA, Chang Sen LQ. Pseudoangiomatous stromal hyperplasia: radiologic-pathologic correlation. J Breast Imaging. 2023:67–72.
4. Virk RK, Khan A. Pseudoangiomatous stromal hyperplasia: an overview. Arch Pathol Lab Med. 2010;134(7):1070–4. https://doi.org/10.5858/2008-0686-RS.1.
5. Barreto DS, Sedgwick EL, Nagi CS, Benveniste AP. Granulomatous mastitis: etiology, imaging, pathology, treatment, and clinical findings. Breast Cancer Res Treat. 2018;171:527–34.
6. Tan H, Li R, Peng W, Liu H, Gu Y, Shen X. Radiological and clinical features of adult non-puerperal mastitis. Br J Radiol. 2013;86:20120657.
7. Joseph K, Luu X, Mor A. Granulomatous mastitis: a New York public hospital experience. Ann Surg Oncol. 2014;21(13):4159–63.
8. Atak T, Sagiroglu J, Eren T, Ozemir IA, Alimoglu O. Strategies to treat idiopathic granulomatous mastitis: retrospective analysis of 40 patients. Breast Dis. 2015;35(1):19–24.
9. Yabanoglu H, Colakoglu T, Belli S, Aytac HO, Bolat FA, Pourbagher A, et al. A comparative study of conservative versus surgical treatment protocols for 77 patients with idiopathic granulomatous mastitis. Breast J. 2015;21(4):363–9.
10. Sansone A, Romanelli F, Sansone M, Lenzi A, Di Luigi L. Gynecomastia and hormones. Endocrine. 2017;55:37–44.
11. Sonnenblick EB, Margolies LR, Szabo JR, et al. Digital breast tomosynthesis of gynecomastia and associated findings—a pictorial review. Clin Imaging. 2014;38:565–70.
12. Tan PH, Lai LM, Carrington EV, Opaluwa AS, Ravikumar KH, Chetty N, et al. Fat necrosis of the breast—a review. Breast. 2006;15:313–8.
13. Winkler NS, Yang WT. Fibrosis. In: Berg WA, Leung JW, editors. Diagnostic imaging: breast. Philadelphia, PA: Elsevier; 2019. p. 568–71.
14. Sickles EA, Herzog KA. Intramammary scar tissue: a mimic of the mammographic appearance of carcinoma. AJR Am J Roentgenol. 1980;135:349–52.
15. Gaur S, Dialani V, Slanetz PJ, Eisenberg RL. Architectural distortion of the breast. AJR Am J Roentgenol. 2013;201(5):W662–70.
16. Hoda SA. Invasive lobular carcinoma. In: Hoda SA, Brogi E, Koerner FC, Rosen PP, editors. Rosen's breast pathology (5th ed.). Wolters Kluwer; 2021.
17. Shin SJ, Desmedt C, Kristiansen G, Reis-Filho JS, and Sasano H. "Invasive lobular carcinoma." WHO classification of tumors: breast tumors (5th ed.) edited by the WHO Classification of Tumors Editorial Board, International Agency for Research on Cancer, 2019.
18. Rakha EA, Allison KH, Bu H, Ellis IO, Foschini MP, Horii R, et al. "Invasive breast carcinoma of no special type." WHO classification of tumors: breast tumors (5th ed.) edited by the WHO Classification of Tumors Editorial Board, International Agency for Research on Cancer, 2019.

Architectural Distortions

7

Reni Butler, Melissa Durand, Sonali Lanjevar, Peter Podany, Liva Andrejeva, and Malini Harigopal

Benign

Radial Scar (RS)/Complex Sclerosing Lesion (CSL)

Radial Scar (RS)/Complex Sclerosing Lesion (CSL): Radial scars, or complex sclerosing lesions, do not represent true scars. Proposed theories for these benign proliferative lesions include inflammation and ischemia [1, 2]. Due to the pseudo-infiltrative appearance of these lesions on histology and stellate/spiculated appearance on radiology they can mimic invasive carcinoma. A small percentage of radial scars can be associated with atypical hyperplasia, in situ or invasive carcinoma. Radial scars and complex sclerosing lesions have a similar mammographic appearance. The distinction between them is based primarily on size, with the latter term reserved for lesions >1 cm. RS/CSLs are categorized as high-risk lesions due to a variable rate of upgrade to malignancy at surgical excision [3]. As a result, standard management recommendations have been to completely excise RS/CSLs diagnosed by core needle biopsy [4]. The presence of atypia in core biopsy samples increases the likelihood of surgical upgrade [4, 5].

- **Clinical Presentation**: Radial scars typically occur in women between 40 and 60 years of age, but they can be seen anytime from the first to tenth decade. They are commonly seen in women, however a single report of radial sclerosing lesion has been reported in the breast of a man [6]. Their incidence in benign breast biopsies is reported between 5% and 10% [7–9]. Most cases (80%) are detected on radiologic examination, and radial scars typically manifest as areas of architectural distortion detected on mammogram [3, 10]. While most RS/CSLs present as asymptomatic lesions detected on screening mammography, a minority of large CSL lesions may produce clinically palpable findings [6].
- **Imaging Findings**:
  - **Mammography**: The mammographic appearance of a RS/CSL is characterized by thin elongated spicules emanating from a lucent center (Figs. 7.1, 7.2 and 7.3).

R. Butler · M. Durand
Department of Radiology and Biomedical Imaging, Yale University, New Haven, CT, USA
e-mail: reni.butler@yale.edu; Melissa.durand@yale.edu

S. Lanjevar
Department of Pathology, Albert Einstein College of Medicine, Bronx, NY, USA

P. Podany · M. Harigopal (✉)
Department of Pathology, Yale University, New Haven, CT, USA
e-mail: peter.podany@yale.edu; malini.harigopal@yale.edu

L. Andrejeva
Department of Radiology and Biomedical Imaging, Yale School of Medicine, New Haven, CT, USA
e-mail: liva.andrejeva@yale.edu

M. Harigopal et al. (eds.), *Radiology Pathology Correlations of Breast Lesions*, https://doi.org/10.1007/978-3-031-65711-5_7

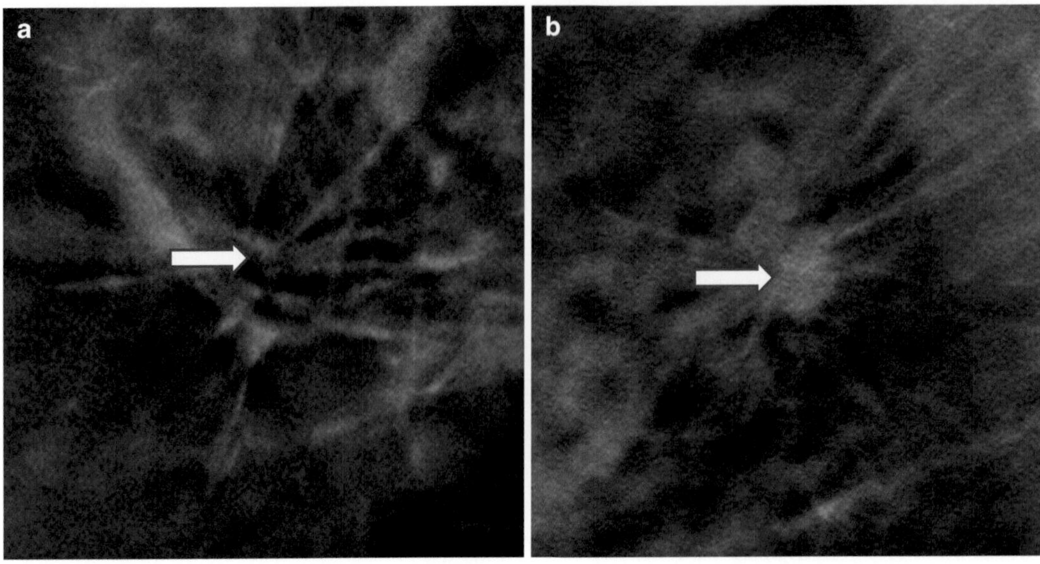

Fig. 7.1 Radial scar (**a**) with "black star" appearance of thin elongated spicules emanating from a lucent center (white arrow). Companion case of invasive ductal carcinoma (**b**) with "white star" appearance of central mass with spiculated margins (white arrow)

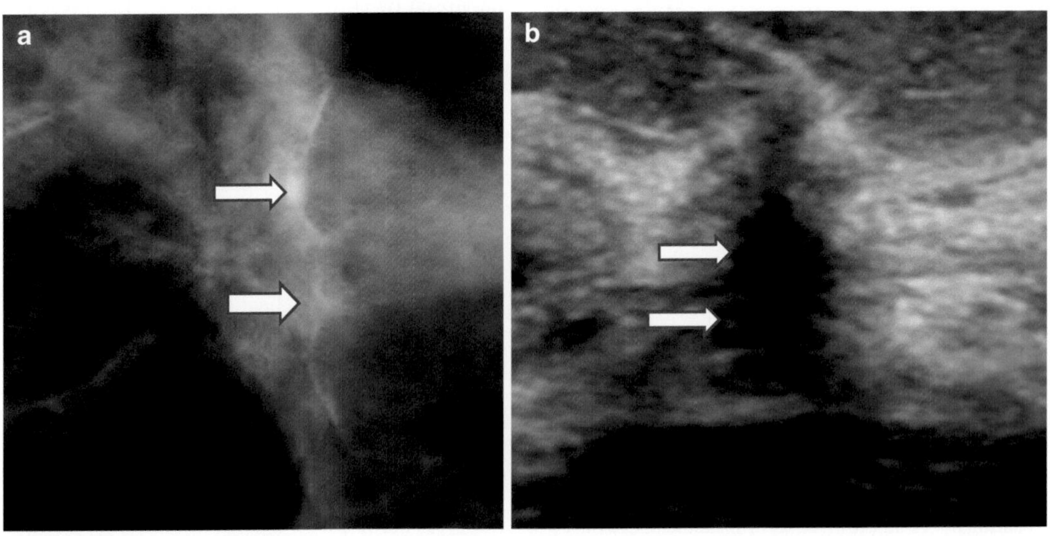

Fig. 7.2 Screening mammogram in a 54-year-old woman. Architectural distortion incidentally detected on screening mammography (**a**) with digital breast tomosynthesis (white arrows). Targeted ultrasound (**b**) shows a focal area of shadowing (white arrows). Percutaneous ultrasound-guided hand-held 14-gauge core needle biopsy revealed a radial scar

This pattern has been described as a "black star", a term intended to aid in the differentiation of these lesions from a malignant spiculated mass which would be expected to produce a "white star". Multiple investigators have reported overlap in these imaging features between benign and malignant lesions, concluding that the "black star" pattern is not a reliable method to exclude

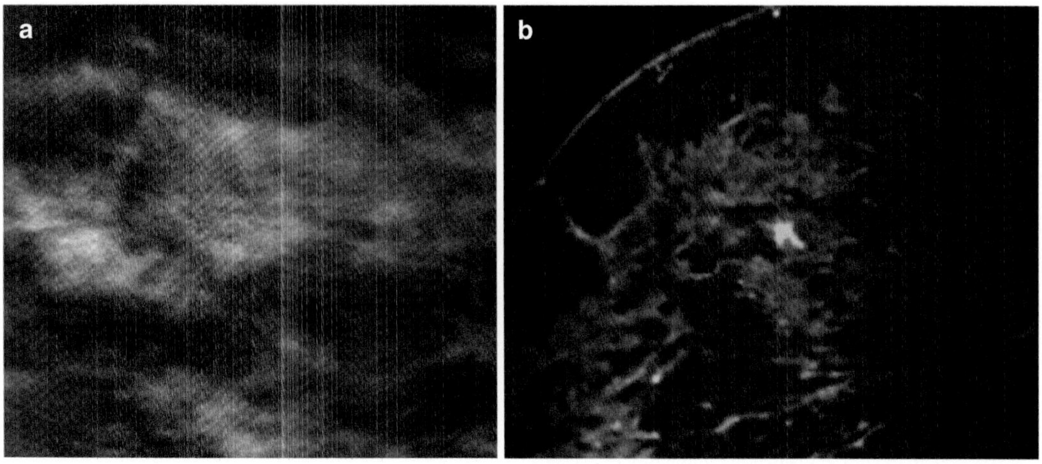

Fig. 7.3 Screening mammogram in a 57-year-old woman. Architectural distortion incidentally detected on a tomosynthesis slice from screening mammography performed with digital breast tomosynthesis (**a**). Targeted ultrasound was negative (not shown). Dynamic contrast-enhanced MRI shows a clumped area of non-mass enhancement (**b**). Percutaneous MRI-guided vacuum-assisted 9-gauge core needle biopsy revealed a complex sclerosing lesion

malignancy and histologic diagnosis is still required [2, 3].

- **US**: RS/CSLs may be sonographically occult or subtle.

  When a sonographic correlate is present the most common appearance is an irregular hypoechoic mass with posterior shadowing.

  RS/CSLs may also present as a hyperechoic or heterogeneous mass, as well as an area of shadowing without a definable mass [11].

  Careful attention to sonographic technique and correlation with mammography are often necessary to identify the subtle presentations of a RS/CSL.
- **MRI**: As with ultrasound, the MRI appearance of a RS/CSL is variable.

  The most common MRI finding is an irregular mass with variable kinetics.

  RS/CSLs may also produce non-mass enhancement in a stellate pattern that mirrors the mammographic finding of architectural distortion.

  Approximately 30% of RS/CSLs show no enhancement on MRI. Multiple studies have reported a high negative predictive value for surgical upgrade to malignancy in these non-enhancing lesions [10–12].
- **BI-RADS**: 4, suspicious for malignancy. Biopsy is recommended for histologic confirmation.
- **Differential Diagnosis**: Postsurgical scar, invasive ductal carcinoma, especially tubular carcinoma; invasive lobular carcinoma.

- **Pathology Findings**:
  - **Gross**: Radial scars when <1 cm in size are less likely to be identified grossly.

    When >1 cm in size, they appear as a stellate mass with central puckering and have an irregular edge.

    Creamy white or yellow streaks of elastosis can be seen emanating from a pale gray central core.

    Dilated cysts may be visible at the periphery of the lesion [3].
  - **Microscopic Histology**: Radial scars show a characteristic central zone of sclerosis and elastosis (nidus) with ducts and angulated glands entrapped within fibroelastotic stroma (Fig. 7.4).

    The ducts and lobules radiate from the sclerotic center and appear to be expanding in a centrifugal manner.

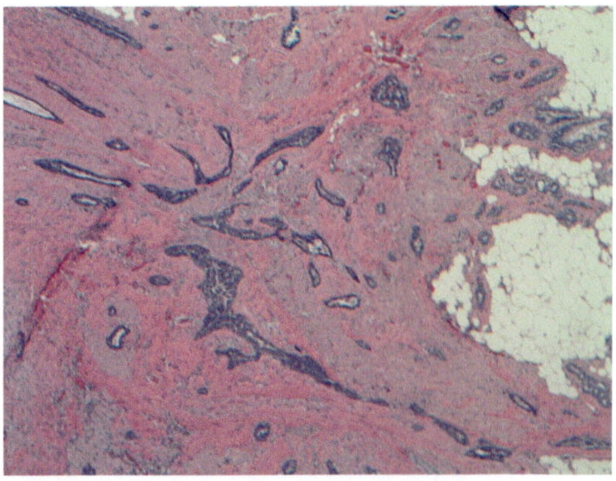

Fig. 7.4 A lumpectomy specimen from a 38-year-old woman with architectural distortion on imaging in her left breast. The breast tissue shows ducts in a sclerotic background in a radiating pattern consistent with a radial scar

In the early phase of development, the central nidus is more cellular and shows myxoid extracellular material [6].

In the later stages, there is more collagen deposition and sclerosis which results in the characteristic stellate configuration with entrapment of glands [6].

Due to a pseudo-infiltrative pattern, they commonly mimic invasive carcinoma and can be distinguished with the aid of myoepithelial markers [11] (Fig. 7.5).

Occasionally benign glands can show perineural infiltration and when found should not be used as a sole criterion for malignancy [12].

Ducts and lobules can be involved by fibrocystic changes, squamous metaplasia, apocrine metaplasia, usual and atypical ductal hyperplasia and rarely by in situ lobular or ductal carcinoma as well as invasive carcinoma (Fig. 7.6).

Invasive carcinoma when identified is typically tubular type, <2 cm and is limited to the periphery of the lesion.

Calcifications when found are seen in areas of adenosis or epithelial hyperplasia.

- **Differential Diagnoses**:

  Tubular carcinoma: The entrapped and angulated glands in radial scars are paucicellular and are embedded in the central sclero-elastotic stroma.

  The entrapped ducts are often compressed and distorted with absent or slit-like lumina. Use of more than one myoepithelial marker is recommended as myoepithelial cells may only be identified around some of the entrapped glands.

  In contrast to radial scars, invasive carcinoma is cellular and arises in the periphery of the lesion, the stroma is desmoplastic and infiltrating glands can be seen in the adjacent benign breast and adipose tissue.

  Accompanying atypical ductal hyperplasia and/or in situ carcinoma is frequently identified. The tubules show loss of myoepithelial cells on staining for myoepithelial markers.

  Low-grade adenosquamous carcinoma: Entrapped glands and ducts in the central fibroelastotic nidus can resemble low-grade adenosquamous carcinoma (LGASC).

  When squamous metaplasia is present LGASC shows an infiltrative pattern of glands and squamous nests with an absence of myoepithelial markers. They have mixed tumor populations of luminal cells, myoepithelial cells, and squamous cells in most cases.

  The presence of lymphoid aggregates in the periphery is characteristic.

  These lesions are typically triple negative.

- **Management**: Palpable RS/CSL, >1 cm should be excised due to higher risk of malignancy. For lesions <1 cm, management depends on the clinical and radiologic findings.

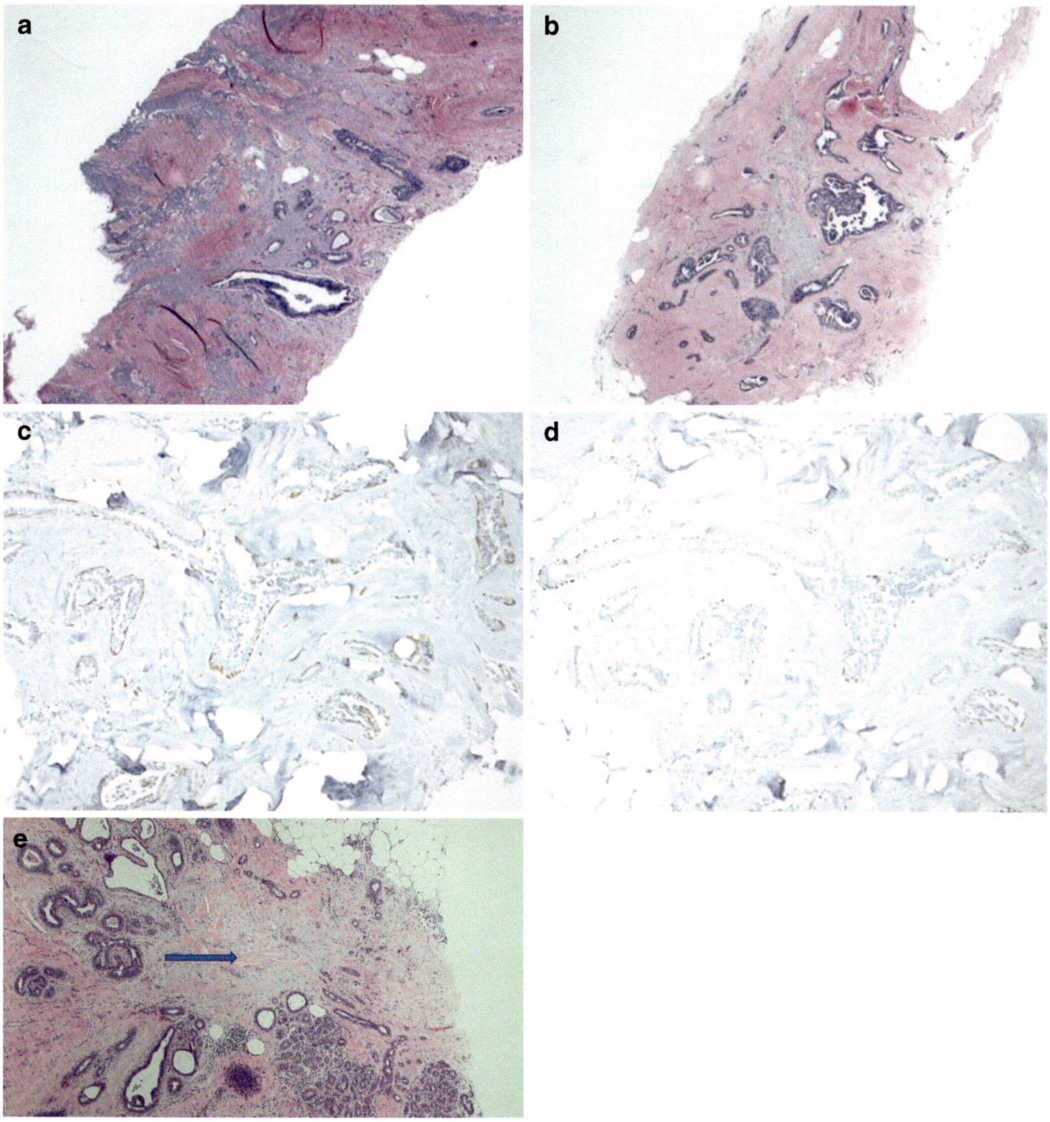

Fig. 7.5 Core needle biopsy with a complex sclerosing lesion with atypical ductal hyperplasia (**a**), which was upgraded to ductal carcinoma in situ (DCIS) at surgical excision. H&E slide of core biopsy showing a portion of radial sclerosing lesion consisting of a central sclerotic zone with collagenized stroma with entrapped small glands and a peripheral zone consisting of cysts and sclerosing adenosis (**b**). Myoepithelial cells are attenuated but preserved around these ducts which can be demonstrated using immunostains for p63 (**c**) and calponin (**d**), which helps distinguish the lesion from invasive carcinoma. Subsequent surgical excision shows a central sclerotic nidus (blue arrow) with peripheral adenosis and a few cystically dilated glands (**e**)

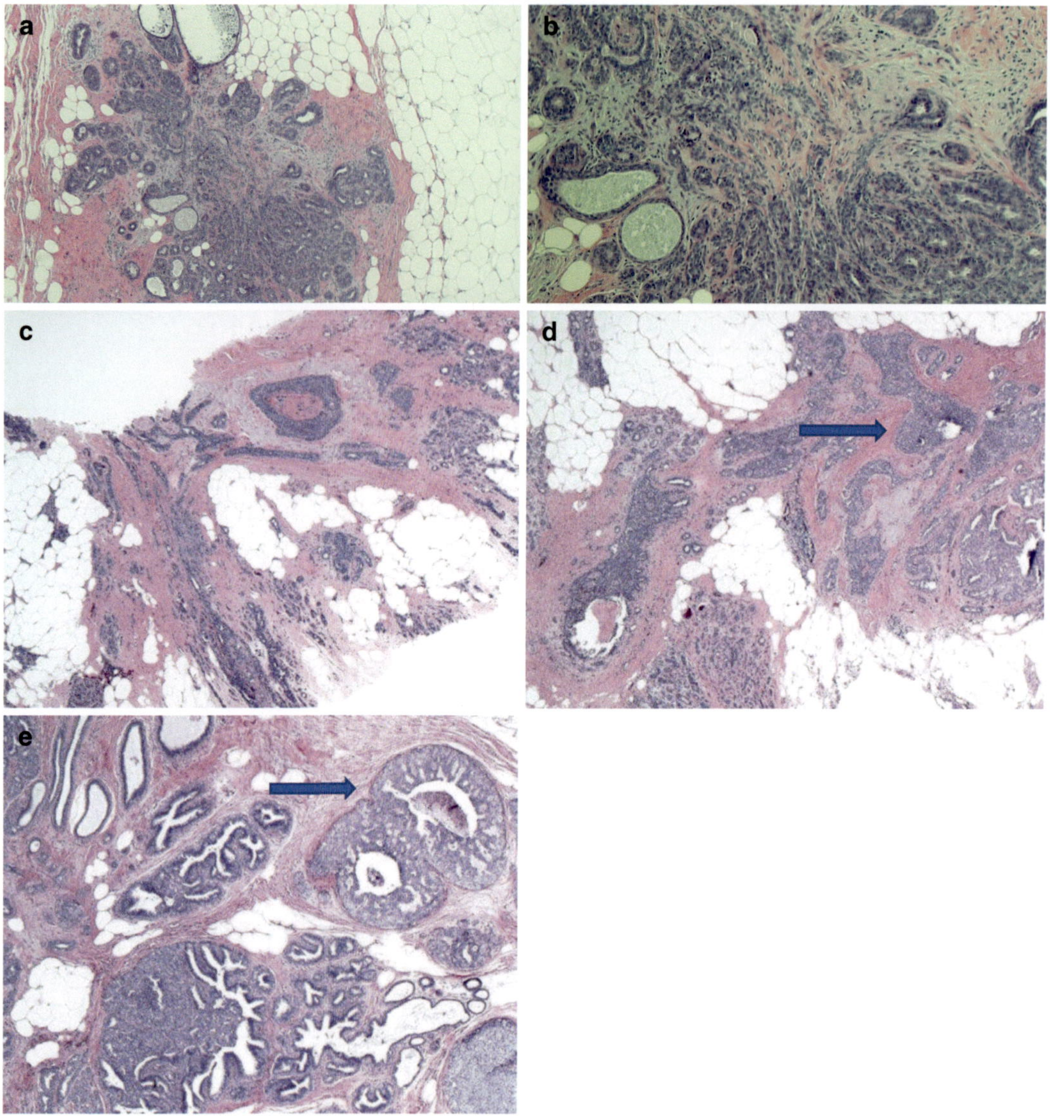

Fig. 7.6 Surgical resection demonstrating a radial scar (**a**, **b**). H&E of the core biopsy showed a complex sclerosing lesion with a central nidus of fibroelastotic stroma with entrapped glands with peripheral benign epithelial proliferations, including adenosis, cysts and usual ductal hyperplasia (**c**). Excisional biopsy showed UDH involving a radial scar (blue arrow in **d**) and DCIS involving a complex sclerosing lesion (blue arrow in **e**)

Postsurgical Scar

Postsurgical Scar: Postsurgical architectural distortion varies in extent according to the surgical procedure. While a benign excisional biopsy may produce a small area of focal distortion, reduction mammoplasty often results in diffuse architectural distortion, most pronounced in the peri-areolar region and inferior breast tissue, corresponding to the surgical incisions. A post-lumpectomy scar is typically more prominent than a benign postsurgical scar since lumpectomy for a malignancy requires wider excision to ensure negative margins and post-lumpectomy radiation treatment produces further scarring (Fig. 7.7).

- **Clinical Presentation**: Typically noted on a screening mammogram with a reported history of postsurgical change. Postsurgical scars

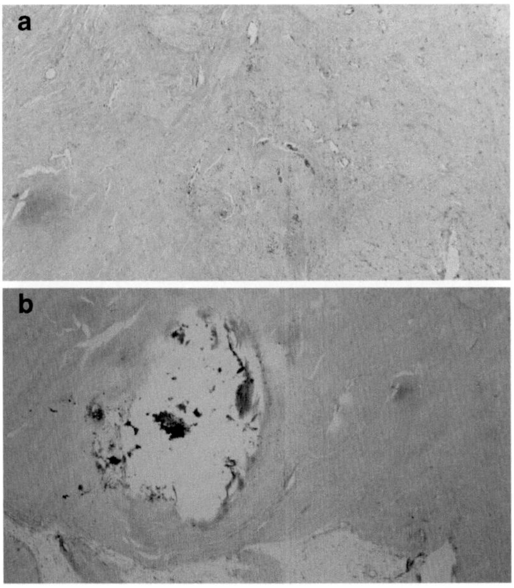

Fig. 7.7 Surgical resection demonstrating a postsurgical scar, (**a**) and a postsurgical scar with calcifications (**b**)

should be documented at the time of the breast imaging study.

- **Imaging Findings**:
  - **Mammography**: Mammographically, postsurgical scars are characterized by the absence of a central mass and may demonstrate a lucent center (Fig. 7.8).
    - Nonetheless, they cannot be reliably distinguished from a malignancy without the appropriate clinical history.
    - Comparison to serial prior mammograms is helpful to assess stability.
    - In the absence of prior mammograms, placement of a skin marker may be helpful to confirm correspondence between the surgical scar and the mammographic distortion.
  - **US**: Postsurgical scars produce a hypoechoic region with posterior shadowing on ultrasound.
    - Real-time scanning to search for extension of the parenchymal scar to the skin surface may be helpful in confirming its benign etiology.
    - As with mammography, the appropriate clinical history is essential for establishing the diagnosis.
  - **MRI**: In the acute postoperative setting of a post-lumpectomy patient with positive surgical margins, MRI may be helpful in identifying residual disease.
    - To this end, postsurgical changes must be distinguished from possible residual malignancy.
    - Benign postsurgical findings include thin rim enhancement outlining the surgical cavity with persistent kinetics. By contrast, residual disease may present as mass or non-mass enhancement, often with plateau, wash-out, or mixed kinetics, along the border of the lumpectomy site.
    - During long-term surveillance of the post-lumpectomy patient, MRI may be helpful in identifying possible recurrence.
      - After approximately 3 years post-lumpectomy, enhancement at the surgical site is no longer seen in most patients [13].
        - Therefore, abnormal enhancement in this region may represent a recurrent breast cancer.
        - However, up to 15% of patients demonstrate continued enhancement at the lumpectomy site for 5 years or more [13].
        - Therefore, it is essential to compare findings to prior MRI examinations. Any areas of new or increasing enhancement in the post-lumpectomy region may indicate a recurrent malignancy.
  - **BI-RADS**: 2, with appropriate clinical history.
  - **Differential Diagnosis**: Radial scar/complex sclerosing lesion; invasive ductal carcinoma, especially tubular carcinoma; invasive lobular carcinoma.
  - **Management**: Core needle biopsy may show fat necrosis or nonspecific findings with fibrosis. Correlation with radiology should be performed to ensure that the mammographic finding of architectural distortion is concordant with histologic findings.

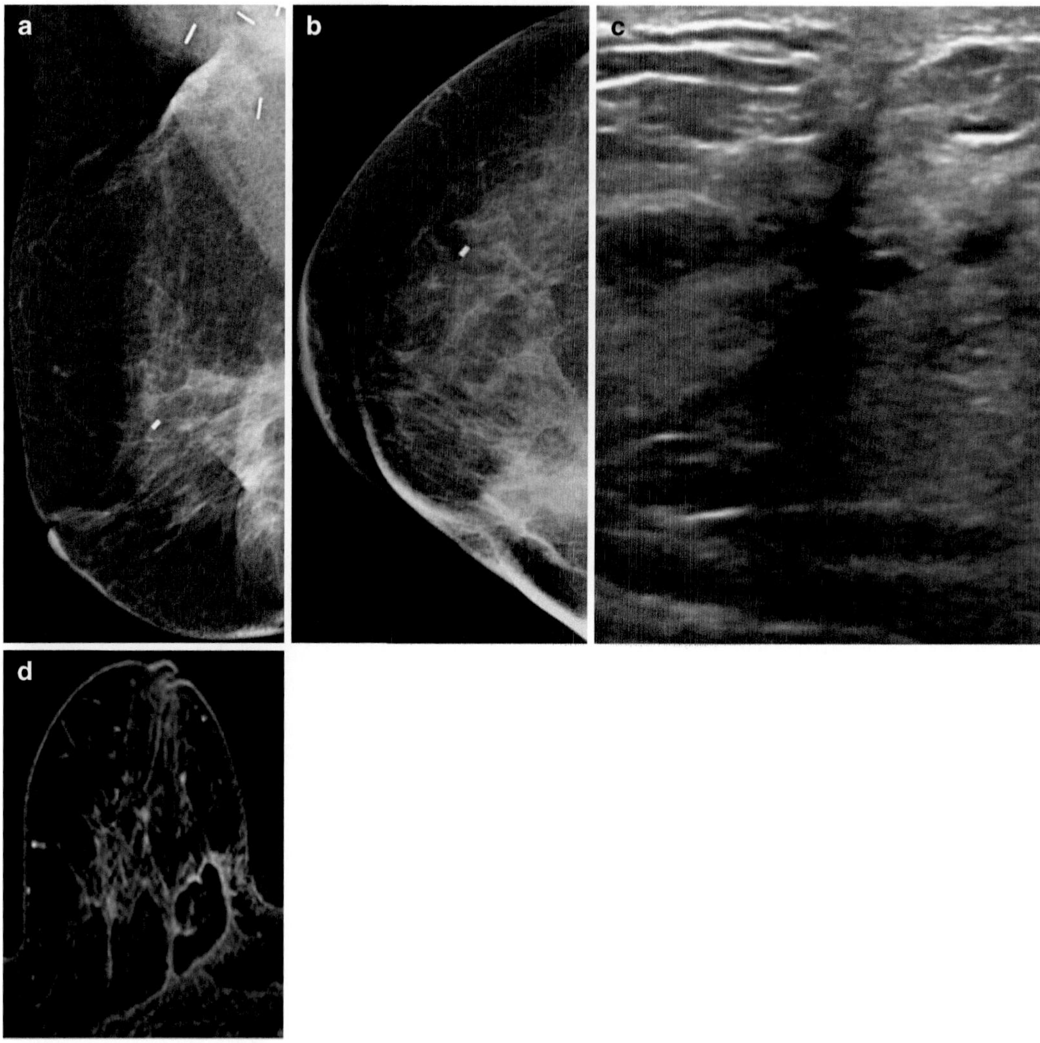

Fig. 7.8 Initial post-lumpectomy imaging in 59-year-old woman performed 5 months after surgical excision of invasive lobular carcinoma. Right MLO (**a**) and CC (**b**) views demonstrate architectural distortion and skin retraction, consistent with post-lumpectomy changes. Ultrasound shows a linear area of shadowing extending to the skin surface, corresponding to the surgical scar (**c**). Post-contrast subtraction MRI demonstrates thin rim enhancement surrounding the lumpectomy cavity (**d**)

Pseudoangiomatous Stromal Hyperplasia

Pseudoangiomatous Stromal Hyperplasia: Pseudoangiomatous stromal hyperplasia (PASH) is a hormonally derived benign myofibroblastic stromal proliferation, incidentally found on core needle biopsies and excision specimens [14–17]. While non-mass forming PASH is commonly seen as an incidental finding, mass forming PASH is well circumscribed, lobulated, and has margins that can be irregular or spiculated raising the differential of fibroadenoma, stromal fibrosis, and phyllodes tumor [18].

- **Clinical Presentation**: PASH is found in 23% of routinely performed core needle biopsies and is seen in a wide age group varying from 3 to 86 years old [19–21]. It commonly affects premenopausal women and is frequently associated with oral contraceptive use [21, 22]. It can increase in size during pregnancy and can result in bilateral gigantic breast enlargement including bilateral axillary tissue. In males it is seen in association with gynecomastia and can be seen in males receiving antiretroviral therapy [23]. Although there is no increased risk of subsequent breast carcinoma, there is one reported case of sarcoma arising in PASH and reports of associated invasive and in situ ductal carcinoma [21, 22, 24, 25].

- **Image Findings**:
  - **Mammography**: PASH can present as a mass or focal asymmetry (Fig. 7.9).
    Typically lacks calcifications.
  - **US**: Appears as a hypoechoic mass.
  - **MRI**: Is a mass or non-mass enhancement [26].
  - **BIRADS**: 2, 3, 4.
  - **Differential Diagnosis**: Fibroadenoma, phyllodes tumor, stromal fibrosis.
- **Pathology Findings**:
  - **Gross**: Nodular PASH is a well circumscribed, lobulated, firm, fibrous lesion and can vary in size from 1 to 10 cm and may contain cysts up to 1 cm in size.
    It may have irregular and spiculated margins.
    Hemorrhage and necrosis are not usually identified.
  - **Microscopic Histology**: PASH consists of a proliferation of myofibroblasts forming slit-like, empty spaces that may mimic vascular channels. These empty slit-like spaces are not lined by true endothelial cells and rarely contain red blood cells (Fig. 7.10).
    PASH can be focal, diffuse or infiltrative, and mainly involves the interlobular stroma. It is often seen admixed with benign ducts and lobules. It can also involve the intralobular stroma.
    The cellular variant of PASH shows poorly formed fascicles and may show only rare clefts or even none. The myofibroblasts show bland nuclear features and lack atypia and mitoses.
    The myofibroblasts of PASH are immunoreactive for CD34, smooth muscle actin, BCL2, and hormone receptors (PR > ER) [15, 16]. They are negative for keratin and endothelial markers.

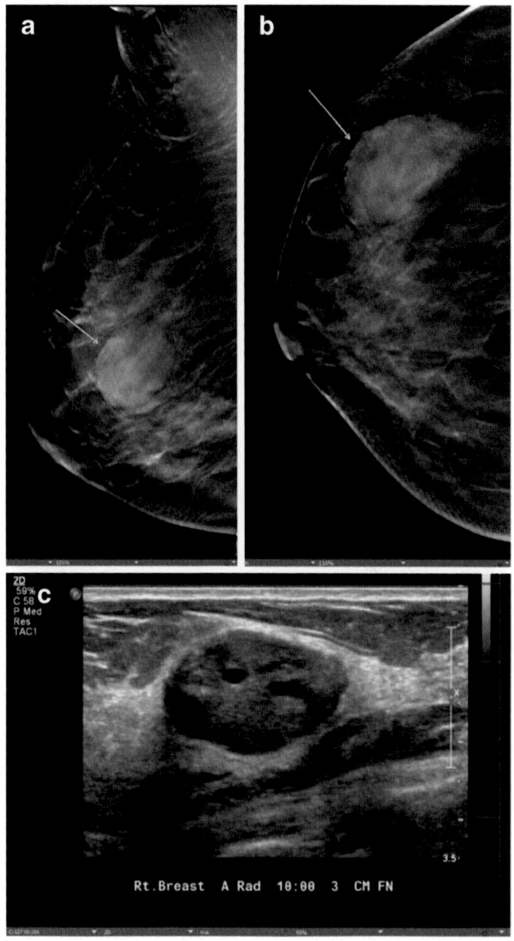

Fig. 7.9 A 41-year-old woman was called back after screening mammography revealed a mass in her right breast (**a**, **b**). On follow-up ultrasound the lesion is hypoechoic and well circuscribed (**c**). The lesion is biopsied to reveal nodular PASH

    Collagenization of the stroma can create a fibroadenoma-like appearance.
    Rare examples of atypical PASH have been described with atypical hyperchromatic nuclei and other rare examples of PASH that show cytoplasmic inclusions like those seen in digital fibromas have been reported.
  - **Differential Diagnoses**: Vascular lesions: Vascular lesions are typically filled with RBCs and are immunoreactive for endothelial-specific markers.
    Myofibroblastoma: Myofibroblastomas are more cellular and lack the clefting seen in PASH. They typically form a

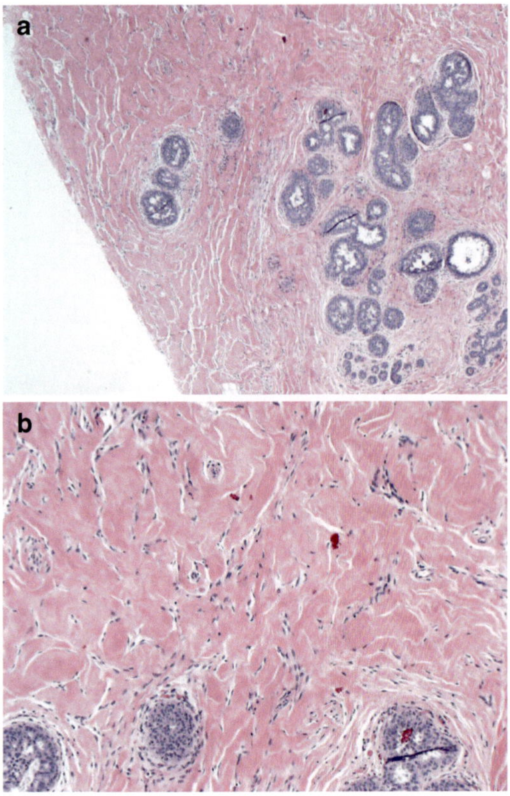

Fig. 7.10 Surgical resection demonstrating myofibroblast-lined slit-like spaces of PASH (**a**, **b**)

solid mass which does not contain normal ducts and acini, as seen in PASH.

Invasive carcinoma: PASH is negative for keratin immunostains.

Fibroepithelial lesions: PASH can be seen as a component of fibroepithelial lesions. Fibroepithelial lesions show proliferation of both epithelial and stromal components, whereas PASH can involve and infiltrate normal ducts and acini.

– **Management**: Incidentally discovered PASH and stable/uncomplicated nodular PASH diagnosed on core biopsies can be managed conservatively. A clinical and radiological follow-up is recommended.

Sclerosing Adenosis

See Chap. 5 for additional information (Figs. 7.11 and 7.12).

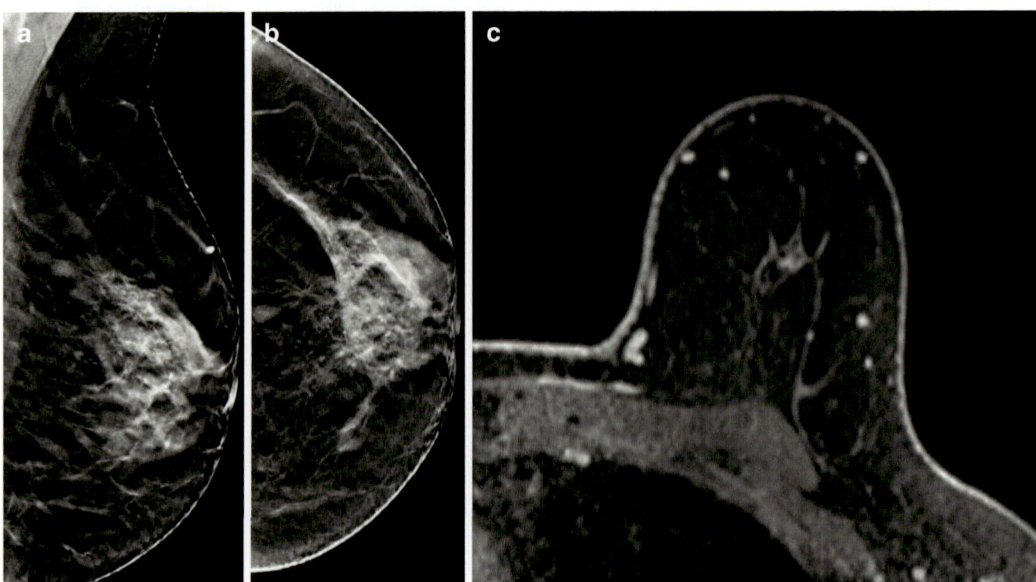

Fig. 7.11 Screening mammogram in a 61-year-old woman. Left MLO (**a**) and CC (**b**) views show focal architectural distortion at 12 o'clock in the left breast. Ultrasound was negative (not shown). Dynamic contrast-enhanced MRI shows a clumped area of non-mass enhancement with persistent kinetics (**c**). Percutaneous stereotactic vacuum-assisted 8-gauge core needle biopsy revealed exuberant sclerosing adenosis

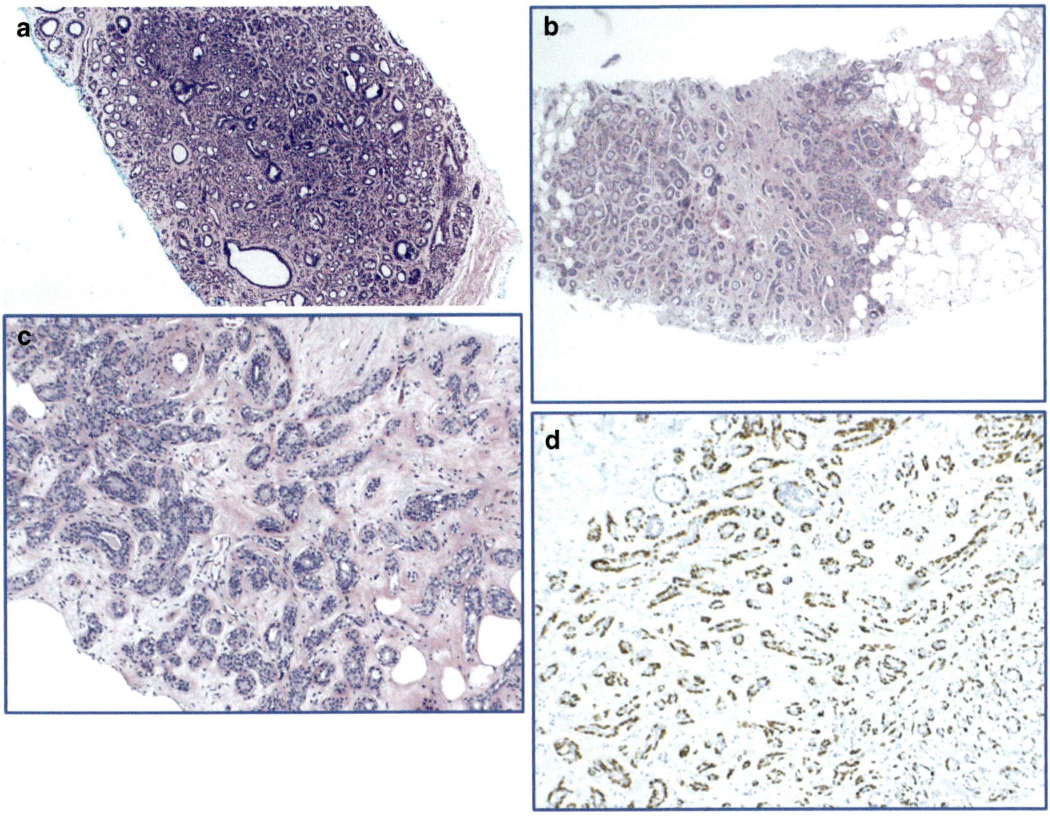

Fig. 7.12 Core needle biopsy with exuberant sclerosing adenosis (**a**). H&E of a core biopsy showed a circumscribed lesion with lobulocentric proliferation of distorted glands compressed by sclerotic stroma (**b**). Higher power magnification showed round to angulated glands in a fibrous collagenized stroma (**c**). Nuclear p63 immunostain demonstrates a preserved myoepithelial cell layer around the adenosis glands (**d**)

Diabetic Mastopathy

See Chap. 5.

Mammary Fibromatosis (Desmoid Tumor)

Mammary Fibromatosis (Desmoid Tumor): Primary breast fibromatosis, or desmoid tumor, is a rare benign neoplasm that accounts for 4% of extra-abdominal desmoid tumors and < 0.2% of all breast tumors [27]. It is a low-grade spindle cell neoplasm composed of fibroblasts infiltrating stroma with variable amounts of collagen. Patients with mammary fibromatosis have a wide age range from 30 to 80 years [27].

- **Clinical Presentation**: It may present as a palpable mass with clinical and imaging features that are indistinguishable from malignancy [28]. Skin retraction may be seen [29]. Although the tumor may be associated with familial adenomatous polyposis syndrome, or Gardner's syndrome, most cases are sporadic. Pathogenesis is linked to activating mutations of CTNNB1 which is associated with increased signaling through the WNT/beta-catenin pathway [30]. A locally invasive tumor prone to recurrence, primary breast fibromatosis is best treated with wide surgical excision.
- **Imaging Findings**:
  - **Mammography**: The typical mammographic presentation of primary breast

fibromatosis is a spiculated mass. When it is characterized by elongated spicules with minimal central density, this tumor mimics the appearance of benign and malignant lesions presenting with architectural distortion [31, 32] (Fig. 7.13).
- **US**: Primary breast fibromatosis most often demonstrates an irregular hypoechoic mass with posterior shadowing on ultrasound. When it is characterized primarily by architectural distortion mammographically, it may only produce an area of shadowing without a discrete mass.
- **MRI**: The most common MRI features are a hypointense or isointense spiculated mass with rapid initial enhancement and persistent kinetic behavior on delayed sequences. Signal intensity on T2-weighted sequences is variable.
- **BI-RADS**: 4, 5.
- **Differential Diagnosis**: Invasive ductal carcinoma, invasive lobular carcinoma, radial scar/complex sclerosing lesion.

• **Pathology Findings**:
  - **Gross**: Grossly the lesion forms a poorly defined mass with a size range from 0.1 to >10 cm [28].
  - **Microscopic Histology**: On histology, there are bland uniform spindle-shaped tumor cells distributed in broad sheets of long interlacing sweeping fascicles with stellate invasive extensions into surrounding adipose tissue and trapping mammary ducts/lobules and skeletal muscle [28–30] (Fig. 7.14).

    Mitoses are usually absent.

    The stroma has localized myxoid areas with focal lymphoid aggregates at the periphery. In longstanding lesions, the stroma is more collagenized with calcification and chondro-osseous metaplasia [30].
  - **Differential Diagnosis**: On core biopsy the differential includes other spindle cell lesions like nodular fasciitis, fibrous scarring from prior trauma, fibromatosis-like metaplastic carcinoma, and phyllodes tumor.

    Immunostains for nuclear beta catenin is present in most cases [28, 30, 33].

    Actin, desmin, and S100 positivity can be seen at least focally in some cells [30]. When a spindle cell lesion is seen on core needle biopsy it is prudent to exclude metaplastic carcinoma with broad spectrum keratins and p63.

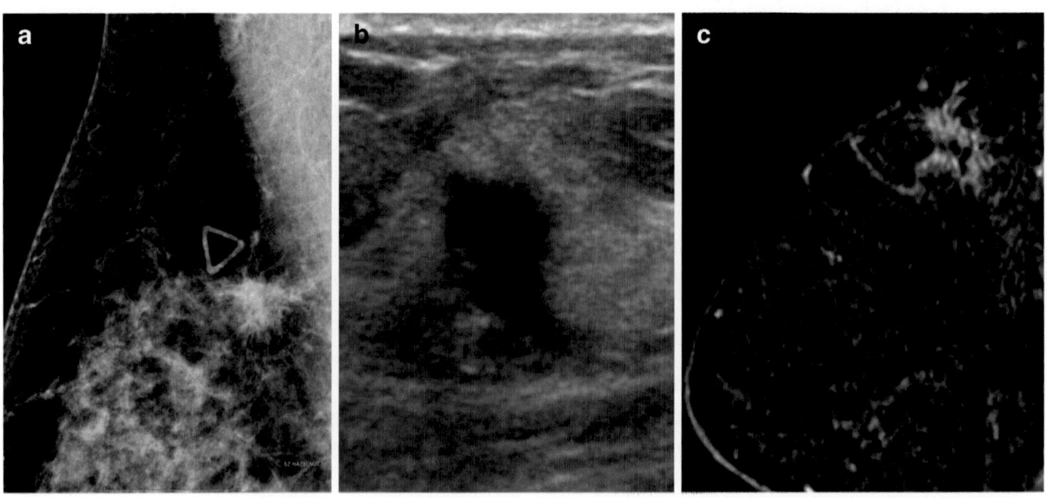

Fig. 7.13 A 45-year-old woman presented with palpable right breast mass. Right MLO view shows a spiculated mass with associated architectural distortion corresponding to the palpable abnormality indicated by a triangular skin marker (**a**). Ultrasound demonstrates an irregular hypoechoic mass with anti-parallel (taller-than-wide) orientation (**b**). Dynamic post-contrast sagittal subtracted image shows an enhancing spiculated mass with associated skin retraction (**c**). Percutaneous ultrasound-guided hand-held 14-gauge core needle biopsy revealed fibromatosis (desmoid tumor), which was confirmed at surgical excision

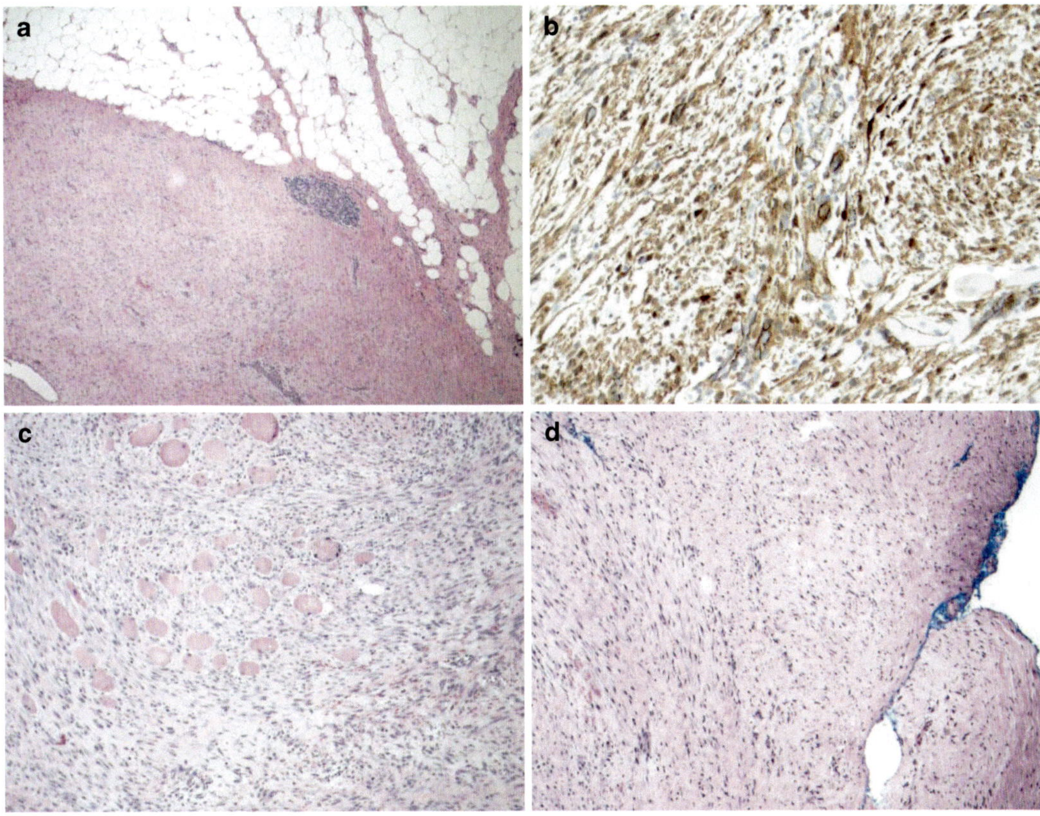

Fig. 7.14 Resection demonstrating fibromatosis with spindle cells invading into adipose with lymphoid aggregates (**a**), and nuclear staining with beta catenin (**b**). Additional sections demonstrating fibromatosis with entrapped muscle fibers and spindle cell morphology (**c**, **d**)

- **Management**: Spindle cell lesions diagnosed on core biopsy following appropriate immunohistochemical workup require excision for definitive diagnosis.

  Local recurrence rates following excision are anywhere between 20% and 30% of cases [28, 30]. However, while recurrences are higher in patients with positive margins they can also be seen in cases with apparently negative margins.

Granular Cell Tumor

See Chap. 5.

Malignant Architectural Distortion

Tubular Carcinoma

See Chap. 5 for text (Figs. 7.15 and 7.16).

Invasive Lobular Carcinoma, Classic and Variants

See Chap. 5 for additional information and pathology.

Invasive Lobular Carcinoma, Classic and Variants: Invasive lobular carcinoma (ILC) is a special histologic type of breast cancer that consti-

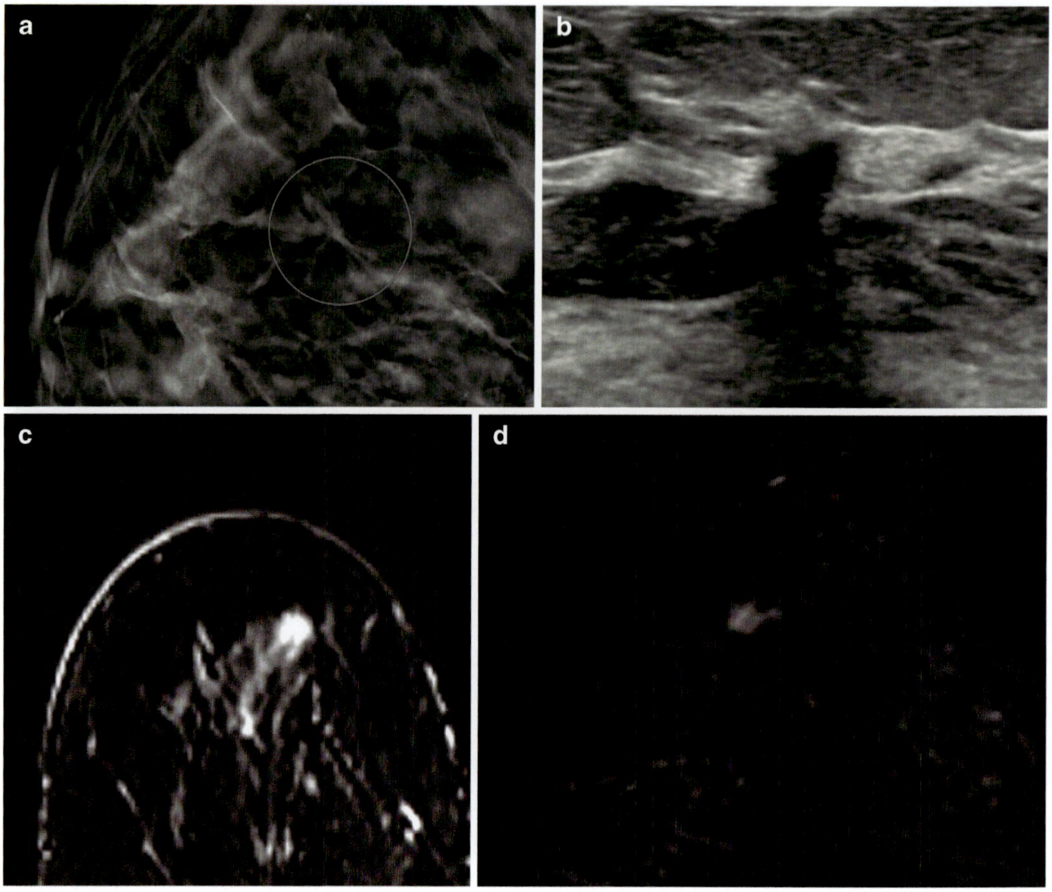

Fig. 7.15 A 50-year-old presented for screening mammogram. Right CC DBT view shows an architectural distortion (circle) with a small central, irregular mass (**a**). Ultrasound confirms a 7-mm irregular, hypoechoic mass (**b**). Additional smaller masses were also seen (not shown). MRI for extent of disease was performed. Axial (**c**) and sagittal (**d**) dynamic post-contrast subtracted images demonstrate a small, irregular, enhancing mass with spiculated margins. The mass was subsequently biopsied revealing a tubular carcinoma

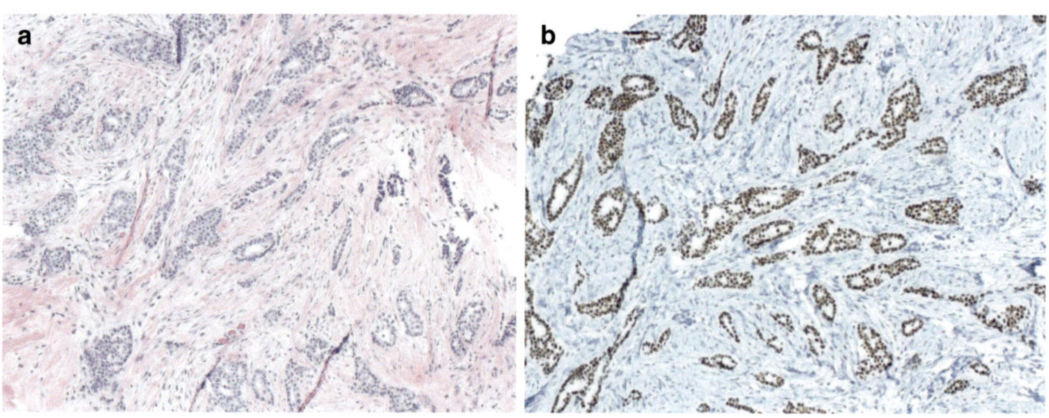

Fig. 7.16 Surgical excision from a 38-year-old woman who was found to have architectural distortion on screening mammogram. Histology showed a well-differentiated invasive carcinoma with tubular features and DCIS (**a**). The tumor is ER positive (**b**)

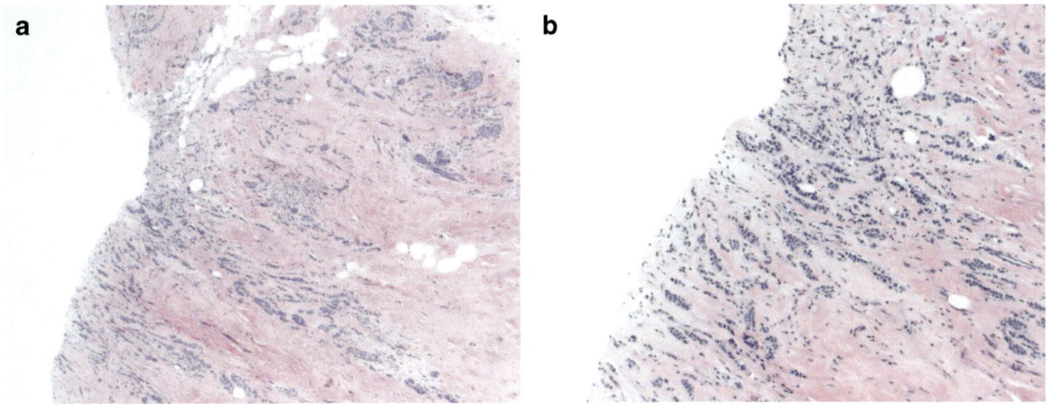

Fig. 7.17 Core needle biopsy from a 48-year-old female with architectural distortion on mammography. Pathology showed invasive lobular carcinoma, classic type with monotonous, discohesive cells present in single files (**a**, **b**)

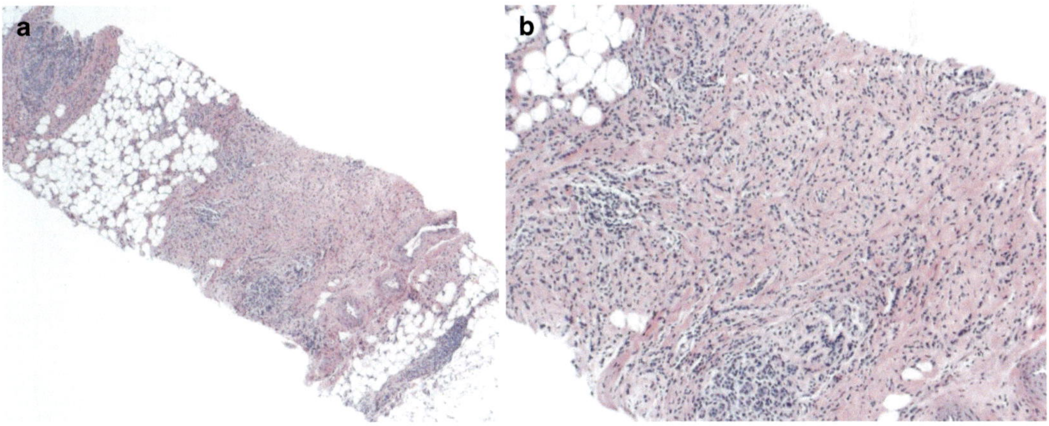

Fig. 7.18 Core needle biopsy with single filing, discohesive tumor cells of invasive lobular carcinoma (**a**, **b**)

tutes 10–15% of all breast cancers [34] (Figs. 7.17 and 7.18). Although ILC is less common than IDC, on imaging it more frequently presents as architectural distortion and comprises up to 25% of all malignancies [34]. Pathologically, ILC may be associated with lobular carcinoma in situ (LCIS). LCIS can be further subdivided into classic, pleomorphic, or florid subtypes [35]. Reported upgrade rates of pleomorphic and florid LCIS at surgical excision after core needle biopsy average ~ 40%, with a range of 25–80% [36–38]. As such, routine excision following core needle biopsy of pleomorphic or florid LCIS is warranted [39].

- **Clinical Presentation**: Invasive lobular carcinoma (ILC) can present as architectural distortion in 11–25% of cases [40–42]. Though typically asymptomatic, presentations may include a palpable lump, shrinking breast, or nipple retraction.
- **Imaging Findings**:
  - **Mammography**: Approximately 25% of ILC will present as architectural distortion, typically without associated calcifications [43] (Figs. 7.19 and 7.20).

    There may be an associated mass or asymmetry.

    Calcifications may be present if there is associated LCIS.

    However, up to 30% may be mammographically occult as the single-file growth that characterizes ILC tends to

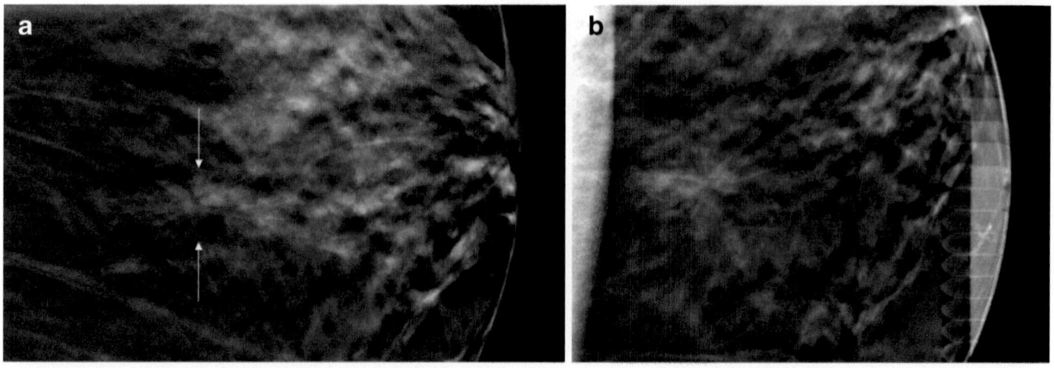

Fig. 7.19 A 73-year-old presented for screening mammogram. Left CC DBT view shows the radiating lines of an architectural distortion with no central mass (**a**, **b**). No ultrasound correlate was found. Tomosynthesis-guided stereotactic biopsy was performed revealing invasive lobular carcinoma

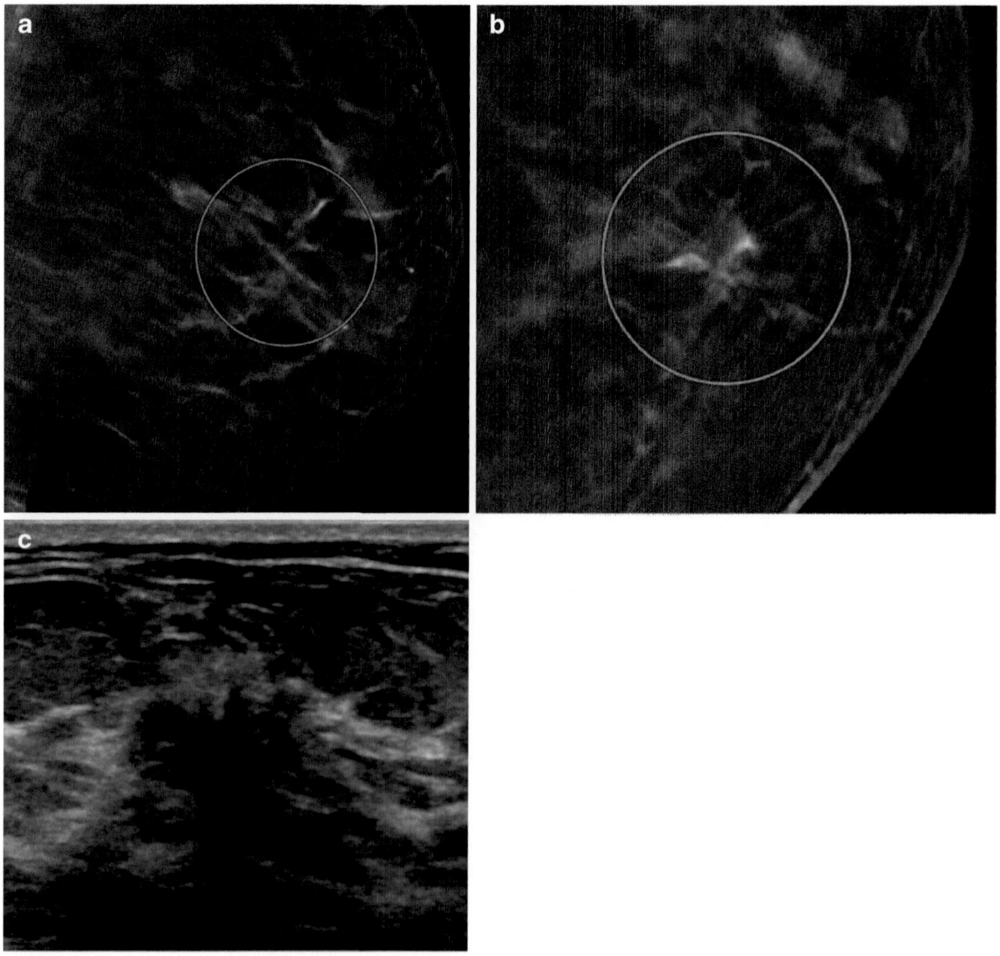

Fig. 7.20 A 46-year-old presenting for diagnostic mammogram follow up due to a known, probably benign left breast mass. Left MLO (**a**) and left CC DBT (**b**) views demonstrate a new architectural distortion. Ultrasound shows an irregular, shadowing mass correlate (**c**). Percutaneous ultrasound-guided 14-gauge core needle biopsy demonstrates invasive lobular carcinoma

permeate rather than displace normal structures [42, 44].
- **US**: Most commonly, ILC will present as an irregular, shadowing, hypoechoic mass on ultrasound.
  However, in cases of architectural distortion found only on digital breast tomosynthesis (DBT), if no sonographic correlate is seen, the positive predictive value of malignancy remains high at 47% and further evaluation and tissue diagnosis remains necessary [45].
- **MRI**: Cases of architectural distortion without a sonographic correlate may be further evaluated by MRI.
  MRI correlation for a subtle mammographic architectural distortion can heighten suspicion and tissue diagnosis may be obtained using mammographic or MRI guidance.
  Most commonly, ILC will present as an irregular enhancing mass, with the distortion correlating with spiculated margins.
- **BIRADS**: 4, 5.
- **Differential Diagnosis**: Invasive ductal carcinoma, radial scar/complex sclerosing lesion, stromal fibrosis, postoperative scar.

Invasive Ductal Carcinoma

Invasive Ductal Carcinoma: Includes the majority of invasive carcinoma in the breast including all adenocarcinomas that do not meet the criteria for special histologic types [46, 47]. Invasive ductal carcinomas (IDCs) are referred to as no special type (NST) or not otherwise specified (NOS) [46, 47]. Median age at diagnosis is around 60 years [46]. All invasive carcinomas whether ductal, lobular or special types arise in the terminal ductal lobular unit [46]. They can be ER and/or PR positive, HER2 positive or triple negative. In younger patients (<40 years) IDC can present as a palpable mass while in older patients it is more commonly detected by screening [48, 49].

- **Clinical Presentation**: Invasive ductal carcinoma is the most common malignancy that can present with architectural distortion. Digital breast tomosynthesis (DBT) has been shown to detect malignant architectural distortion 2–3 times more often than conventional digital mammography [41, 50]. Careful comparison with prior studies is essential to identify subtle changes.
- **Imaging Findings**:
  - **Mammography**: Thin, radiating lines without a central mass will be seen with primary architectural distortion on conventional mammography (Fig. 7.21).
    With DBT and careful inspection, a central mass can sometimes be found.
    The presence of calcifications can increase suspicion for malignancy.
    Alternatively, IDC can appear as a spiculated mass with associated architectural distortion.
    If no ultrasound or MRI correlate is seen and there is no surgical history, stereotactic-guided biopsy (either conventional or tomosynthesis-guided) is recommended.
  - **US**: IDC typically is shown as a hypoechoic irregular mass with spiculated and/or angular margins. Identification of an ultrasound correlate can permit ultrasound-guided biopsy.
  - **MRI**: If an ultrasound correlate is not seen and mammographic architectural distortion is subtle, MRI can be employed for further characterization. The presence of an irregular, enhancing mass on MRI can confirm suspicion and provide additional means for tissue diagnosis.
  - **BIRADS**: 4, 5.
  - **Differential Diagnosis**: Radial scar/complex sclerosing lesion, stromal fibrosis, fat

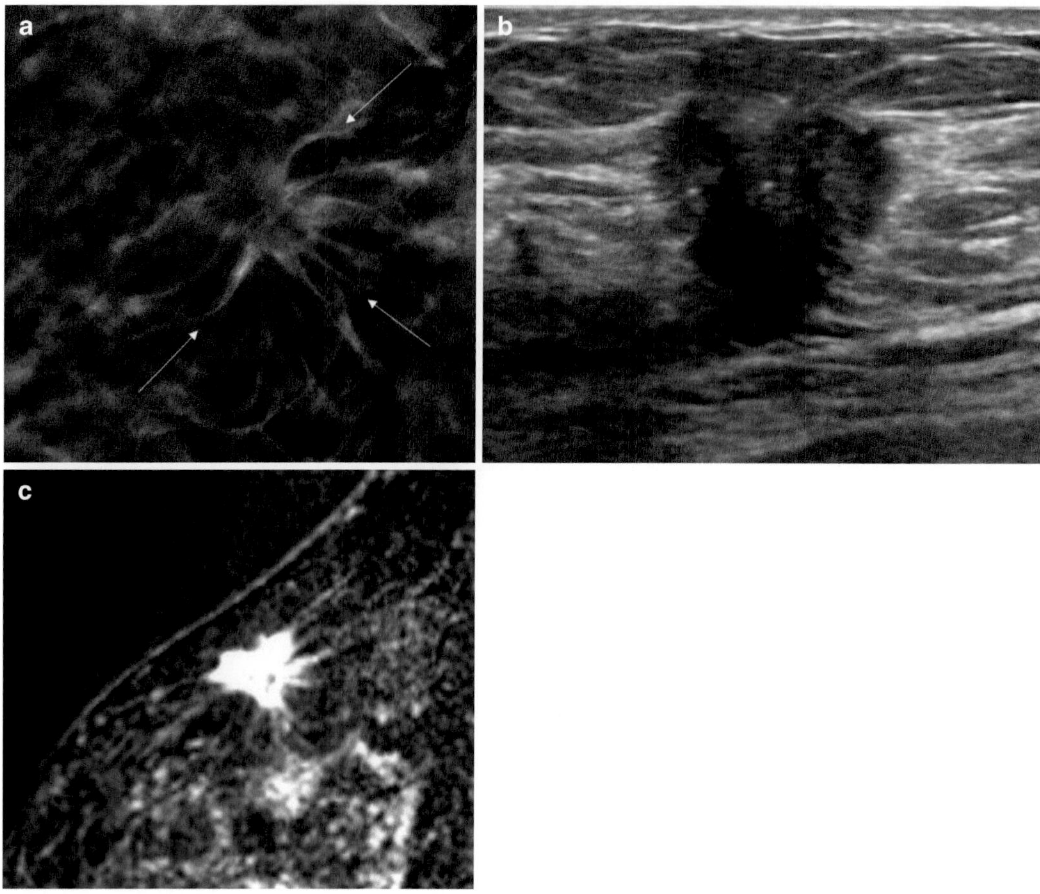

Fig. 7.21 A 35-year-old presented with a palpable mass. Right CC DBT diagnostic mammogram shows in irregular mass with long radiating lines of architectural distortion (**a**). Ultrasound confirms a solid, irregular mass (**b**). Given the patient's young age at presentation, MRI for extent of disease was performed. Sagittal dynamic post-contrast subtracted image demonstrates an irregular mass with spiculated margin (**c**), correlating with mammography and ultrasound. Surgical core biopsy was performed revealing invasive ductal carcinoma

necrosis, postoperative scar, invasive lobular carcinoma.

- **Pathology Findings**:
  - **Gross**: Firm to hard mass with gritty sensation when cut.

    The borders may be well defined or stellate and irregular.

    Sometimes when cells infiltrate diffusely no mass can be visualized.
  - **Microscopic Histology**: Histology can be variable depending on whether the glands form tubules with open lumens or tumor cells infiltrate as solid nests and cords [46] (Fig. 7.22).

    Invasive carcinoma can infiltrate diffusely into the breast adipose tissue without eliciting a desmoplastic reaction.

    Depending on the differentiation the nuclei may be low grade, intermediate or high grade.

    Cytoplasm can be moderate or abundant and granular.

    Mitoses may be low or easily found depending on the grade of the tumor.
  - **Differential Diagnosis**: Sclerosing adenosis, microglandular adenosis, DCIS, invasive lobular carcinoma, epithelial displacement, metastatic carcinomas.
  - **Management**: Core needle biopsy diagnosis of invasive versus in situ carcinoma will dictate whether the patient will require sen-

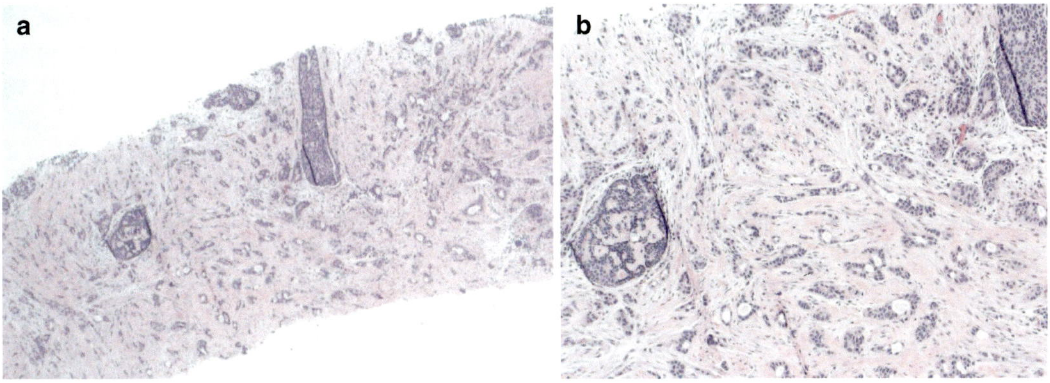

Fig. 7.22 Core needle biopsy from a 48-year-old woman with architectural distortion of the left breast on screening mammography. The biopsy showed a well-differentiated invasive ductal carcinoma (**a**). On high power, the tubule formation with angulated contours invading the breast stroma can be seen (**b**)

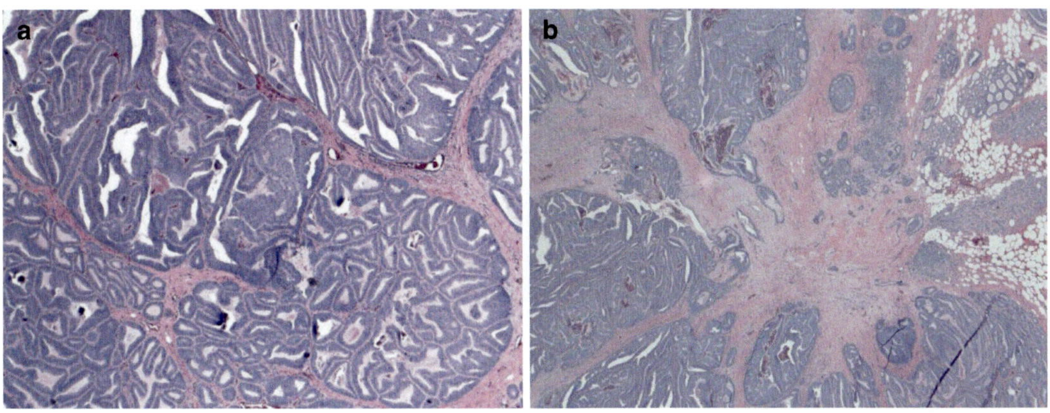

Fig. 7.23 A 41-year-old women with architectural distortion on screening mammogram. Core biopsy revealed atypical ductal hyperplasia bordering on DCIS. Surgical excision confirmed DCIS, grade 2, ER+/PR+, with no invasive component (**a**). DCIS involving a radial scar was also seen in the same excision specimen (**b**)

tinel node biopsy [48]. Some invasive carcinomas have the growth pattern of cribriform DCIS and can be diagnosed accurately by using ancillary immunohistochemical stains for myoepithelial markers [30, 47]. Due to the limitation of sampling in core needle biopsy there may be a few glands entrapped in a desmoplastic stroma that cannot be investigated further due to depletion of tissue on deeper levels. In such situations additional sampling to confirm the diagnosis of malignancy is needed for management as some may need mastectomy versus neoadjuvant therapy.

Ductal Carcinoma In Situ

See Chap. 8 for additional text.

***Ductal Carcinoma* In Situ**: DCIS less frequently presents as an architectural distortion on imaging, representing 1.1–18.5% of all malignancies [40, 42] (Fig. 7.23).

- **Clinical Presentation**: Ductal carcinoma in situ (DCIS) begins in the terminal ductal lobular unit and is a precursor of invasive cancer. It accounts for 20–25% of all screen-detected cancers and 5% of symptomatic cancers [42]. Overall, 20–25% of DCIS will upgrade to invasive cancer on surgical excision [42]. However, DCIS presenting as architectural distortion mammographically, has only been found to upgrade to invasive carcinoma in 3.0% of cases [40].
- **Imaging Findings**:
  - **Mammography**: DCIS presents as architectural distortion in 1.5–11% of cases [42, 51] (Figs. 7.24 and 7.25).

    Most commonly, DCIS presents as calcifications on mammography (80%), or as a mass (12%) with or without calcifications (10%) [42].
  - **US**: The sensitivity of ultrasound for DCIS is 50% as most cases present as calcifications, which can be difficult to discern sonographically [42].

    Ultrasound may be useful to evaluate if an associated mass is present, which could permit ultrasound-guided biopsy.
  - **MRI**: MRI can be utilized to identify extent of disease and to aid in identification of a possible invasive component.

    Linear or segmental clumped non-mass enhancement is the most common MRI presentation of DCIS [42, 52–54].
  - **BIRADS**: 4, 5.
  - **Differential Diagnosis**: Invasive ductal carcinoma, invasive lobular carcinoma, radial scar/complex sclerosing lesion, stromal fibrosis.

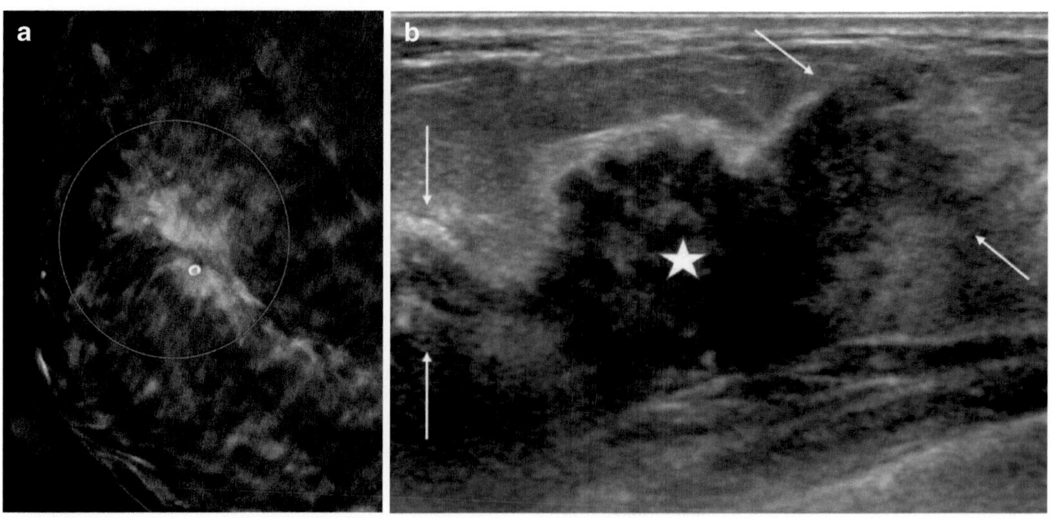

Fig. 7.24 A 49-year-old patient presented for screening mammogram. Right MLO DBT view (**a**) shows a focal asymmetry with associated architectural distortion (circle). Ultrasound (**b**) shows an irregular mass with irregular margins (star). Arrows indicate the extensions of irregular tissue from the mass that are correlates for the mammographic architectural distortion seen in (**a**). Percutaneous ultrasound-guided hand-held 14-gauge core needle biopsy of the finding shown in (**b**) revealed atypical ductal hyperplasia bordering on DCIS

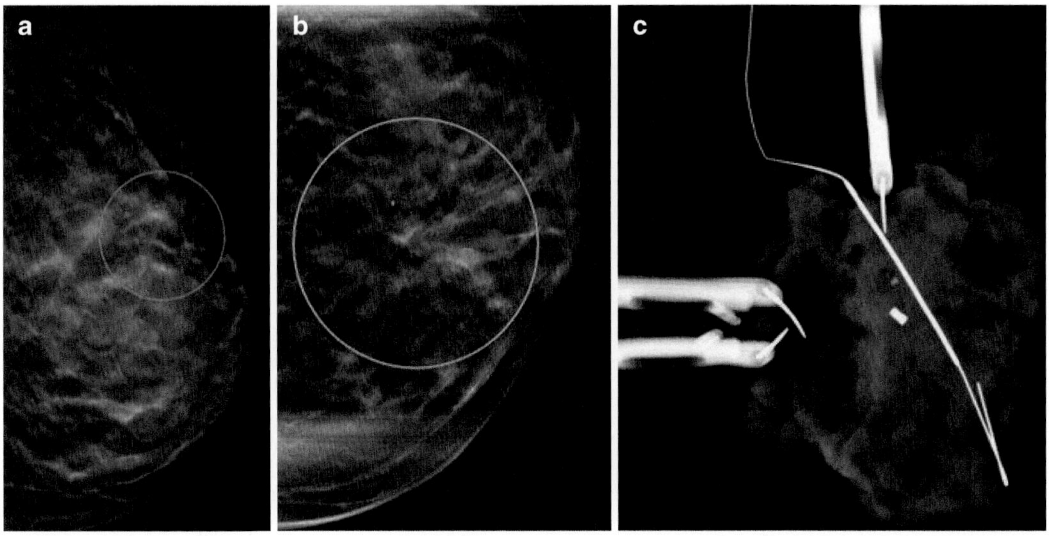

Fig. 7.25 A 46-year-old female was recalled from screening due to an area of architectural distortion in the left breast. On mammography there was a high-density area of focal asymmetry with architectural distortion in the 12 o'clock position of the left breast (**a**, **b**). On ultrasound fibrocystic changes were present, but no suspicious sonographic correlate was identified. The distortion was graded as BI-RADS 4, suspicious of malignancy; a tomosynthesis-guided biopsy was recommended and performed, with 12 core samples obtained with a 9-gauge vacuum-assisted device. Pathology yielded nodular adenosis involved by atypical apocrine adenosis. Given the presence of atypia, a needle localization and surgical excision were performed (**c**) and yielded 2 cm of intermediate to high nuclear grade DCIS with close margins, ADH, and a CSL

References

1. Wellings SR, Alpers CE. Subgross pathologic features and incidence of radial scars in the breast. Hum Pathol. 1984;15(5):475–9.
2. Alleya QD, Smetherman DH, Farr, GH., Cederbom GJ. Radial scar of the breast: radiologic-pathologic correlation in 22 cases. BREAST IMAGING, volume 19.
3. Cohen MA, Newell MS. Radial scars of the breast encountered at core biopsy: review of histologic, imaging, and management considerations. AJR Am J Roentgenol. 2017;209(5):1168–77.
4. Kennedy M, Masterson AV, Kerin MF. Pathology and clinical relevance of radial scars: a review. J Clin Pathol. 2003;56(10):721–4.
5. Shin SJ. A comprehensive guide to core needle biopsies of the breast. Springer International Publishing Switzerland; 2016.
6. Hoda SA, Rosen PP, Brogi E, Koerner F, Rosen PP. Rosen's breast pathology. Lippincott Williams & Wilkins; 2020.
7. Berg JC, et al. Breast cancer risk in women with radial scars in benign breast biopsies. Breast Cancer Res Treat. 2008;108(2):167–74.
8. Jacobs TW, et al. Radial scars in benign breast biopsy specimens and the risk of breast cancer. N Engl J Med. 1999;340(6):430–6.
9. Sanders ME, et al. Interdependence of radial scar and proliferative disease with respect to invasive breast carcinoma risk in patients with benign breast biopsies. Cancer. 2006;106(7):1453–61.
10. Londero V, Zuiani C, Linda A, Girometti R, Bazzocchi M, Sardanelli F. High-risk breast lesions at imaging-guided needle biopsy: usefulness of MRI for treatment decision. AJR Am J Roentgenol. 2012;199(2):W240–W50.
11. Cohen MA, Sferlazza SJ. Role of sonography in evaluation of radial scars of the breast. AJR Am J Roentgenol. 2000;174(4):1075–8.
12. Linda A, Zuiani C, Londero V, Cedolini C, Girometti R, Bazzocchi M. Magnetic resonance imaging of radial sclerosing lesions (radial scars) of the breast. Eur J Radiol. 2012;81(11):3201–7.
13. Drukteinis J, Gombos E, Raza S, Chikarmane S, Swami A, Birdwell R. MR imaging assessment of the breast after breast conservation therapy: distinguishing benign from malignant lesions. Radiographics. 2012;32(1):219–34.
14. Anderson C, Ricci A Jr, Pedersen CA, Cartun RW. Immunocytochemical analysis of estrogen and progesterone receptors in benign stromal lesions of the breast. Evidence of hormonal etiology in pseudoangiomatous hyperplasia of mammary stroma. Am J Surg Pathol. 1991;15(2):145–9. Epub 1991/02/11

15. Powell CM, Cranon ML, Rosen PP. Pseudoangiomatous stromal hyperplasia (APSH). A mammary stromal tumor with myofibroblastic proliferation. Am J Surg Pathol. 1995;19(3):270–7. Epub 1995/03/01
16. Virk RL, Khan A. Pseudoangiomatous stromal hyperplasia: an overview. Arch Pathol Lab Med. 2010;134(7):1070–4. Epub 2010/07/01
17. Abdull GB. Pseudoangiomatous stromal hyperplasia of the breast. Arch Pathol Lab Med. 2009;133(8):1335–8. /Epub 2009/08/06
18. Jones KN, Glazebrook KN, Reynolds C. Pseudoangiomatous stromal hyperplasia: imaging findings with pathologic and clinical correlation. AJR Am J Roentgenol. 2010;195(4):1036–42. Pub 2010/09/23
19. Ibrahim RE, Scitto CG, Weidner N. Pseduoangiomatous hyperplasia of mammary stroma. Some observations regarding its clinicopathologic spectrum. Cancer. 1989;63(6):1154–60. Epub 1989/03/15
20. Shehata BM, Fishman I, Collings MH, et al. Pseudoangiomatous stromal hyperplasia of the breast in a pediatric patient: an underrecognized entity. Pediatr Dev Pathol. 2009;12:450–4.
21. Bownman E, Opera G, Okoli J, Gundry K, Rizzo M, Gabram-Mendola S, et al. Pseudoangiomatous stromal hyperplasia (APSH) of the breast: a series of 24 patients. Breast J. 2012;18(3):242–7. Epub 2012/05/16
22. Ferreira M, Albarracin CT, Resetkova E. Pseudoangiomatous stromal hyperplasia tumor: a clinical, radiologic and pathologic study of 26 cases. Mod Pathol. 2008;21(2):201–7. Epub 2007/12/18
23. Badve S, Sloane JP. Pseudoangiomatous hyperplasia of male breast. Histopathology. 1995;26(5):463–6. 1995/05/01
24. Degnim AC, Frost MH, Rdisky DC, Anderson SS, Viekrant RA, Boughey JC, et al. Pseudoangiomatous stromal hyperplasia and breast cancer risk. Ann Surg Oncol. 2010;17(12):3269–77. EPub 2010/06/23
25. Nassar H, Elieff MP, Kronz JD, Argani P. Pseudoangiomatous stromal hyperplasia (PASH) of the breast with foci of morphologic malignancy: a case of PASH with malignant transformation? Int J Surg Pathol. 2010;18(6):564–9. Epub 2008/07/10
26. Raj SD, Sahani VG, Adrada BE, Scoggins ME, Albarracin CT, Woodtichartpreecha P, Posleman Monetto FE, Whitman GJ. Pseudoangiomatous stromal hyperplasia of the breast: multimodality review with pathologic correlation. Curr Probl Diagn Radiol. 2017;46(2):130–5.
27. WHO Classification of Tumors Editorial Board. Breast tumours. WHO classification of tumors. 5th ed. Lyon, France: IARC; 2019.
28. Glazebrook KN, Reynolds CA. Mammary fibromatosis. AJR Am J Roentgenol. 2009;193(3):856–60.
29. Rosen Y, Papasozomenos SC, Gardner B. Fibromatosis of the breast. Cancer. 1978;41(4):1409–13.
30. Schmitt SJ, Collins LC. Biopsy interpretation of the breast. 3rd ed. Wolters Kluwer Health; 2018.
31. Boland MR, Nugent T, Nolan J, O'Mahony J, O'Keeffe S, Gillham CC, Maguire A, Geraghty J, McCartan D, Evoy D, Prichard RS, McDermott EW, Alazawi D, Boyle TJ, Connolly EM. Fibromatosis of the breast: a 10-year multi-institutional experience and review of the literature. Breast Cancer. 2021;28(1):168–74.
32. Liu H, Zeng H, Zhang H, Wang H, Cheng Z, Hu Y, Wu Z. Breast fibromatosis: imaging and clinical findings. Breast J. 2020;26(11):2217–22.
33. Kuba MG, Lester SC, Giess CS, Bertagnolli MM, Wieczorek TJ, Brock JE. Fibromatosis of the breast: diagnostic accuracy of core needle biopsy. Am J Clin Pathol. 2017;148(3):243–50.
34. Lakhani S, Rakha E, Simpson PT. Invasive lobular carcinoma. In: Lakhani S, Ellis IO, Schnitt SJ, et al., editors. WHO classification of tumors of the breast. Lyon, France: IARC Press; 2012.
35. Hicks DG, Susan C. Lester: diagnostic pathology breast. 2nd ed. Expert Consultation; 2016.
36. Schnitt SJ, et al. American registry of pathology expert opinions: the spectrum of lobular carcinoma in situ: diagnostic features and clinical implications. Ann Diagn Pathol. 2020;45:151481.
37. Nakhlis F, et al. Evaluating the rate of upgrade to invasive breast cancer and/or DCIS following a Core biopsy diagnosis of non-classic LCIS. Ann Surg Oncol. 2019;26:55–61.
38. Kuba M, et al. Morphologic subtypes of lobular carcinoma in situ diagnosed on core needle biopsy: clinicopathologic features and findings at follow up excision. Mod Pathol. 2021; published online
39. American Society of Breast Surgeons Consensus Guidelines, copyright 2018.
40. Bahl M, Baker JA, Kinsey EN, Ghate SV. Architectural distortion on mammography: correlation with pathologic outcomes and predictors of malignancy. AJR Am J Roentgenol. 2015;205(6):1339–45.
41. Freer PR, Niell B, Raffery EA. Preoperative tomosynthesis-guided needle localization of mammographically and sonographically occult breast lesions. Radiology. 2015;275(2):377–83.
42. Berg W, Leung J. Diagnostic imaging: breast. 3rd ed. Philadelphia, PA: Elsevier; 2019.
43. Harvey J, March. *Making the diagnosis*: a practical guided to breast imaging. Philadelphia, PA: Elsevier; 2013.
44. Durand MA, Wang S, Hooley RJ, et al. Tomosynthesis-detected architectural distortion: management algorithm with radiologic-pathologic correlation. Radiographics. 2016;36(2):311–21.
45. Da Silva L, Parry S, Reid L, et al. Aberrant expression of E-cadherin in lobular carcinomas of the breast. Am J Surg Pathol. 2008;32(5):773–83.
46. Ellis I, Collins L, Ichhara S, et al. Invasive carcinoma of no special type (NST). In: Lakhani S, Ellis IO, Schnitt SJ, et al, eds. WHO classification of tumors of the breast. 4th Lyon, France: IARC Press;2012.

47. Weigelt B, Horlings HM, Kreike B, et al. Refinement of breast cancer classification by molecular characterization of histological special types. J Pathol. 2008;216(2):141–50.
48. Cady B, Stone MD, Schuler JG, et al. The new era in breast cancer: invasion, size and nodal involvement dramatically decreaing as a result of mammographic screening. Arch Surg. 1996;131(3):301–8.
49. Haakinson DJ, et al. A significant number of women present with palpable breast cancer even with normal mammogram within 1 year. Am J Surg. 2010;20(6):712–7.
50. Partyka L, Lourenco AP, Maniero MB. Detection of mammographically occult architectural distortion on digital breast tomosynthesis screening: initial clinical experience. AJR Am J Roentgenol. 2014;203(1):216–22.
51. Shaheen R, Schimmelpenninck CA, Stoddart L, Raymond H, Slanetz PJ. Spectrum of diseases presenting as architectural distortion on mammography: multimodality radiologic imaging with pathologic correlation. Semin Ultrasound CT MR. 2011;32(4):351–62.
52. Schnall MD, Blume J, Bluemke D, et al. Radiology. 2006;238:42–53.
53. Uematsu T, Kasami M. AJR Am J Roentgenol. 2012;198:1223–30.
54. Tozaki M, Igarashi T, Fukuda K. AJR Am J Roentgenol. 2006;187:313–21.

Calcifications

8

Kamaljeet Singh, Laura Sheiman, Brigid Killelea, Kirstyn Brownson, and Liva Andrejeva

Benign Calcifications

Coarse Calcifications (Degenerating Fibroadenoma)

Degenerating Fibroadenoma: Over time, fibroadenomas (FAs) may undergo so-called degenerating changes, like hyalinization of the stroma, and develop internal calcifications. These may initially manifest as round calcifications (equal or greater than 0.5 mm), or may appear indeterminate and even prompt biopsy, but then become increasingly coarse over time, ultimately becoming large and somewhat irregular, and are then referred to as "popcorn" calcifications. Such calcifications are generally easily recognized as benign. These are frequently seen incidentally on screening mammography, but, if large, the patient may present with a palpable mass. These can be solitary or multiple, uni- or bilateral [1].

- **BI-RADS**: 3, if presenting early on as round calcifications, or 3, if presenting as "popcorn" calcifications.

Pathology Findings: The calcifications in FA are usually found in postmenopausal women. With aging, the stromal component of the fibroadenoma shows loss of cellularity, hyalinization, and an increase in the stromal fibrous portion. The calcifications are identified in the hyalinized stroma of these FA. These calcifications are phosphate-type and easily identified on the hematoxylin-stained sections.

Differential Diagnosis: Fat necrosis.

Management Recommendations: No intervention is needed if appearance is typical [2]. Surgical excision is recommended to exclude malignancy when the lesion is symptomatic or rapidly growing. Large fibroadenomas may need to be resected due to patient symptoms or if the imaging appearance of the lesion creates concern for sampling error on core needle biopsy. Emotional distress in the setting of a breast mass and aesthetic concerns are patient-driven

K. Singh (✉)
Department of Pathology and Laboratory Medicine, Brown University and Women and Infants Hospital of RI, Providence, RI, USA
e-mail: kamaljeet_singh@brown.edu

L. Sheiman
Department of Radiology and Biomedical Imaging, Yale University, New Haven, CT, USA
e-mail: laura.sheiman@yale.edu

B. Killelea
Department of Surgery, Brigham and Women's Hospital, Boston, MA, USA
e-mail: brigidkillelea@gmail.com

K. Brownson
Department of Surgery, University of Utah, Salt Lake City, UT, USA
e-mail: Kirstyn.Brownson@hci.utah.edu

L. Andrejeva
Department of Radiology and Biomedical Imaging, Yale School of Medicine, New Haven, CT, USA
e-mail: liva.andrejeva@yale.edu

M. Harigopal et al. (eds.), *Radiology Pathology Correlations of Breast Lesions*,
https://doi.org/10.1007/978-3-031-65711-5_8

reasons why surgical removal of fibroadenomas may be performed. Given the exceptionally low likelihood of malignancy, surgical excision should be used judiciously and offered only after thorough patient education. Alternative management suitable for smaller (<4 cm), biopsy-proven fibroadenomas is cryoablation.

Concordant and Discordant Scenarios

Case 1

Clinical History: A 70-year-old female presenting for screening mammography (Figs. 8.1 and 8.2).

BI-RADS: 2, benign findings.

Pathology Findings: The FA showed phosphate-type calcifications in the stroma (Figs. 8.3 and 8.4).

Case 2

Clinical History: A 64-year-old female presents for screening mammography (Figs. 8.5 and 8.6).

BI-RADS: 2, benign finding (Figs. 8.7 and 8.8).

BI-RADS: 4, suspicious finding. An US-guided biopsy was recommended and performed. The patient subsequently underwent a lumpectomy.

Pathology Findings: An invasive breast carcinoma (no special type) was identified. An FA

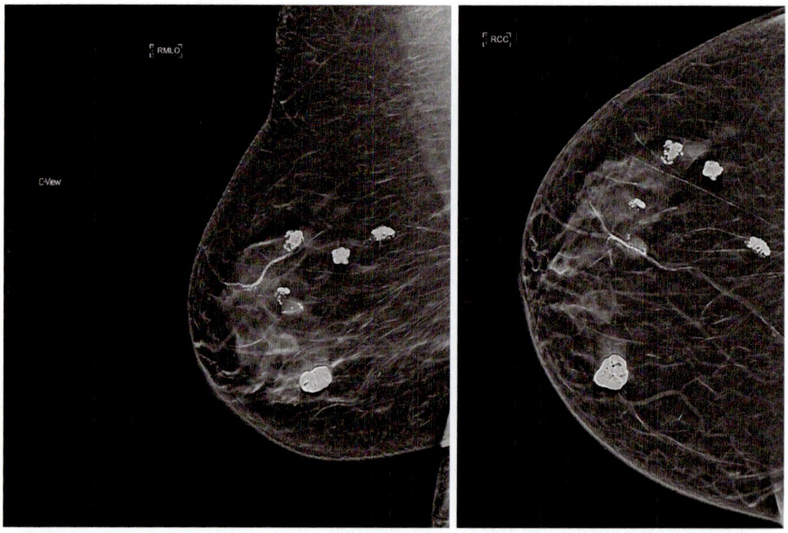

Figs. 8.1 and 8.2 **MG findings**: Multiple large, coarse calcifications, typical of multiple degenerated fibroadenomas

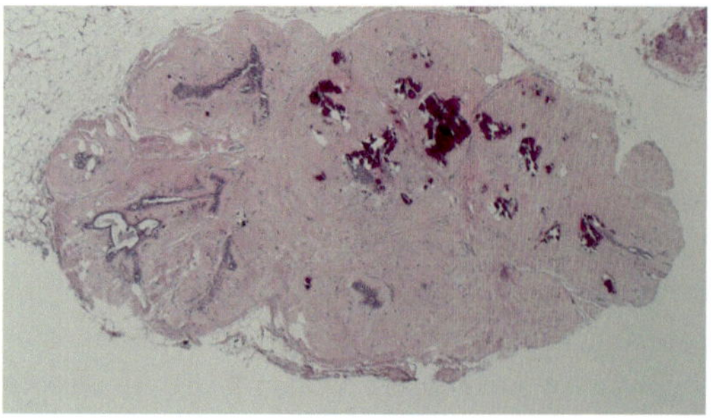

Fig. 8.3 (H&E, 2×) Fibroadenoma with stromal phosphate-type calcifications

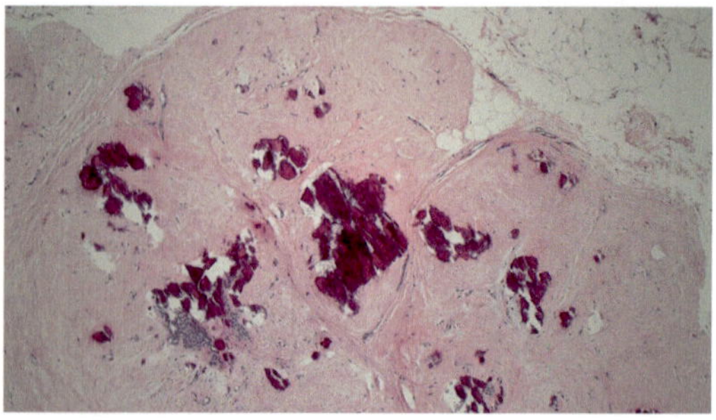

Fig. 8.4 (H&E, 10×) Fibroadenoma with stromal phosphate-type calcifications

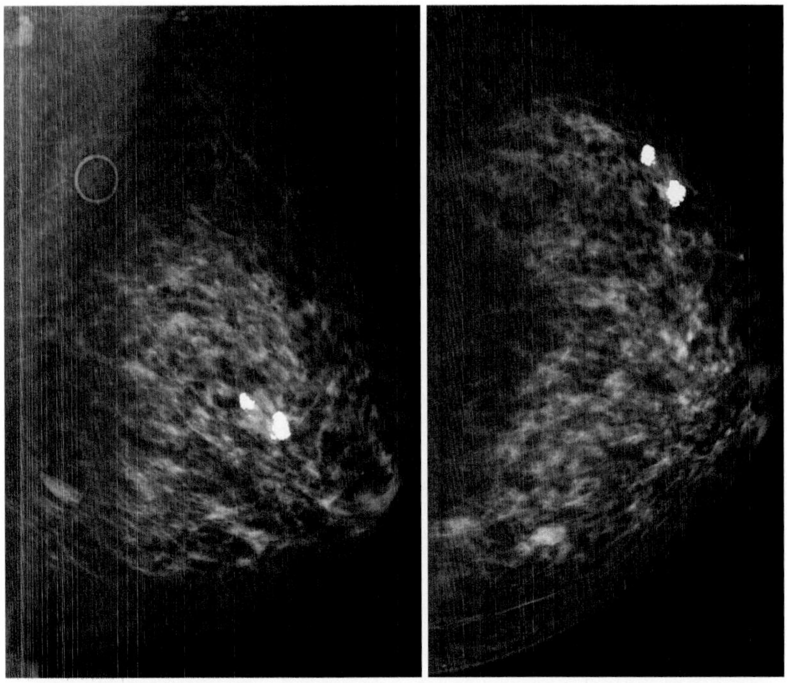

Figs. 8.5 and 8.6 MG: Prior mammogram demonstrated large, coarse heterogeneous calcifications consistent with degenerating fibroadenomas

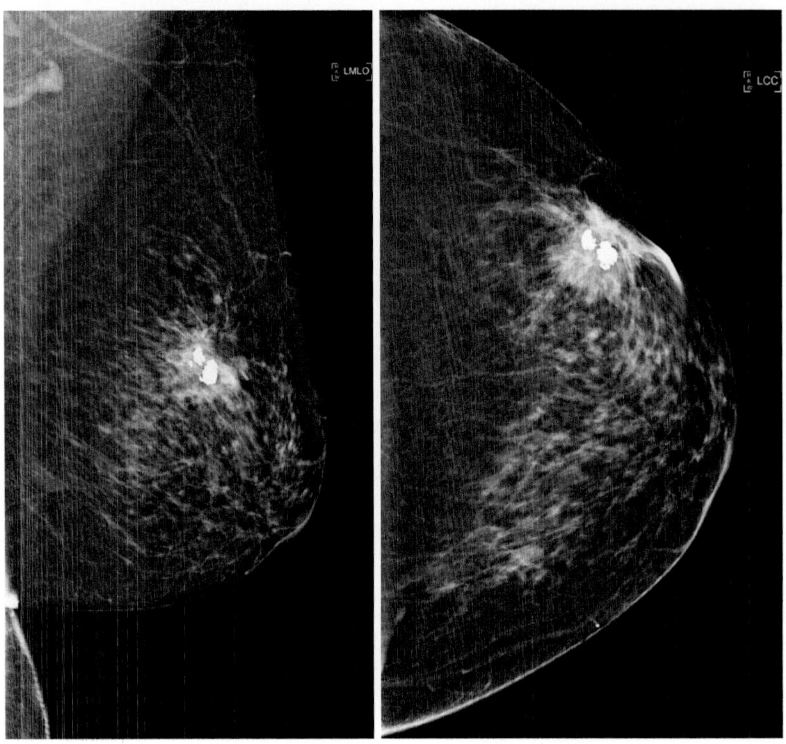

Figs. 8.7 and 8.8 The current mammogram demonstrates an irregular mass with a spiculated margin engulfing the coarse benign calcifications

with calcifications was present in the vicinity. The calcifications were present in the hyalinized stroma of the FA (Fig. 8.9).

Case 3

Clinical History: A 61-year-old female with known stable benign coarse calcifications, likely degenerating fibroadenomas and fibroadenomatoid change, is recalled from screening mammography due to new calcifications in the right breast (Figs. 8.10 and 8.11).

BI-RADS: 4, suspicious. A stereotactic biopsy yielded grade 3, DCIS, cribriform and solid pattern. The patient subsequently underwent a lumpectomy, which yielded DCIS adjacent to a fibroadenoma.

Pathology Findings (Fig. 8.12):

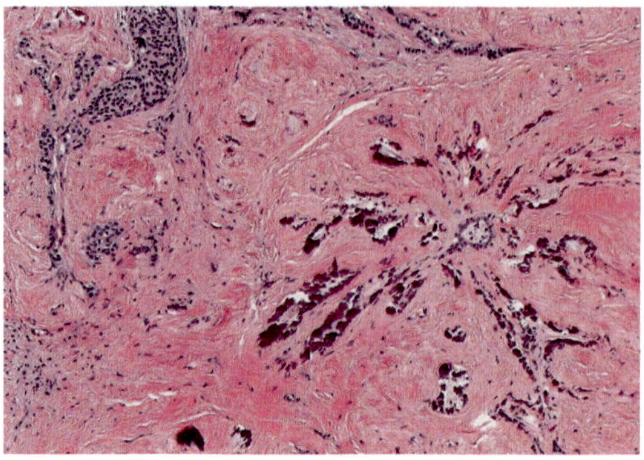

Fig. 8.9 (H&E, 10×) Invasive ductal carcinoma present adjacent to fibroadenoma, with associated calcifications

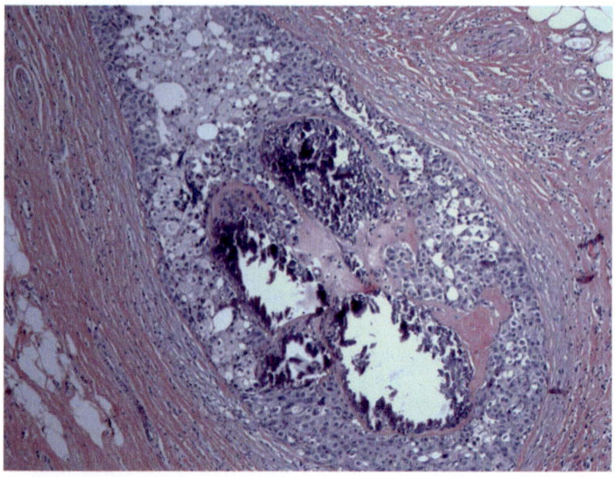

Fig. 8.12 (H&E 10×) Ductal carcinoma in situ, intermediate nuclear grade with associated calcifications

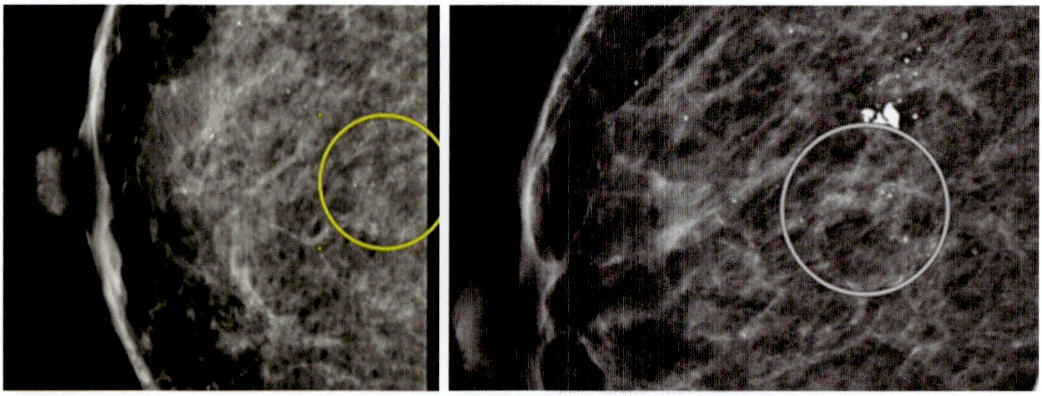

Figs. 8.10 and 8.11 **MG findings**: Coarse heterogeneous calcifications in a ductal distribution adjacent to the stable, benign coarse calcifications likely due to a degenerating fibroadenoma. Although early calcifying fibroadenomatoid change may present as somewhat heterogeneous calcifications [3, 4] these calcifications were completely new since the prior mammogram 2 years ago, and did not have an appearance suggestive of degenerating fibroadenoma/fibroadenomatoid change

Large Rod-Like Calcifications

Imaging Findings: Large, smooth, rod-like, >0.5 mm in diameter (sometimes also referred to as cigar-shaped) calcifications occurring in a ductal distribution, sometimes in the setting of duct ectasia. Occasionally, these can also have a thinner, needle-like appearance. These are usually incidental findings on screening mammography and are seen in a ductal distribution. These may involve a single duct or be segmental, regional or diffuse, and frequently bilateral.

- **BI-RADS**: 2, benign.
- **Differential Diagnosis**: DCIS presenting as coarse calcifications.

Pathology Findings: The calcifications are present in association with sclerosed ducts. The phosphate-type calcifications are identified in the sclerosed and hyalinized stroma of large ducts. The duct often shows marked periductal fibrosis. The duct may also show obliterated lumen.

Concordant and Discordant Scenario

Case 1

Clinical History: A 50-year-old female presenting for screening mammography (Figs. 8.13 and 8.14).

BI-RADS: 2, benign findings.

Management Recommendations: No intervention is needed if appearance is typical, but caution is needed when the finding is new, unilateral, and involves a small area within the distribution of a single duct system.

Pathology Findings (Fig. 8.15):

Case 2

Clinical History: A 50-year-old female presented for screening mammography, with increased calcifications seen in the left breast. On the prior mammogram report, these were described as benign secretory calcifications (Figs. 8.16 and 8.17).

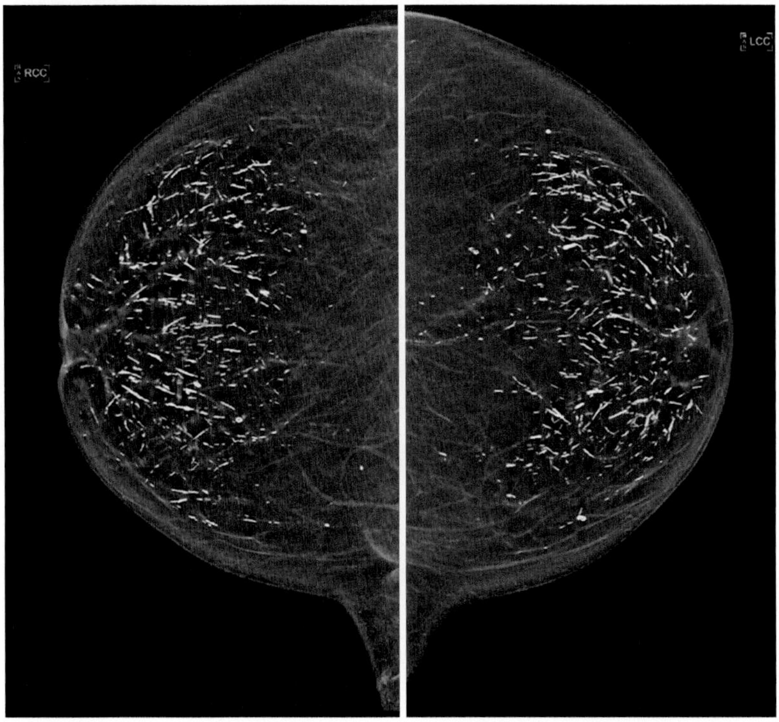

Figs. 8.13 and 8.14 **MG findings**: Coarse, diffuse, bilateral rod-like calcifications in a ductal distribution

BI-RADS: 4, suspicious. A stereotactic biopsy was performed and yielded DCIS.

Pathology Findings (Figs. 8.18 and 8.19):

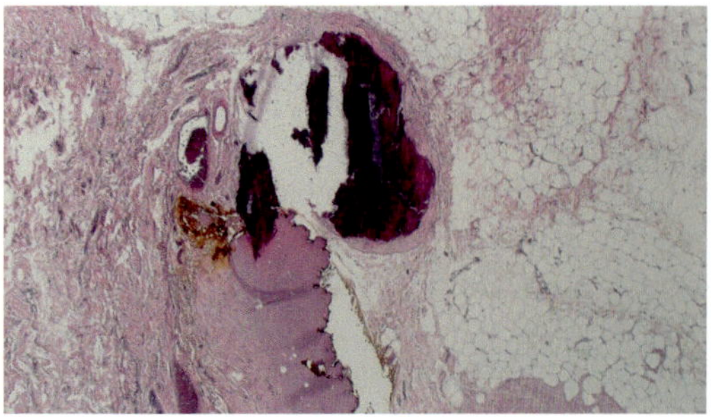

Fig. 8.15 (H&E, 4×) Fibrous stroma with large phosphate-type calcification

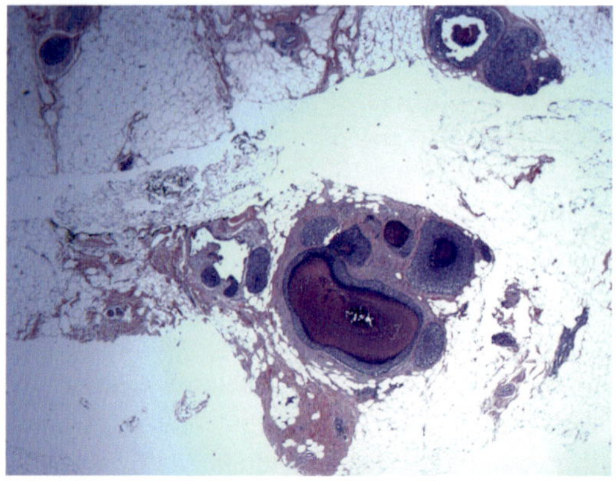

Fig. 8.18 (H&E, low power). Ductal carcinoma in situ, high nuclear grade with comedo necrosis and associated calcifications

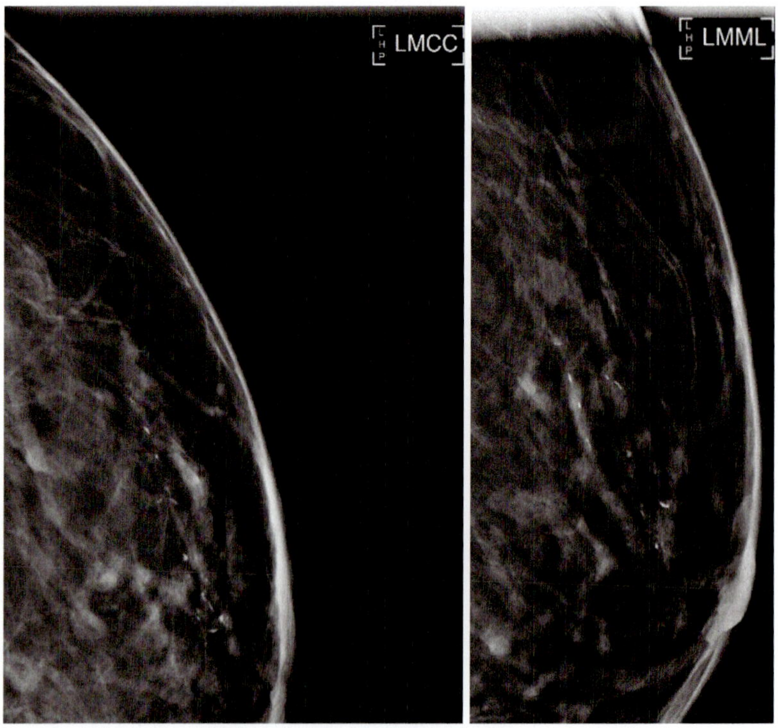

Figs. 8.16 and 8.17 **MG findings**: Magnification views reveal that some of these ductal-distribution calcifications have a rod-like shape, but others are pleomorphic and branching

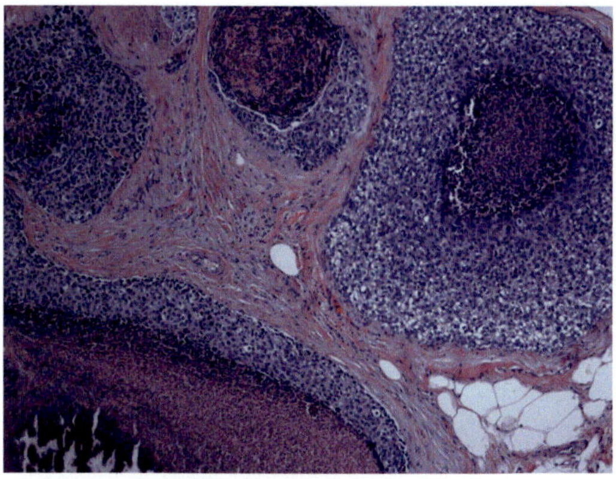

Fig. 8.19 (H&E, 10×). Ductal carcinoma in situ, high nuclear grade with comedo necrosis and associated calcifications

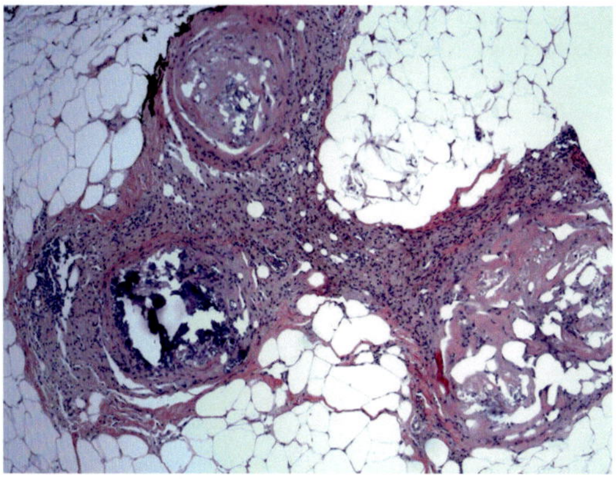

Fig. 8.20 (10×, H&E) Phosphate-type calcifications associated with fat necrosis. Calcifications are embedded in fibrous tissue with mild chronic inflammation

Dystrophic Calcifications: Fat Necrosis

Imaging Findings: Fat necrosis commonly manifests as calcifications at the site of prior surgery or trauma, and these can widely range in size and appearance. Initially, these calcifications can appear fine and linear and it is therefore crucial to correlate the imaging findings with patient history. In the setting of prior oncologic surgery, fat necrosis can mimic a recurrence, and vice versa. However, late-stage fat necrosis frequently manifests with large, irregular calcifications, which may be palpable.

- **BI-RADS**: 2, if late: large and coarse calcifications; or 3, 4, if early and fine.

Differential Diagnosis: Degenerating fibroadenoma.

Pathology Findings: On H&E, the fat necrosis (Fig. 8.20) contains fibroadipose tissue with variable amount of lymphoplasmacytic inflammation, lipogranulomas and fibrosis. Giant cell, and rare eosinophils may be present. Neutrophil infiltrate is unusual in fat necrosis. Calcifications associated with fat necrosis are phosphate-type. Postradiation fat necrosis can also present with calcifications.

Concordant and Discordant Scenario

Case 1

Clinical History: A 64-year-old female with history of dermatomyositis and lumpectomy several years ago, now presenting with a palpable mass in the upper outer quadrant of the right breast (Figs. 8.21 and 8.22).

BI-RADS: 2, benign finding.

Follow-up: Although the finding was benign, the patient found this area very uncomfortable and wanted an excision.

Management Recommendations: No intervention is needed if appearance is typical.

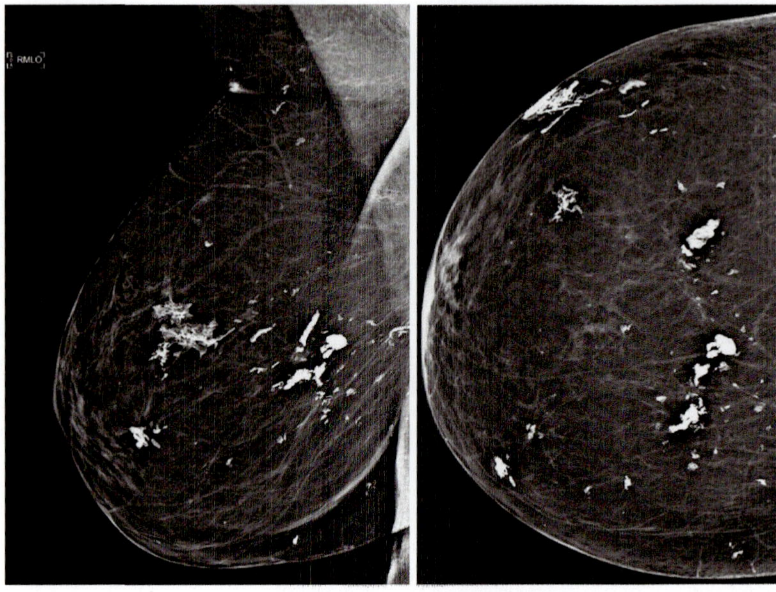

Figs. 8.21 and 8.22 **MG findings**: Multiple large, coarse irregular calcifications, consistent with fat necrosis. The palpable finding correlates with a large, irregular calcification beneath the skin surface, also consistent with fat necrosis

Milk of Calcium Calcifications

Imaging Findings: Milk of calcium (MOC) calcifications occurs due to the precipitation of calcium oxalate crystals within the acini of the breast lobules. These calcifications are unique because their shape changes between the CC view and the true lateral view. On the CC view, MOC calcifications appear amorphous, but on the true lateral view, they form crescents, as the calcifications layer in the dependent aspect of dilated acini.

- **BI-RADS**: 2, benign finding, if all/nearly all calcifications are observed to layer on the lateral magnification view; BI-RADS 3, probably benign, if not all calcifications are observed to layer. BI-RADS 4, suspicious, if suspicious appearing calcifications coexist with MOC calcifications [5, 6].

Differential Diagnosis: If all calcifications layer, this is an "Aunt Minnie" for benign MOC calcifications. However, MOC calcifications frequently coexist with other processes, including benign processes such as fibrocystic changes and sclerosing adenosis, high-risk benign findings such as atypical ductal hyperplasia and lobular carcinoma in situ, as well as malignant processes, such as DCIS.

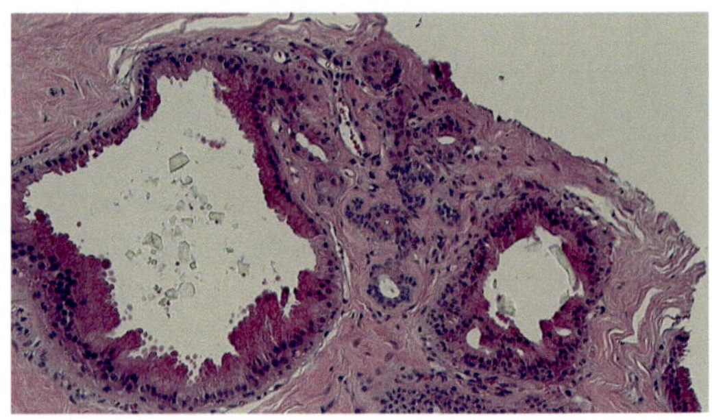

Fig. 8.23 (H&E, 10×) Various angulated shapes and sizes of pale yellow refractile calcium oxalate calcifications present inside the apocrine cysts

Pathology Findings: The MOC calcifications (Fig. 8.23) are present in apocrine cysts. The calcifications are pale yellow crystalline deposits usually identified inside apocrine cysts. These calcifications can be present in the stroma adjacent to the cysts or the dense inflammation, likely related to cyst rupture (Fig. 8.24).

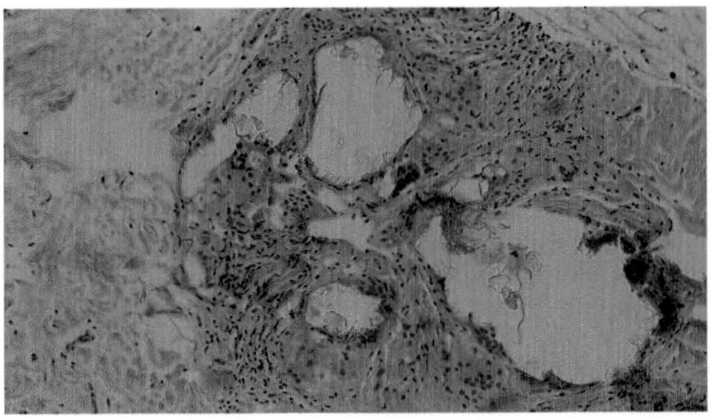

Fig. 8.24 Calcium oxalate calcifications (10×, H&E) embedded in the fibrous stroma with associated foreign body-type giant cells

Concordant and Discordant Scenario

Case 1

- **Clinical History**: A 45-year-old asymptomatic female presents for screening mammography (Figs. 8.25 and 8.26).

BI-RADS: 2, benign finding.

Pathology Findings: The calcifications are oxalate type. The calcifications are present in association with benign ducts (Figs. 8.27 and 8.28).

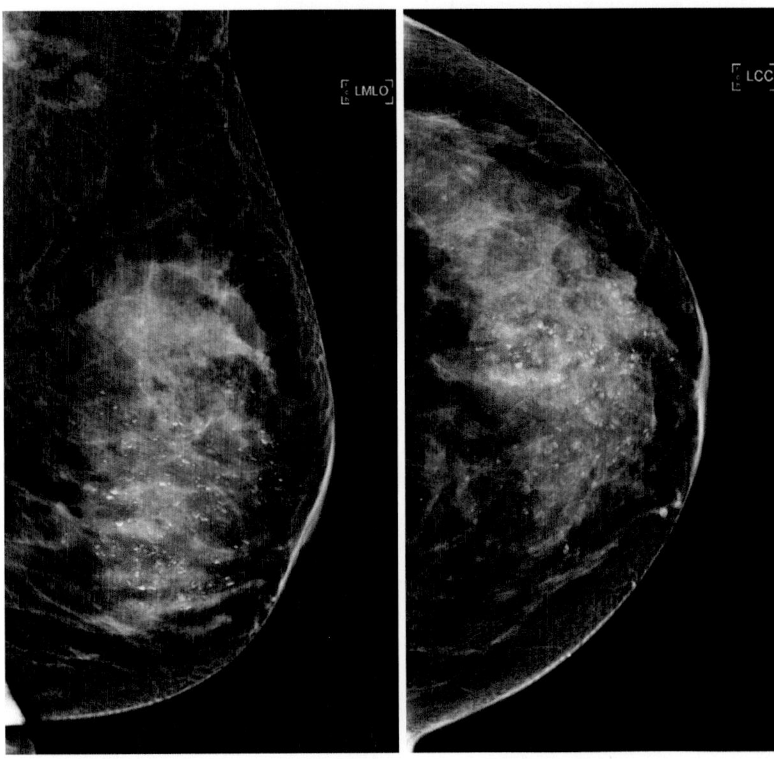

Figs. 8.25 and 8.26 **MG findings**: Diffuse calcifications that layer on the lateral view and are amorphous on the CC view, typical for MOC calcifications

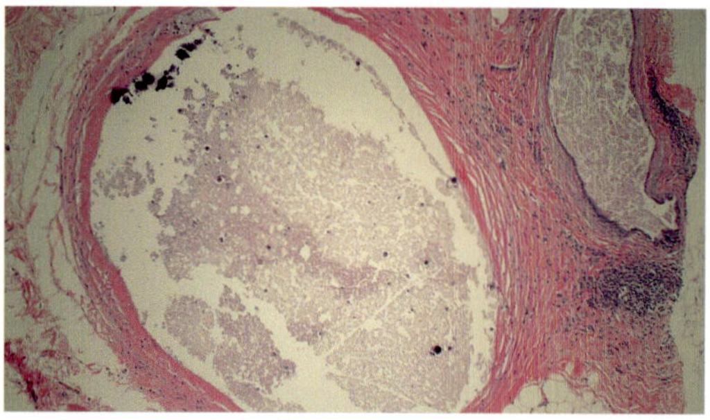

Fig. 8.27 (H&E, 10×) Oxalate- and phosphate-type calcifications (inter-mixed) present in association with benign ducts

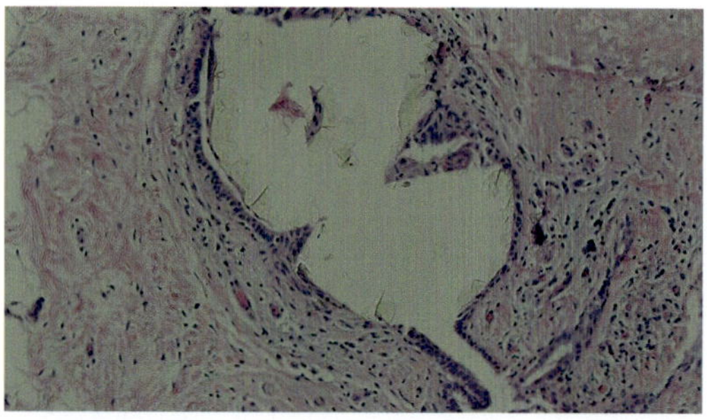

Fig. 8.28 (H&E, 10×) Oxalate-type calcifications (intermixed) present in association with a duct

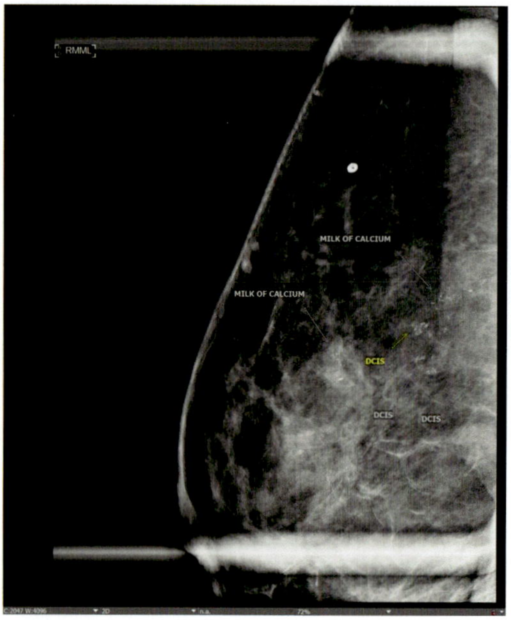

Fig. 8.29 **MG findings**: Lateral magnification views demonstrate several groups of calcifications that layer, and are typical for MOC calcifications. However, there are adjacent groups of pleomorphic calcifications

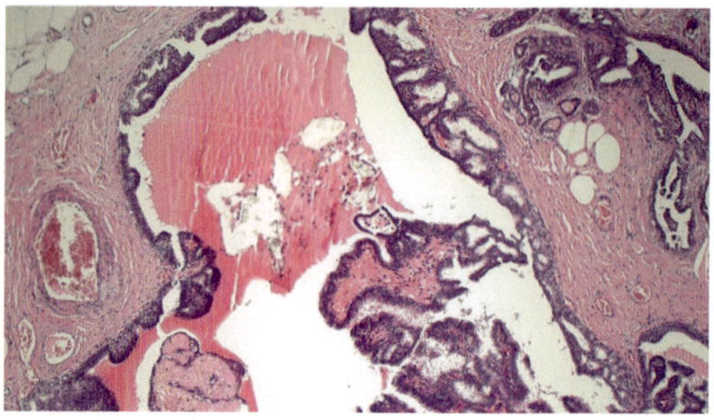

Fig. 8.30 (H&E, 10×) Ductal carcinoma in situ, low nuclear grade with associated calcium oxalate-type calcifications

Case 2

Clinical History: A 40-year-old female presented for baseline screening mammography. Multiple groups of calcifications were noted in the right breast, upper outer quadrant. The patient returned for diagnostic mammography (Fig. 8.29).

BI-RADS: 4, suspicious finding. A stereotactic biopsy was performed and yielded DCIS. The patient subsequently underwent a right mastectomy.

Pathology Findings (Fig. 8.30):

Amorphous Calcifications

Imaging Findings: Amorphous calcifications tend to be small, <0.1 mm in size, with individual shapes difficult to characterize. These calcifications can be faint and resemble ground chalk. They form within microcysts within the terminal ductal lobular unit. The management of these calcifications usually depends on the distribution: diffuse calcifications, particularly when bilateral and symmetric, may generally be considered benign, while grouped, asymmetric calcifications usually warrant a biopsy.

- **BI-RADS**: 2, benign, if diffuse, bilateral and symmetric; BI-RADS: 4, suspicious, if grouped and asymmetric.
- **Differential Diagnosis**: If diffuse: fibrocystic changes, sclerosing adenosis. If grouped and asymmetric: atypical ductal hyperplasia, atyp-

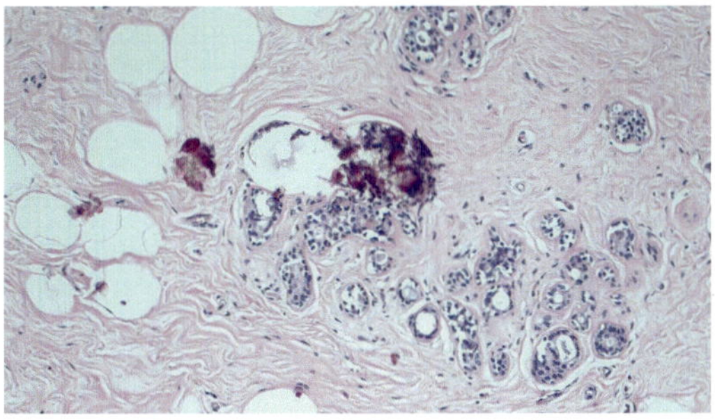

Fig. 8.31 (H&E, 10×). Oxalate- and phosphate-type calcifications associated with benign lobule

ical lobular hyperplasia, lobular carcinoma in situ, DCIS, IDC.

Pathology Findings (Fig. 8.31):

Concordant and Discordant Scenario

Case 1

Clinical History: A 38-year-old female with a strong family history of breast cancer presents for screening mammography (Figs. 8.32 and 8.33).

BI-RADS: 4, suspicious findings. Given strong family history of breast cancer, this finding was deemed suspicious and a stereotactic biopsy was recommended, which was performed and yielded adenosis and stromal fibrosis.

Pathology Findings (Fig. 8.34):

Case 2

Clinical History: A 45-year-old female underwent screening mammography. Multiple areas of grouped calcifications and dilated ducts were noted in the left breast, and the patient was asked to return for diagnostic mammography with magnification views and ultrasound (Figs. 8.35, 8.36 and 8.37).

BI-RADS: 4, suspicious findings. Stereotactic biopsies of 3 areas in the left breast were recommended, which yielded papilloma with ADH (5 o'clock), DCIS (7 o'clock), and severely atypical intraductal proliferation adjacent to and involving a sclerosing papillary lesion (7 o'clock).

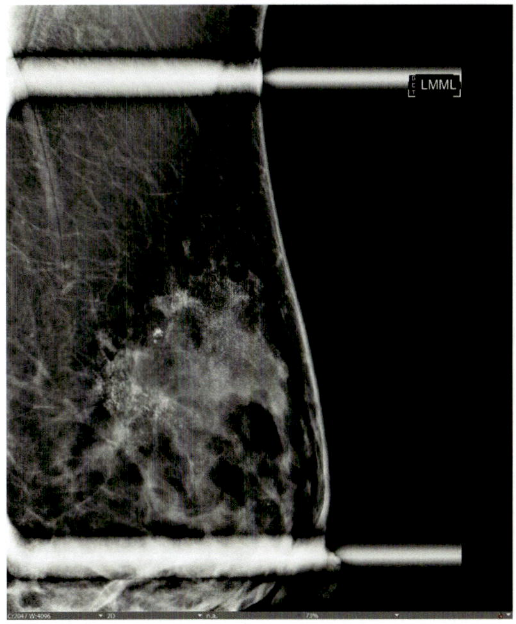

Fig. 8.32 Grouped calcifications are seen in the left breast, and the patient is asked to return for diagnostic evaluation with magnification views

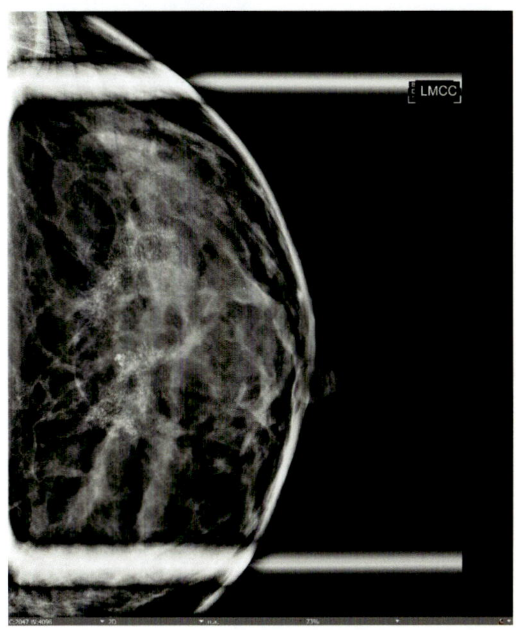

Fig. 8.33 MG: magnification views demonstrate segmental, amorphous calcifications

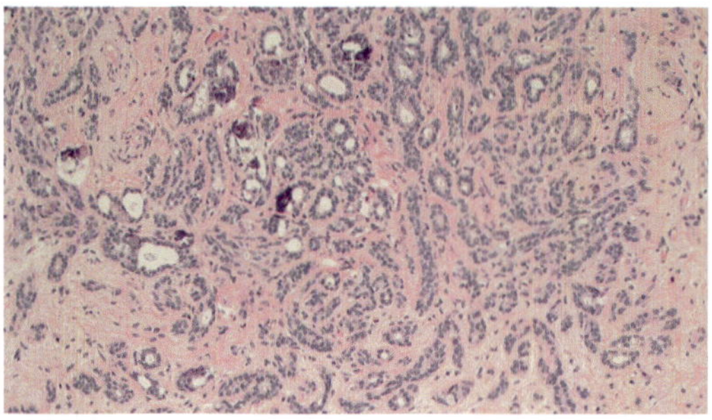

Fig. 8.34 (H&E, 10×) Sclerosing adenosis with associated calcifications

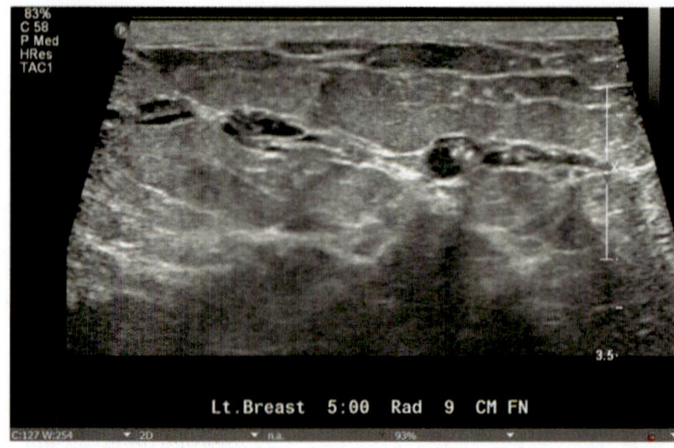

Fig. 8.37 US: multiple areas of dilated ducts containing calcifications

Figs. 8.35 and 8.36 MG: multiple groups of amorphous calcifications in a ductal distribution and dilated ducts

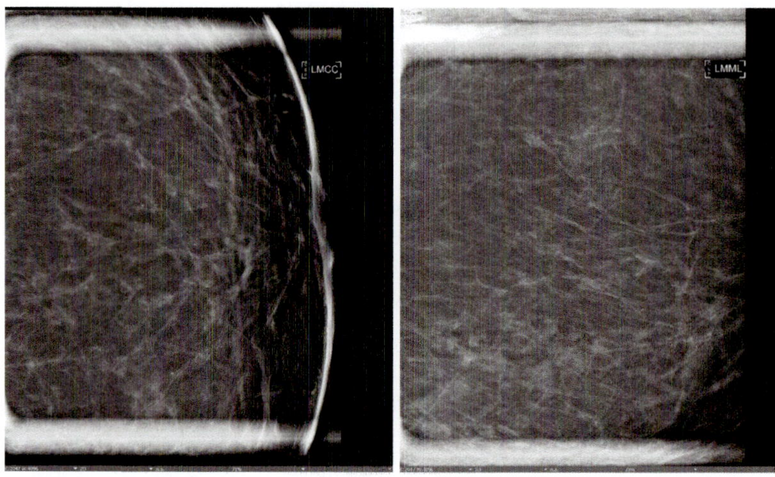

Follow-up: Given the extent of the disease, mastectomy was recommended, but the patient strongly wished to attempt breast conservation. The patient underwent a multi-wire localization and partial mastectomy with oncoplastic reduction of both breasts. Final pathology yielded DCIS with multiple papillomas (Fig. 8.38).

Pathology Findings (Fig. 8.39):

Case 3

Clinical History: A 45-year-old female presents for screening mammography. New grouped calcifications are found in the left breast. The patient returned for magnification views (Figs. 8.40–8.42).

BI-RADS: 4, suspicious findings. A stereotactic biopsy of two groups was recommended and performed, yielding ADH.

Pathology Findings (Fig. 8.43):

Follow-up: The patient underwent needle localization and excision, which yielded ADH and LCIS.

Management: ADH significantly increases a patient's lifetime risk of breast cancer. It can be difficult to distinguish from low-grade DCIS on core needle biopsy (CNB) alone, because the two entities appear pathologically similar and are distinguished from one another by lesion size and/or number of involved ducts. When ADH is found on CNB, there is a possibility of finding DCIS or invasive carcinoma in the vicinity of the CNB site upon surgical excision. Therefore, it is the standard of care to surgically excise ADH. However, in the literature, the actual rates of upgrade of ADH to DCIS or invasive cancer upon excision is variable. Nomograms for estimating the likeli-

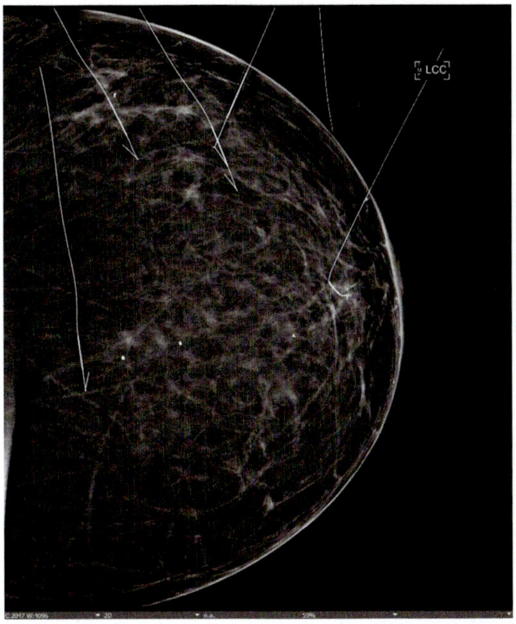

Fig. 8.38 MG showing multiwire localization before partial mastetctomy

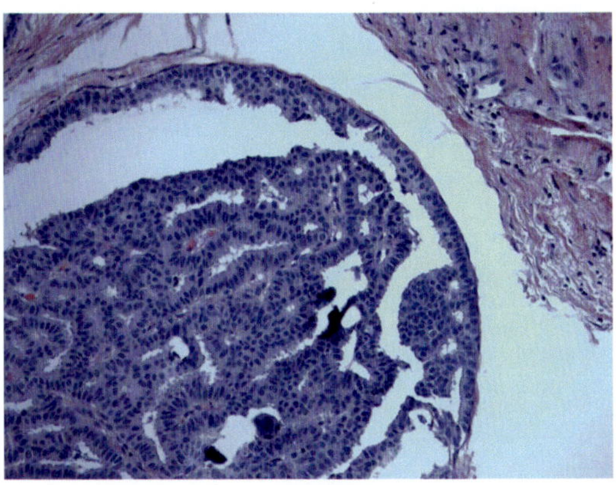

Fig. 8.39 (H&E, 10×) Ductal carcinoma in situ low nuclear grade involving a papilloma

hood of upgrade to malignancy have been created to help guide decision making. If the calcifications are completely removed by CNB and radiologic-pathologic concordance is established, omission of surgical excision can be considered in favor of close imaging and clinical follow-up [7–10].

Case 4

Clinical History: A 48-year-old premenopausal female underwent screening mammography, which showed segmental calcifications in the left breast. She returned for diagnostic mammography with magnification views (Figs. 8.44 and 8.45).

US: Screening ultrasound was performed, as the patient has dense breast tissue, and no associated ultrasound abnormality is seen (Fig. 8.46).

BI-RADS: 4, suspicious of malignancy; a stereotactic biopsy was recommended and performed, which yielded ADH and FEA.

Follow-up: The patient underwent a needle localized excisional biopsy of the most suspi-

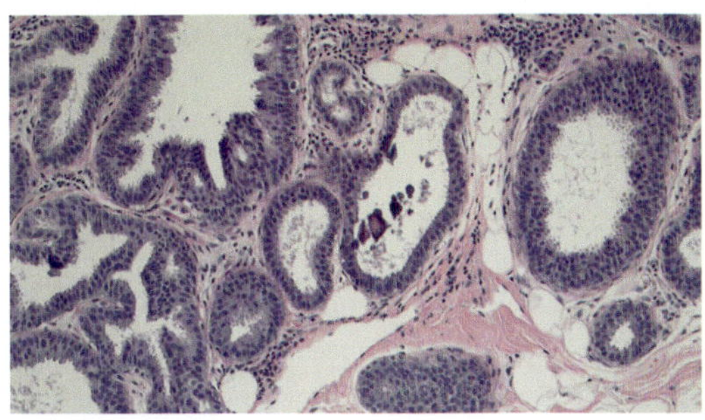

Fig. 8.43 (H&E, 10×) Atypical ductal hyperplasia associated with calcifications. ADH is arising in a setting of flat epithelial atypia

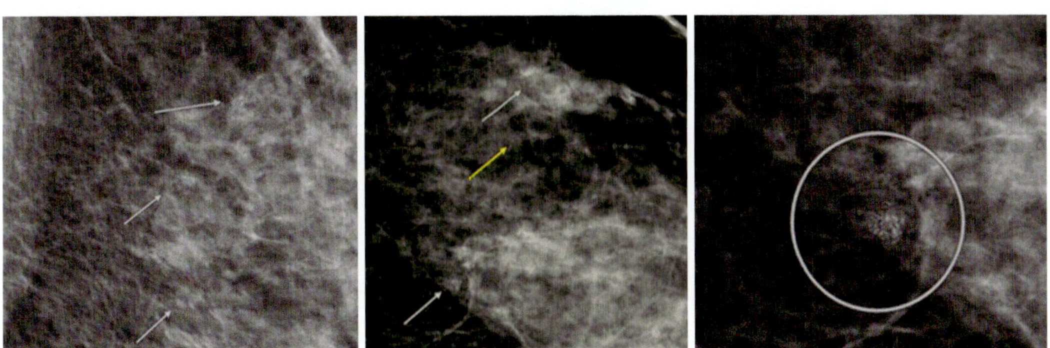

Figs. 8.40–8.42 **MG**: multiple small groups of amorphous calcifications are seen in the left breast

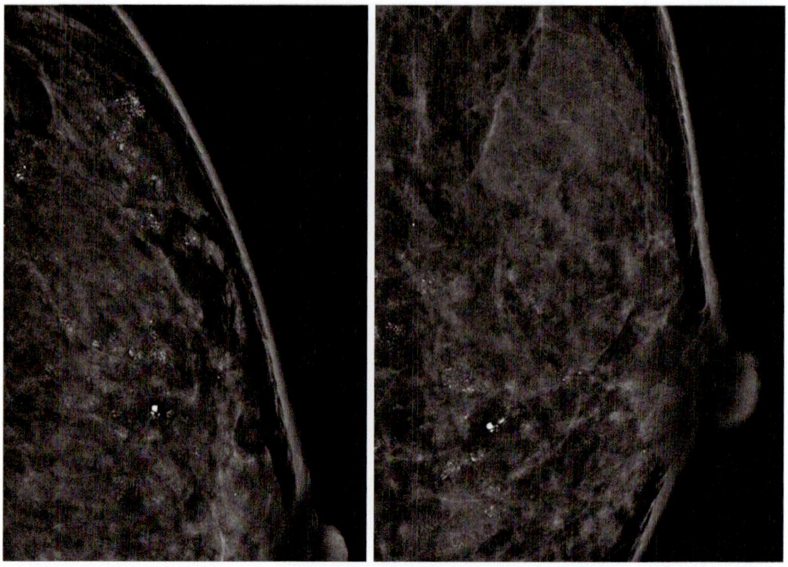

Figs. 8.44 and 8.45 **MG**: segmental amorphous calcifications are demonstrated in the lateral aspect of the left breast

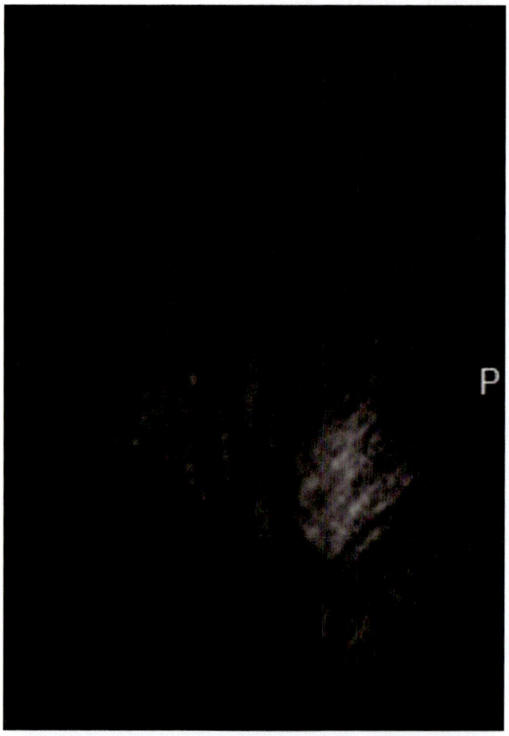

Fig. 8.46 **MRI**: given the extent of calcifications, a breast MRI was requested by the treating surgeon. This demonstrated segmental, clumped non-mass enhancement with delayed persistent kinetics

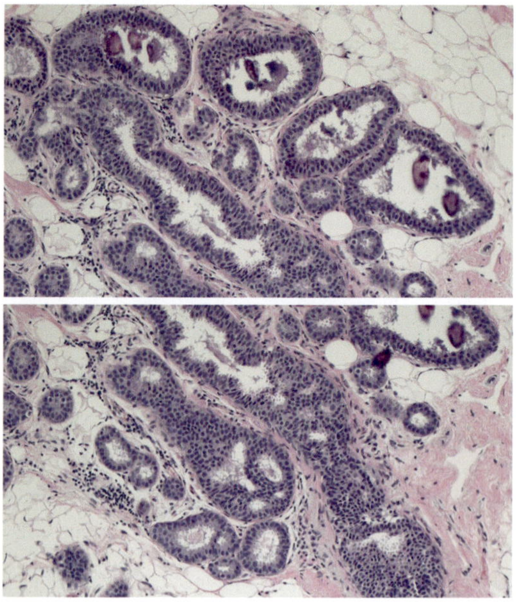

Figs. 8.47 and 8.48 (H&E, 10×). Atypical ductal hyperplasia and flat epithelial atypia with associated calcifications

cious area of calcifications, which also yielded ADH and FEA. The patient was counseled regarding her increased risk of breast cancer, and offered chemoprevention. However, she declined this and opted for annual surveillance with mammography and MRI.

Pathology Findings (Figs. 8.47 and 8.48):

Case 5

Clinical History: A 55-year-old female presented for screening mammography, and new

Figs. 8.49 and 8.50 **MG**: grouped, amorphous calcifications in the left breast

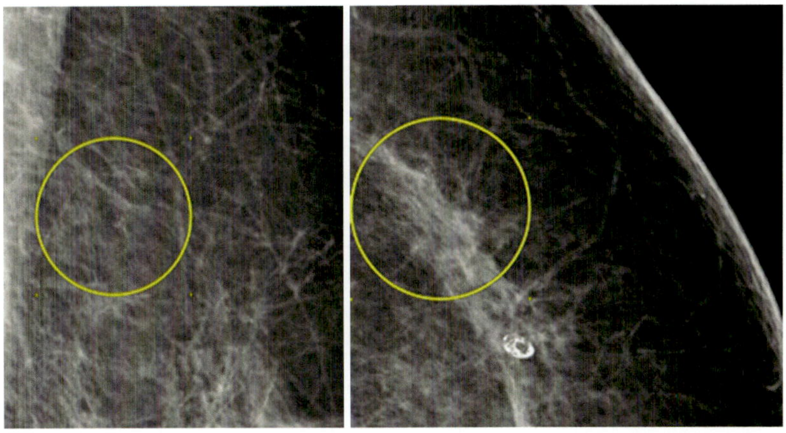

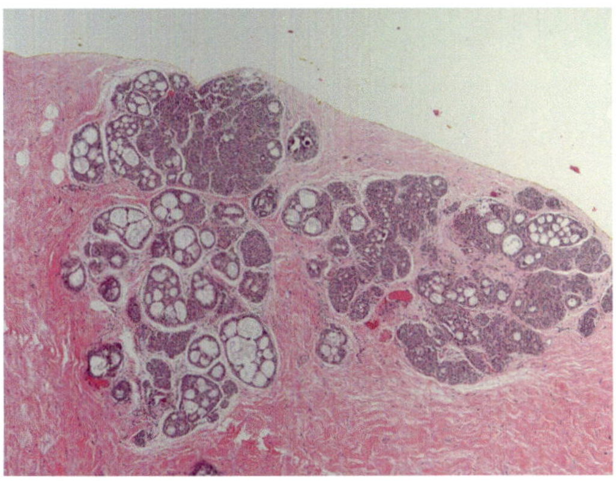

Fig. 8.51 (H&E, 2×) Pseudocribrifrom architecture of collagenous spherulosis with secondary involvement by lobular neoplasia

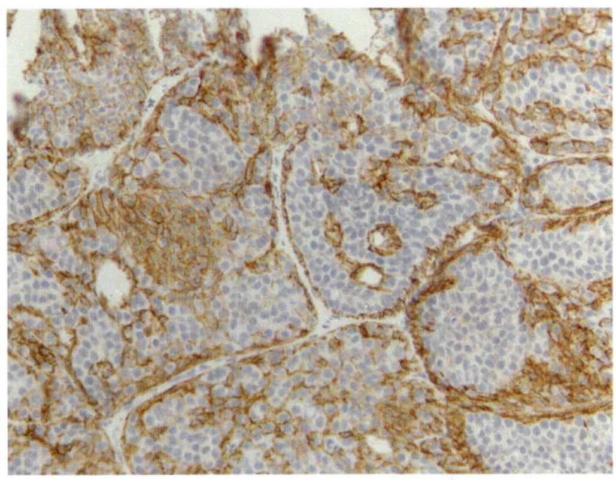

Fig. 8.52 (IHC, 10×). E-cadherin immunohistochemistry showing loss of membranous staining in lobular neoplasia cells. Residual myoepithelial cells at the periphery and the luminal ductal cells show intact membranous staining

grouped calcifications were noted in the left breast. She returned for a diagnostic evaluation with magnification views (Figs. 8.49 and 8.50).

BI-RADS: 4, suspicious of malignancy. A stereotactic biopsy was recommended and performed, yielding ALH and collagenous spherulosis with associated calcifications.

Pathology Findings (Figs. 8.51 and 8.52):

Follow-up: The patient was counseled regarding her elevated risk of breast cancer given the diagnosis of ALH. Chemoprevention was offered, but the patient declined this, instead opting for annual surveillance with mammography and possibly MRI.

Management: The upgrade risk for ALH, when deemed concordant with imaging findings, is estimated to be low (around 3%). Therefore, when found on CNB, it can be observed with clinical and imaging surveillance. Surgical excision is recommended if the result is deemed discordant, or if other high-risk lesions are present. ALH signals an elevated lifetime risk of developing breast cancer, and the patients should be offered risk-modulating endocrine therapy and close surveillance [11].

Coarse Heterogeneous Calcifications

Imaging Findings: Coarse heterogeneous calcifications are irregularly shaped, and are smaller than dystrophic calcifications, ranging in size from 0.5 to 1 mm. Both benign and malignant etiologies can manifest with coarse heterogeneous calcifications, and management of these is based on the patient's surgical or trauma history as well as distribution of the calcifications. Early fat necrosis at a site of surgery yielding benign pathology, or at a site of prior breast trauma can manifest as coarse heterogeneous calcifications. Multiple bilateral groups of coarse heterogeneous calcifications are likely benign. However, a new group of coarse heterogeneous calcifications is suspicious and biopsy should be considered.

- **BI-RADS**: 3, probably benign, if occurring in a surgical site/area of prior trauma, or if these are multiple and bilateral. BI-RADS 4, suspicious, if occurring in a site of prior lumpectomy, or if a new group of calcifications.

Differential Diagnosis: Benign processes: fibroadenomas, fibroadenomatoid change, fibrosis, fat necrosis, papilloma. High-risk processes: papilloma with atypia. Malignant processes: DCIS.

Concordant or Discordant Scenario

Case 1

Clinical History: A 50-year-old female presents for screening mammography, and increased calcifications are noted in the right breast. The patient returned for diagnostic mammography with magnification views (Figs. 8.53 and 8.54).

BI-RADS: 4, suspicious. A stereotactic biopsy was recommended and yielded DCIS.

Pathology Findings (Fig. 8.55):

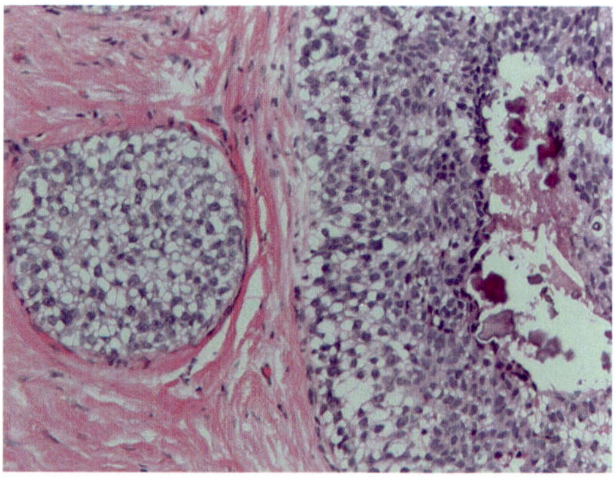

Fig. 8.55 (H&E, 20×) Ductal carcinoma in situ, intermediate nuclear grade with solid pattern and comedo necrosis and associated phosphate-type calcifications

Case 2

Clinical History: A 75-year-old female presented for screening mammography, and new coarse, heterogeneous calcifications are noted in the left breast. She returned for diagnostic mammography (Figs. 8.56 and 8.57).

BI-RADS: 4, suspicious. A stereotactic biopsy was recommended and performed, yielding a well-differentiated mucinous carcinoma with

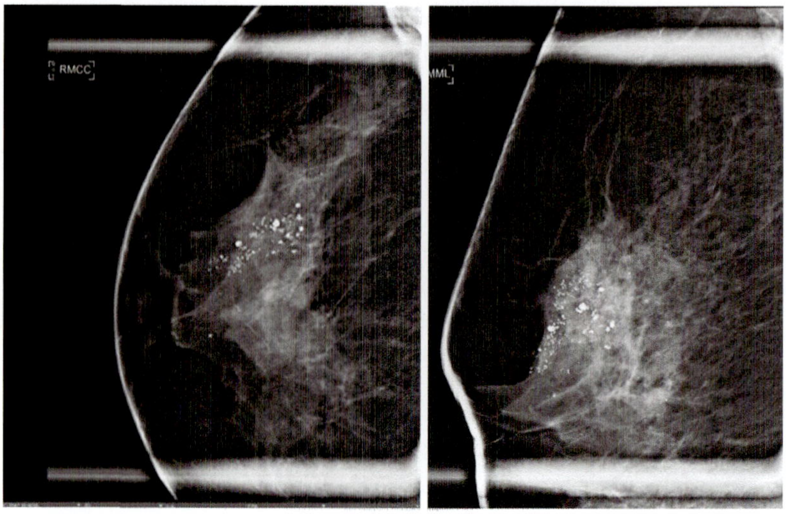

Figs. 8.53 and 8.54 **MG**: coarse heterogeneous calcifications in a segmental distribution. Although some of the calcifications appear coarse, interspersed are heterogeneous, suspicious-appearing calcifications

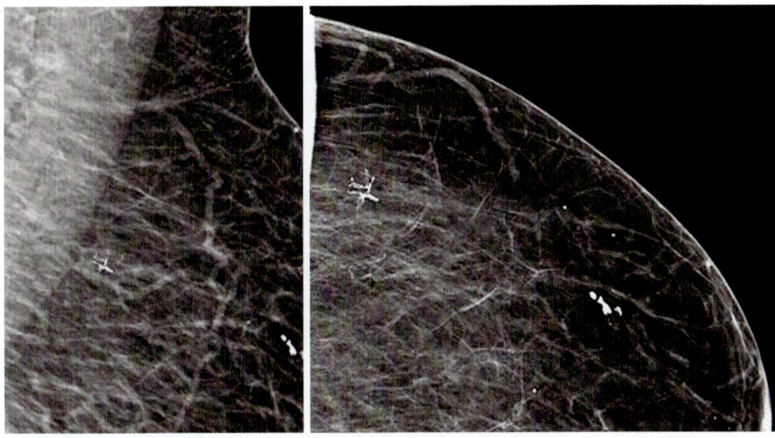

Figs. 8.56 and 8.57 **MG**: coarse heterogeneous, bizarrely shaped, grouped calcifications. Other benign appearing, stable coarse heterogeneous calcifications are present more anteriorly in the breast. However, the new group appeared suspicious

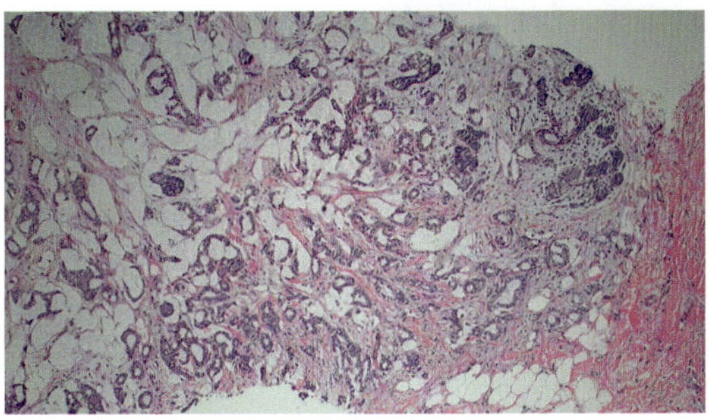

Fig. 8.58 (H&E, 4×) Invasive ductal carcinoma with mucinous features histologic grade 1

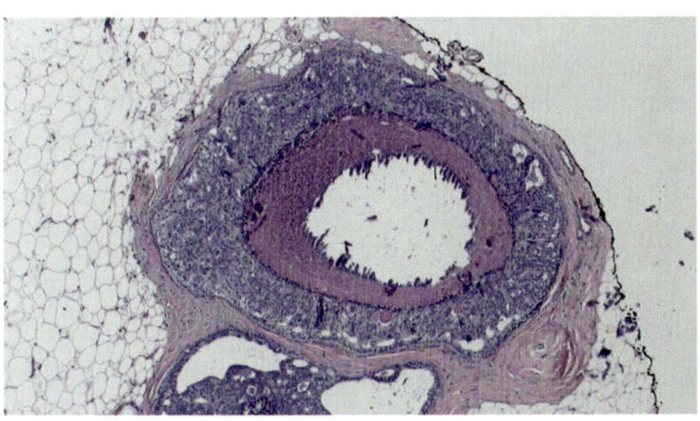

Fig. 8.59 (H&E, 4×) Ductal carcinoma in situ intermediate nuclear grade with cribriform pattern comedo necrosis and associated phosphate-type calcifications

DCIS, grade 2, and ADH. The patient subsequently underwent a lumpectomy.

Pathology Findings (Figs. 8.58 and 8.59):

Case 3

Clinical History: A 28-year-old female presents for evaluation of a palpable lump in the right breast (Figs. 8.60 and 8.61).

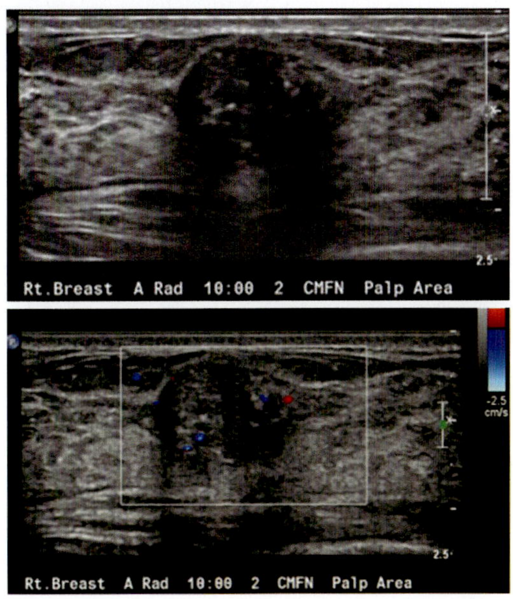

Figs. 8.60 and 8.61 **US findings**: round mass with a partially circumscribed, but partially indistinct margin, and a combined pattern of posterior features (partial enhancement and partial shadowing). A few echogenic foci are seen within, thought to be calcifications within a likely fibroadenoma

BI-RADS: 4a, low suspicion of malignancy. An US-guided biopsy was recommended and performed, yielding a well-differentiated IDC with extensive mucinous features and grade 2 DCIS, with coarse calcifications present near the invasive carcinoma.

The patient returned for a bilateral mammogram to fully assess both breasts before surgery (Figs. 8.62 and 8.63).

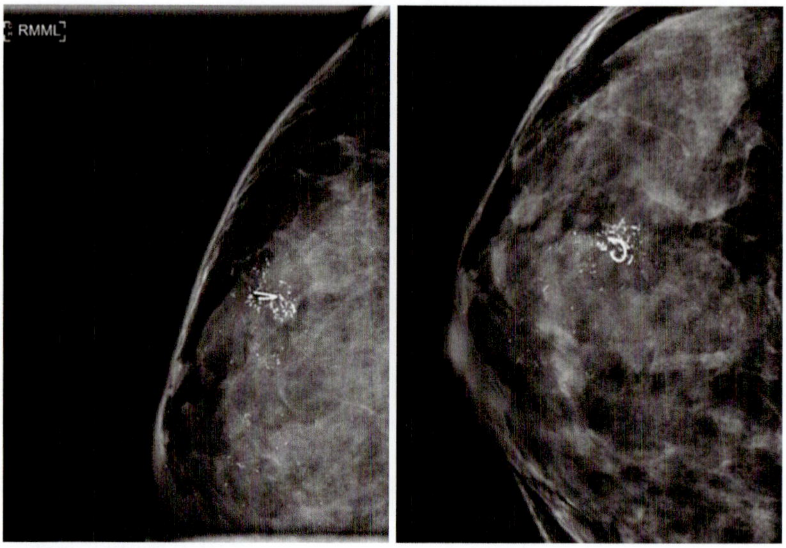

Figs. 8.62 and 8.63 **MG findings**: coarse, heterogeneous calcifications in a segmental distribution extending toward the nipple, with associated biopsy marking clip

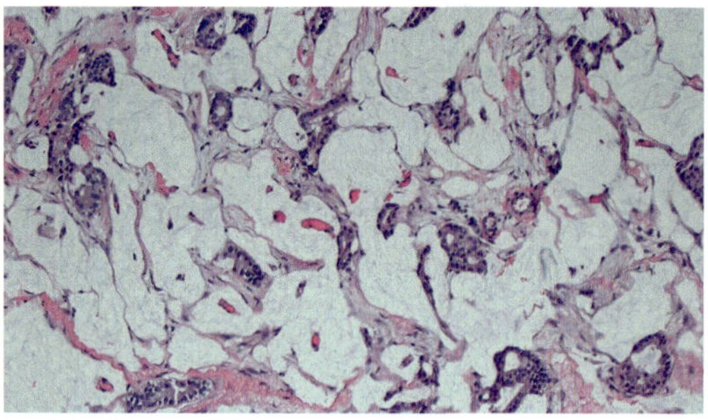

Fig. 8.64 (H&E, 10×) Mucinous carcinoma. The invasive carcinoma cells are floating in dissecting acellular mucin pool

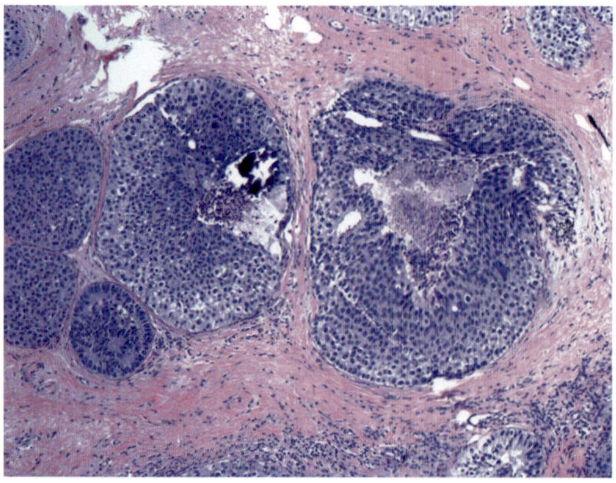

Fig. 8.65 (H&E, 10×) Ductal carcinoma in situ intermediate nuclear grade with solid and cribriform patterns, comedo necrosis, and associated calcifications

Follow-up: The patient underwent a right mastectomy and sentinel lymph node biopsy. This demonstrated a moderately differentiated invasive mucinous carcinoma and 4 cm of grade 2 DCIS.

Pathology Findings (Figs. 8.64 and 8.65):

Pleomorphic Calcifications

Imaging Findings: Pleomorphic calcifications are characterized as having different sizes and different shapes, with individual calcifications typically smaller than 0.5 mm. Pleomorphic calcifications are almost always suspicious and a biopsy should be performed. The biopsy results should be carefully assessed for concordance. If a small group of well-sampled pleomorphic calcifications yields a benign result, this may be concordant, but if a benign result is obtained from sampling segmental pleomorphic calcifications, a repeat needle biopsy or an excisional biopsy should be considered [12].

- **BI-RADS**: 4, suspicious of malignancy. Stereotactic needle biopsy should be performed. In dense breast tissue, US evaluation should also be strongly considered, particularly if the breast tissue is dense, to assess for any associated masses that may be obscured by the dense breast tissue. In cases of segmental calcifications or long areas of linear calcifications, the sampling of more than one area (anterior and posterior, for example), should be considered to assess whether the grade of disease is uniform throughout the entire area of abnormality.

Differential Diagnosis: Benign processes: fibroadenomatoid change, sclerosis adenosis, early fat necrosis. High-risk benign: ADH. Malignant: DCIS, IDC.

Concordant or Discordant Scenario

Case 1

Clinical History: A 48-year-old female underwent screening mammography, with segmental calcifications seen in the left breast. She returned for diagnostic mammography, which demonstrated pleomorphic segmental calcifications. An ultrasound of the area of calcifications demonstrated no associated masses or other definite abnormalities (Figs. 8.66 and 8.67).

BI-RADS: 4, suspicious. A stereotactic biopsy was recommended and performed, which yielded ADH and FEA.

Follow-up: This was deemed possibly discordant and a wire localization and excisional biopsy was recommended. Prior to the excisional biopsy, the patient underwent an MRI of the breasts (Fig. 8.68).

Follow-up: The patient underwent an excisional biopsy, which yielded ADH and FEA. Due to the patient's small breast size and the extent of the calcifications, additional excisions would yield poor cosmetic results. The patient is at significantly elevated risk of breast cancer in the future and should be screened annually with mammography and MRI (Figs. 8.69 and 8.70).

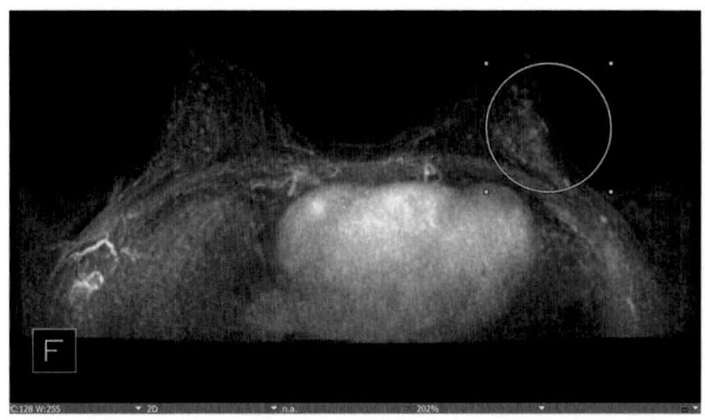

Fig. 8.68 **MRI findings**: non-mass enhancement in a segmental distribution, corresponding to that of mammographic calcifications, with homogeneous, persistent enhancement, but no suspicious masses

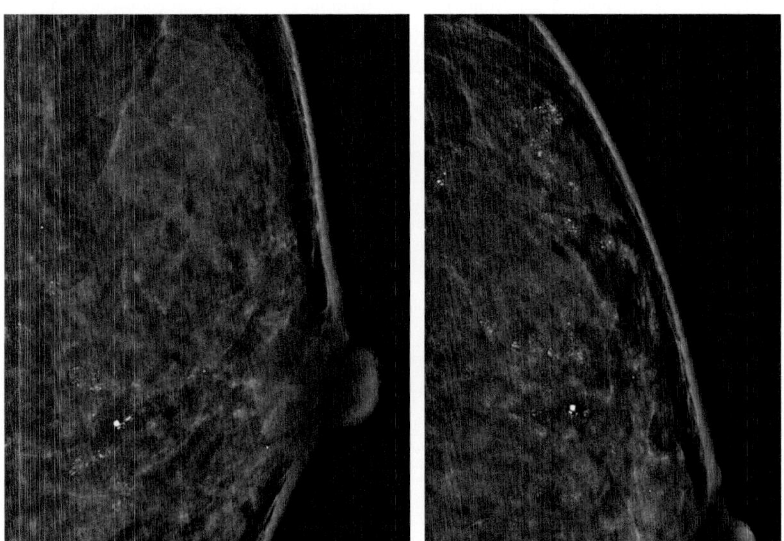

Figs. 8.66 and 8.67 **MG findings**: pleomorphic segmental calcifications in the left breast

Case 2

Clinical History: A 38-year-old female presented for diagnostic mammography due to a palpable area in the left axilla. No abnormality was seen in the left breast or axilla on mammography or ultrasound, but suspicious calcifications were seen in the right breast (Figs. 8.71, 8.72 and 8.73).

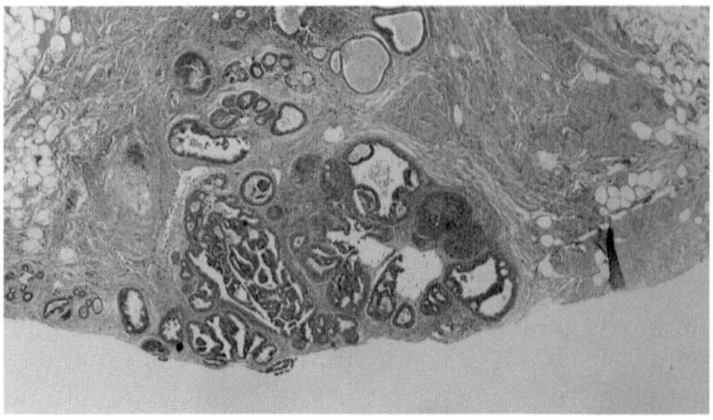

Fig. 8.69 (H&E, 4×) Atypical ductal hyperplasia arising in a background of flat epithelial atypia

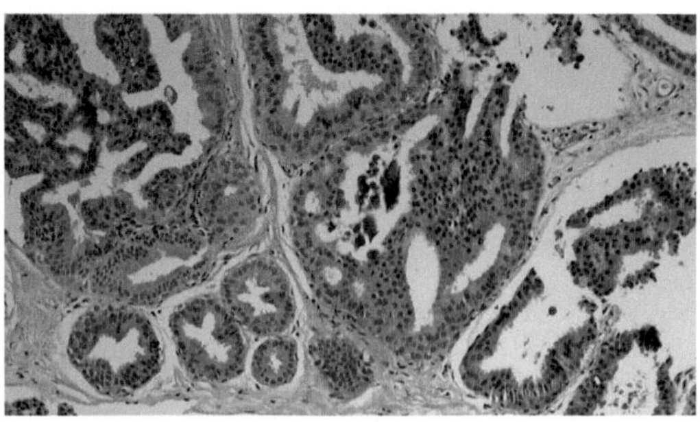

Fig. 8.70 (H&E, 10×) Atypical ductal hyperplasia comprising of low-nuclear grade monomorphic intraductal epithelial proliferation forming rigid structures including bridges and cribriform spaces. Calcifications are present with ADH

- **BI-RADS**: 5, highly suggestive of malignancy. A US-guided biopsy was performed, which yielded DCIS, grade 2. The patient underwent a lumpectomy, which yielded DCIS.

Follow-up: On an annual mammogram 3 years after the lumpectomy, the patient was found to have two small groups of pleomorphic calcifications anterior to the lumpectomy site (Figs. 8.74, 8.75 and 8.76).

BI-RADS: 4, suspicious findings.

Pathology Findings: A stereotactic biopsy was performed and yielded IDC, moderately differentiated. The patient underwent a bilateral mastectomy. The right mastectomy yielded DCIS, but no residual IDC.

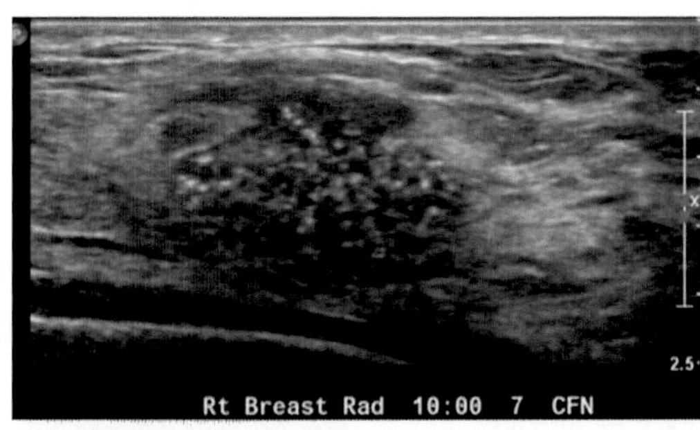

Fig. 8.73 **US**: calcifications are also visible sonographically

Figs. 8.71 and 8.72 **MG**: large group of pleomorphic calcifications in the right breast, upper outer quadrant

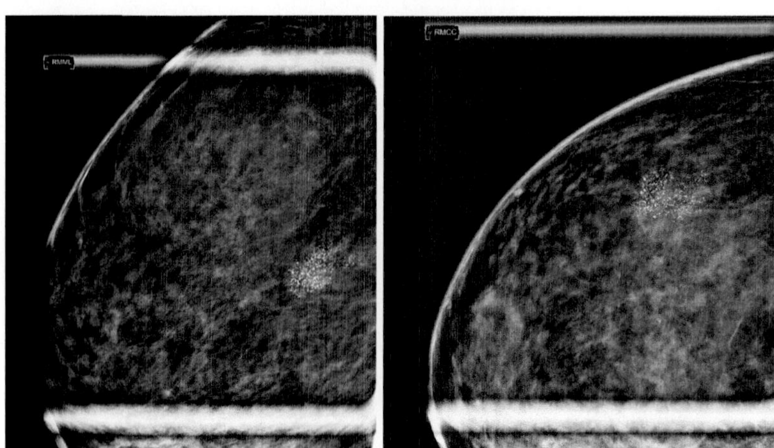

Case 3

Clinical History: A 72-year-old female presented for screening mammography. A small, new group of calcifications was noted in the left breast. The patient returned for additional evaluation with magnification views (Figs. 8.77 and 8.78).

BI-RADS: 4, suspicious of malignancy. A stereotactic biopsy was recommended and performed, yielding Invasive Lobular Carcinoma and LCIS.

Pathology Findings (Fig. 8.79):

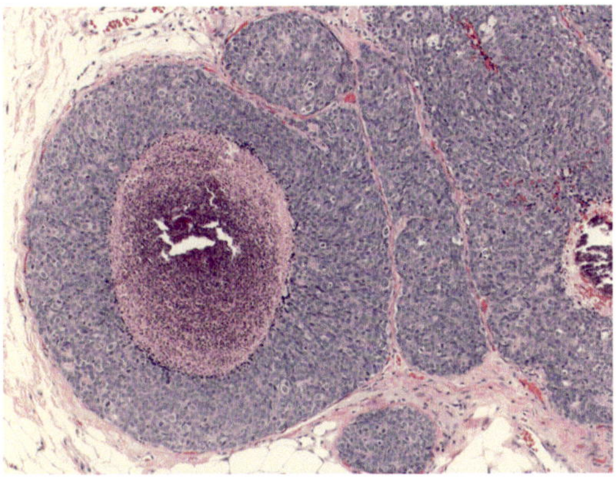

Fig. 8.74 (H&E, 10×) Ductal carcinoma in situ, intermediate nuclear grade with solid pattern, comedo necrosis, and associated calcifications

Case 4

Clinical History: A 63-year-old female underwent screening mammography, which revealed a small new group of calcifications in the right breast. She returned for diagnostic evaluation with magnification views (Figs. 8.80 and 8.81).

BI-RADS: 4, suspicious finding.

Pathology: A stereotactic biopsy was recommended and performed, yielding LCIS and ALH. The patient underwent a needle localization and excision, yielding LCIS with pleomorphic features (Figs. 8.82 and 8.83).

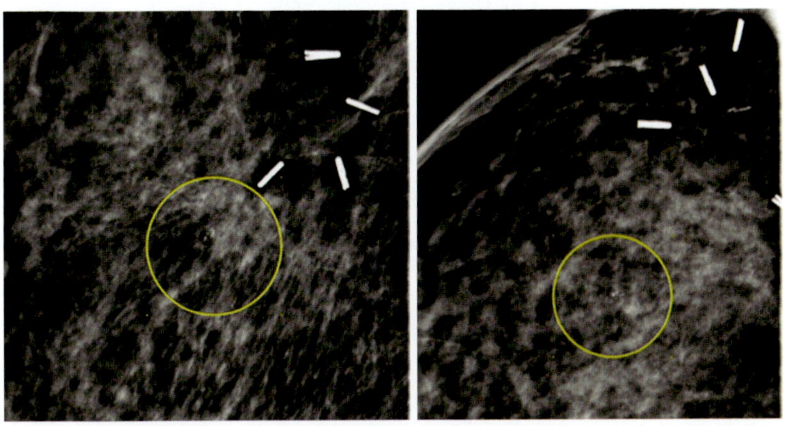

Figs. 8.75 and 8.76 **MG findings**: grouped pleomorphic calcifications anterior to the lumpectomy site

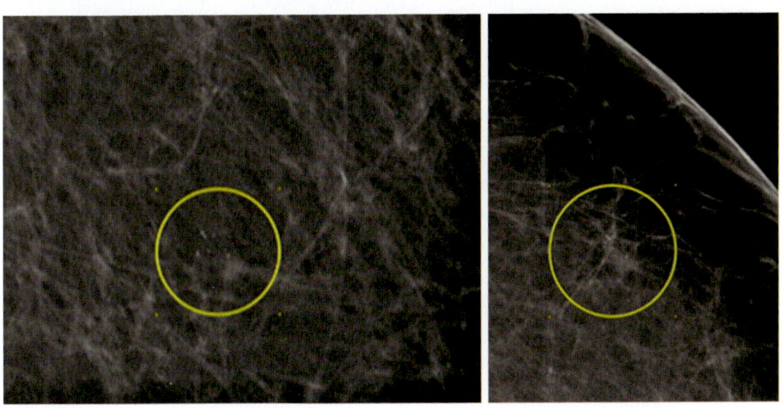

Figs. 8.77 and 8.78 **MG**: grouped, pleomorphic calcifications in the left breast with an associated faint focal asymmetry

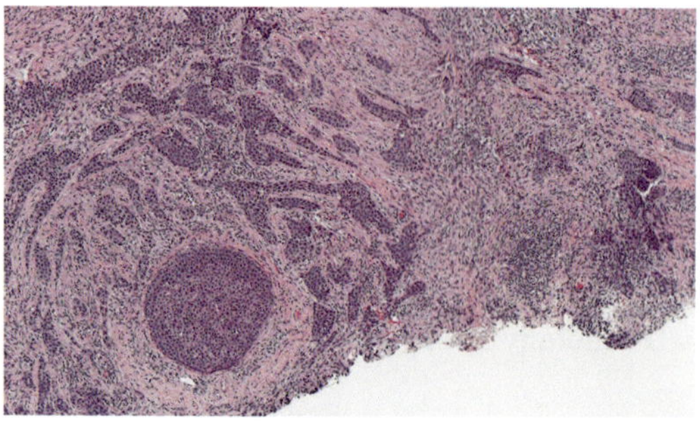

Fig. 8.79 (**H&E, 10×**) Invasive lobular carcinoma histologic grade 2 with associated florid lobular carcinoma in situ

Management: LCIS is no longer classified as pTis. The presence of LCIS signals an increased lifetime risk of breast cancer estimated at 11.3% at 10 years and 19.8% at 20 years. Two decades ago, women with the diagnosis of LCIS were offered prophylactic mastectomy, but now the degree of risk is determined to not be sufficient to warrant prophylactic mastectomy, thus it is no longer recommended. The upgrade risk of LCIS that is deemed concordant with imaging findings is low, estimated around 3%. Therefore, when classic LCIS is encountered on core needle biopsy (CNB), it can be observed with clinical and imaging surveillance. Non-classic forms of LCIS (pleomorphic and florid) should be surgically excised to negative margins.

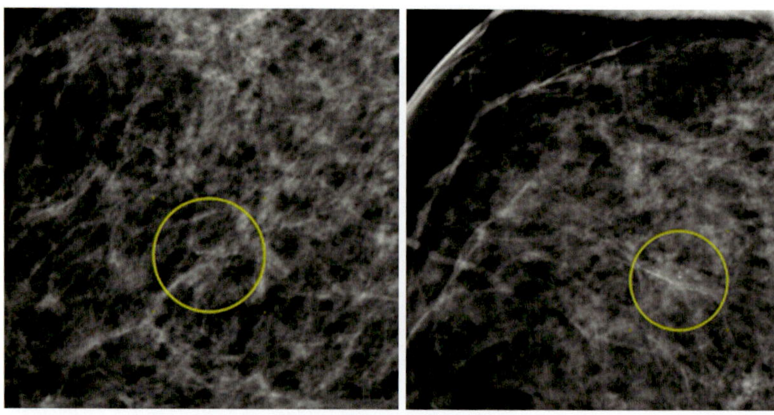

Figs. 8.80 and 8.81 **MG**: small group of pleomorphic calcifications in the right breast

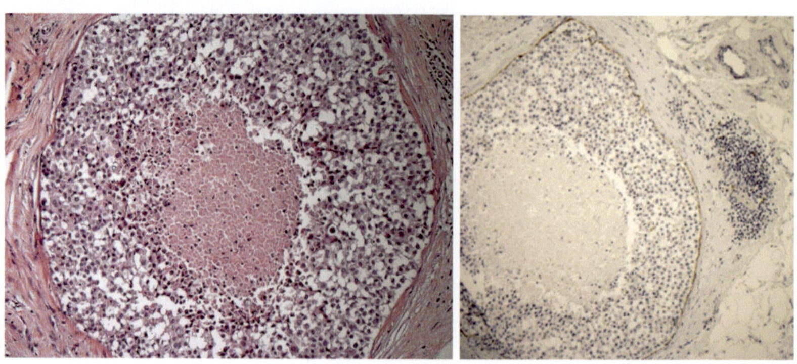

Figs. 8.82 and 8.83 Pleomorphic lobular carcinoma in situ (H&E, 10×) and E-cadherin IHC. The E-cadherin IHC shows loss of membranous staining in the tumor cells, confirming lobular phenotype. The nuclear atypia is similar to high nuclear grade DCIS

Fine Linear and Fine Linear Branching Calcifications

Imaging Findings: Fine linear and fine linear branching calcifications are nearly pathognomonic for malignancy, particularly DCIS. These calcifications follow the course of the ducts, and may be associated with a slightly dilated duct that is visible mammographically. These calcifications nearly always require a biopsy.

- **BI-RADS**: 4, suspicious of malignancy. A stereotactic biopsy is usually recommended.

Differential Diagnosis: Although typically associated with DCIS, occasionally early vascular calcifications, particularly when only involving one aspect of the vessel wall, as well as finer secretory calcifications, can mimic suspicious fine linear branching calcifications.

Concordant or Discordant Scenario

Case 1

Clinical History: An 81-year-old female presented for screening mammography. A small group of linear calcifications was detected, and the patient returned for diagnostic magnification views (Figs. 8.84 and 8.85).

BI-RADS: 4, suspicious.

Pathology Findings: A stereotactic biopsy was recommended and performed, yielding DCIS, grade 3. The patient then underwent a lumpectomy, which yielded DCIS, grade 2 (Fig. 8.86).

Management: The management of DCIS should be made with patient and multidisciplinary input, given that pure DCIS does not pose an immediate risk to the patient's life. Management of DCIS aims to ensure that there is no concomitant invasive cancer, prevent progression of DCIS to invasive cancer, and to decrease the risk of future breast malignancies. Surgical excision is the standard of care for DCIS, in the form of lumpectomy or mastectomy, depending on extent of involvement of the breast by disease and patient preferences. In patients undergoing lumpectomy, 2 mm margins are recommended. Given that pure DCIS does not have the ability to metastasize, sentinel lymph node biopsy (SLNB) is not usually performed at time of surgical excision. Most patients who undergo a lumpectomy for the treatment of DCIS are recommended to

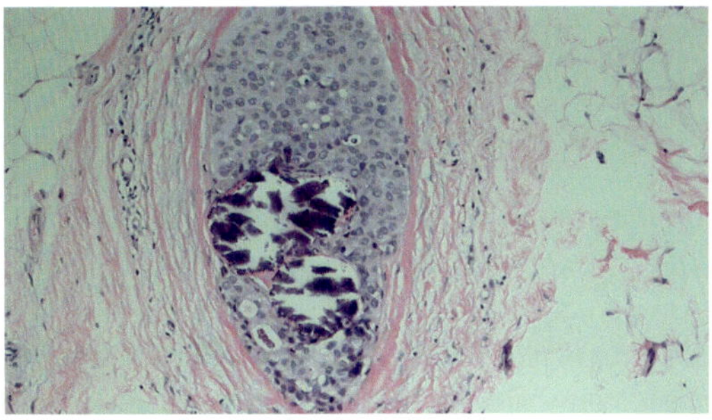

Fig. 8.86 (H&E, 20×). Ductal carcinoma in situ, intermediate nuclear grade (grade 2). The duct is distended by cohesive neoplastic epithelial cells with associated calcifications

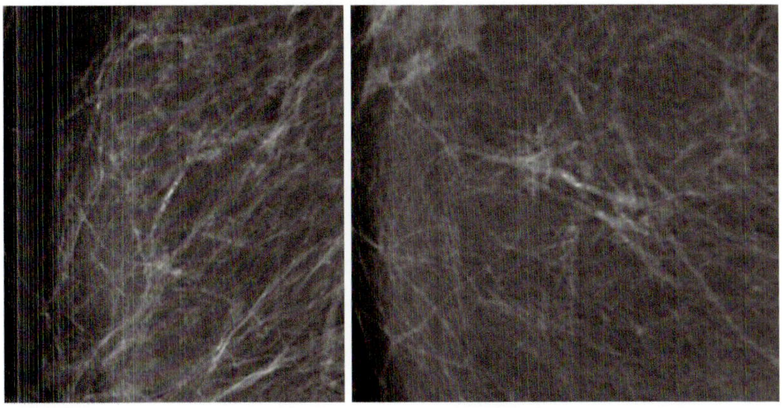

Figs. 8.84 and 8.85 MG findings: fine linear branching calcifications within a slightly dilated duct

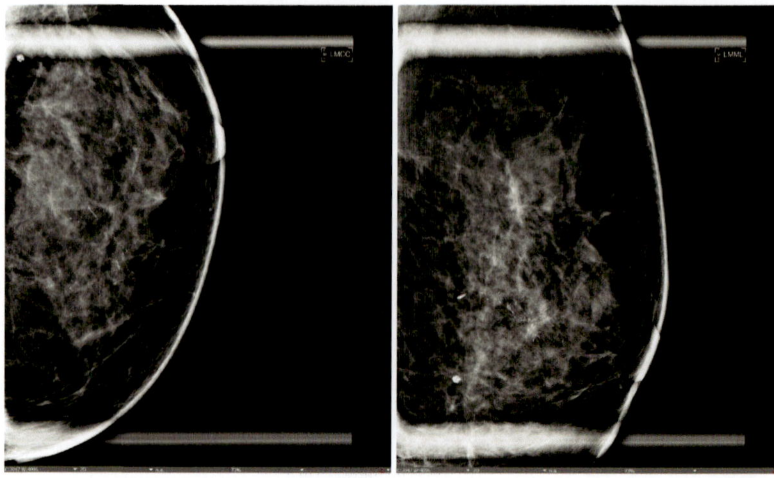

Figs. 8.87 and 8.88 **MG** findings: linear branching calcifications in the central aspect of the breast, posterior to the nipple

receive radiation therapy following surgery to decrease their risk of recurrence. Models to predict the risk of local recurrence, such as the Van Nuys Prognostic Indicator, have been developed and may assist with patient treatment decision making. Most patients diagnosed with estrogen receptor (ER) and progesterone receptor (PR) positive DCIS are recommended to receive treatment of endocrine therapy to decrease their risk of future breast cancer after lumpectomy. Patients who undergo mastectomy due to extent of disease or patient preference do not require radiation therapy. Patients who undergo double mastectomy are not recommended for treatment with endocrine therapy. The Comparison of Operative versus Monitoring and Endocrine Therapy (COMET) trial is investigating the role of active surveillance (clinical and imaging monitoring plus endocrine therapy) rather than surgical excision for the treatment of low-grade DCIS [13–17].

Case 2

Clinical History: A 55-year-old female, status post left lumpectomy and radiation therapy several years ago presents for annual screening mammography. New calcifications were noted in the left breast, and the patient was asked to return for diagnostic mammography with magnification views (Figs. 8.87 and 8.88).

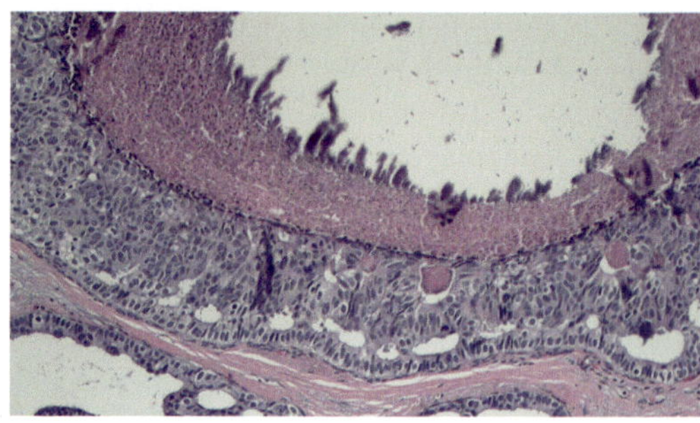

Fig. 8.89 (**H&E, 20×**) Ductal carcinoma in situ, an intermediate nuclear grade with cribriform pattern, associated comedo necrosis and calcification

BI-RADS: 4, suspicious findings.

Pathology Findings: A stereotactic biopsy was recommended and performed, yielding DCIS, grade 2. The patient then underwent a simple left mastectomy, yielding DCIS, grade 2 (Fig. 8.89).

References

1. Demetri-Lewis A, Slanetz P, Eisenberg RL. Breast calcifications: the focal group. AJR. 2012; 198:W325–W343.
2. American Society of Breast Surgeons. Official statement. Management of fibroadenomas. 2008. https://www.breastsurgeons.org/docs/statements/Management-of-Fibroadenomas.pdf.

3. Kamal M, Evans AJ, Denley H, et al. Fibroadenomatoid hyperplasia: a cause of suspicious microcalcification on mammographic screening. AJR. 1998;171:1331–4.
4. Lai KC, Slanetz PJ, Eisenberg RL. Linear breast calcifications. AJR. 2012;199:W151–7.
5. Sickles EA, Abele JS. Milk of calcium within tiny benign breast cysts. Radiology. 1981;141:655–8.
6. Imbriaco M, Riccardi A, Sodano A, Panza M. Milk-of-calcium in breast microcysts with adjacent malignancy. AJR. 1999;173:1137–8.
7. Khoury T, Chen X, Wang D, Kumar P, Qin M, Liu S, Turner B. Nomogram to predict the likelihood of upgrade of atypical ductal hyperplasia diagnosed on a core needle biopsy in mammographically detected lesions. Histopathology. 2015;67(1):10.
8. American Society of Breast Surgeons. Official statement. Consensus guideline on concordance assessment of image-guided breast biopsies and management of borderline or high-risk lesions. 2016. https://www.breastsurgeons.org/docs/statements/Consensus-Guideline-on-Concordance-Assessment-of-Image-Guided-Breast-Biopsies.pdf.
9. Murray MP, Luedtke C, Liberman L, Nehhozina T, Akram M, Brogi E. Classic lobular carcinoma in situ and atypical lobular hyperplasia at percutaneous breast core biopsy: outcomes of prospective excision. Cancer. 2013;119(5):1073.
10. Marshall LM, Hunter DJ, Connolly JL, Schnitt SJ, Byrne C, London SJ, Colditz GA. Risk of breast cancer associated with atypical hyperplasia of lobular and ductal types. Cancer Epidemiol Biomarkers Prev. 1997;6(5):297.
11. Wong SM, King T, Boileau JF, Barry WT, Golshan M. Population-based analysis of breast cancer incidence and survival outcomes in women diagnosed with lobular carcinoma in situ. Ann Surg Oncol. 2017;24(9):2509.
12. Chen PH, Ghosh ET, Slanetz PJ, Eisenberg RL. Segmental breast calcifications. AJR. 2012;199:W532–42.
13. Yamada T, Mori N, Watanabe M, et al. Radiologic-pathologic correlation of ductal carcinoma en situ. Radiographics. 2010;30:1183–98.
14. Morrow M, Van Zee KJ, Solin LJ, Houssami N, Chavez-MacGregor M, Harris JR, Horton J, Hwang S, Johnson PL, Marinovich ML, Schnitt SJ, Wapnir I, Moran MS. Society of Surgical Oncology-American Society for Radiation Oncology-American Society of Clinical Oncology consensus guideline on margins for breast-conserving surgery with whole-breast irradiation in ductal carcinoma in situ. Ann Surg Oncol. 2016;23(12):3801.
15. American Society of Breast Surgeons. Official statement. Consensus guideline on the management of the axilla in patients with invasive/in-situ breast cancer. 2019. https://www.breastsurgeons.org/docs/statements/Consensus-Guideline-on-the-Management-of-the-Axilla.pdf.
16. Silverstein MJ, Lagios MD. Choosing treatment for patients with ductal carcinoma in situ: fine tuning the University of Southern California/Van Nuys Prognostic Index. J Natl Cancer Inst Monogr. 2010;2010(41):193–6.
17. Hwang ES, Hyslop T, Lynch T, Frank E, Pinto D, Basila D, Collyar D, Bennett A, Kaplan C, Rosenberg S, Thompson A, Weiss A, Partridge A. The COMET (comparison of operative versus monitoring and endocrine therapy) trial: a phase III randomized controlled clinical trial for low-risk ductal carcinoma in situ (DCIS). BMJ Open. 2019;9(3):e026797.

MRI Breast Findings

9

Mohan Narasimhamurthy, Sophia R. O'Brien, Liva Andrejeva, and Anupma Nayak

Since its inception in the 1990s, breast magnetic resonance imaging (MRI) has emerged as a valuable tool for screening and diagnosing breast cancers [1]. At present, breast MRI is widely utilized for a number of clinical indications including high-risk screening in women with strong risk for developing breast cancer (>20% lifetime risk), assessment of extent of malignant disease for surgical planning, evaluation of response to neoadjuvant therapy, and further characterization of indeterminate lesions detected on mammography and ultrasound. Breast MRI is a highly sensitive imaging technique with reported sensitivity ranging between 94% and 100% for diagnosing invasive cancers [2]; however, the considerable overlap in the appearance of benign and malignant lesions results in lower specificity (75–85%) warranting unnecessary breast core biopsies that end up on pathologists' desks [3]. Therefore, it is essential for practicing pathologists to be cognizant of the radiology lexicon used in relation to breast MRI and to understand the radiologic-pathologic correlates for appropriate interpretation of such biopsy specimens. The purpose of this chapter is to apprise practicing pathologists with current indications for breast MRI (Table 9.1) and review the imaging patterns of common breast lesions encountered in MRI-guided breast core biopsies.

M. Narasimhamurthy
Pathology and Laboratory Medicine, Pennsylvania Hospital, University of Pennsylvania Health System, Philadelphia, PA, USA
e-mail: mohana.sopanahallinarasimhamurthy@pennmedicine.upenn.edu

S. R. O'Brien
Diagnostic Radiology and Breast Imaging, Perelman School of Medicine, Hospital of the University of Pennsylvania, Philadelphia, PA, USA
e-mail: Sophia.obrien@pennmedicine.upenn.edu

L. Andrejeva
Department of Radiology and Biomedical Imaging, Yale School of Medicine, New Haven, CT, USA
e-mail: liva.andrejeva@yale.edu

A. Nayak (✉)
Pathology and Laboratory Medicine, Perelman School of Medicine, Hospital of the University of Pennsylvania, Philadelphia, PA, USA
e-mail: Anupma.nayak@pennmedicine.upenn.edu

M. Harigopal et al. (eds.), *Radiology Pathology Correlations of Breast Lesions*,
https://doi.org/10.1007/978-3-031-65711-5_9

Table 9.1 Indications for breast MRI

High-risk screening in women with >20% lifetime risk for developing breast cancer
Diagnostic work-up of inconclusive findings in conventional mammogram and ultrasound
Search for mammographically occult lesions, for example: • Metastatic axillary lymph node • Paget's disease of the nipple without any mammographic evidence of a primary malignancy in breast
Preoperative staging to assess the extent of disease for surgical planning
Evaluation of response to therapy after neoadjuvant therapy
Postsurgical follow-up: • Assess residual disease after lumpectomy with positive margins • Evaluate for suspected recurrence • Screening tool after breast-conserving therapy
Assessment of breast implant integrity (non-contrast breast MRI with implant-specific sequences)

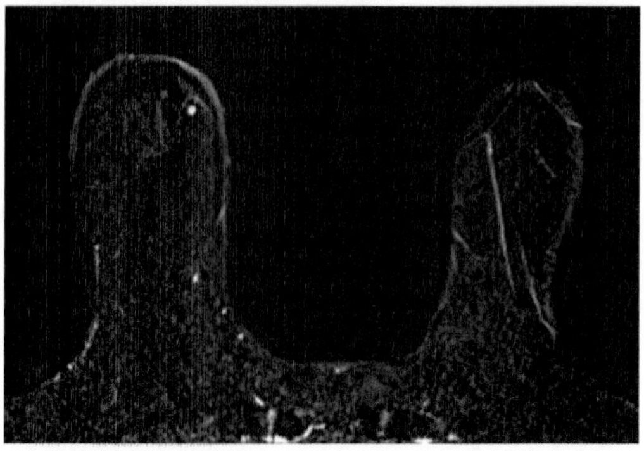

Fig. 9.1 Axial T1-weighted post-contrast subtraction image demonstrating a 3-mm focus of enhancement in the anterior right breast

Interpretation of Breast MRI

Breast MRI is invariably performed using dedicated breast coils and dynamic contrast-enhancement methods after administration of intravenous gadolinium-based contrast agents. Pulse sequences vary by site but typically include T1-weighted images acquired in pre- and post-contrast phases, T2-weighted sequences, and sometimes diffusion-weighted imaging to evaluate the morphologic and functional features of the lesion. Contrast is necessary for demonstrating cancers. Without contrast, the sensitivity of MRI is too low to be useful. Breast density and background parenchymal enhancement (BPE), the physiologic enhancement of normal fibroglandular tissues, is assessed for all patients. Higher BPE can make interpretation of images more difficult and has been shown to lead to a higher abnormal interpretation rate, though some studies have shown that it does not measurably affect cancer detection rate, sensitivity, or specificity of breast MRI [4].

Radiologists broadly classify breast MRI lesions into three groups, as defined below, based on morphology and abnormal enhancement which depends upon multiple factors including cellularity, microvessel density, and vascular permeability.

Focus (foci when multiple) is a punctate enhancement (<5 mm) that is too small to characterize and has no pre-contrast correlate (Fig. 9.1). These lesions are typically stable on follow-up and are considered part of the typical background enhancement pattern in the breast. A new focus that appears as a dominant, asymmetric finding not in keeping with the overall pattern of background parenchymal enhancement is often sampled or followed closely. Multiple scattered foci, especially if bilateral, can generally be dismissed.

Mass is a three-dimensional lesion that occupies space within the breast and can be round, oval, or irregularly shaped. As in mammography and ultrasound, margins, as well as shape, are important predictors of malignancy. Figure 9.2a shows an oval-shaped mass with circumscribed margins that is typically a benign feature. Figure 9.2b shows a mass with spiculated margins, typically a feature of malignancy. The enhancement patterns of the mass can be (a) homogeneous—uniform and confluent throughout the mass (Fig. 9.3a), (b) heterogeneous—non-uniform and varying within the mass (Fig. 9.3b), (c) rim pattern—enhancement around the periphery of the mass (Fig. 9.3c), and (d) dark internal septations (Fig. 9.3d).

Non-mass enhancement (NME) denotes areas of enhancement without a clear space-occupying lesion present. Areas of NME are fur-

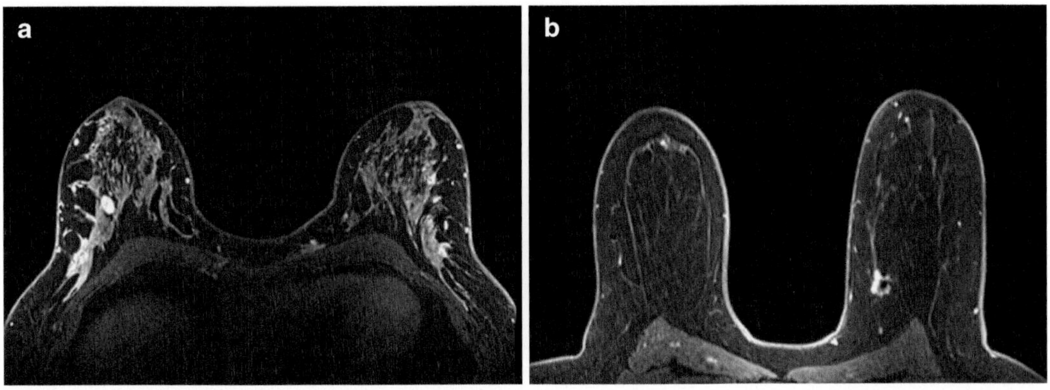

Fig. 9.2 (**a**) Axial T1-weighted non-fat saturated post-contrast image demonstrating a 1.0-cm circumscribed enhancing mass in the outer right breast at posterior depth. (**b**) Axial T1-weighted non-fat saturated post-contrast image demonstrating a 1.5-cm irregularly shaped spiculated mass in the inner left breast at posterior depth. There is an internal susceptibility artifact from a biopsy clip. Pathology revealed estrogen receptor (ER) positive, progesterone receptor (PR) positive, human epidermal growth factor 2 (HER 2)-negative invasive ductal carcinoma

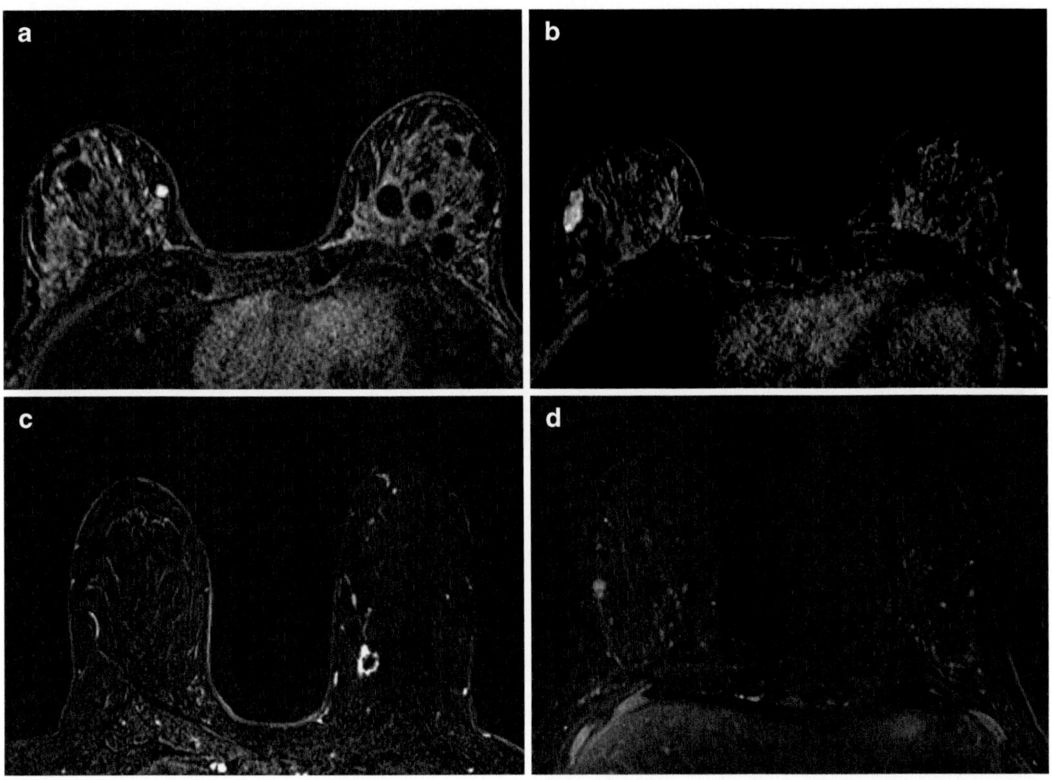

Fig. 9.3 (**a**) Axial T1-weighted post-contrast subtraction image demonstrating a 5-mm homogeneously enhancing mass. There is marked, symmetric BPE and multiple non-enhancing cysts bilaterally. (**b**) Axial T1-weighted post-contrast subtraction image demonstrating a 1.2-cm heterogeneously enhancing mass in the outer right breast. (**c**) Axial T1-weighted post-contrast subtraction image demonstrating rim enhancement of an irregular spiculated mass in the inner left breast at posterior depth, biopsy-proven ER/PR+ HER2− invasive ductal carcinoma. (**d**) Axial T1-weighted post-contrast subtraction image demonstrating an 8-mm oval, circumscribed mass with internal non-enhancing septations in keeping with a fibroadenoma

ther described according to distribution patterns as focal (Fig. 9.4a), linear (Fig. 9.4b), segmental (Fig. 9.4c), regional (Fig. 9.4d), and diffuse (Fig. 9.4d). Diffuse distribution is generally benign, whereas segmental or linear distribution suggests a higher risk of malignancy. Once identified, non-mass enhancement is further assessed to see whether it is bilaterally symmetric or if it is asymmetric. In general, asymmetric findings are more likely to be cancer than are symmetric findings. The internal enhancement pattern of non-mass enhancement is also classified as homogeneous, heterogeneous, clumped, or clustered ring (Fig. 9.4e).

Table 9.2 summarizes the common morphologic features of benign and malignant breast

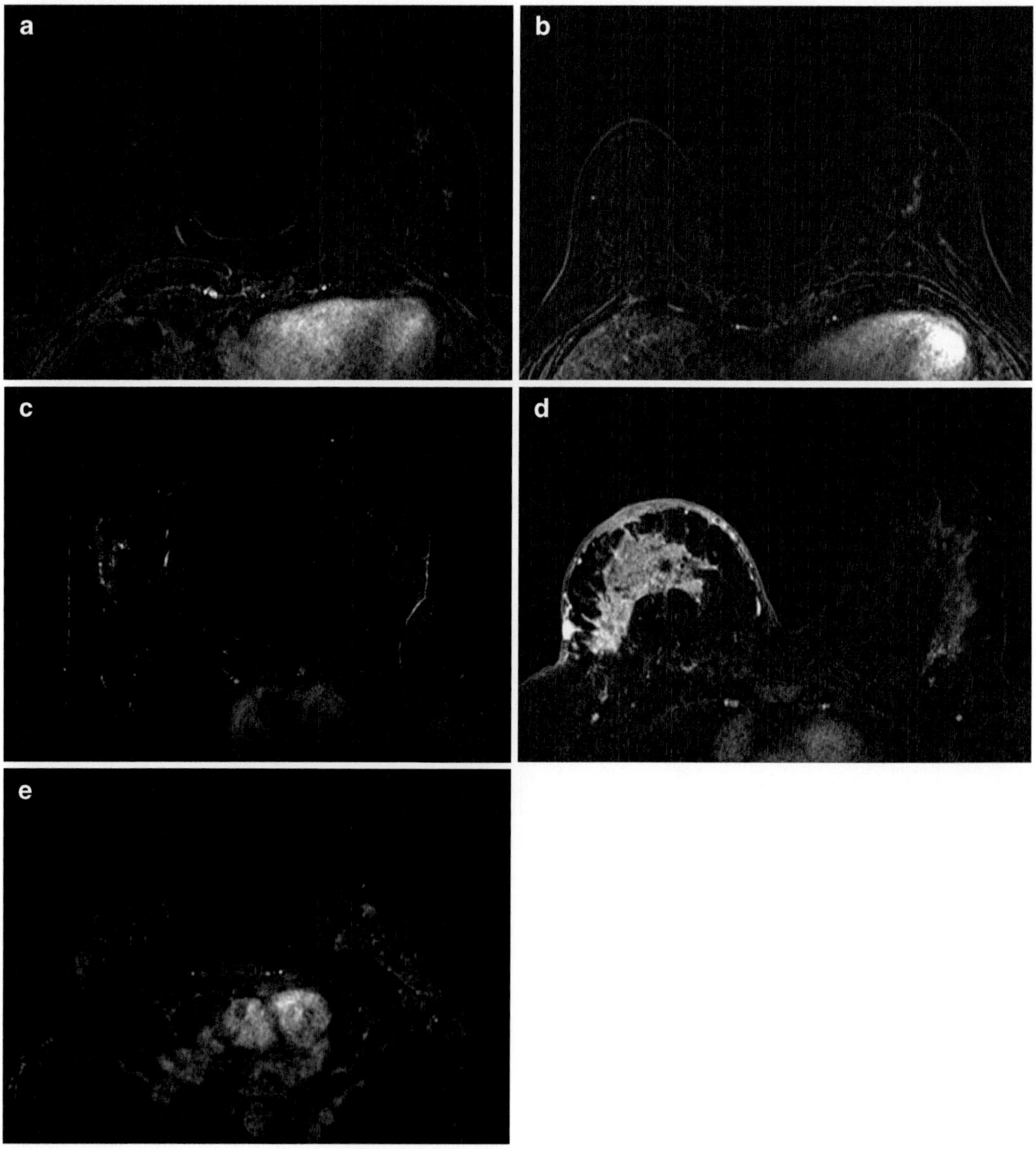

Fig. 9.4 (**a**) Axial T1-weighted post-contrast subtraction imaging demonstrating two areas of focal NME seen in the left breast. (**b**) Linear NME seen in the central left breast. (**c**) Segmental NME seen in the outer right breast. (**d**) Regional NME in the left breast and diffuse NME in the right breast (there is associated skin thickening on the right; this patient has biopsy-proven ER/PR+ HER2− invasive carcinoma with mixed ductal and lobular features). (**e**) Focal clustered ring enhancement with internal septations seen in the central right breast at anterior depth

Table 9.2 Morphologic features suggestive of benign and malignant breast lesions on breast MRI

Features suggestive of benign lesions	Features suggestive of malignant lesions
No or minimal enhancement	Rapid/bright enhancement
Center enhances first	Rim enhancement
Homogeneous enhancement	Heterogeneous enhancement
Circumscribed or mildly lobulated margin	Spiculated or irregular margins
Oriented parallel to Cooper's ligaments	Oriented perpendicular to Cooper's ligaments
Diffuse distribution	Linear, linear-branching or segmental enhancement
Non-enhancing internal septations	Clumped or clustered ring enhancement
Symmetric	Asymmetric

lesions on MRI. In general, benign lesions are either non-enhancing or show minimal enhancement with center enhancing first. A homogeneously enhancing mass favors benignity, while a rapidly/brightly enhancing mass, with rim enhancement or enhancing septations or heterogeneous pattern, is usually suspicious for malignancy. As with mammography, masses with spiculated or irregular borders are suspicious, while circumscribed, oval, or lobulated masses are frequently benign. Masses oriented parallel to Cooper's ligaments suggest benign lesions, whereas lesions traversing Cooper's ligaments are abnormal and suggest invasive ductal cancer. Non-enhancing dark internal septations in circumscribed, oval, or lobulated masses are almost always benign fibroadenomas, although they can be seen in mucinous cancers as well. A ductal, linear, or segmental pattern of clumped enhancement is suspicious for ductal carcinoma in situ (DCIS); however, it may also be seen in benign fibrocystic change (FCC), atypical ductal hyperplasia or duct ectasia. Clustered ring enhancement is often a feature of DCIS.

As mentioned previously, achieving high specificity with breast MRI is difficult because of considerable overlap between the appearance of benign and malignant lesions. Some benign breast lesions enhance more avidly than normal breast parenchyma and therefore mimic breast cancer. For example, fibroadenoma, intraductal papilloma, and fibrocystic change (FCC) also enhance to a greater degree than normal surrounding breast parenchyma. Dynamic enhancement kinetic curves (DCE) created by perfusion and diffusion gradients of contrast material from the blood vessels to the extracellular space can be utilized to improve the distinction between benign and malignant lesions, but their utility is limited. The kinetic curve has two parts—the initial perfusion phase (within 2 min of contrast injection or before the curve shape begins to change) and the second delayed diffusion phase (after 2 min or after the curve starts to change). The 2013 ACR BI-RADS MRI lexicon further classifies the initial kinetic curve based on increase in signal intensity as—*slow*, an increase of signal intensity <50% than baseline; *medium*, an increase of signal intensity 50–100% higher than baseline; or *fast*, an increase of signal intensity >100% higher than baseline. The delayed kinetic curves are classified as either *persistent* (signal intensity increases by at least 10% of the initial-phase signal intensity); *plateau* (signal intensity does not change from the initial phase); or *washout* (signal intensity decreases by at least 10% of the initial-phase signal intensity). In general, benign lesions usually show slow initial rise curve and a persistent delayed-phase curve, whereas malignant lesions have a fast initial curve with a washout kinetic curve in the delayed phase (Fig. 9.5a, b). Table 9.3 summarizes common false-positives and false-negatives seen on breast MRI.

Benign Lesions

Fibrocystic changes (FCC) refer to a spectrum of benign histologic findings, including cysts, apocrine metaplasia, adenosis, ductal epithelial hyperplasia, and stromal fibrosis (Fig. 9.6a). FCC is often a nonspecific incidental finding in breast core biopsies.

MRI Findings

- MRI appearance of FCC depends on whether the process is focal or diffuse and also on the components of fibrocystic changes.

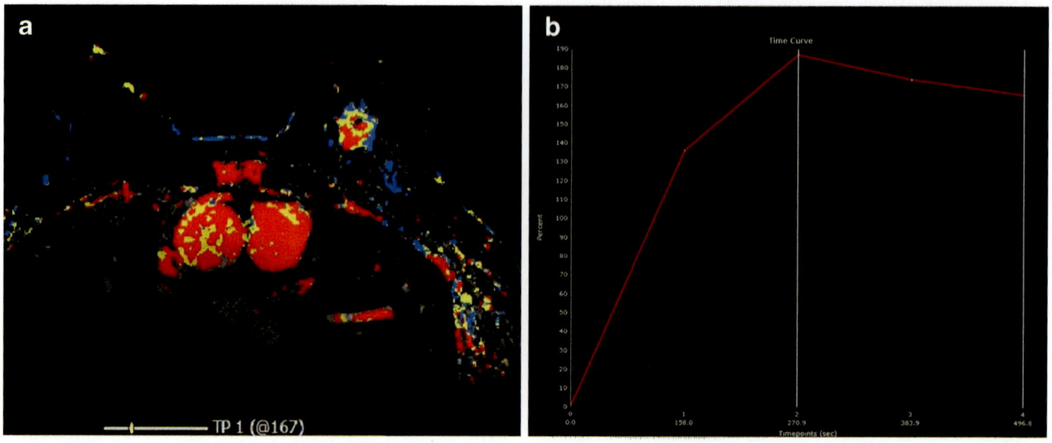

Fig. 9.5 (**a**) Demonstrates an axial post-contrast subtracted MRI image with computer-aided detection parametric mapping from a patient with a known left breast IDC displaying a mixture of washout and plateau kinetics within the malignant mass. (**b**) Shows a plot of signal intensity (SI) of the lesion over time following intravenous contrast injection, demonstrating a decrease of SI of more than 10% after peaking, consistent with a washout (type III) enhancement pattern

Table 9.3 Common false-positives and false-negatives on breast MRI

False-positives	False-negatives
Hormone-related enhancement	Non-enhancing DCIS
Focal stromal fibrosis	Non-enhancing invasive lobular carcinoma
Radial scar with spiculated margin	Residual tumors post-chemotherapy
Surgical scar with irregular margin	Gradually enhancing tumor in a background of bright benign parenchymal enhancement
Cystic papillary apocrine metaplasia (FCC)	
Intraductal papilloma	
Fibroadenoma especially hyalinized	
Fat necrosis	
Intramammary lymph nodes without a fatty hilum	

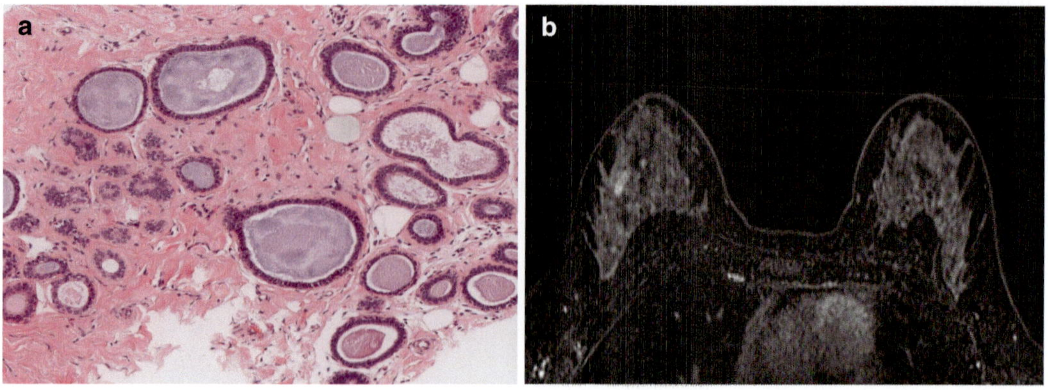

Fig. 9.6 A 37-year-old woman with BRCA1 mutation presents for a high-risk screening MRI. (**a**) Biopsy revealed fibrocystic changes consisting of cystically dilated ducts and stromal fibrosis [H&E stain; 10×] presenting as NME. (**b**) Axial T1-weighted fat-saturated post-contrast subtraction image demonstrates linear NME in the upper outer right breast, subsequently biopsied

- FCC has a wide spectrum of morphologic and kinetic features on MRI that may overlap with features suggesting malignancy.
- It may appear as a prominent non-mass-like enhancement in regional, focal, or segmental distribution (Fig. 9.6b), or may appear as a mass with spiculated or circumscribed margins (Fig. 9.7a–c).
- The enhancement in the initial phase of the kinetic curve may range from slow to rapid, and may vary between persistent, plateau, or washout enhancement during the delayed phase.
- The knowledge of MRI appearance of individual components of FCCs is essential to decipher the underlying components of fibrocystic changes and to differentiate from malignancy.

Cystic apocrine metaplasia belongs to the spectrum of FCC consisting of a discrete cluster of closely packed cysts lined by single or multiple layers of metaplastic apocrine epithelium arranged in mounds or papillae with fibrovascular cores (Fig. 9.8a). Recent studies correlating the histologic features with MRI findings have reported an increased prevalence of apocrine lesions in MRI-guided core biopsies. The reported detection rate varies from 7% to as high as 25% in MRI-guided biopsies [5–7], in contrast to low detection rate of 2–4% in stereotactic biopsies [8, 9].

MRI Findings

- The cystic apocrine metaplasia lesions present as hyperintense lesions on T2 images, as linear non-mass enhancement (Fig. 9.8b–d) or a focus (Fig. 9.8e).

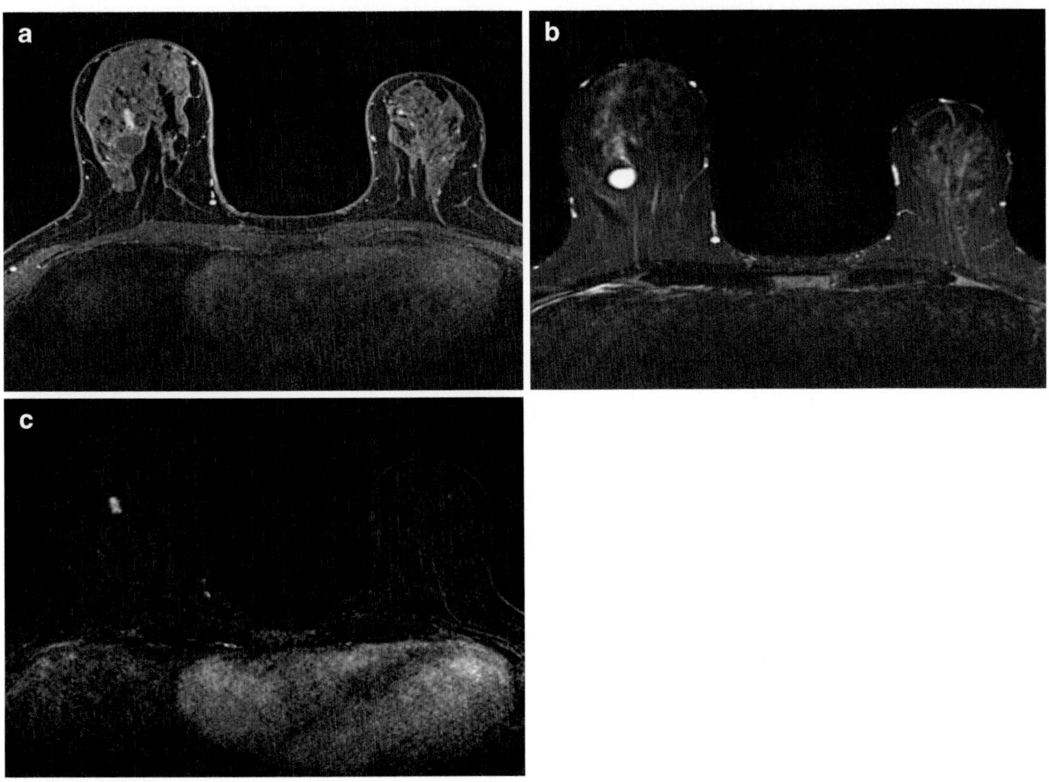

Fig. 9.7 Another 61-year-old woman with a history of left breast lobular carcinoma in situ, now with a 1.1-cm oval enhancing mass seen in the lower central breast. (**a**) High-resolution post-contrast T1 imaging demonstrates indistinct margins. (**b**) On T2-weighted imaging the lesion was isointense with an incidental hyperintense simple cyst seen posteriorly. (**c**) Subtraction imaging demonstrates the mass is a dominant finding in the breast. Patient subsequently underwent MR-guided core biopsy revealing fibrous breast tissue with fibrocystic changes and focal florid duct hyperplasia

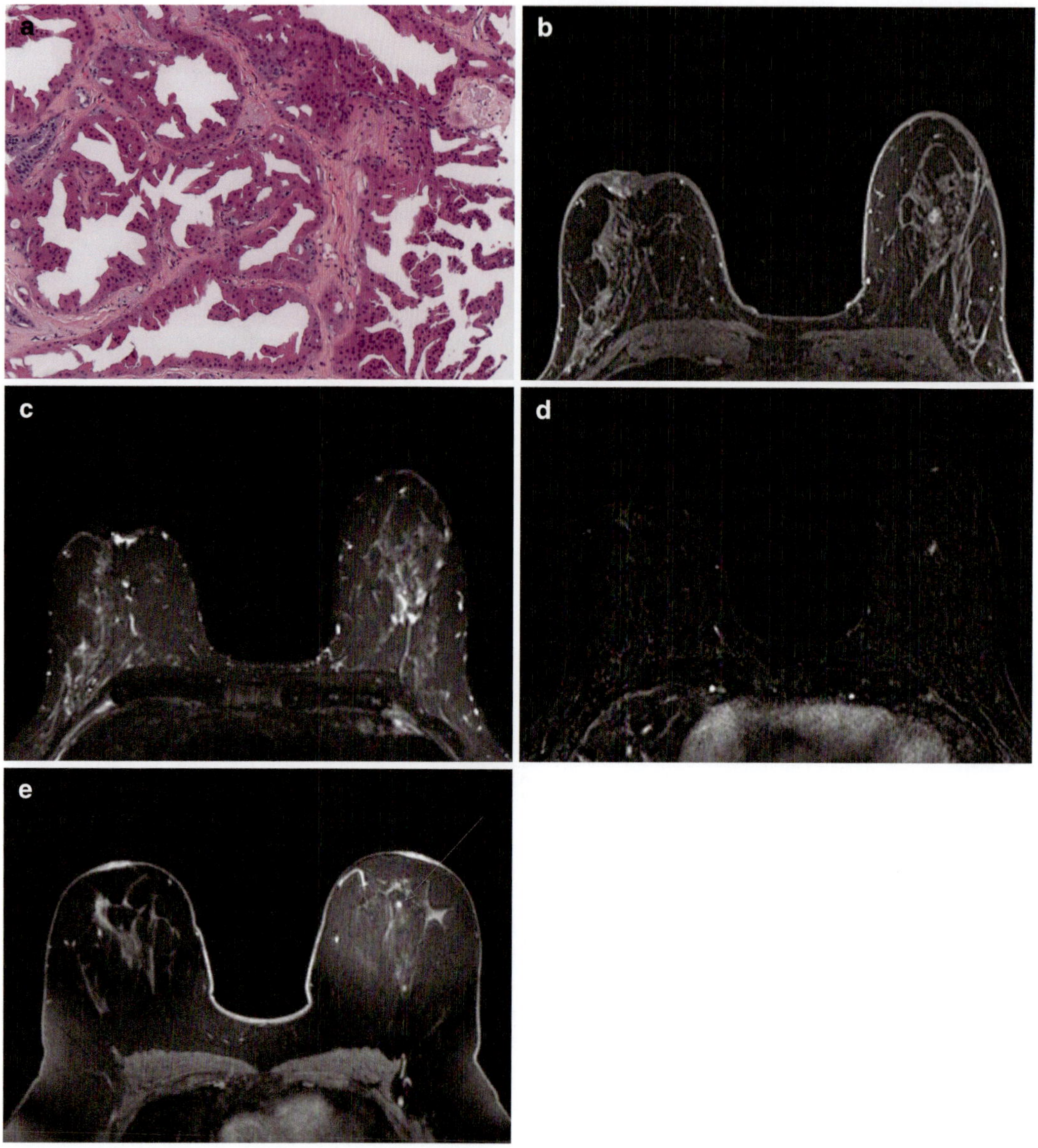

Fig. 9.8 A 57-year-old woman with history of right breast cancer status post-breast conservation therapy and left breast atypical ductal hyperplasia (ADH) on concurrent surgical excisional biopsy. MRI obtained for surveillance. (**a**) The MRI-guided core biopsy demonstrated a nodular focus of cystic-papillary apocrine metaplasia, with cystically dilated duct spaces lined by apocrine cells [H&E stain; 10×]. (**b**) High-resolution T1 post-contrast imaging demonstrates 6-mm linear non-mass enhancement (NME) in the central left breast. (**c**) T2-weighted imaging demonstrates T2 iso- or hypointensity in the region of the linear NME. (**d**) Subtraction imaging demonstrates this is a dominant finding. The patient subsequently underwent MR-guided core biopsy revealing cystic papillary apocrine metaplasia (CPAM) and other fibrocystic changes containing calcifications. (**e**) Another patient with biopsy-proven CPAM presenting as 3-mm focus of enhancement in the left breast (arrow) on axial T1-weighted post-contrast imaging

- They may present as masses with circumscribed (smooth or lobulated) margins.
- The kinetic pattern is usually mixed, with plateau kinetics being most common. However, a significant proportion of cases may exhibit washout kinetics leading to a core biopsy procedure.

Pseudoangiomatous stromal hyperplasia (PASH) is a benign myofibroblastic proliferative lesion, predominantly seen in premenopausal and perimenopausal females, and that frequently presents as a nonspecific incidental finding, with a reported range from 9% to 23% [10, 11]. Rarely, it may present as a palpable mass. Histologically, it is characterized by anastomosing slit-like spaces resembling small blood vessels that are either acellular or lined by spindle-shaped stromal cells (Fig. 9.9a).

MRI Findings

- On MRI, PASH has a wide-ranging appearance, but it most commonly appears as a region of non-mass enhancement (Fig. 9.9b–d).
- Other patterns include mass (Fig. 9.9e) and foci.
- No definitive imaging characteristic reliably identifies PASH.

Radial scar/Complex sclerosing lesions (RS/CSL) are benign sclerosing lesions histologically characterized by a central fibroelastotic core surrounded by radiating ducts and lobules exhibiting fibrocystic and proliferative changes (Fig. 9.10a). They are often confused with invasive cancer in imaging as well as histology. Mammographic and sonographic features of radial scars have been described in previous chapters.

MRI Findings

- The MRI features of RS/CSL are nonspecific and variable in the reported literature.
- Few studies have reported non-mass enhancement in linear or clumped distribution showing early rapid enhancement with plateau or delayed washout kinetics (type 2 or 3 curves) as the most frequent abnormality (Fig. 9.10b) [12, 13].
- On the contrary, others have found a mass lesion with irregular morphology, the most frequent appearance of radial scar on MRI (Fig. 9.10c) [14].
- Unfortunately, MRI does not help to distinguish between RS/CSL with or without associated atypia/malignancy [15].

Intraductal papillomas are benign intraductal lesions formed by arborizing finger-like fronds of fibrovascular stalks lined by a layer of myoepithelial cells and one or multiple layers of proliferative luminal epithelium (Fig. 9.11a). They may be solitary or multiple. Solitary intraductal papillomas are often centrally located and arise from subareolar large lactiferous ducts. Multiple intraductal papillomas arise from the terminal duct and lobular unit (TDLU) and are usually peripherally located. The imaging features of central and peripheral papillomas are essentially similar. Papillomas, when smaller than 5 mm in size, may be occult on conventional mammography or US. MRI has a high sensitivity but low specificity for detecting papillary tumors [16–19].

MRI Findings

- Papillomas mostly appear as a homogeneously enhancing mass with circumscribed or irregular margins, and are frequently associated with an ectatic duct. They demonstrate iso- to slightly hyper-signal intensity than surrounding fibroglandular breast parenchyma on T1-weighted pre-contrast images and fat-suppressed T2-weighted images (Fig. 9.11b, c). Signal hyperintensity is most likely due to hemorrhage and periductal fibrosis commonly associated with papillomas.
- Less frequently, they may appear as a complex solid and cystic mass.
- Rarely, they may have heterogeneous or peripheral rim enhancement mimicking a malignant lesion [20].
- Post-contrast, they may enhance rapidly, with variable persistent, plateau, or washout kinetics in the delayed phase.

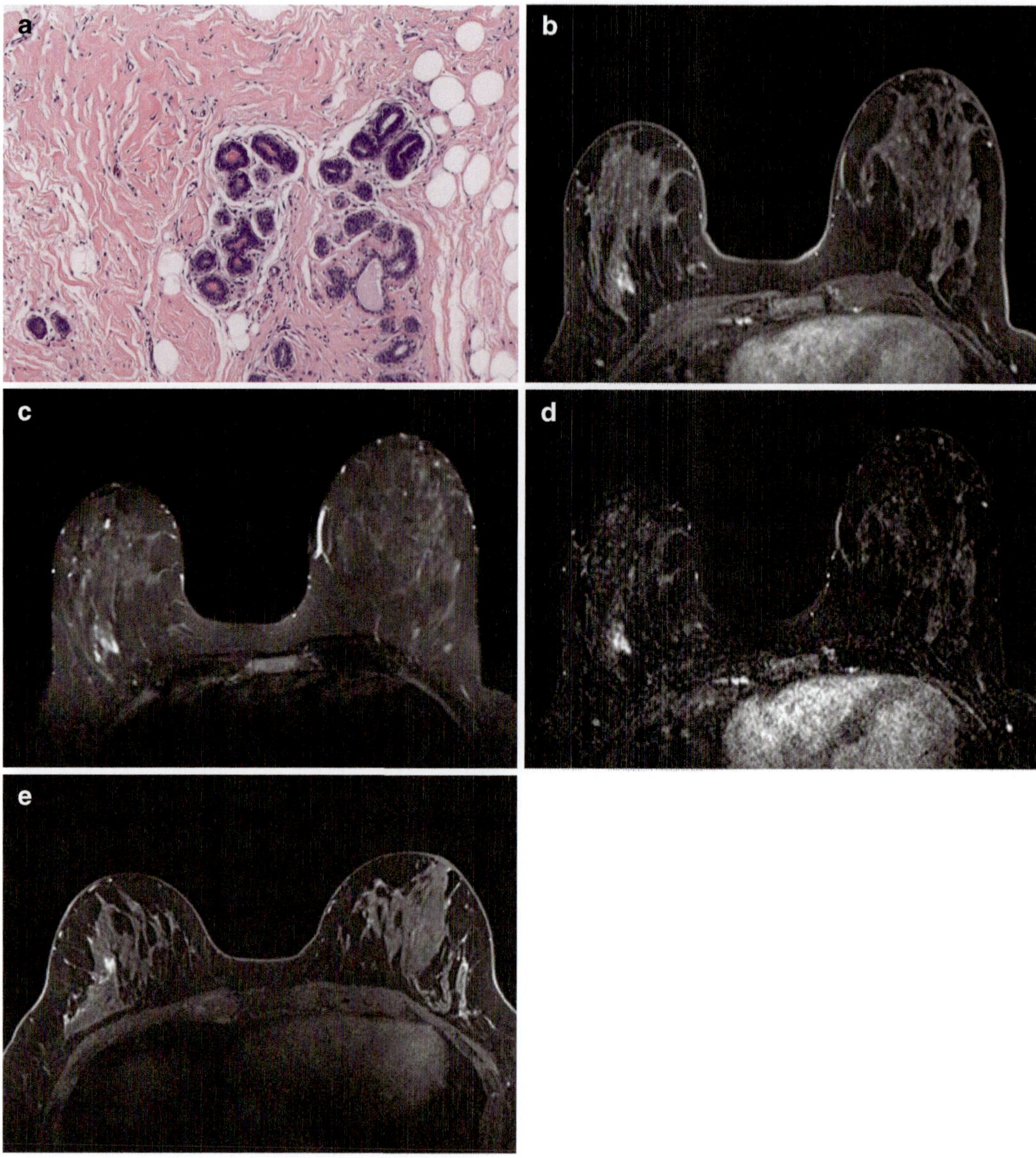

Fig. 9.9 A 37-year-old woman with a history of abnormal mammogram (probably benign lesion in the posterior right breast) presents for an MRI. (**a**) The core biopsy shows breast tissue with dense collagenous stroma with prominent slit-like spaces lined by stromal cells mimicking thin capillaries (pseudoangiomatous stromal hyperplasia aka PASH) [H&E section; 10×]. (**b**) Post-contrast T1 imaging demonstrates clumped and linear non-mass enhancement (NME) in the lower central right breast at posterior depth. (**c**) T2-weighted imaging demonstrates T2 hyperintensity. (**d**) Axial subtraction imaging demonstrates that this is a dominant finding. Of note, this finding did not correlate with the abnormal mammographic lesion. Patient subsequently underwent MR-guided core biopsy revealing benign breast tissue with nodular fibrocystic changes with rare calcifications, focal florid duct hyperplasia, and pseudoangiomatous stromal hyperplasia (PASH). (**e**) High-resolution post-contrast T1 imaging demonstrates an 8-mm irregular enhancing mass with indistinct margins in the central right breast in another 36-year-old woman with history of acute lymphoblastic leukemia and total body irradiation at age 16 now presents for high-risk screening breast MRI, core biopsy of which revealed fibrous breast tissue with PASH

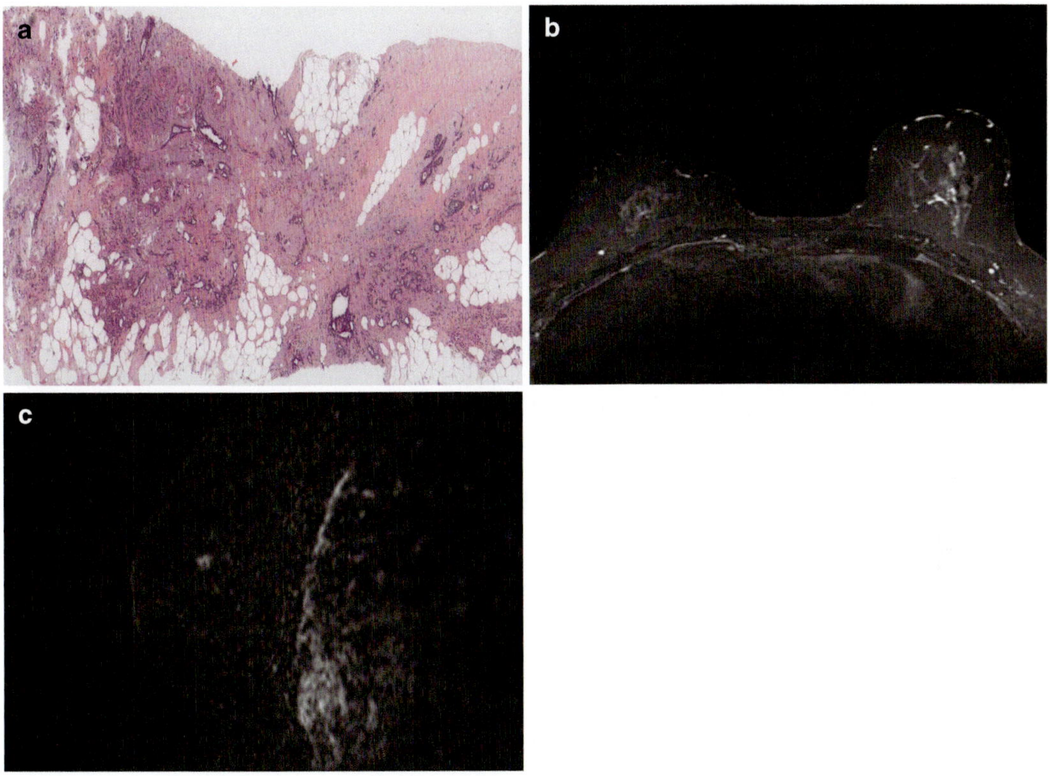

Fig. 9.10 A 58-year-old woman with history of right breast cancer post-breast conservation therapy, presenting for surveillance imaging with MRI. (**a**) A case of radial scar with central fibroelastotic scar and radiating compressed tubules [H&E section; 4×] presenting as linear non-mass enhancement on surveillance MRI. (**b**) T1 imaging demonstrates 17-mm linear non-mass enhancement in the upper central left breast. (**c**) Subtraction imaging demonstrates 9 mm of clumped mass-like enhancement in the upper central right breast at middle depth. Bilateral MR-guided biopsies revealed radial scars with calcifications on both sides

- Washout kinetics similar to malignant lesions are less common, but not rare, hence mandating a core biopsy for a definitive diagnosis.
- Unfortunately, there are no definitive morphologic or kinetic features on MRI that can predict the upgrade of papillomas to malignancy to help in triaging surgery [21].

Duct ectasia is a dilation of the major lactiferous ducts, with occasional involvement of peripheral smaller ducts, caused by obstruction of the ducts by accumulated secretions or an intraductal mass. The proteinaceous or hemorrhagic secretions may calcify or leak in the surrounding stroma causing secondary chronic inflammation and periductal fibrosis (Fig. 9.12a).

MRI Findings

- On MRI, ectatic ducts frequently appear as non-enhancing, fluid-filled, branching tubular structures draining toward the nipple. Frequently, the duct fluid is hyperintense on T1-weighted images because of its proteinaceous or hemorrhagic nature (Fig. 9.12b).
- Rarely, ectatic ducts may show signal intensities similar to that of water (hypointense on T1-weighted images and hyperintense on T2-weighted sequences).
- Focal enhancement within the dilated duct lumen triggers suspicion for intraductal papilloma or carcinoma and results in a core biopsy.
- Chronic inflammation and periductal fibrosis secondary to leakage of fluid into stroma may present as periductal enhancement.

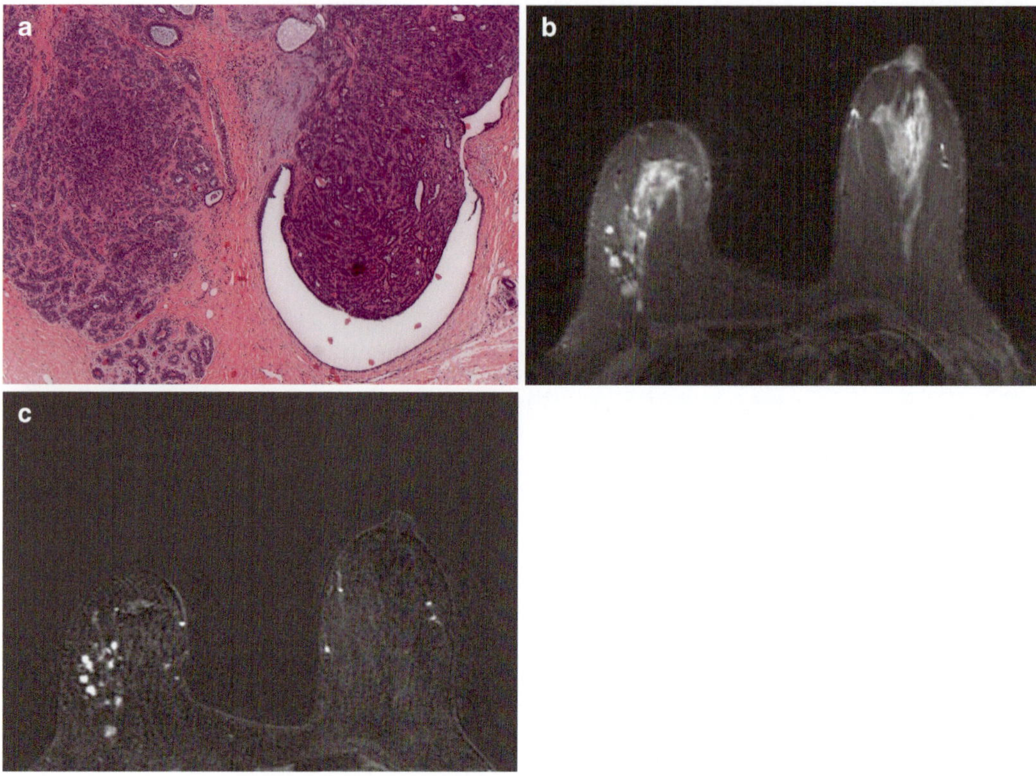

Fig. 9.11 A 66-year-old woman presents for breast MRI for further evaluation of multiple subcentimeter masses in her outer right breast. (**a**) Sclerosing duct papilloma [H&E section; 4×] with dilated duct containing complex adenotic mass with papillary fibrovascular cores lined by luminal epithelial and basal myoepithelial cell layer, presenting as a 5-mm enhancing mass on screening MRI. (**b**) On axial T2-weighted imaging some of the masses have corresponding T2-hyperintensity while others are T2-hypointense. (**c**) Axial subtraction imaging demonstrates multiple subcentimeter enhancing masses in a regional distribution in the outer right breast at posterior depth spanning approximately 5 cm in the anterior-posterior dimension

Fat necrosis, a common benign breast finding caused by trauma, surgery, or radiation, is a mimicker of malignancy on imaging and often leads to a core biopsy. The imaging features of fat necrosis are variable and depend upon its histologic stage. Histologically, in the early phase, it is characterized by disrupted fat accompanied by hemorrhage and fat-engulfing macrophages (Fig. 9.13a, b). As the lesion progresses, the inflammatory cellular debris and necrotic fat may become cystic and surrounded by a peripheral rim of fibrosis. In the later phases, the fibrosis replaces the central necrotic fat giving rise to a scar which may or may not be associated with dystrophic calcification.

MRI Findings

- On MRI, fat necrosis frequently presents as a rim-enhancing mass with irregular margins and central non-enhancing fat (Fig. 9.13c, d). Its appearance varies widely depending upon the amount of fat and the extent of inflammation and fibrosis.
- Fibrosis is responsible for the mass effect and architectural distortion, and the degree of inflammation determines the degree of enhancement. Although a thin rim of enhancement is more common, the rim may also be thick, irregular, or spiculated.
- A fat-fluid level (Fig. 9.13e) or thin enhancing internal septations may be identified within the central fat collection.

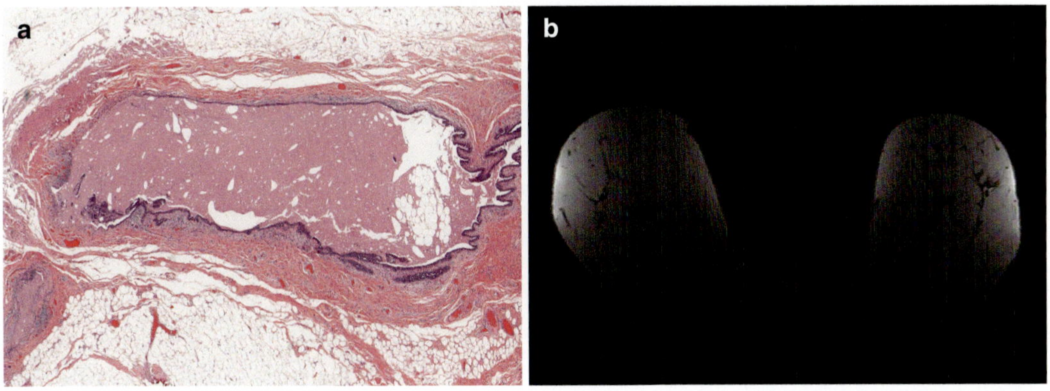

Fig. 9.12 A 65-year-old woman with newly diagnosed right breast ductal carcinoma presents for staging breast MRI. The contralateral breast showed a non-mass enhancement. (**a**) MRI-guided core biopsy [H&E section, 10×] shows portions of dilated ducts with amorphous secretions, prominent periductal fibrosis, and chronic inflammation representing duct ectasia. (**b**) Axial non-contrast T1-weighted imaging of the left breast reveals focally dilated ducts with peripheral non-mass enhancement and debris

- The kinetics may vary from slow to rapid initially, with persistent, plateau, or even washout delayed patterns. Due to this overlap in the kinetic patterns, a biopsy is sometimes needed to distinguish it from malignant lesions on imaging.
- Besides presenting as an enhancing mass lesion, fat necrosis may also appear as an enhancing focus, or clumped non-mass enhancement when it contains a nominal amount of fat (Fig. 9.13f).

Parenchymal scar is another common pathologic finding in MRI-guided core biopsies (Fig. 9.14a) as MRI is increasingly being used in surveillance of patients with personal history of cancer post-lumpectomy.

MRI Findings

- Similar to mammography, surgical scar on MRI appears as architectural distortion with long spicules radiating from the surgical bed (Fig. 9.14b, c).
- Surgical scars tend to enhance within the first 6 months due to accompanying seroma, fat necrosis, and inflammatory granulation tissue. Though persistent enhancement beyond 5 years has been reported, they generally do not enhance more than 18 months after surgery. Hence, MRI is more useful in detection of delayed recurrences in the lumpectomy bed. Delayed appearance of enhancement generally warrants a diagnostic core biopsy to exclude residual tumor or recurrence.

Postradiation changes include edema, vascular dilatation, capillary, and microvascular damage, and thickening of the skin and breast parenchyma (Fig. 9.15a, b).

MRI Findings

- On MRI, the irradiated breast tissue shows intense patchy or diffuse non-mass enhancement coupled with edema and diffuse thickening of skin during the first 6–9 months after radiation (Fig. 9.15c). After that, these changes begin to subside and by 18 months postradiation, the treated breast shows prominent decrease in size and parenchymal enhancement, compared with those in the untreated breast (Fig. 9.15d).
- Sometimes, postradiation changes can appear as focal abnormalities which are suspicious (Fig. 9.15e).
- Any increase in parenchymal enhancement beyond 18 months (mass or non-mass) is indicative of recurrence and merits a core biopsy.

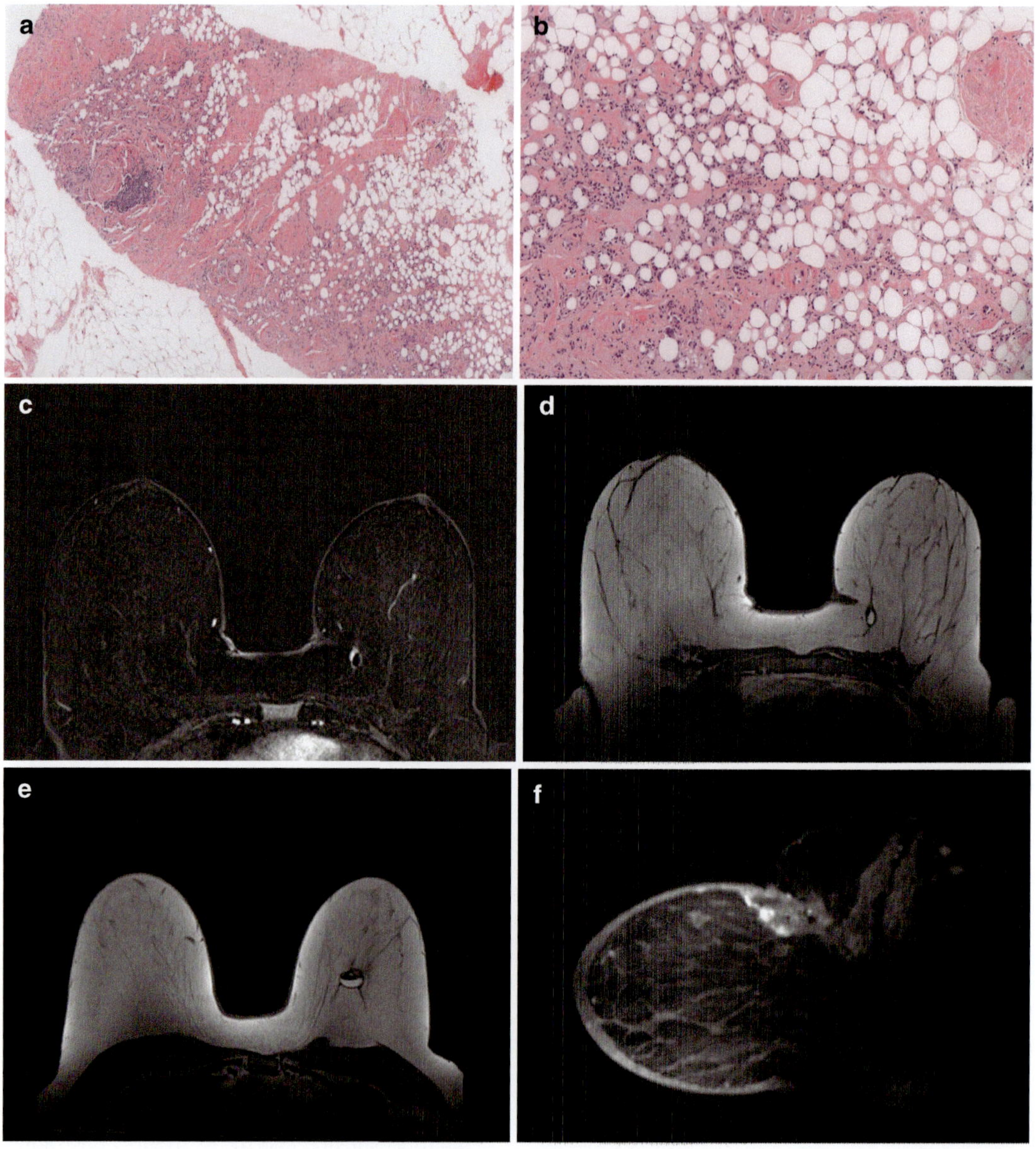

Fig. 9.13 A 57-year-old woman with bilateral breast pain presents for breast MRI. (**a**, **b**) MRI-guided core biopsy demonstrating fat necrosis, adipocytes surrounded by foamy histiocytes and chronic inflammatory cells [H&E section, 4×, 10×]. (**c**) Axial T1-weighted post-contrast subtraction imaging demonstrates a rim-enhancing lesion in the inner left breast at posterior depth with (**d**) internal fat seen on axial T1-weighted pre-contrast imaging in keeping with fat necrosis. (**e**) An additional lesion seen in the central left breast demonstrates a fat fluid level on axial T1-weighted non-contrast imaging. These findings are in keeping with fat necrosis. (**f**) Clumped, nodular, non-mass enhancement seen on sagittal post-contrast T1-weighted fat suppressed image along the anterior margin of a lumpectomy bed in an 81-year-old with history of left breast cancer post-breast conservation planning. Subsequent MRI-guided breast biopsy revealed fat necrosis

Granulomatous mastitis is a benign inflammatory disease of unclear etiology. It is more common in women in the reproductive age group, with a history of recent pregnancy, lactation, and hyperprolactinemia [22]. Histologically, it is characterized by lobulocentric chronic granulomatous inflammation without associated necrosis (Fig. 9.16a). Patients usually present with clinical

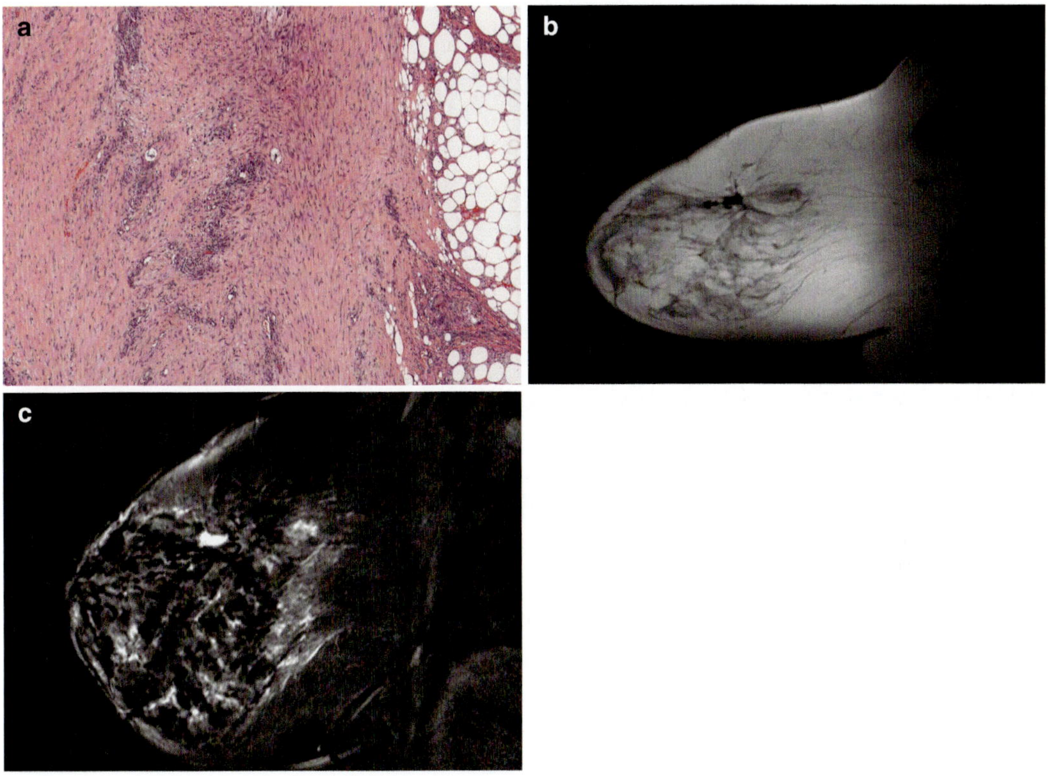

Fig. 9.14 A 56-year-old woman with newly diagnosed DCIS in the left breast and history of DCIS in the right breast post-lumpectomy and radiation 6-years prior who presents for staging MRI. (**a**) MRI-guided core biopsy shows fibrosis and hemosiderin macrophages. (**b**) Sagittal T1-weighted non-fat saturated non-enhanced image of the right breast demonstrating the postsurgical changes from prior lumpectomy. (**c**) Sagittal T1-weighted post-contrast subtraction imaging of the right breast demonstrating linear enhancement anterior to the lumpectomy bed. Subsequent MRI-guided biopsy revealed parenchymal scar

signs and symptoms, including palpable mass, pain, nipple discharge, skin changes, and enlarged axillary nodes. The clinical and imaging findings often overlap with those of malignancy and therefore a diagnostic core biopsy is warranted.

MRI Findings

- Granulomatous mastitis may present as both non-mass enhancement (NME) and enhancing masses with circumscribed margins and rim enhancement.
- NME is often in segmental or regional distributions and is associated with clustered ring enhancement (Fig. 9.16b, c).
- Most cases have benign persistent enhancement kinetics, although rapid initial enhancement and washout on delayed kinetic curves simulating breast carcinomas can also be seen.
- Architectural distortion, focal skin thickening, skin retraction, and nipple retraction are additional features noted in these patients.
- Rarely, the skin thickening or enhancement can be diffuse, mimicking an inflammatory breast carcinoma.
- In general, MRI is not so helpful in distinguishing granulomatous mastitis from cancer due to a significant overlap in imaging features [23, 24].

Diabetic mastopathy is a rare breast condition predominantly seen in women with type 1 insulin-dependent diabetes. Clinically, patients present with a nontender, palpable, firm to hard mass in one or both breasts, suggesting malignancy. Histologically, it is characterized by dense keloid-like fibrosis, with prominence of epitheli-

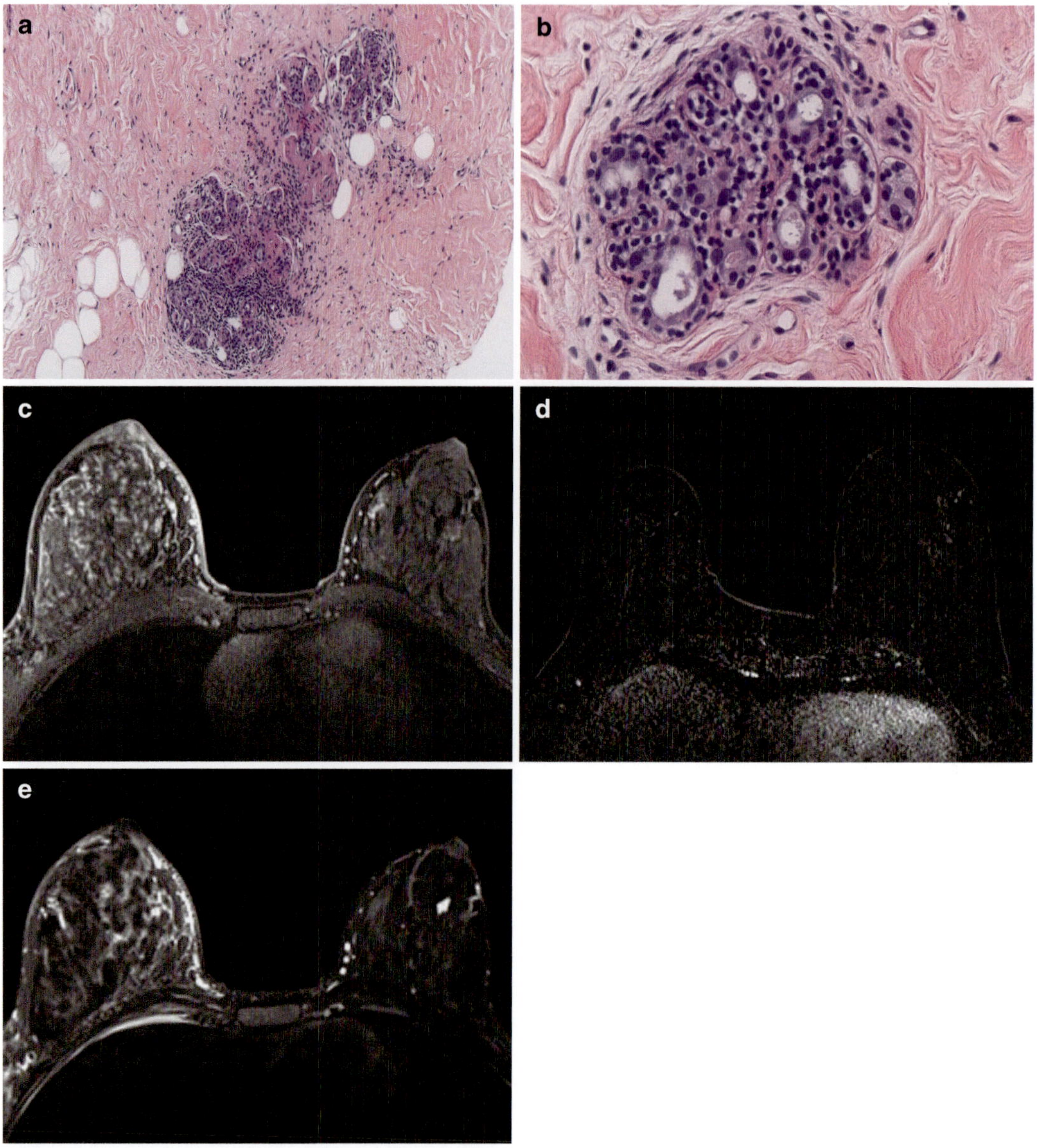

Fig. 9.15 A 53-year-old woman with history of right breast DCIS post whole breast radiation, completed 4 months prior to surveillance breast MRI. (**a**, **b**) MRI-guided core biopsy shows terminal duct lobular units with cells exhibiting random nuclear atypia and intralobular fibrosis [H&E section, 4×, 10×]. (**c**) Axial T1-weighted post-contrast imaging demonstrates patchy non-mass enhancement and diffuse skin thickening of the right breast as well as parenchymal edema. Another 68-year-old woman with a remote history of right breast cancer post right lumpectomy and whole breast radiation presents for surveillance breast MRI. (**d**) Axial T1-weighted post-contrast subtraction imaging demonstrates asymmetrically small right breast in keeping with treatment history as well as asymmetric background parenchymal enhancement, mild on the left and minimal on the right, in keeping with history of right breast radiation. (**e**) There is a 3-mm focus of enhancement in the upper central left breast seen on axial subtraction. MRI-guided biopsy revealed findings of postradiation change

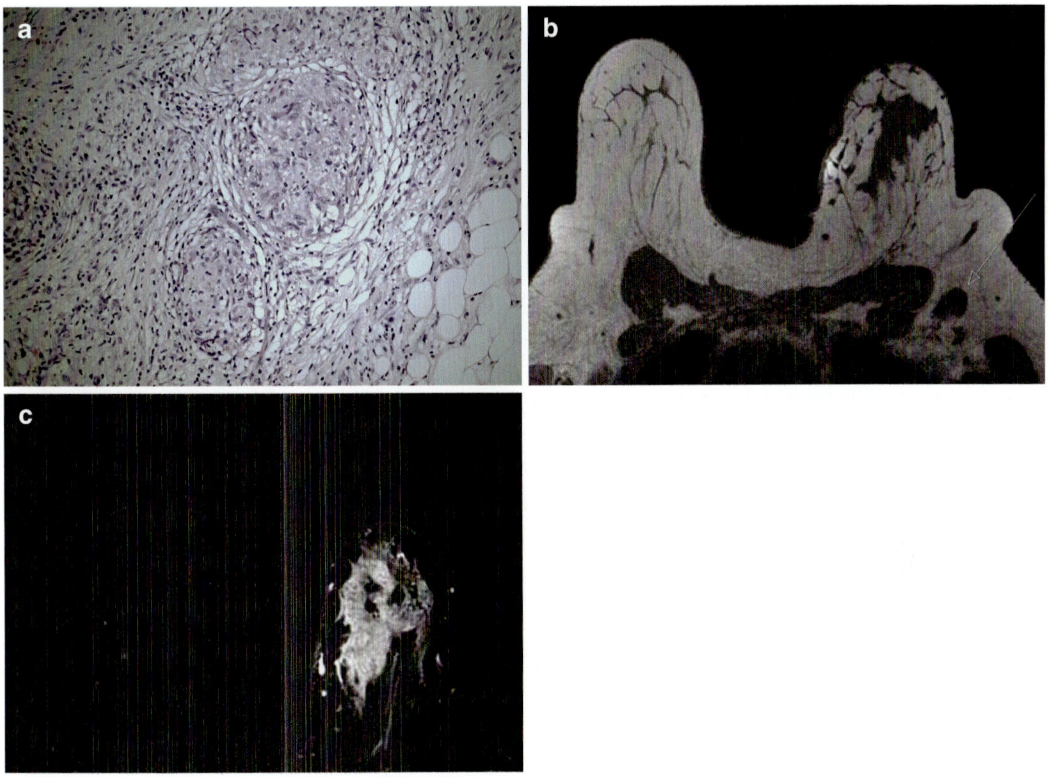

Fig. 9.16 A 34-year-old woman presented with a left breast lump. (**a**) The biopsy showed lobulocentric granulomas and chronic inflammation. Abnormal findings on diagnostic work-up with mammography and ultrasound; MRI obtained for better characterization and assessment of overall disease. (**b**) Axial T1-weighted pre-contrast imaging demonstrates regional, confluent enhancement of the left breast spanning above and below the nipple and over 6 cm in the medial-lateral dimension with diffuse skin thickening, nipple retraction, and abnormal left level 1 axillary nodes (one shown, arrow) with cortical thickening and loss of the fatty hilum. (**c**) Axial T1-weighted post-contrast subtraction image demonstrating regional, confluent enhancement of the breast. Biopsy was recommended which demonstrated granulomatous mastitis

oid fibroblasts, and perilobular and perivascular lymphocytic infiltration (Fig. 9.17a).

MRI Findings

- On MRI, diabetic mastopathy typically shows homogeneous, low enhancement, and glandular distortion (Fig. 9.17b–d) [25, 26].

Intramammary lymph nodes (IMLN) are lymph nodes within the breast tissue (Fig. 9.18a). They may enlarge secondary to inflammatory conditions of the skin or also as a reaction to metastatic involvement.

MRI Findings

- Normal intramammary lymph nodes appear as a small (<10 mm) oval reniform-shaped mass with a suggestion of a central notch and homogeneous enhancement, most commonly in the upper outer quadrants.
- Abnormal metastatic nodes enhance heterogeneously and present with mass with circumscribed margins and loss of normal reniform shape (Fig. 9.18b).

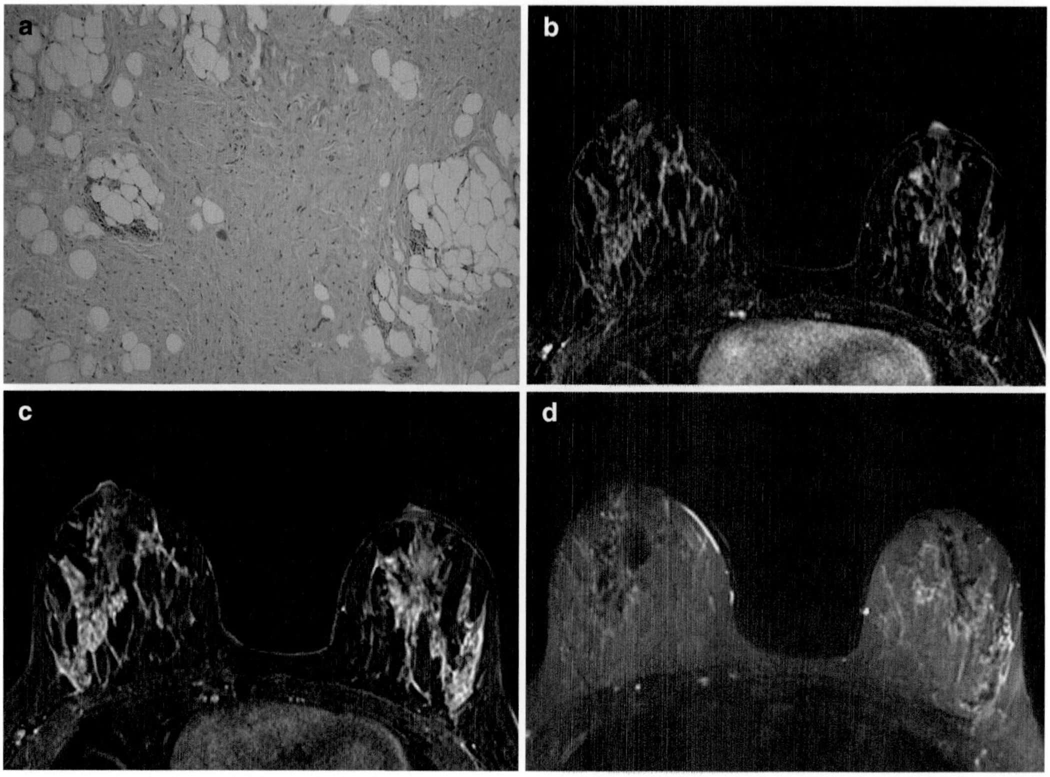

Fig. 9.17 A 28-year-old woman with a history of bilateral breast lumps and pain, long-standing insulin-dependent diabetes. (**a**) MRI-guided biopsy shows dense stromal fibrosis with perivascular lymphocytic infiltrate (H&E, 10×). Axial T1-weighted fat-saturated post-contrast subtraction images. (**b**) Early and (**c**) delayed time points demonstrate bilateral, confluent, progressively enhancing areas of breast parenchyma with associated T2 hypointensity (**d**) in many areas suggestive of fibrosis. The overall imaging appearance and history is most in keeping with diabetic mastopathy

High-Risk Lesions

Atypical ductal hyperplasia (ADH) is a high-risk proliferative lesion with cytological atypia, which exhibits some, but not all, of the cytological and architectural features of ductal carcinoma in situ (DCIS) (Fig. 9.19a). A meta-analysis of 22 studies by Heller and Moy showed ADH to be the most common high-risk lesion detected on MRI and to have the highest upgrade rate to a carcinoma on subsequent excision among all high-risk lesions [21]; however, no morphologic or kinetic features of the MRI were specific to upgrade.

MRI Findings

- ADH may appear as areas of non-mass enhancement in a focal, linear, segmental, or regional distribution (Fig. 9.19b, c) or masses with rapid homogeneous enhancement (Fig. 9.19d, e).
- Features of invasive carcinoma such as irregular shape, spiculated margins, rim enhancement is not usually seen with ADH.

Flat epithelial atypia (FEA), characterized by enlarged TDLU and lined by a variable number of layers of atypical cuboidal to columnar cells with cytologic atypia (Fig. 9.20a), often presents with grouped calcifications on breast imaging.

MRI Findings

- FEA may rarely present with non-mass enhancement on MRI (Fig. 9.20b).
- As with ADH, there are no specific MRI features predictive of its diagnosis or of subsequent upgrade on excision.

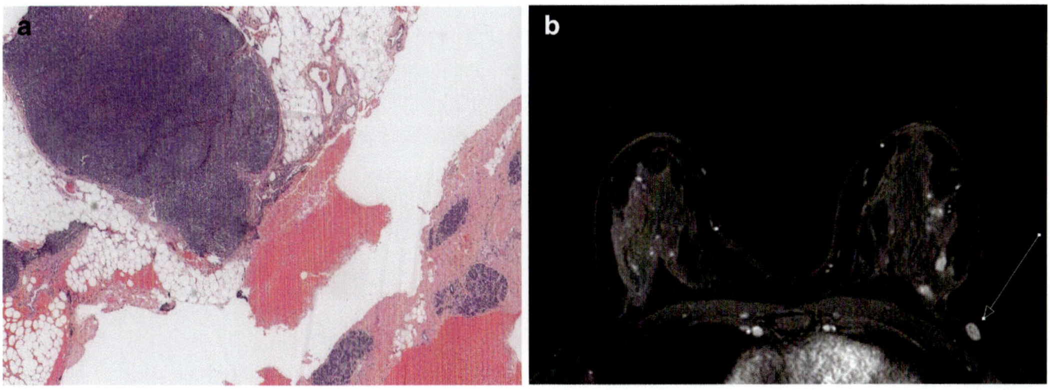

Fig. 9.18 (**a**) An abnormal intramammary lymph node can be seen in this 42-year-old woman's left axillary tail. The patient presented with two palpable lumps in the left breast, subsequently biopsied with pathology revealing malignancy, now presenting for staging breast MRI. MRI-guided core biopsy shows a fragment of reactive lymphoid tissue with adjacent benign breast parenchyma [H&E section, 10×]. (**b**) There are multiple enhancing satellite masses seen in the left breast on Axial T1-weighted post-contrast imaging as well as a 1.2-cm ovoid enhancing mass in the left axillary tail (arrow) in keeping with an abnormal intramammary lymph node. This node has lost its reniform shape and no longer has a normal fatty hilum. Surprisingly, the core biopsy performed showed a benign lymph node

Lobular neoplasia, including atypical lobular hyperplasia (ALH) and lobular carcinoma in situ, is characterized by proliferation of discohesive epithelial cells within the TDLU that may or may not expand the acini (Fig. 9.21a). Lobular neoplasia is usually a clinically occult lesion with no known distinguishing radiologic features.

MRI Findings

- There is very limited data on MRI features specific for lobular neoplasia.
- In our experience, they dominantly present as NME (Fig. 9.21b–d), and rarely as a mass or a focus.
- The majority show enhancement kinetics favoring a benign pattern, with persistent enhancement in the delayed phase.
- When appearing as a mass lesion, they demonstrate medium or rapid enhancement kinetics in the early phase, with mixed persistent, plateau, and washout kinetics in late phase.

Malignant Lesions

Ductal carcinoma* in situ *(DCIS) encompasses a heterogeneous group of low-, intermediate-, and high-grade intraductal proliferation of neoplastic epithelial cells confined to the ductal-lobular system without extension beyond the basement membrane (Fig. 9.22a, b). The majority (approximately 90%) of DCIS cases present with abnormal calcifications on screening mammography, with the remaining 10% presenting as mass-forming lesions on imaging [27]. MRI has emerged as a highly sensitive imaging tool for identifying DCIS and assessing the extent of DCIS for surgical planning [28, 29].

MRI Findings

- Pure DCIS lesions usually present as NME, followed by enhancing mass, no enhancement and as a focus of enhancement [30–32].
- In contrast, mixed invasive and DCIS lesions predominantly manifest as an enhancing mass in three-fourth of cases.
- The most common enhancement pattern is clumped internal enhancement, followed by heterogeneous, homogeneous, reticular, and punctate enhancement. Enhancement distribution is most commonly segmental, followed by focal, diffuse, linear-ductal, and regional.
- High-grade DCIS more frequently manifests as an enhancing mass (Fig. 9.22c–e) when

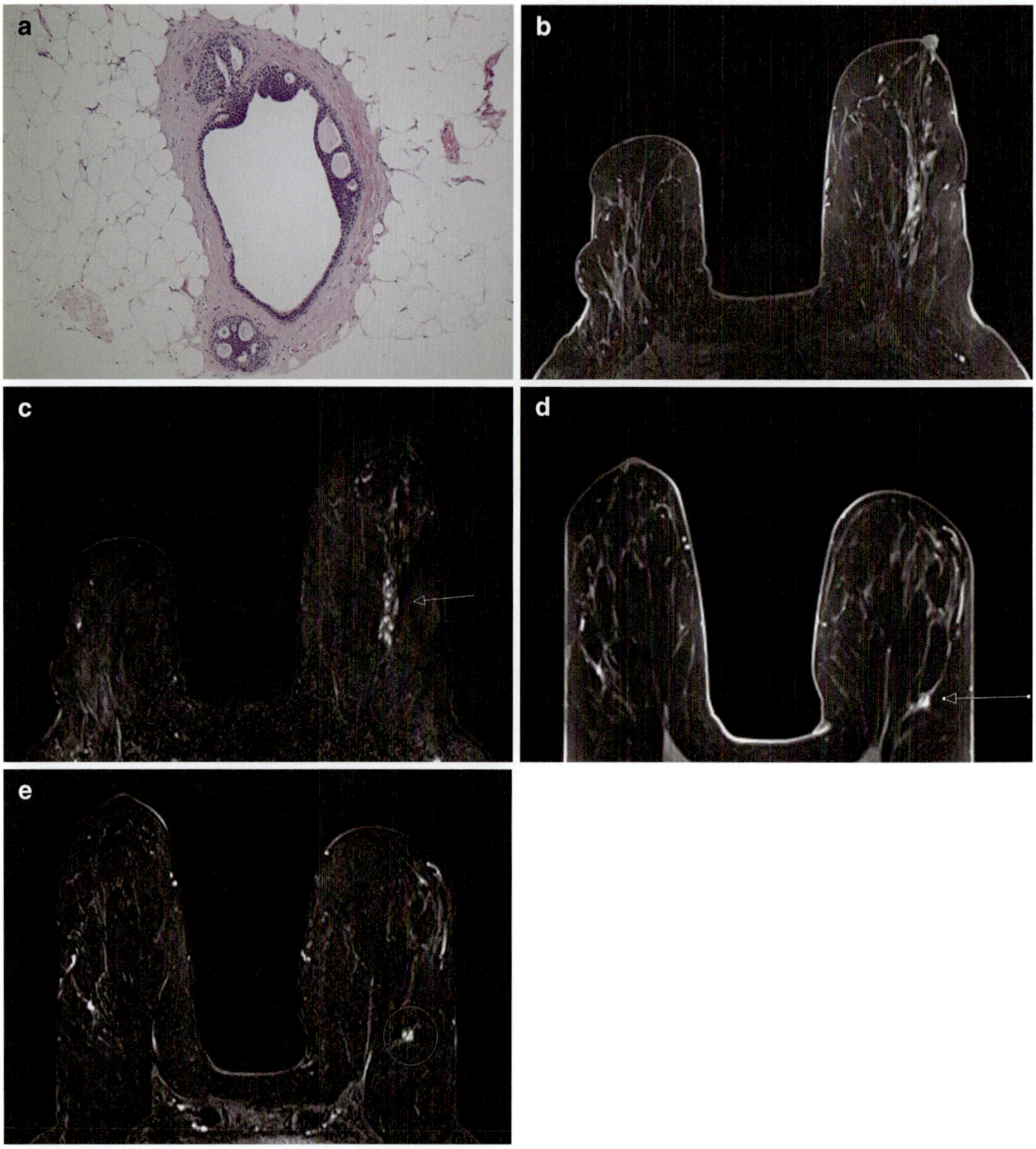

Fig. 9.19 A 76-year-old woman presents for staging breast MRI in the setting of newly diagnosed right breast cancer (not shown). (**a**) Axial T1-weighted post-contrast imaging demonstrates linear non-mass enhancement in the central right breast at middle depth better seen on (**b**) axial T1-weighted post-contrast subtraction imaging (arrow). Subsequent MRI-guided biopsy revealed atypical ductal hyperplasia. Another 62-year-old woman presents for staging breast MRI in the setting of newly diagnosed left breast cancer (not shown). (**c**) Axial T1-weighted post-contrast imaging and (**d**, **e**) axial T1-weighted post-contrast subtraction imaging demonstrates a heterogeneously enhancing mass in the outer left breast at posterior depth (arrow and circle). Subsequent MRI-guided biopsy revealed atypical ductal hyperplasia

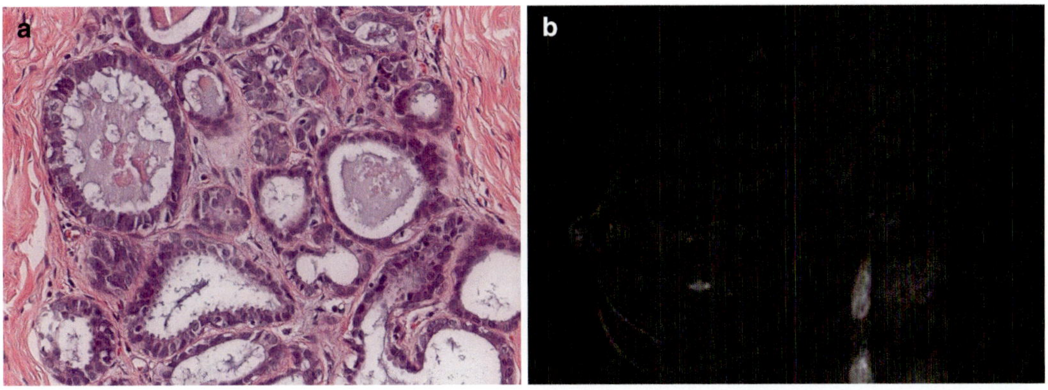

Fig. 9.20 (**a**) MRI-guided core biopsy demonstrates dilated acini lined by many layers of atypical cells [H&E section, 10×]. Focal linear NME (**b**) seen in the lower central left breast on sagittal T1-weighted post-contrast subtraction imaging in a 65-year-old woman who presented for a staging breast MRI after new diagnosis of right breast cancer. Subsequent MRI-guided biopsy demonstrated flat epithelial atypia

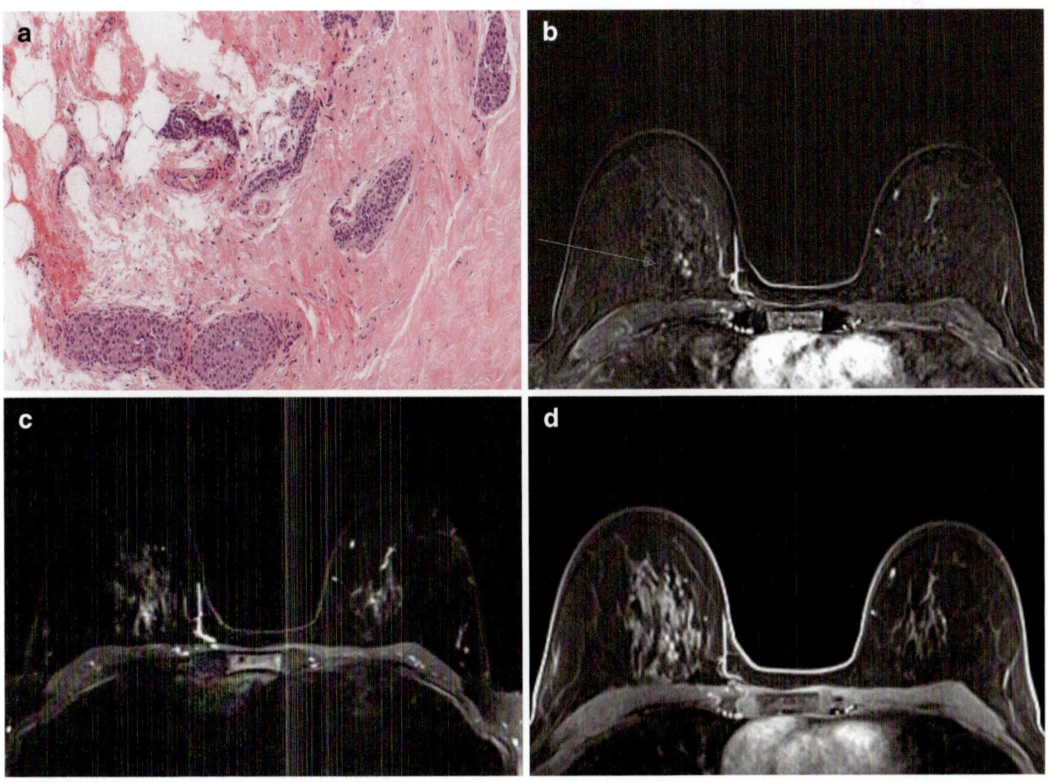

Fig. 9.21 A 67-year-old woman with elevated lifetime risk of breast cancer (27%) presents for screening breast MRI. (**a**) MRI-guided core biopsy shows terminal duct lobules filled and expanded by discohesive, bland and uniform cells, representing lobular carcinoma in situ [H&E section, 10×]. (**b**) Clumped non-mass enhancement is seen in the inner right breast at posterior depth on axial T1-weighted pre-contrast imaging with associated T2-hyperintensity seen on axial T2-weighted imaging. (**c**) The enhancement is less conspicuous on the axial T1-weighted post-contrast sequence. (**d**) Subsequent MRI-guided biopsy demonstrated pleomorphic LCIS

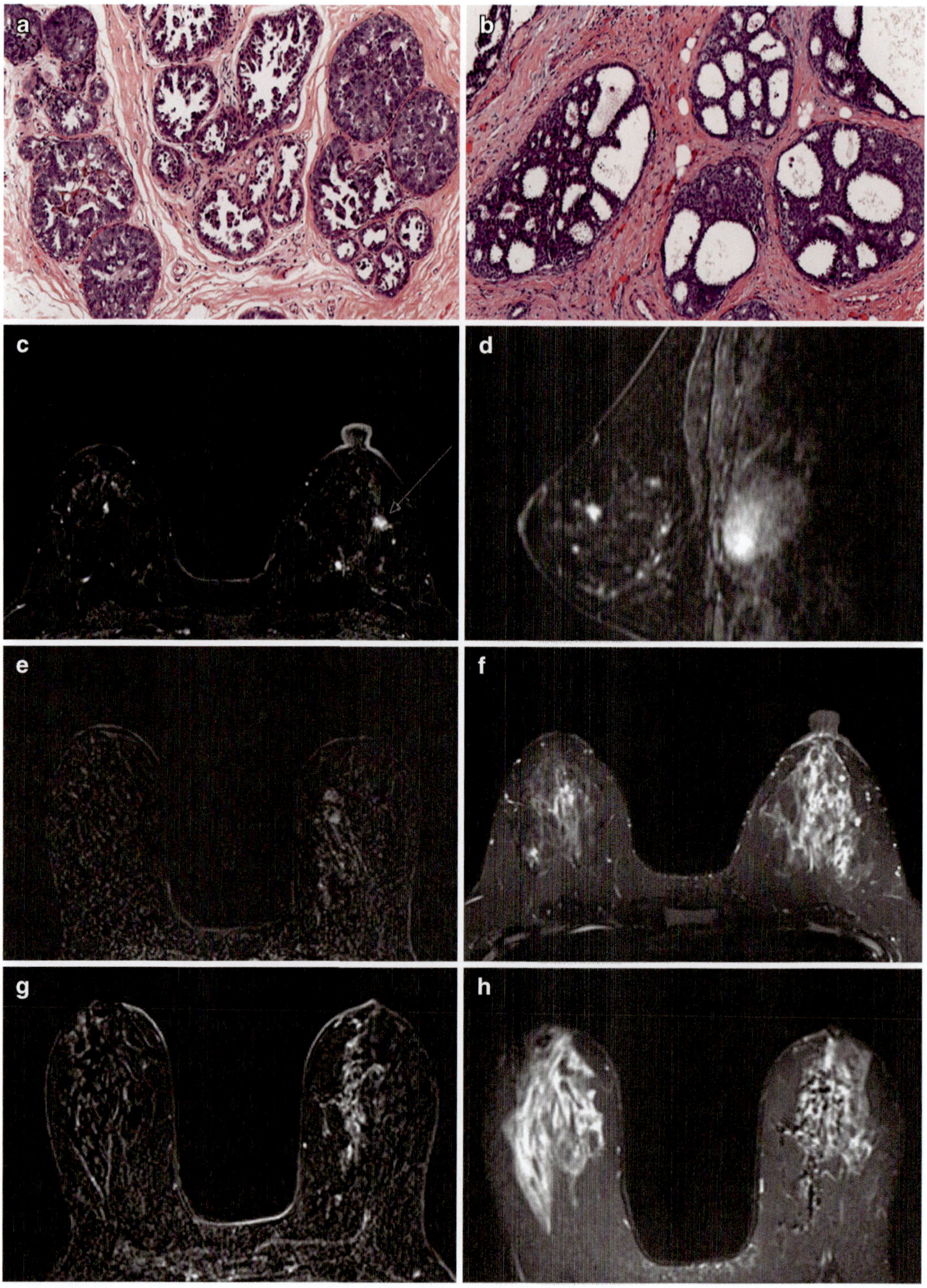
a
b
c
d
e
f
g
h

Fig. 9.22 Breast MRI done to assess the extent of disease in a young 35-year-old woman with biopsy-proven diagnosis of DCIS, revealed another area of non-mass enhancement in linear distribution suspicious for DCIS. (**a**) The core biopsy confirmed the DCIS, high nuclear grade, diagnosis with presence of dilated ducts lined by highly atypical cells in micropapillary pattern. (**b**) The core biopsy shows low-grade nuclei features. Of note, this area was not visible on mammography due to absence of associated calcifications [H&E section, 10×]. (**c**) Axial and (**d**) sagittal T1-weighted post-contrast subtraction imaging demonstrates an irregular enhancing mass in the outer left breast at middle depth with ill-defined margins (arrow). (**e**) There is no associated T2-hyperintensity seen on axial T2-weighted imaging. Subsequent MRI-guided biopsy revealed high-grade DCIS with necrosis. The smaller, circumscribed enhancing mass in the posterior left breast more medially was also sampled, revealing papilloma without atypia. (**f**) Breast MRI of a 69-year-old woman without mammographic or sonographic correlate demonstrates segmental clumped non-mass enhancement in the left inner breast on axial T1-weighted post-contrast subtraction imaging. (**g**) Demonstrates progressive enhancement on delayed subtraction imaging. (**h**) Axial T2-weighted imaging demonstrates correlated T2-hypointensity. Subsequent MRI-guided biopsy demonstrated intermediate-grade DCIS

compared with intermediate- or low-grade DCIS whereas low-grade DCIS frequently shows NME (Fig. 9.22f–h) or no enhancement [30].

Invasive ductal carcinoma, not otherwise specified (IDC-NOS) is the most common type of breast cancer (Fig. 9.23a), comprising approximately 65–75% of all breast carcinomas.

MRI Findings

- IDC-NOS most commonly presents as an enhancing mass with spiculated margins on MRI (Fig. 9.23b, c).
- IDC-NOS can also manifest as non-mass enhancement (Fig. 9.23d, e) or as a focus. When presented with non-mass enhancement, the distribution is variable, and internal enhancement can be heterogeneous, clumped, or stippled.

Invasive lobular carcinoma (ILC) accounts for 10–15% of breast carcinomas and is histologically characterized by fibrous tissue with infiltrating linear strands of small uniform cells with occasional intracytoplasmic vacuoles (Fig. 9.24a). A significant number of ILCs are isointense relative to fibroglandular breast parenchyma and remain occult on mammography (20–40%). They do not always form masses because of inherent inability to elicit a desmoplastic response, and only a minority are associated with microcalcifications. Additionally, the incidence of multifocal, multicentric, and bilateral disease is higher with ILC. Hence, breast MRI serves as a useful adjunct to mammography and ultrasound in detection of occult ILCs. It is more accurate in demonstrating the extent of disease when compared to mammography and ultrasound, and therefore, it is frequently utilized for preoperative staging and surgical planning (lumpectomy vs. mastectomy) in patients diagnosed with ILCs [33, 34].

MRI Findings

- On breast MRI, ILC most frequently presents as a solitary, irregular or angular enhancing mass with spiculated or ill-defined margins (Fig. 9.24b).
- Other presentations include a dominant mass lesion surrounded by multiple small enhancing foci (Fig. 9.24c, d), multiple small enhancing foci connected with enhancing strands and septa, architectural distortions, enhancing septa without a dominant focus, and regional or focal heterogeneous non-mass enhancement.
- In approximately 20% of cases, they present with diffuse infiltration of parenchyma and are visualized as an asymmetric, non-mass enhancement (Fig. 9.24e).

Mucinous carcinoma or colloid carcinoma account for approximately 2% of all invasive breast carcinomas characterized by extracellular mucin pools with floating neoplastic cells (Fig. 9.25a) and are associated with relatively better prognosis.

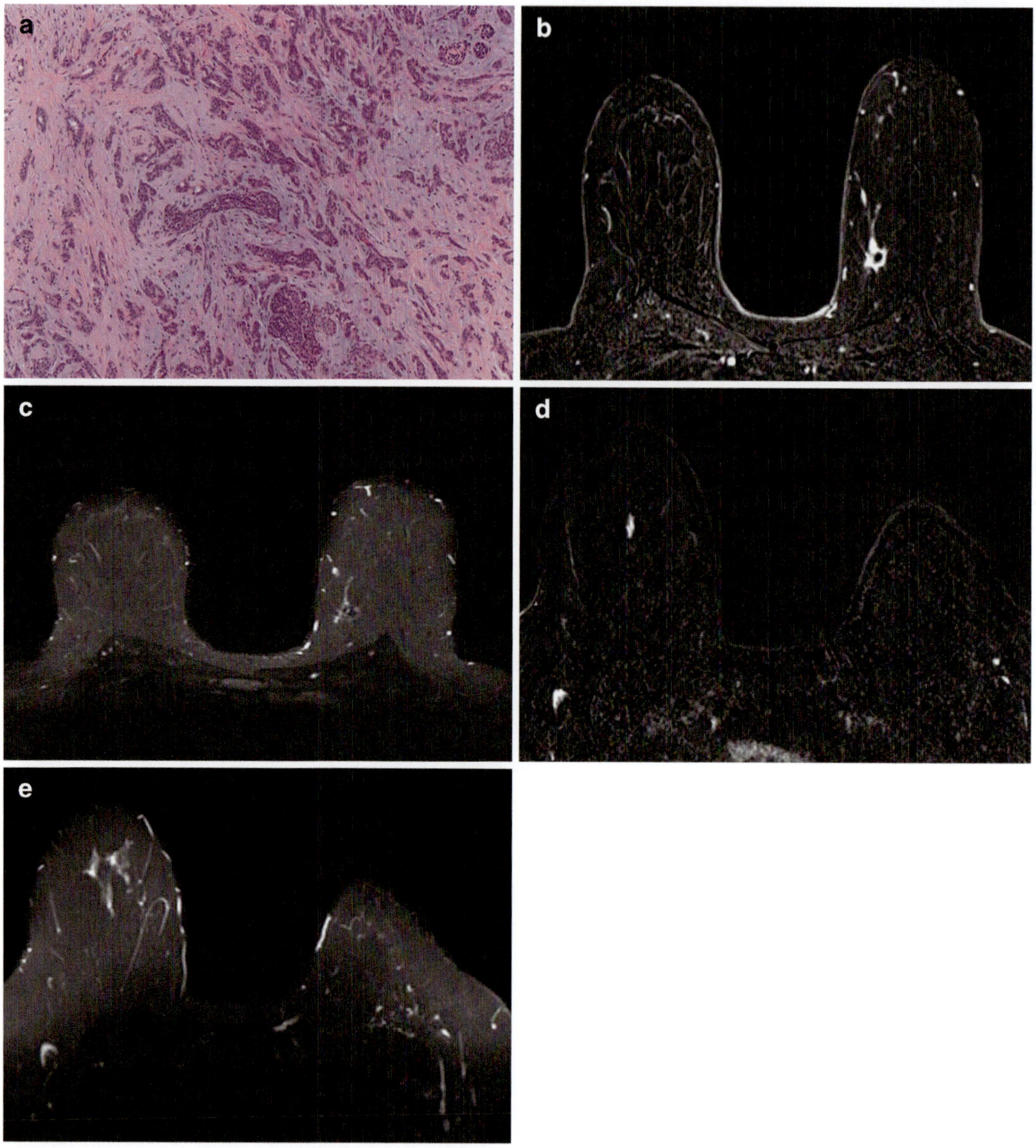

Fig. 9.23 A 52-year-old woman with newly diagnosed left-breast ER/PR+ HER2− invasive ductal carcinoma presents for staging breast MRI. (**a**) H&E section (10×) shows fibrous stroma with irregular nests and tubules of neoplastic cells. (**b**) Axial T1-weighted post-contrast subtraction imaging demonstrates a spiculated mass in the left inner breast at posterior depth with heterogeneous rim-enhancement reflecting patient's biopsy-proven IDC. (**c**) Axial T2-weighted imaging demonstrates largely T2-hypointensity of the mass. Another 69-year-old woman with a history of left breast cancer post-breast conservation therapy presents for surveillance breast MRI. (**d**) The axial T1-weighted post-contrast subtraction imaging demonstrated linear non-mass enhancement which is iso-intense on axial T2-weighted imaging. (**e**) Subsequent MRI-guided biopsy demonstrated IDC

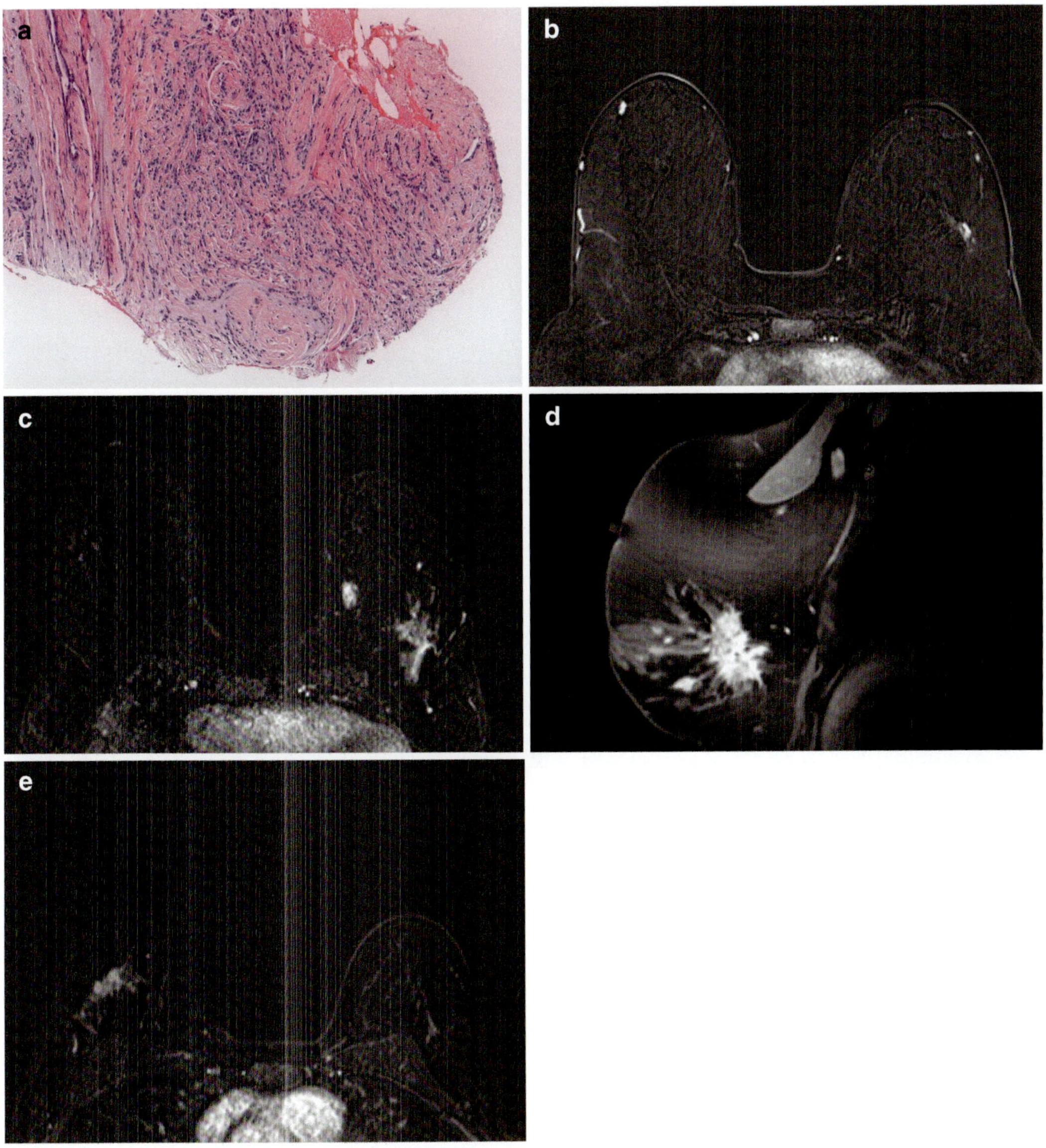

Fig. 9.24 A 67-year-old woman presents with a palpable mass. (**a**) H&E section (10×) shows fibrous tissue infiltrating linear strands of small uniform cells with occasional intracytoplasmic cytoplasmic vacuoles. (**b**) Staging MRI demonstrates a spiculated mass in the outer left breast on axial T1-weighted post-contrast subtraction imaging. Another 65-year-old woman with newly diagnosed left breast invasive lobular carcinoma presents for staging breast MRI. (**c**) Axial T1-weighted post-contrast subtraction imaging and (**d**) sagittal T1 post-contrast imaging demonstrates a large spiculated mass in keeping with the patient's index malignancy as well as several surrounding enhancing masses and foci suspicious for satellite lesions. (**e**) A 48-year-old woman with newly diagnosed right breast invasive lobular carcinoma presents for staging breast MRI. Axial T1-weighted post-contrast subtraction imaging demonstrates clumped non-mass enhancement in the central right breast reflecting the patient's biopsy-proven ILC

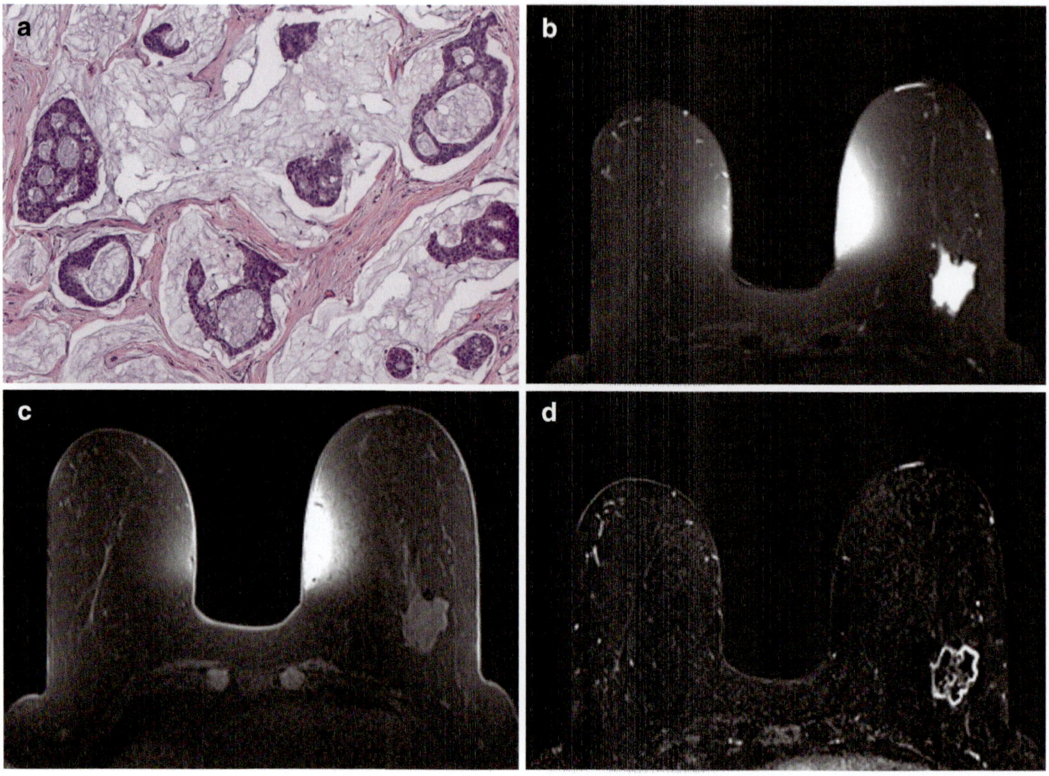

Fig. 9.25 A 67-year-old woman with biopsy-proven left breast mucinous carcinoma presents for staging MRI. (**a**) H&E section (10×) shows clusters of neoplastic cells floating in abundant extracellular mucin. (**b**) Axial T1-weighted pre-contrast imaging demonstrates an irregular mass in the outer left breast at posterior depth reflecting patient's known malignancy with susceptibility artifact anteriorly in keeping with biopsy clip. (**c**) Axial T2-weighted imaging shows marked, homogeneous T2-hyperintensity of the mass, a common MRI characteristic of mucinous breast cancers. (**d**) Axial T1-weighted post-contrast subtraction imaging demonstrates heterogeneous, rim-enhancement of the lesion

MRI Findings

- Mucinous carcinomas can present as circumscribed (mimicking benign breast lesions such as, fibroadenomas and benign cysts) or irregular masses with variable signal intensity on fat saturated T1-weighted images; significantly high signal intensity on fat saturated T2-weighted images; and gradual and progressive enhancement on kinetics.
- The enhancement pattern varies from homogeneous to heterogeneous depending upon the amount of extracellular mucin and cellularity within the tumor.
- Hypercellular or mixed mucinous carcinomas often show lobulated or irregular borders and a peripheral rim of heterogeneous enhancement suspicious for malignancy (Fig. 9.25b–d).
- The presence of enhancing internal septations favor the diagnosis of mucinous carcinoma over fibroadenoma; however, this is a rare finding.

Metaplastic carcinoma constitutes less than 5% of breast carcinomas, and is characterized by nonglandular metaplastic components, including squamous cell, spindle cell, and heterologous mesenchymal growth patterns (Fig. 9.26a).

MRI Findings

- Metaplastic carcinomas illustrate isointense or hypointense signals on T1-weighted images

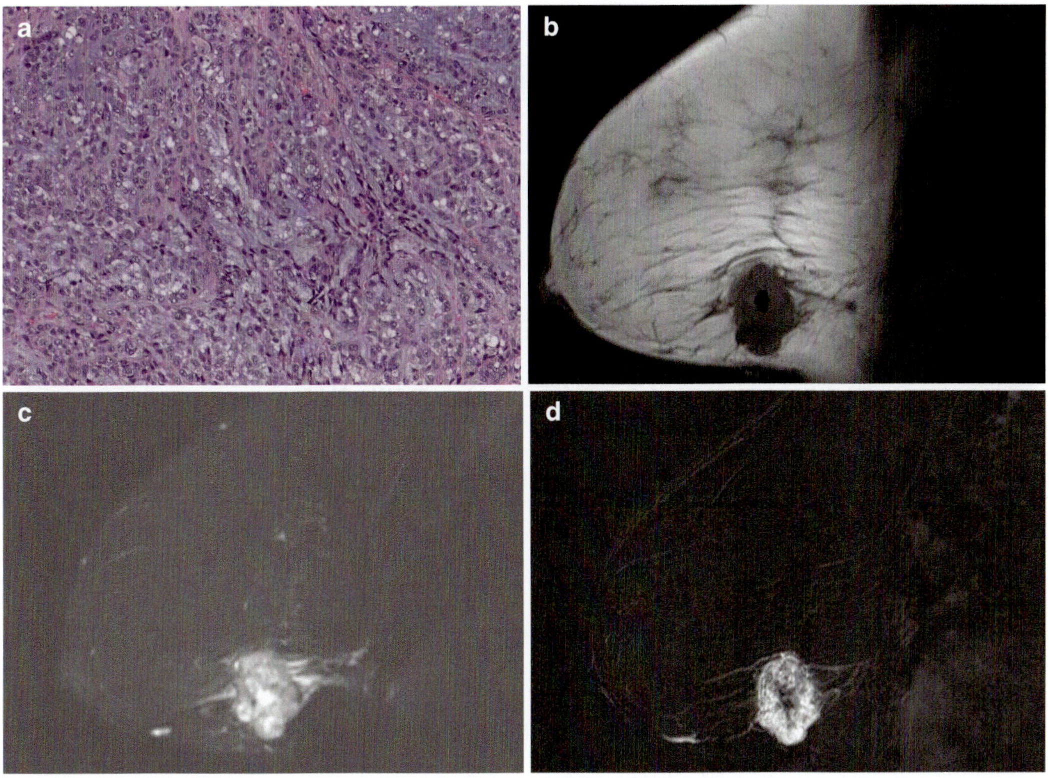

Fig. 9.26 Incidentally detected mass in a 60-year-old woman while being evaluated for pulmonary embolism. (**a**) The biopsy shows a tumor with extensive chondroid differentiation [H&E, 10×]. She presents for staging breast MRI. (**b**) Sagittal T1 non-fat saturated pre-contrast image demonstrates a 3.7 × 2.8 cm irregular mass in the inferior left breast at posterior depth which is isoechoic to the surrounding, minimal fibroglandular tissue. The internal susceptibility artifact (dark spot) reflects a biopsy clip. (**c**) On sagittal T2 imaging the mass demonstrates high T2 signal intensity, some of which represents internal necrosis. (**d**) Sagittal T1-weighted fat-saturated post-contrast subtraction imaging demonstrates heterogeneous enhancement of the mass with an internal area of non-enhancement, in keeping with necrosis

(Fig. 9.26b) when compared with normal glandular tissue, similar to that seen in invasive duct carcinoma, NOS.
- T2 hyper signal, similar to that seen in mucinous carcinomas, is a common finding because of extensive tumor necrosis frequently observed in these tumors (Fig. 9.26c, d).

Evaluation of Response to Therapy After Neoadjuvant Therapy

Neoadjuvant therapy is the standard of treatment these days for triple negative, HER2 overexpressing, locally advanced and inflammatory breast cancers. MRI has emerged as the most precise modality to assess tumor response to neoadjuvant therapy and to plan surgery.

MRI Findings

- Changes in tumor size, volume, and enhancement patterns predict the extent of treatment response and can be categorized into complete (Fig. 9.27a, b), partial (Fig. 9.27c, d), or non-response to therapy (Fig. 9.27e, f). However, residual disease may be overestimated or underestimated at MRI.
- The sensitivity of MRI for depiction of residual disease is 63–88% and the specificity is 54–91% [35].
- Treatment-related fibrosis, necrosis, and residual benign masses may result in overesti-

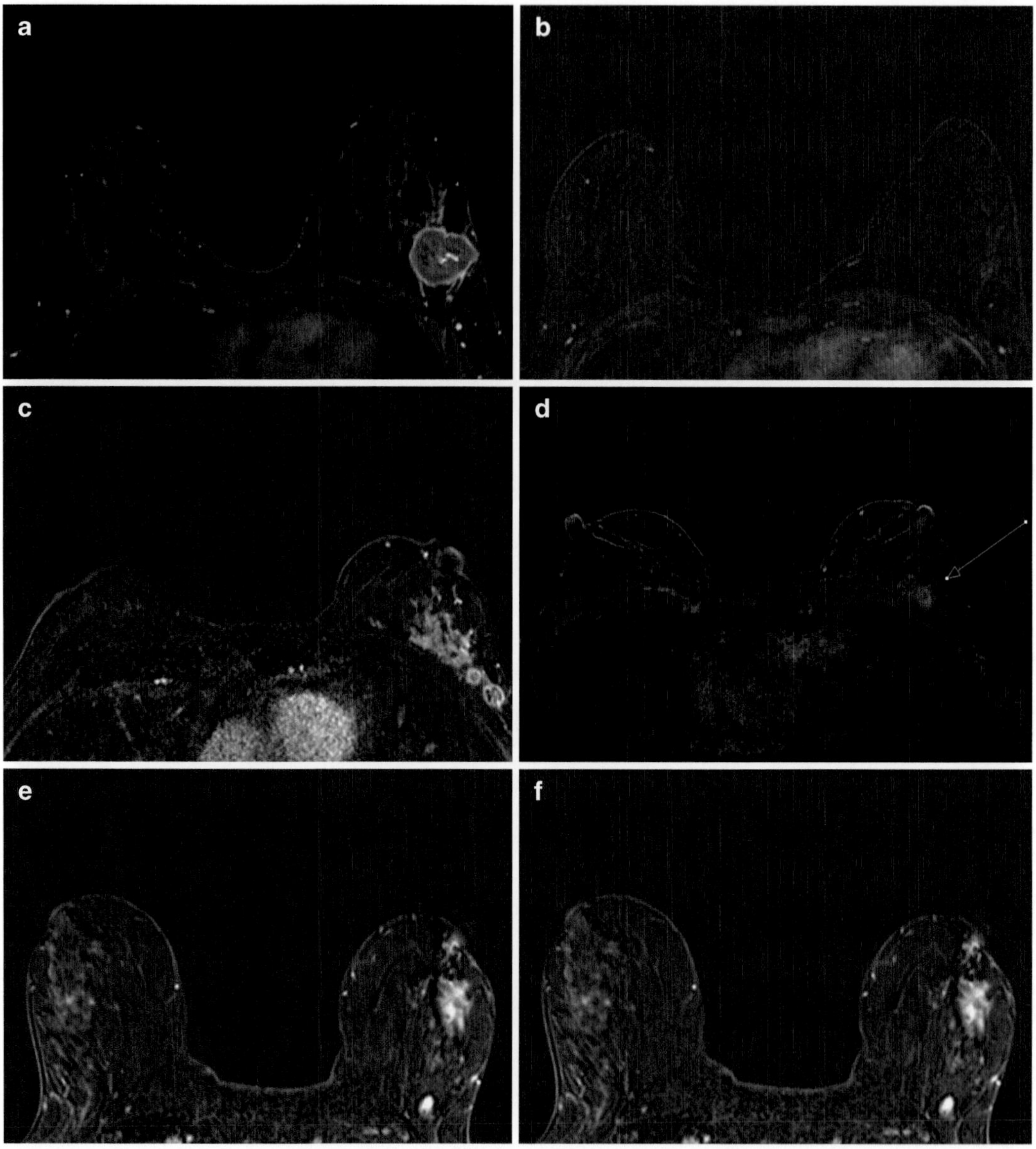

Fig. 9.27 A 47-year-old woman with left breast triple negative cancer seen on axial T1-weighted post-contrast subtraction imaging (**a**) demonstrates complete imaging response to neoadjuvant chemotherapy with total resolution of previously seen enhancing mass on post-chemotherapy axial T1-weighted post-contrast subtraction (**b**). Another 52-year-old woman with left breast invasive ductal carcinoma seen as (**c**) confluent enhancing masses and non-mass enhancement in the upper outer left breast on axial T1-weighted post-contrast subtraction imaging demonstrates marked partial response to neoadjuvant chemotherapy with residual, small, mildly enhancing masses seen (**d**; arrow). A 61-year-old woman with left breast multifocal metaplastic triple-negative breast cancer demonstrates no response to neoadjuvant chemotherapy with essentially unchanged index malignancy and satellite lesion seen in the left breast on axial T1-weighted post-contrast subtraction imaging pre-chemotherapy (**e**) and post-chemotherapy (**f**)

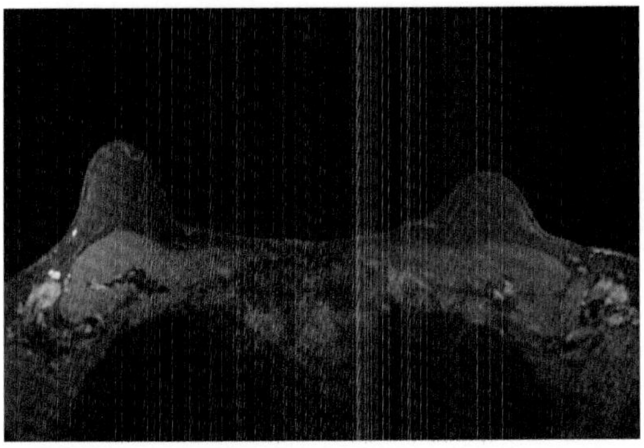

Fig. 9.28 Axial T1 pre-contrast non-fat saturated image demonstrating an enlarged abnormally enhancing oval right level 1 axillary lymph node with loss of reniform shape

mation of residual disease, whereas non-mass lesions, invasive lobular carcinoma, hormone receptor-positive tumors, non-concentric shrinkage patterns, the use of antiangiogenic therapy, and late-enhancing tumor foci may result in underestimation of residual disease.

- The MRI sensitivity to detect persistent lymph node involvement in the post-neoadjuvant setting is 61–72% [36]. Lymph nodes are considered normal when they are symmetric, are homogeneously enhancing, and have a thin cortex and preserved fatty hilum with reniform shape. Any of the following findings is abnormal: cortical thickening, loss of the fatty hilum, round shape, irregular margin, heterogeneous cortex, and surrounding edema (Fig. 9.28a).

Assessment of Breast Implant Integrity.

Breast MRI is an effective imaging modality to evaluate the integrity of breast implants because of its high spatial resolution, lack of ionizing radiation, and ability to enhance or suppress signals from water, silicone, and fat [37]. Screening for implant rupture is recommended by the FDA in asymptomatic patients with silicone implants starting 5 years after implant placement and every 2–3 years subsequently; however, per the American College of Radiology (ACR) Appropriateness Criteria, imaging screening in asymptomatic patients with silicone implants is not recommended. Instead, the ACR Appropriateness Criteria recommends evaluation with non-contrast breast MRI in women with silicone implants and a suspected complication, such as implant rupture. Unlike standard breast MRI, evaluation for implant rupture includes silicone-specific sequences and does not require intravenous contrast material. Implants are recognized as "foreign" by the body and over time develop peripheral, benign fibrous tissue or "capsule". This capsule is soft, flexible, and not clinically apparent. When a silicone implant ruptures but the outer fibrous capsule does not, it is called an "intracapsular rupture". This can be seen as the "linguine sign"—multiple long folds of the implant shell are seen with silicone on either side of the folds (Fig. 9.29a). Free silicone in the breast or axilla is not seen with intracapsular rupture since it is still contained within the fibrous capsule. When the fibrous capsule is also ruptured, it is called an "extracapsular rupture". In this instance, the contour of the implant is often abnormal on physical exam and free silicone can be seen on imaging. Free silicone shows isointensity or low signal intensity on fat suppressed T1-weighted MRI and high signal intensity on water suppressed T2-weighted MRI (Fig. 9.29b, c). Silicone granulomas may show enhancement similar to that of breast cancer leading to core biopsy. The presence of free silicone in the breast parenchyma or the axillary lymph nodes is suggestive of rupture.

Contrast is used for evaluating other implant-related complications, for example, recurrence of breast cancer, breast implant-associated anaplastic large cell lymphoma (BIA-ALCL), peri-implant seroma/hematoma or superimposed infection. Pathologists should consider these diagnoses when evaluating a breast core biopsy from a patient with breast implant. The most common imaging finding for BIA-ALCL is recurring seroma adjacent to the implant (Fig. 9.29d), followed by a soft-tissue enhancing mass mimicking breast cancer. Seromas appear as fluid signal intensity on breast MRI images with all sequences, whereas hematomas

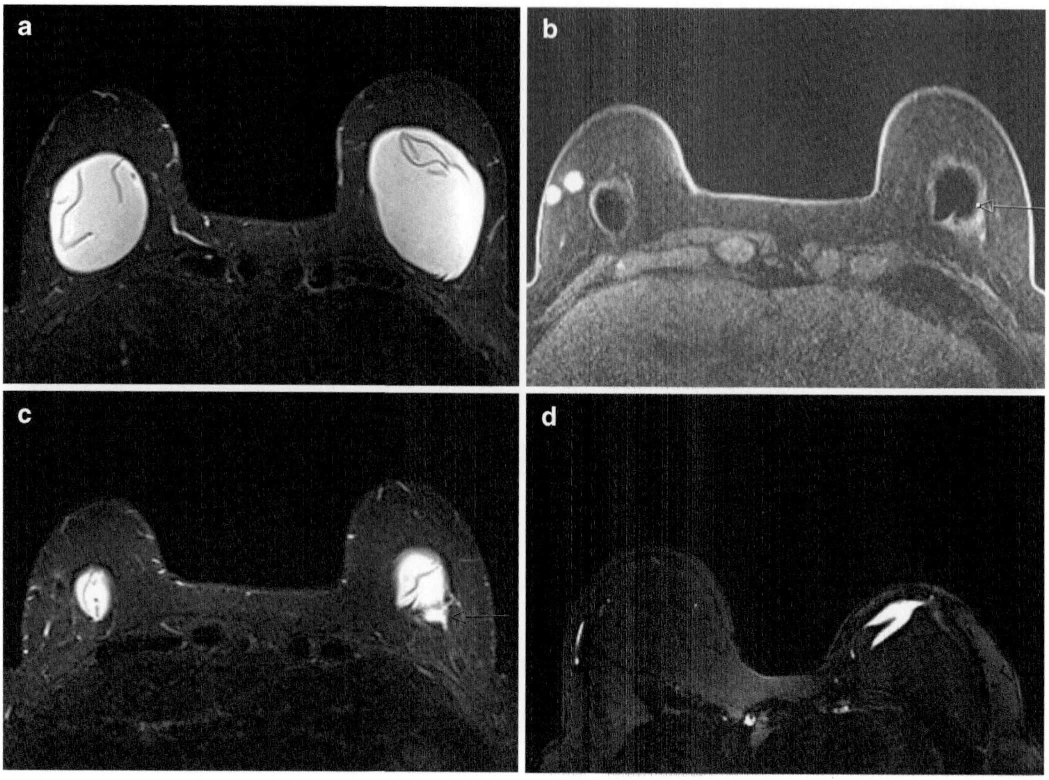

Fig. 9.29 (**a–c**) A 62-year-old woman with bilateral subpectoral saline implants originally placed more than 30 years ago. Patient states the implants feel "hardened". (**a**) Bilateral "linguine" sign is seen on axial T2-weighted non-contrast imaging, with silicone seen on both sides of multiple capsular folds. (**b**) Axial T1-weighted fat-suppressed imaging demonstrates hypointense collection (arrow), with intensity that of the intracapsular silicone, directly adjacent to the outer capsule of the implant (difficult to see on this series) in keeping with free silicone. Two high-intensity foci are seen in the right breast reflecting benign susceptibility artifacts from postsurgical changes/clips. (**c**) On axial T2-weighted imaging the pericapsular collection demonstrates high T2-signal (arrow), again following that of the intracapsular silicone, again in keeping with free silicone. The line of the peripheral capsule just anterior to the collection is better seen on this sequence. (**d**) A 51-year-old woman with a peri-implant fluid collection adjacent to the left breast implant, seen on axial T2-weighted sequence as a T2-bright collection anterior to the implant. This finding was present on the patient's imaging for at least 3 years and is a nonspecific finding, though concerning for a breast implant-associated anaplastic large cell lymphoma in the setting of a textured implant. (**e, f**) A 59-year-old woman with left breast invasive ductal carcinoma post-lumpectomy with positive margins and subsequent resection. MRI performed 1-month post resection reveals (**e**) axial T2-weighted images demonstrated a T2 hyperintense collection in her left breast with (**f**) peripheral enhancement in keeping with a hematoma. This patient's hematoma is not associated with a breast implant but the imaging findings of a peri-implant hematoma would be the same. (**g–i**) A 63-year-old woman presents with left breast swelling, pain, and hardness. (**g**) Axial T1 fat-saturated post-contrast subtraction imaging demonstrates peripheral capsular enhancement on the left. (**h**) Axial T2-weighted imaging demonstrates T2 intense fluid posterior to the left breast implant as well as prominent left axillary lymph nodes. This clinical presentation and constellation of MRI findings is in keeping with a peri-implant infection; however, implant-associated anaplastic large cell lymphoma cannot be entirely excluded. This patient underwent US-guided peri-implant fluid aspiration with benign findings and responded to antibiotics, confirming infection as the etiology. Of note, there are few radial folds in this patient's silicone implants, which are a benign, normal finding and not indicative of implant rupture. (**i**) A different slice of the axial T2-weighted imaging demonstrates that there is a single radial fold in each implant which is perpendicular to the capsule with fluid intensity seen in the infold in the left breast (if this were capsular rupture, silicone-intensity fluid would be seen on both sides of the fold)

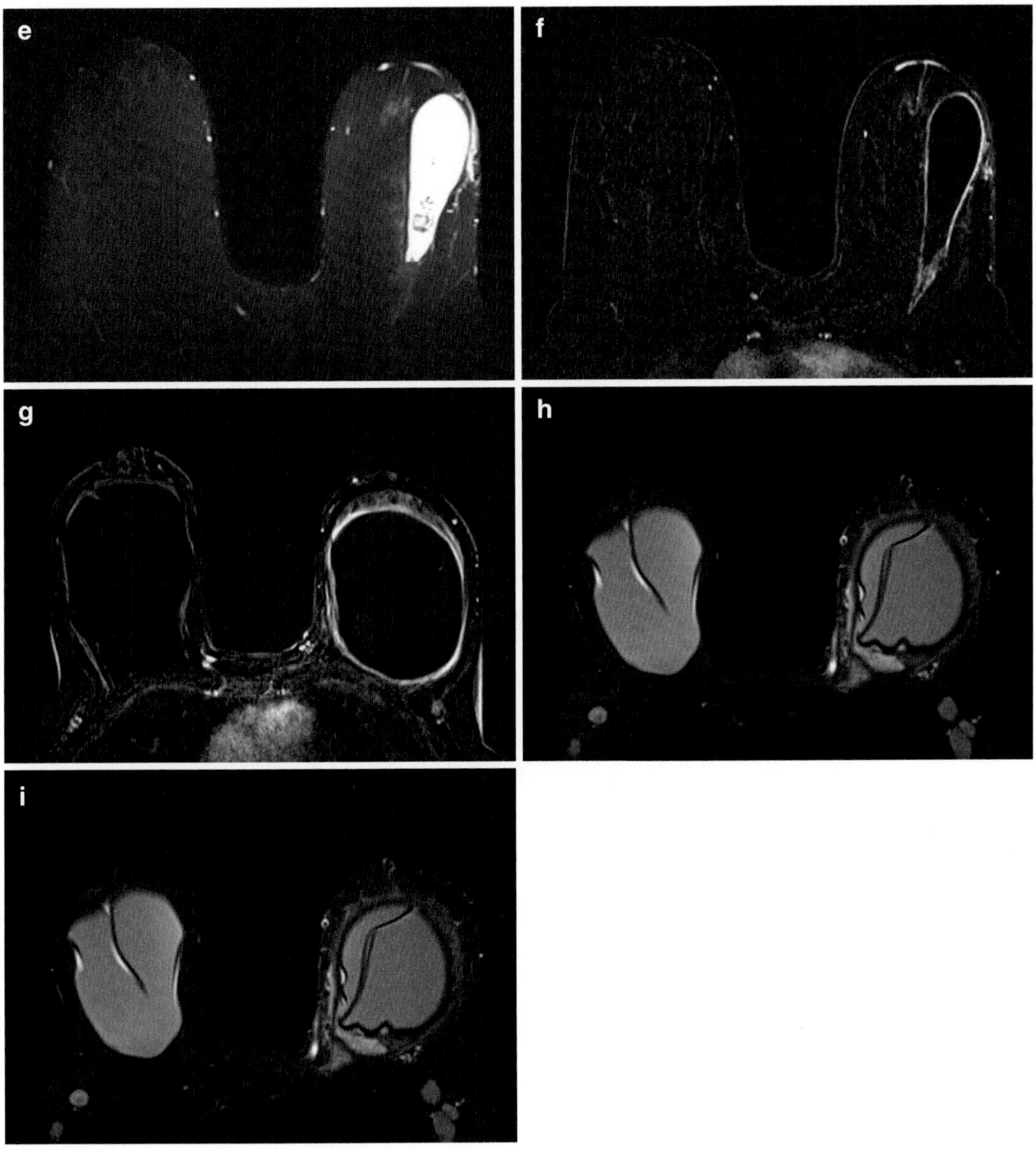

Fig. 9.29 (continued)

show heterogeneous signal intensity at MRI, depending on the age of the hematoma. Early hematomas show no enhancement unlike late hematomas which present with rim enhancement secondary to an inflammatory reaction (Fig. 9.29e, f). Infection can be associated with complex fluid collections, skin thickening, edema, and capsular enhancement on imaging (Fig. 9.29g, i).

To conclude, MRI is a highly sensitive breast imaging modality for detection of malignant breast lesions; however, the considerable overlap in the appearance of benign and malignant lesions results in higher false-positive rate than other modalities with subsequent benign breast core biopsies. Therefore, pathologists should be aware of these features to reliably interpret the breast core biopsy from MRI lesions.

References

1. Saslow D, et al. American Cancer Society guidelines for breast screening with MRI as an adjunct to mammography. CA Cancer J Clin. 2007;57(2):75–89. https://doi.org/10.3322/canjclin.57.2.75.
2. Liberman L, et al. Breast lesions detected on MR imaging: features and positive predictive value. AJR Am J Roentgenol. 2002;179(1):171–8. https://doi.org/10.2214/ajr.179.1.1790171.
3. Torous VF, et al. Histopathologic correlates of nonmass enhancement detected by breast magnetic resonance imaging. Arch Pathol Lab Med. 2021;145(10):1264–9. https://doi.org/10.5858/arpa.2020-0266-OA.
4. Sippo DA, et al. Impact of background parenchymal enhancement on diagnostic performance in screening breast MRI. Acad Radiol. 2020;27(5):663–71. https://doi.org/10.1016/j.acra.2019.06.020.
5. diFlorio-Alexander RM, et al. Breast MRI-detected cystic apocrine metaplasia: imaging features with microvessel analysis and histologic correlation. AJR Am J Roentgenol. 2015;204(1):211–8. https://doi.org/10.2214/AJR.14.12869.
6. Ginter PS, Winant AJ, Hoda SA. Cystic apocrine hyperplasia is the most common finding in MRI detected breast lesions. J Clin Pathol. 2014;67(2):182–6. https://doi.org/10.1136/jclinpath-2013-201804.
7. Siziopikou KP, Jokich P, Cobleigh M. Pathologic findings in MRI-guided needle core biopsies of the breast in patients with newly diagnosed breast cancer. Int J Breast Cancer. 2011;2011:613285. https://doi.org/10.4061/2011/613285.
8. Kushwaha AC, O'Toole M, Sneige N, Stelling CB, Dryden MJ. Mammographic-pathologic correlation of apocrine metaplasia diagnosed using vacuum-assisted stereotactic core-needle biopsy: our 4-year experience. Am J Roentgenol. 2003;180(3):795–8. https://doi.org/10.2214/ajr.180.3.1800795.
9. Warner JK, Kumar D, Berg WA. Apocrine metaplasia: mammographic and sonographic appearances. Am J Roentgenol. 1998;170(5):1375–9. https://doi.org/10.2214/ajr.170.5.9574619.
10. Kelten Talu C, Boyaci C, Leblebici C, Hacihasanoglu E, Bozkurt ER. Pseudoangiomatous stromal hyperplasia in core needle biopsies of breast specimens. Int J Surg Pathol. 2017;25(1):26–30.
11. Ibrahim RE, Sciotto CG, Weidner N. Pseudoangiomatous hyperplasia of mammary stroma. Some observations regarding its clinicopathologic spectrum. Cancer. 1989;63(6):1154–60.
12. Pediconi F, et al. Radial scars of the breast: contrast-enhanced magnetic resonance mammography appearance. Breast J. 2005;11(1):23–8. https://doi.org/10.1111/j.1075-122X.2005.21530.x.
13. Baum F, Fischer U, Füzesi L, Obenauer S, Vosshenrich R, Grabbe E. The radial scar in contrast media-enhanced MR mammography. Rofo. 2000;172(10):817–23. https://doi.org/10.1055/s-2000-7894.
14. Linda A, Zuiani C, Londero V, Cedolini C, Girometti R, Bazzocchi M. Magnetic resonance imaging of radial sclerosing lesions (radial scars) of the breast. Eur J Radiol. 2012;81(11):3201–7. https://doi.org/10.1016/j.ejrad.2012.01.038.
15. Alsharif S, Aldis A, Subahi A, Khoury ME, Mesurolle B. Breast MRI does not help differentiating radial scar with and without associated atypia or malignancy. Can Assoc Radiol J. 2021;72(4):759–66. https://doi.org/10.1177/0846537120930360.
16. Eiada R, Chong J, Kulkarni S, Goldberg F, Muradali D. Papillary lesions of the breast: MRI, ultrasound, and mammographic appearances. AJR Am J Roentgenol. 2012;198(2):264–71. https://doi.org/10.2214/AJR.11.7922.
17. Daniel BL, Gardner RW, Birdwell RL, Nowels KW, Johnson D. Magnetic resonance imaging of intraductal papilloma of the breast. Magn Reson Imaging. 2003;21(8):887–92. https://doi.org/10.1016/s0730-725x(03)00192-9.
18. Bhattarai N, Kanemaki Y, Kurihara Y, Nakajima Y, Fukuda M, Maeda I. Intraductal papilloma: features on MR ductography using a microscopic coil. AJR Am J Roentgenol. 2006;186(1):44–7. https://doi.org/10.2214/AJR.04.1600.
19. Kurz KD, Roy S, Saleh A, Diallo-Danebrock R, Skaane P. MRI features of intraductal papilloma of the breast: sheep in wolf's clothing? Acta Radiol. 2011;52(3):264–72. https://doi.org/10.1258/ar.2011.100434.
20. Wang W, et al. MRI characteristics of intraductal papilloma. Acta Radiol. 2015;56(3):276–83. https://doi.org/10.1177/0284185114526590.
21. Heller SL, Moy L. Imaging features and management of high-risk lesions on contrast-enhanced dynamic breast MRI. AJR Am J Roentgenol. 2012;198(2):249–55. https://doi.org/10.2214/AJR.11.7610.
22. Pluguez-Turull CW, et al. Idiopathic granulomatous mastitis: manifestations at multimodality imaging and pitfalls. Radiographics. 2018;38(2):330–56. https://doi.org/10.1148/rg.2018170095.
23. Al-Khawari HAT, Al-Manfouhi HA, Madda JP, Kovacs A, Sheikh M, Roberts O. Radiologic features of granulomatous mastitis: radiology of GM. Breast J. 2011;17(6):645–50. https://doi.org/10.1111/j.1524-4741.2011.01154.x.
24. Dursun M, et al. Multimodality imaging features of idiopathic granulomatous mastitis: outcome of 12 years of experience. Radiol Med. 2012;117(4):529–38. https://doi.org/10.1007/s11547-011-0733-2.
25. Tuncbilek N, Karakas HM, Okten O. Diabetic fibrous mastopathy: dynamic contrast-enhanced magnetic resonance imaging findings. Breast J. 2004;10(4):359–62. https://doi.org/10.1111/j.1075-122X.2004.21382.x.
26. Wong KT, Tse GMK, Yang WT. Ultrasound and MR imaging of diabetic mastopathy. Clin Radiol.

2002;57(8):730–5. https://doi.org/10.1053/crad.2002.0936.
27. Yamada T, et al. Radiologic-pathologic correlation of ductal carcinoma in situ. Radiographics. 2010;30(5):1183–98. https://doi.org/10.1148/rg.305095073.
28. Lehman CD. Magnetic resonance imaging in the evaluation of ductal carcinoma in situ. J Natl Cancer Inst Monogr. 2010;2010(41):150–1. https://doi.org/10.1093/jncimonographs/lgq030.
29. Menell JH, Morris EA, Dershaw DD, Abramson AF, Brogi E, Liberman L. Determination of the presence and extent of pure ductal carcinoma in situ by mammography and magnetic resonance imaging. Breast J. 2005;11(6):382–90. https://doi.org/10.1111/j.1075-122X.2005.00121.x.
30. Jansen SA, Newstead GM, Abe H, Shimauchi A, Schmidt RA, Karczmar GS. Pure ductal carcinoma in situ: kinetic and morphologic MR characteristics compared with mammographic appearance and nuclear grade. Radiology. 2007;245(3):684–91. https://doi.org/10.1148/radiol.2453062061.
31. Liu H, Peng W. MRI morphological classification of ductal carcinoma in situ (DCIS) correlating with different biological behavior. Eur J Radiol. 2012;81(2):214–7. https://doi.org/10.1016/j.ejrad.2010.12.084.
32. Greenwood HI, Heller SL, Kim S, Sigmund EE, Shaylor SD, Moy L. Ductal carcinoma in situ of the breasts: review of MR imaging features. Radiographics. 2013;33(6):1569–88. https://doi.org/10.1148/rg.336125055.
33. Parvaiz MA, et al. Breast MRI in invasive lobular carcinoma: a useful investigation in surgical planning? Breast J. 2016;22(2):143–50. https://doi.org/10.1111/tbj.12566.
34. Mann RM. The effectiveness of MR imaging in the assessment of invasive lobular carcinoma of the breast. Magn Reson Imaging Clin N Am. 2010;18(2):259–76. https://doi.org/10.1016/j.mric.2010.02.005.
35. Lobbes MBI, et al. The role of magnetic resonance imaging in assessing residual disease and pathologic complete response in breast cancer patients receiving neoadjuvant chemotherapy: a systematic review. Insights Imaging. 2013;4(2):163–75. https://doi.org/10.1007/s13244-013-0219-y.
36. Reig B, et al. Breast MRI for evaluation of response to neoadjuvant therapy. Radiographics. 2021;41(3):665–79. https://doi.org/10.1148/rg.2021200134.
37. Noreña-Rengifo BD, et al. MRI for evaluation of complications of breast augmentation. Radiographics. 2022;42(4):929–46. https://doi.org/10.1148/rg.210096.

Lesions of Nipple and Axilla

10

Liva Andrejeva, Jayalakshmi Venkateswaran, Ramapriya Vidhun, Brigid Killelea, Kirstyn Brownson, and Kamaljeet Singh

Dermatitis

Dermatitis: Dermatitis of the nipple and areolar skin can have variable etiology: allergic contact dermatitis, irritant contact dermatitis, a minor manifestation of atopic dermatitis, or nummular dermatitis. The etiology includes breastfeeding, friction with jogging, and contact with irritants. Dermatitis can mimic Paget disease. Therefore lack of response to topical treatment warrants tissue sampling and exclusion of Paget disease.

L. Andrejeva
Department of Radiology and Biomedical Imaging, Yale School of Medicine, New Haven, CT, USA
e-mail: liva.andrejeva@yale.edu

J. Venkateswaran · R. Vidhun
Department of Pathology and Laboratory Medicine, Danbury Hospital, Danbury, CT, USA
e-mail: jayalakshmi.venkateswaran@nuvancehealth.org; Ramapriya.vidhun@wchn.org

B. Killelea
Department of Surgery, Brigham and Women's Hospital, Boston, MA, USA
e-mail: brigidkillelea@gmail.com

K. Brownson
Department of Surgery, University of Utah, Salt Lake City, UT, USA
e-mail: Kirstyn.Brownson@hci.utah.edu

K. Singh (✉)
Department of Pathology and Laboratory Medicine, Brown University and Women and Infants Hospital of RI, Providence, RI, USA
e-mail: kamaljeet_singh@brown.edu

- **Clinical Presentation**: Patients are often of reproductive age and lactating, but dermatitis is also reported in adolescents and older females and males. It can be unilateral or involve bilateral nipples. The typical clinical findings are erythema and scaling. Acute eczema presents with erythema, papules, and plaques with vesicles, oozing, crusting, and erosions [1]. Chronic eczema has a dry, scaly appearance with hyperpigmentation and lichenification.
- **Imaging Findings**: If unilateral, dermatitis of the nipple is the diagnosis of exclusion, particularly in a middle-aged or older patient without a prior significant history of dermatitis or eczema. Clinical signs and symptoms overlap in dermatitis, nipple eczema, and Paget disease of the nipple. The patient may experience pruritus, erythema, scaling, crusting, fissures, vesicles, erosions, and lichenification. The patient with such findings should undergo mammography and sonography.
  - **Mammogram**: May be normal, or the affected nipple may appear more prominent when compared to the other side.
  - **US**: May be normal, or the affected nipple may appear thickened and hypervascular compared to the unaffected side.
  - **MRI**: Nonspecific asymmetric enhancement of the affected nipple/areola, when compared to the unaffected side.
  - **BIRADS**: 2 or 4, depending on mammographic and sonographic appearance.

M. Harigopal et al. (eds.), *Radiology Pathology Correlations of Breast Lesions*,
https://doi.org/10.1007/978-3-031-65711-5_10

  - **Differential Diagnosis**: Paget disease.
- **Pathology Findings**:
  - **Gross**: The macroscopic appearance can mimic Paget disease.
  - **Microscopic Findings**: The epidermis often shows a spongiotic reaction pattern characterized by the widening of intercellular space and elongated intercellular bridges. Exocytosis is present. Parakeratosis and serum accumulation are present. The presence of eosinophils indicates allergic/contact dermatitis. Irregular acanthosis is present in subacute dermatitis. Psoriasiform hyperplasia with hyperkeratosis and hypergranulosis is present in chronic dermatitis. The upper dermis shows edema, perivascular mononuclear infiltrate, and fibrosis.
  - **Differential Diagnosis**: Allergic contact dermatitis, psoriasis, Paget disease.
- **Management**: Conservative management, including topical steroids.

Case 1

Clinical Findings: A 56-year-old postmenopausal female presents with an enlarged, erythematous, pruritic left nipple (Figs. 10.1 and 10.2).

BI-RADS: 4, suspicious finding; a punch biopsy by a breast surgeon was recommended and performed.

Pathology Findings: Biopsy yielded benign skin with dermal foreign body giant cell reaction and chronic inflammation (Fig. 10.3).

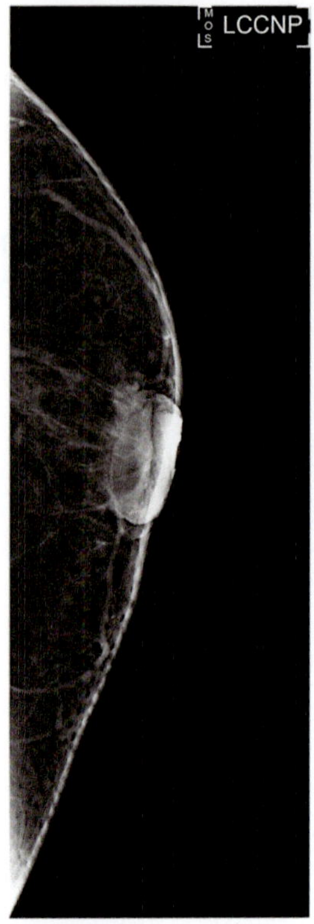

Fig. 10.1 **MMG findings**: The left nipple is enlarged compared to the right nipple, and the technologist had difficulty obtaining a nipple-in-profile view. No other suspicious findings are demonstrated in the left breast

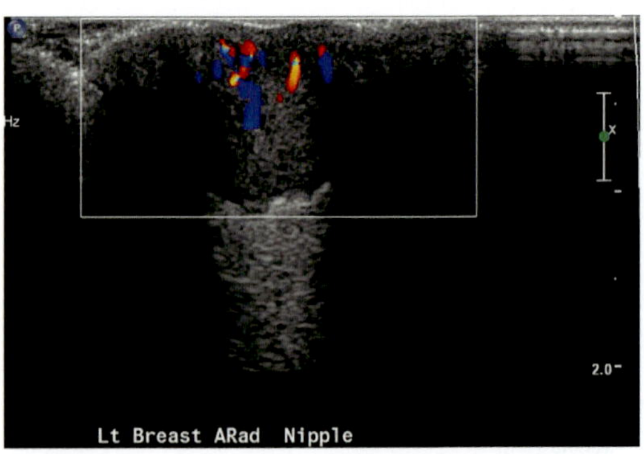

Fig. 10.2 **USG findings**: Markedly thickened, hypervascular nipple

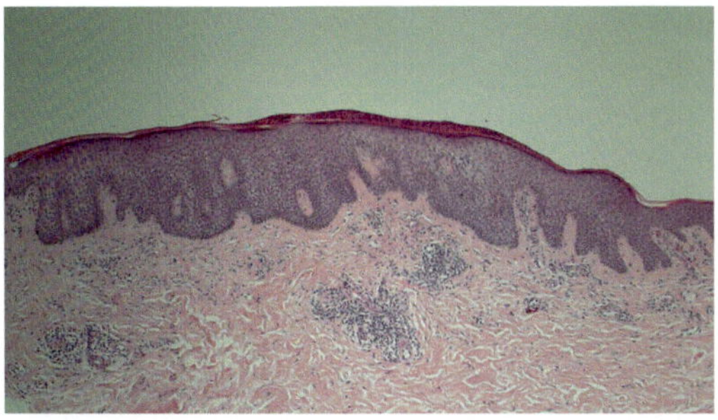

Fig. 10.3 Dermatitis of nipple skin (H&E, 10×). The epidermis is hyperplastic and shows parakeratosis. Dermis contains perivascular mononuclear inflammatory cell infiltrate

Mammary Duct Ectasia

Mammary Duct Ectasia (MDE): Mammary duct ectasia, also known as mastitis obliterans, "varicocele of breast" and periductal mastitis, is characterized by dilatation of the larger subareolar ducts and the dilatation is accompanied by variable degree of periductal chronic inflammation and periductal fibrosis. Patients are often peri- or postmenopausal and smokers. The radiological workup and tissue sampling may be needed to confirm the diagnosis and exclude a malignancy.

- **Clinical Presentation**: The patient may be asymptomatic, or experience pain, nipple discharge (clear, cloudy, or bloody), nipple retraction and a mass. The mass is typically described as a subareolar worm-like doughy, painless and irregular palpable lesion. The etiology of MDE is not known. MDE has been associated with cigarette smoking, squamous metaplasia of ducts, and hyperprolactinemia.
- **Imaging Findings**: Patients are often asymptomatic; the MDE can present with various imaging findings. Nipple retraction, retroareolar duct dilation, or calcfications are often present [2–4].
  - **Mammogram**: MDE may manifest as (usually) bilateral retroareolar duct dilatation that appear as tubular structures. Intraductal secretory (rod-like) calcifications may be present.
  - **US**: Dilated retroareolar ducts that often measure more than 2 mm in diameter, may demonstrate wall thickening and may contain mobile internal echoes and debris.
  - **MRI**: High T1 signal on non-fat saturated T1 pre-contrast images indicates proteinaceous/hemorrhagic/fat containing fluid, which is usually hyperintense on T2WI. Wall enhancement may be present after contrast administration, in cases of concomitant inflammation.
  - **BIRADS**: 2–4; benign when asymptomatic and bilateral; If unilateral findings, a solitary dilated duct, associated suspicious calcifications or worrisome symptoms (single duct spontaneous clear or bloody discharge) require further evaluation.
  - **Differential Diagnosis**: Benign: normal variant, plasma cell mastitis, SMOLD, CGM, mastitis, early abscess, papilloma. Malignant: DCIS, albeit an unusual presentation.
- **Pathology Findings**:
  - **Gross**: No distinct macroscopic findings.
  - **Microscopic Findings**: Large subareolar ducts show dilatation and periductal lymphoplasmacytic infiltrate. The ducts frequently contain inspissated intraductal secretions often associated with foamy histiocytes and periductal fibrosis. The ducts can show luminal obliteration with fibrosis leading to a "garland-pattern" on the histology. The central part of the ducts shows fibrosis and there is a linear array of smaller lumen in the peripheral part of the duct. In late stages the duct can undergo complete obliteration of the lumen with fibrosis. The duct lining epithelium can also show squamous metaplasia.
  - **Differential Diagnosis**: Cysts, ectatic ducts, squamous metaplasia of large ducts. A clinicopathologic correlation can help to render a definite diagnosis of duct ectasia. Cysts are derived from terminal duct lobules. Ectatic ducts are common in breast tissue and form part of the fibrocystic

changes. Ectatic ducts often lack the histologic hallmarks of the chronicity—plasma cells and periductal fibrosis.

- **Management**: The preferred treatment is circumareolar incision and removal of the affected duct and fistula tract (if present).

Case 1

Clinical Findings: A 56-year-old female with a palpable right breast mass (Figs. 10.4, 10.5, and 10.6)

US-guided bx showed mammary duct ectasia (Figs. 10.7, 10.8, and 10.9).

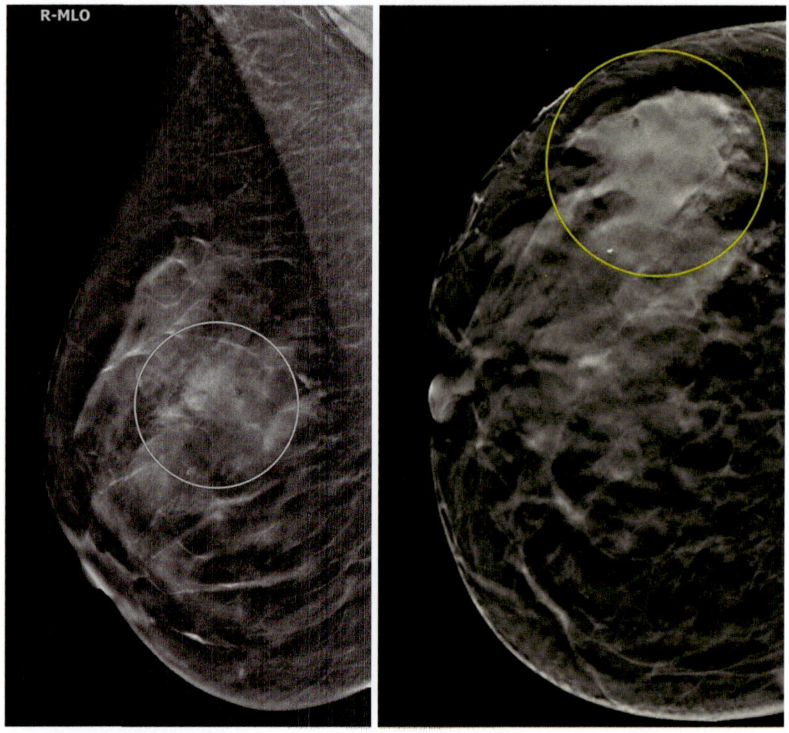

Figs. 10.4 and 10.5 MMG findings: Mammography demonstrates a focal asymmetry with an indistinct margin in the palpable area

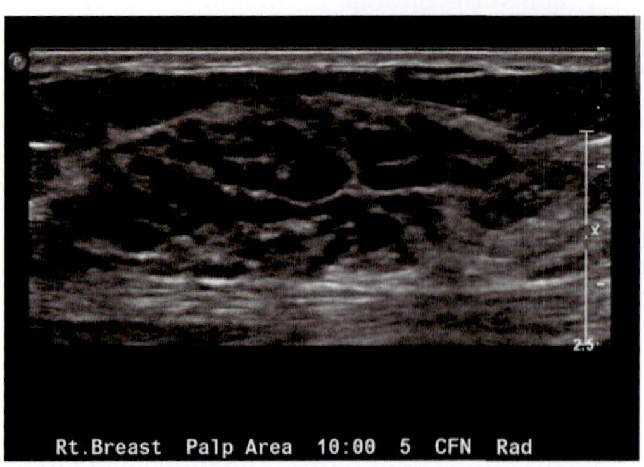

Fig. 10.6 USG findings: US demonstrates multiple serpiginous, dilated ducts

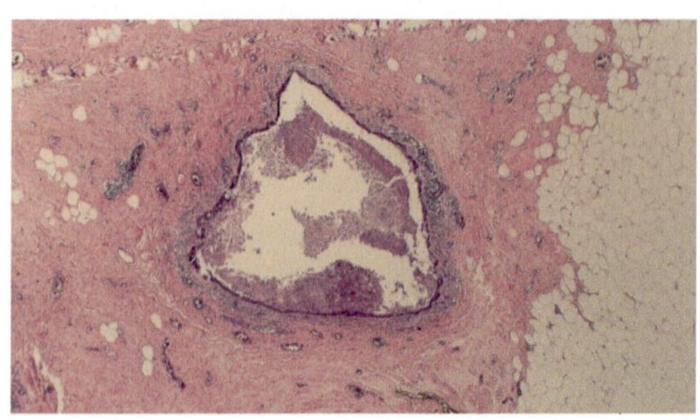

Fig. 10.7 Duct ectasia (H&E, 4×). Dilated duct with inspissated secretions and periductal chronic inflammation

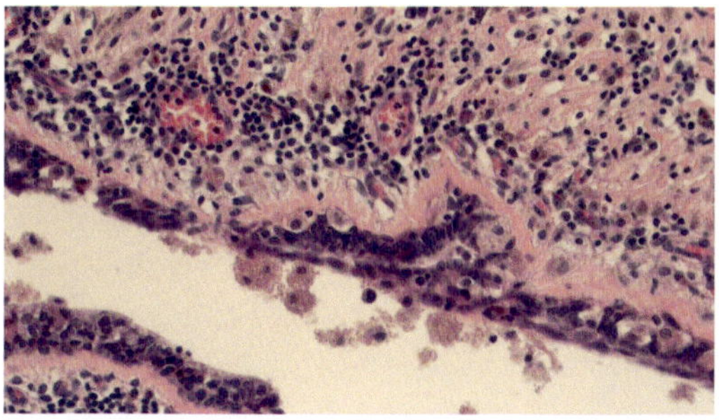

Fig. 10.8 Duct ectasia (H&E, 20×). Periductal fibrosis and chronic inflammation

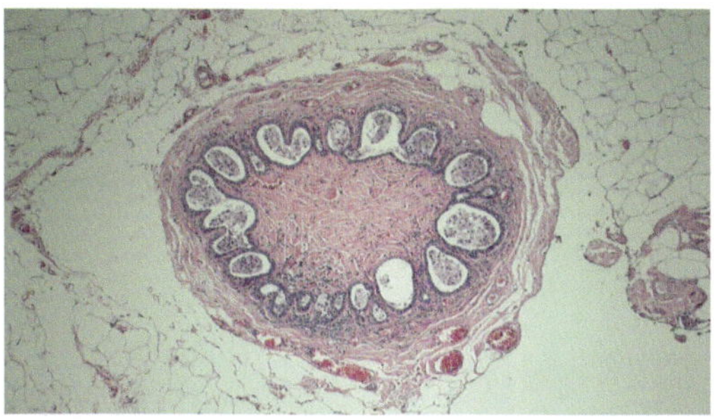

Fig. 10.9 Duct ectasia (H&E, 10×). Obliterated duct with central fibrosis and residual epithelial-lined spaces ("garland" pattern)

Squamous Metaplasia of Lactiferous Ducts

Squamous Metaplasia of Lactiferous Ducts (SMOLD): The squamous epithelium lining the lactiferous duct orifices abruptly transitions to glandular luminal and myoepithelial cells. SMOLD results from squamous metaplasia of the deeper lactiferous ductal epithelium. Squamous metaplasia and keratinization of lactiferous ducts results in the formation of keratin plugs that lead to duct obstruction, occasionally resulting in inflammation and infection. SMOLD can lead to retroareolar abscess, nipple discharge, periareolar fistulae and nipple retraction (Zuska disease) [5, 6].

- **Clinical Presentation**: SMOLD usually occurs in fourth to fifth decade in female smokers. SMOLD can lead to retroareolar abscess, nipple discharge, periareolar fistulae, and nipple retraction (Zuska disease).
- **Imaging Findings**:
  - **Mammogram**: Variable appearance. May appear normal in early stages or in dense breast tissue. Trabecular thickening and skin thickening (particularly in the periareolar region) may be present. When an abscess has formed, an oval, round, or irregular retroareolar mass may be seen. Associated axillary adenopathy may be present.
  - **US**: Oval, round or irregular retroareolar collection, usually with marked internal echoes, and with increased peripheral vascularity. The fluid is usually very viscous and may be difficult to aspirate. Axillary adenopathy may be present.
  - **MRI**: Enhancement of the retroareolar duct walls, sinus tracts, enhancement of abscess walls, as well as the edges of the sinus tracts and periareolar/nipple skin may be present.
  - **BIRADS**: 2, 3, or 4 depending on imaging appearance and clinical history. It is important to correlate with history of smoking and symptomatology. May be indistinguishable from LABC or IBC and tissue sampling may be necessary.
  - **Differential Diagnosis**: Benign: puerperal mastitis (in the correct clinical setting of lactation), non-puerperal mastitis (spontaneous or iatrogenic), hematoma/seroma, galactocele (in the setting of lactation), granulomatous mastitis. Malignant: retroareolar breast cancer, inflammatory breast cancer, locally advanced breast cancer.
- **Pathology Findings**:
  - **Gross**: There is no distinct macroscopic appearance. Grossly the skin may be erythematous and contain vague mass-forming subareolar lesion. In late-stage fistula may be present.
  - **Microscopic Findings**: The lactiferous ducts show squamous metaplasia. Keratin debris fill and dilates the larger ducts. Duct disruption with associated inflammatory

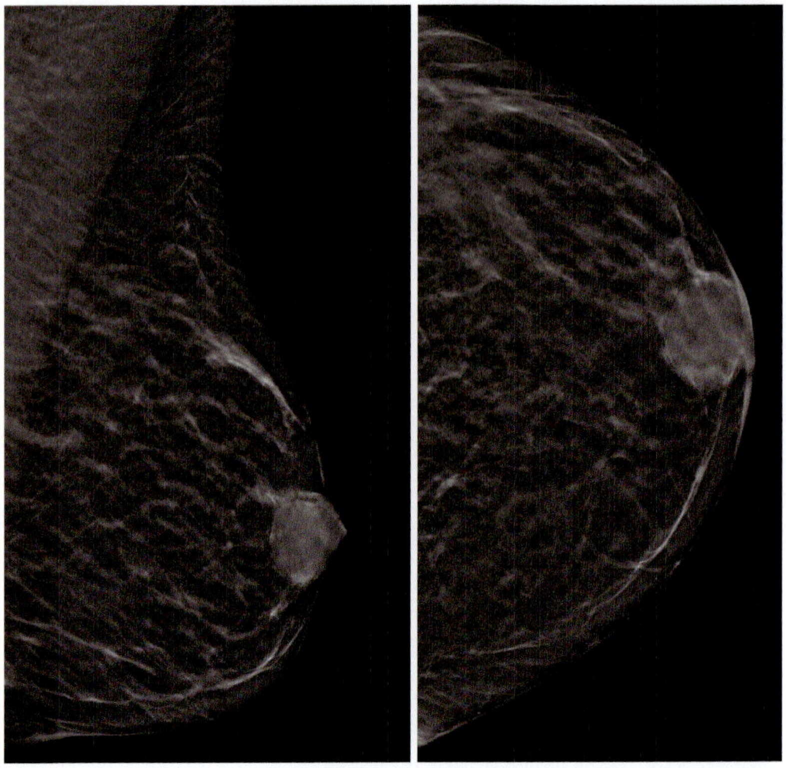

Figs. 10.10 and 10.11 **MG findings**: Circumscribed retroareolar breast mass

reaction including acute and chronic inflammatory infiltrate, foreign body giant cells, and keratin granulomas can be present. Granulation tissue-lined fistula tract formation is present in later stages.

- **Differential Diagnosis**: Mastitis, granulomatous mastitis, and galactocele.
  - Mastitis: The histological findings mimic mastitis. Presence of keratin granulomas can mimic granulomatous mastitis. Subareolar location and squamous metaplasia indicate SMOLD.

- **Management**: Per ASBrS Choosing Wisely® recommendations, percutaneous aspiration of an abscess should first be attempted prior to taking the patient for surgery for incision and drainage. In the setting of devitalized tissue, abscess recalcitrant to repeat aspirations, and surgical site infections, incision and drainage is warranted. Antibiotics with *Staphylococcus aureus* coverage should be prescribed and tailored according to culture results. Smokers should be counselled to quit smoking to improve outcomes [7, 8].

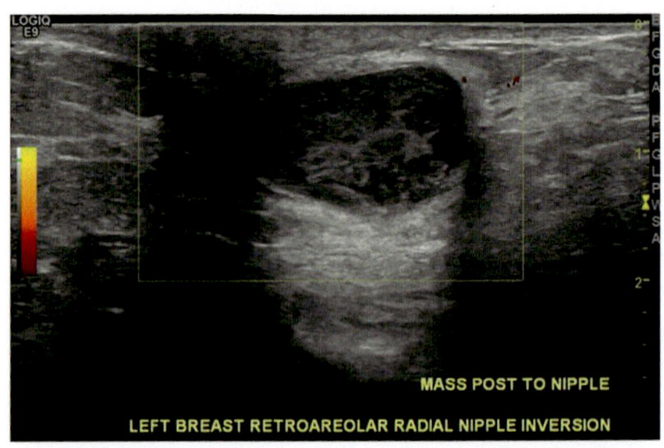

Fig. 10.12 **US findings**: Circumscribed retroareolar complex fluid collection without internal or increased peripheral vascularity, with posterior acoustic enhancement

Case 1

Clinical History: A 44-year-old female, smoker, presents with an increasing, slightly painful left retroareolar breast mass and nipple inversion (Figs. 10.10, 10.11, and 10.12).

BI-RADS: 4a, low likelihood of malignancy; thought to be retroareolar abscess, with aspiration recommended. However, at attempted aspi-

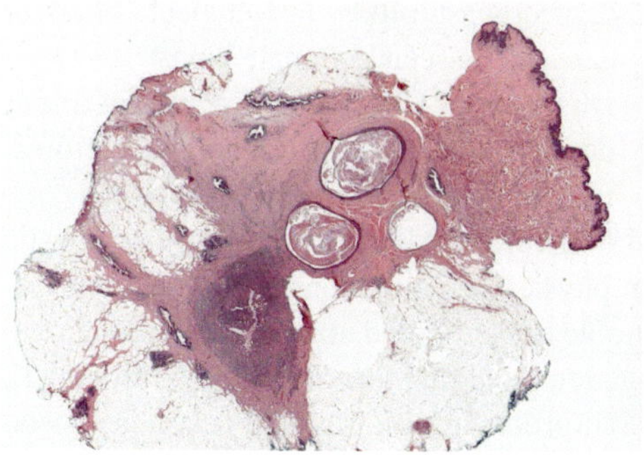

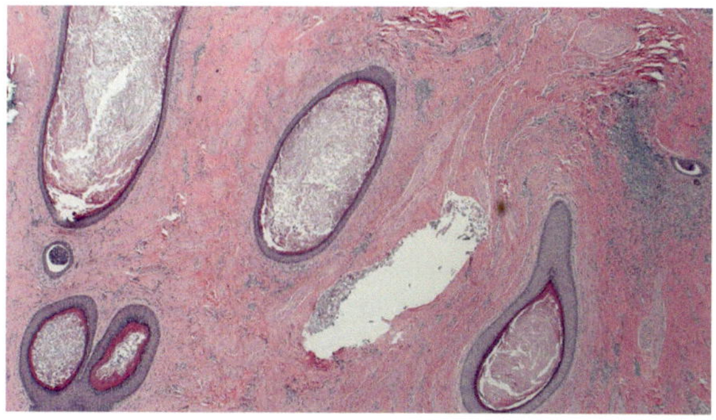

Figs. 10.13 and 10.14 Squamous metaplasia of lactiferous ducts, SMOLD (H&E 2× and 4×). The subareolar large ducts show keratinized stratified squamous epithelium and keratinous debris. One of the cyst is disrupted and accompanied by inflammatory infiltrate

ration, almost no fluid could be obtained, possibly due to the viscosity of the fluid.

An US-guided biopsy was performed, which yielded SMOLD (Figs. 10.13 and 10.14).

Gynecomastia

Gynecomastia: Gynecomastia (GM) is defined as enlargement of male breast with mass formation, with or without pain and tenderness. Histologically GM is comprised of benign proliferation of glandular breast tissue. GM in infancy and puberty are common and resolve spontaneously in majority of cases. The main etiologic factor appears to be increased production and/or activity of estrogen or decreased production and/or activity of testosterone. Systemic disorders resulting in such hormonal imbalances may include obesity, hyperthyroidism, hypogonadism, cirrhosis, chronic renal failure, chronic pulmonary disease. About 25% of cases are drug-induced and the common offending drugs include finasteride, anabolic steroids, digitalis, spironolactone, metronidazole. The etiology remains unknown in about 40% of cases [9–15].

- **Clinical Presentation**: GM may be uni- or bilateral. The GM has a trimodal age distribution—neonatal, pubertal, and elderly age groups. Usual location is subareolar and superior to the nipple in males. GM clinically presents as a palpable, tender, firm, mobile, disc-shaped tissue.
- **Imaging Findings**:
  - **Mammogram**: Three patterns of gynecomastia are described: early nodular: a round, subareolar mass; late dendritic: subareolar, flame-shaped mass with projections into the posterior adipose tissue; diffuse glandular: dense parenchyma within an enlarged breast, mimicking the appearance of the female breast. The latter type is typically seen in the setting of exogenous estrogen exposure (prostate CA treatment, transgender patients) [15].
  - **US**: The earlier forms of gynecomastia resemble the appearance of the breast bud in puberty: a retroareolar, mass-like hypoechoic area with hypoechoic projections posteriorly.
  - **MRI**: Similar to fibroglandular breast tissue on all sequences.
  - **BIRADS**: Usually 2. Evaluate tissue carefully for associated suspicious masses that suggest breast cancer.
  - **Differential Diagnosis**: Benign: diabetic mastopathy. Malignant: male breast cancer.
- **Pathology Findings**:
  - **Gross**: Soft rubbery or firm tan white tissue that forms a discrete or a vague mass lesion.
  - **Microscopic Findings**: Microscopically, three distinct patterns of proliferative

changes are observed—florid, intermediate, and fibrous.
  - o Florid pattern is seen during early phases of GM. It is characterized by irregular branching ducts with mild to moderate epithelial hyperplasia, accompanied by cellular edematous stroma. Micropapillary architecture may be prominent.
  - o Intermediate pattern shows mixture of florid and fibrous patterns.
  - o Fibrous pattern predominates once the GM is present for more than 12 months. Ducts display inconspicuous epithelial proliferation and stoma is hyalinized paucicellular [13].
- – Ductal epithelial proliferation shows usual ductal hyperplasia like intermix of luminal and myoepithelial cells. Metaplastic changes (apocrine, squamous, and lactational) have been reported in the ducts of GM. Atypical ductal hyperplasia and ductal carcinoma in situ can also arise in GM.
- – Gynecomastia-like histological changes can also be seen in female breast.
- – **Differential Diagnosis**: Lipomastia (pseudogynecomastia), mammary hamartoma, fibroadenoma, and myofibroblastoma.

• **Management**: All patients with gynecomastia on physical examination without any demonstrable cause, should undergo hormonal investigation including determination of blood LH, FSH, prolactin, testosterone, oestradiol, beta-hCG, T4, and TSH. Additional workup is needed in a setting of rapid change in breast size, breast skin changes, firm breast mass, testicular mass, hepatomegaly, headache, galactorrhea, and eunuchoid stature. With equivocal clinical examination, breast imaging may be used. In suspicious lesions, core needle biopsy should be sought directly.

Case 1

Clinical Findings: A 38-year-old male with palpable right breast tissue (Figs. 10.15, 10.16, 10.17, and 10.18).

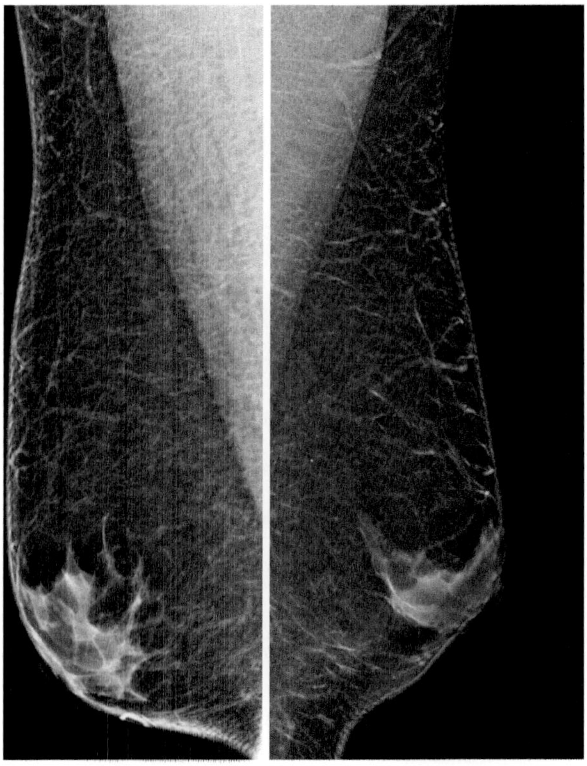

Figs. 10.15 and 10.16 **MG findings**: No specific abnormality was identified

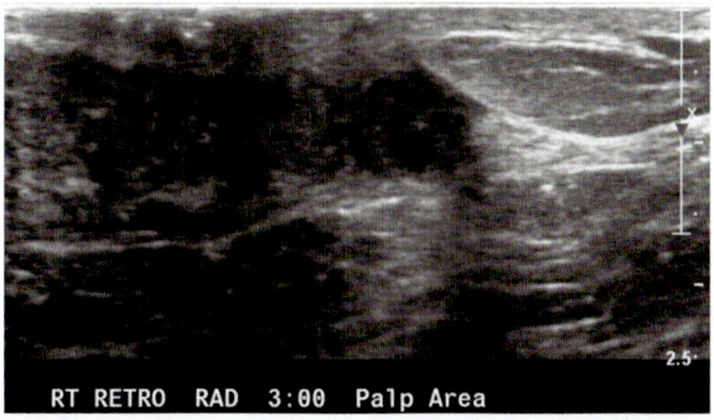

Fig. 10.17 US: No definite mass lesion was identified

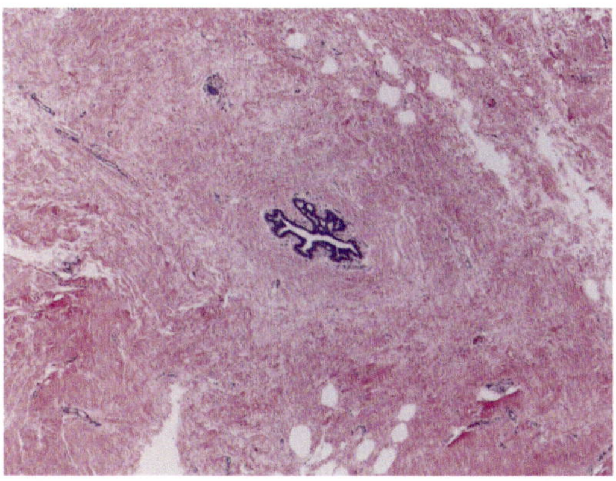

Fig. 10.18 Male breast (H&E, 4×) with gynecomastia. The tissue comprised of duct with usual ductal hyperplasia (no lobules) and fibrous tissue

Nipple Adenoma

Nipple Adenoma (NA): Nipple adenoma is a benign epithelial proliferative lesion arising from lactiferous ducts comprising of usual ductal hyperplasia, benign ducts and fibrotic or sclerotic stromal connective tissue. Histological features are similar to intraductal papilloma with usual ductal hyperplasia and sclerosis; therefore, although not preferred term by WHO, it also known as florid papillomatosis of nipple. Clinical features of NA overlap with Paget disease. Histologically the microscopic infiltrative border and florid proliferative can raise concern for atypia or malignancy. Rarely, NA can be associated with coexisting malignant epithelial proliferation.

- **Clinical Presentation**: It is most commonly seen in fifth to sixth decade but can be seen in women of any age. It also occurs in men. The presentation may simulate Paget disease of the nipple. The patient may present with soreness, ulceration, or swelling of the nipple, and sometimes with bloody nipple discharge.
- **Imaging Findings**:
  - **Mammogram**: Commonly, the mammogram is normal, but asymmetric nipple enlargement may be present [16].
  - **US**: An US evaluation may demonstrate a hypoechoic or isoechoic, hypervascular mass within the nipple.
  - **MRI**: MRI evaluation may demonstrate an avidly enhancing mass within the nipple [17].
  - **BIRADS**: 2, 3, or 4, depending on radiographic appearance.
  - **Differential Diagnosis**: Intraductal papilloma, Paget disease, invasive CA, DCIS.
- **Pathology Findings**:
  - **Gross**: Ill-defined firm irregular subareolar nodule with or without nipple erosion or ulceration is typical finding.
  - **Microscopic Findings**: Microscopically, there is a fairly circumscribed and compact proliferation of the benign ducts and stroma. It is centered around the large subareolar lactiferous duct of the nipple and it can involve and erode overlying epidermis:
    - There is an adenosis-like pattern of the proliferating ducts intermixed with papillomatosis and usual ductal hyperplasia. The stroma is fibrotic and can show sclerosis [18]
    - The ducts are lined by myoepithelial cell and contain epithelial proliferation with histological features of usual ductal hyperplasia. NA with florid UDH may show necrosis and thus mimic in situ carcinoma. An IHC panel of keratin 5/6 and estrogen receptor can aid in confirming UDH: mosaic pattern cytoplasmic staining with keratin 5/6 and variable mild to strong nuclear staining [19].

- **Differential Diagnosis**: Syringomatous tumor and Paget disease.
  - Syringomatous tumor can occur in nipple. The epithelial component of syringomatous tumor is composed of small rounded infiltrative epithelial cell nests and it involves areolar smooth muscle. No epidermal component is present.
  - Paget disease is histologically distinct from NA.
- **Management**: NA is benign and does not mandate surgical excision. Histopathologic confirmation is needed to exclude malignancy. If the lesions are symptomatic and concerning to the patients, excision may be performed. Excision of the entire nipple is not required. NA can recure if it is incompletely excised [20].

Case 1

Clinical History: A 52-year-old female with a pruritic mass within the right nipple.

MG: Normal (Figs. 10.19 and 10.20).

BI-RADS: 4, suspicious finding.

A surgical biopsy was recommended and performed, yielding a nipple adenoma (Fig. 10.21).

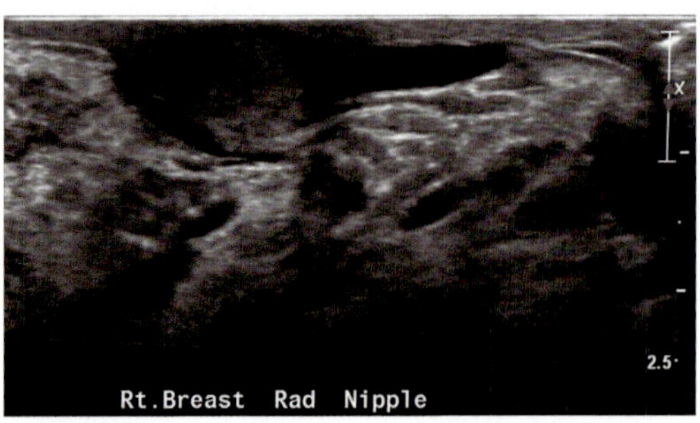

Fig. 10.19 **US**: Hypoechoic, vascular mass within the left nipple

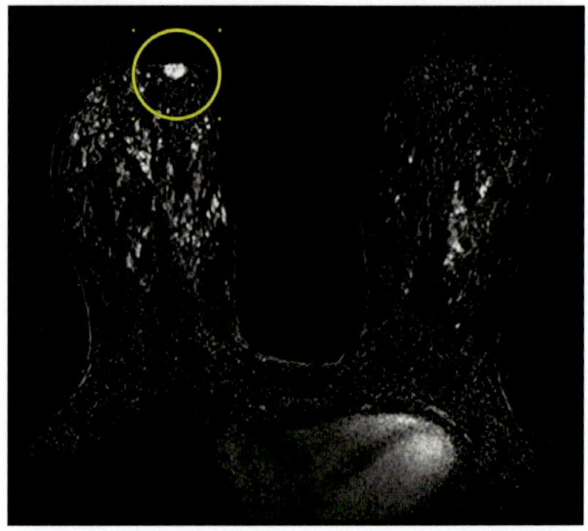

Fig. 10.20 **MRI**: Uniformly avidly enhancing mass within the nipple

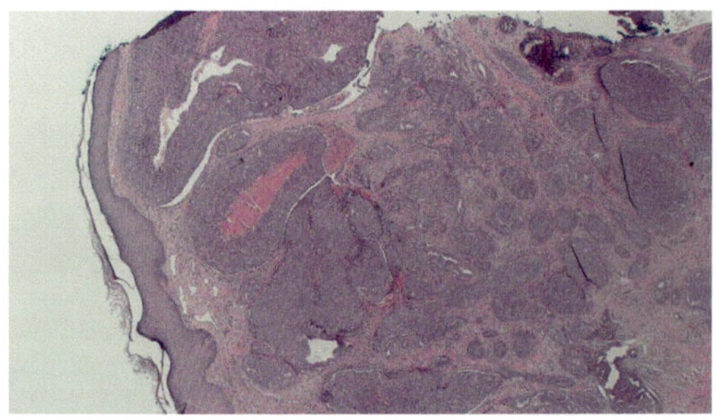

Fig. 10.21 Nipple adenoma (H&E, 4×). The subepidermal breast tissue shows usual ductal hyperplasia with central sclerotic focus. The epithelial proliferation involves a large duct of the nipple and overall histological changes are reminiscent of an intraductal papilloma with sclerosis

Intraductal Papilloma

Intraductal Papilloma: Intraductal papillomas (IDPs) are benign epithelial proliferative lesions that arise within a duct either in central (subareolar) or peripheral (small ducts near lobules) breast tissue. IDP is composed of fibrous papillae containing vessels (fibrovasular projections) that are surfaced by myoepithelial- and luminal-type epithelial cells. Central IDPs can present with nipple discharge or as a mass, peripheral IDP are often clinically and radiologically occult. Atypical and neoplastic epithelial proliferation including a spectrum of ductal and lobular hyperplasia and carcinoma in situ can arise in IDP or secondarily involve IDP [21–24].

- **Clinical Presentation**: IDPs are seen in a wide age range but occur predominantly in 30–50 years old women. Central IDPs arise in large subareolar lactiferous duct, and can present with bloody or clear nipple discharge or a subareolar mass. Patients may occasionally be able to identify a "trigger point" on their breast, which, when pressed, may result in nipple discharge. Peripheral papillomas are usually occult but they can present with calcifications or mass. Small papillomas may be mammographically occult, and detected incidentally on screening ultrasound in asymptomatic patients, but larger papillomas may present as a mass, with margins ranging from circumscribed to indistinct. Punctate, amorphous, or coarse heterogeneous calcifications may be present. A dilated duct may be present [25]. The patient's symptoms of bloody or clear nipple discharge may prompt evaluation with ductography [26].
- **Imaging Findings**:
  - **Mammogram**: May be occult, or may present with as a mass lesion, with margins ranging from circumscribed to indistinct. Papillomas may contain punctate, amorphous, or coarse heterogeneous calcifications.
  - **US**: Intraductal, vascular mass. The segment of the duct surrounding the mass may be dilated.
  - **Ductography**: Intraluminal mural-based filling defect with lobulated borders, duct that abruptly terminates due to obstruction by the intraductal mass.
  - **MRI**: Enhancing intraductal mass that frequently demonstrates contrast washout on delayed images within a fluid filled, dilated duct.
  - **BIRADS**: 3 or 4. Can be designated as probably benign if a small intraductal mass without associated suspicious findings is detected on routine screening ultrasound. However, an imaging guided needle biopsy and/or surgical excision are warranted if the patient is symptomatic or associated suspicious findings are present.
  - **Differential Diagnosis**: Tumefactive debris within an ectatic duct, intraductal epithelial proliferation, adenoma, atypical papilloma, DCIS, encapsulated papillary carcinoma.
- **Pathology Findings**:
  - **Gross**: The large-duct papillomas are seen as circumscribed nodules in a cystically dilated space.
  - **Microscopic Findings**: The fibrovascular stalks of the IDPs are usually thick and fibrous with myoepithelial cell layer and luminal cell lining. Thin and petit papillary fronds may exist but are more frequently seen with coexisting atypia. The myoepithelial cell layer is present at the interface of the papillary frond and the fibrous tissue with oval shape slightly hyperchromactic nuclei arranged parallel to the basement membrane. The epithelium shows variable extent of usual ductal hyperplasia ranging from minimal proliferation to areas of florid UDH with or without central comedo-type necrosis.
  - Apocrine metaplasia and cystic change are common. Squamous metaplasia is not common but can be seen secondary to infarction. IDP can show solid pattern of growth with stromal collagen deposition, also known as sclerosis. Sclerotic areas can show phosphate-type calcification.

- Infarction and hemorrhage can be present, which can be spontaneous or secondary to core biopsy.
- Peripheral papillomas are microscopic and often less than 3 mm in size. Peripheral IDPs are more commonly present as incidental finding in breast core needle biopsy performed for a separate target lesion, therefore warranting a radiology-pathology correlation.
- Papillomatosis is loosely used terminology usually applied in a setting of multiple peripheral papillomas.
- **Differential Diagnosis**: Breast tissue can show a variety of papillary lesions. IDP is a benign papillary breast lesion that can be managed conservatively following radiology pathology correlation. Therefore, IDP needs to be differentiated from atypical and malignant papillary lesions, especially in core needle biopsy.
  - Papilloma with atypical ductal hyperplasia/DCIS: The IDP can harbor foci of ADH/DCIS. The histological findings of ADH involving IDP are similar to ADH outside the papilloma. ADH foci comprise of monotonous low nuclear grade epithelial proliferation with rigid architecture. In IDP, ADH span of more than 3 mm qualifies for low nuclear grade DCIS.
  - Encapsulated papillary carcinoma (EPC), solid papillary carcinoma (SPC), and papillary DCIS: Unlike IDP EPC, SPC, and papillary DCIS are composed of pure population of low to intermediate nuclear grade (often ER positive) neoplastic cells with papillary architecture. Myoepithelial cells are absent in the papillary cores and absent (EPC and SPC) or retained (papillary DCIS) at the lesion stromal interface.
  - Tall cell carcinoma with reverse polarity (TCCRP): TCCRP is recently identified favorable histologic type of triple-negative carcinoma that can show overlapping histological features with sclerotic IDP. Distinct histological features including reverse polarity of tall columnar cell lining the papillae and absent IHC staining with myoepithelial makers (p63 and smooth muscle myosin heavy chain) confirms the diagnosis.
  - Adenomyoepithelioma (AME): AME shows histological overlap with IDP. AME and IDP both are composed of epithelial and myoepithelial cells. AME can have an intraductal origin and show papillary architecture. The clinical behavior of AME is uncertain which may present with recurrences and distant metastases. Histological distinction between AME and IDP can be difficult and sometime impossible. Multi-nodular appearance, peripheral location, prominent sebaceous or squamous metaplasia, and inconsistent myoepithelial immunophenotype favors AME over IDP. A subset of AME show *HRAS* mutations.
  - Nipple adenoma: NA is nipple-based benign proliferative lesion which can have papillary architecture.
  - IDP with lobular neoplasia: Lobular neoplasia can involve IDP. Loss of membranous E-cadherin and cytoplasmic staining of p120 IHC can distinguish lobular neoplasia foci from ductal hyperplasia in IDP.

- **Management**: Incidentally detected, small IDP without associated suspicious radiologic findings may be followed with observation. Symptomatic lesions should be sampled with imaging guidance, usually followed by surgical excision. Alternatively, symptomatic lesions could be excised without a preceding imaging-guided needle biopsy. IDPs with atypia must be excised. Vacuum-assisted removal may be an alternative to surgical excision for benign lesions without atypia.

Case 1

Clinical Findings: A 56-year-old female with a palpable mass within the right nipple.

MMG Findings: Normal (Figs. 10.22 and 10.23).

BI-RADS: 4, suspicious (Figs. 10.24 and 10.25).

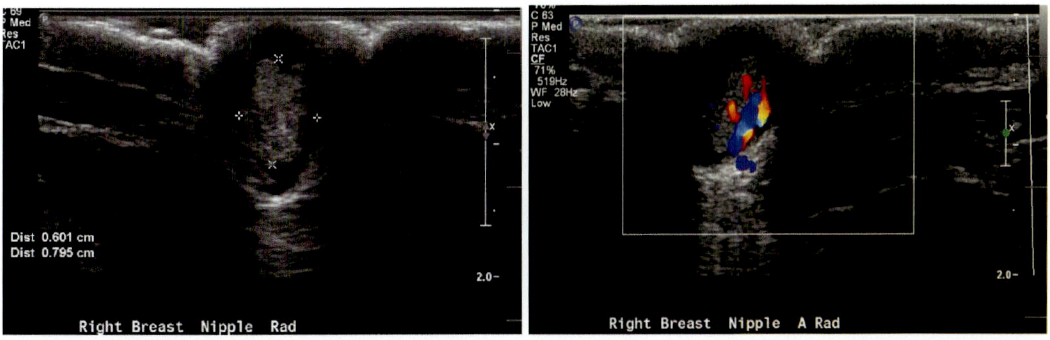

Figs. 10.22 and 10.23 **USG findings**: Mass with a prominent central vascular stalk, with frond-like projections within a dilated lactiferous duct within the nipple

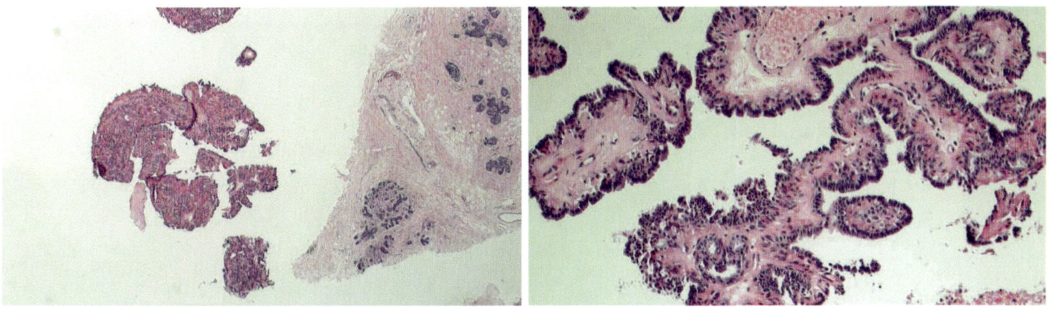

Figs. 10.24 and 10.25 Core needle biopsy tissue with intraductal papilloma (H&E, 4× and 10×). Detached loose papillary fragments and benign breast tissue (upper panel). Papillae are lined by layers of luminal and basal myoepithelial cells

Syringomatous Tumor of Nipple

Syringomatous Tumor of Nipple (STN): Syringomatous tumor is also known as syringomatous adenoma or infiltrating syringomatous adenoma of nipple. It is a rare benign tumor occurring in the nipple that histologically resembles eccrine duct syringoma of the skin. It is a locally infiltrative tumor that involves lactiferous sinus and areolar smooth muscle [27, 28].

- **Clinical Presentation**: Average age at diagnosis is 40 years, the age range is between 11 and 67 years. STN presents as a nipple mass or a subareolar dermal nodule with variable pain, erythema, nipple distortion, and nipple discharge. Rare cases are reported in male nipple.
- **Imaging Findings**: STN are difficult to detect by mammogram because of superficial location and presence within the dense smooth muscle.
- **Pathology Findings**:
  - **Gross**: Firm poorly defined mass in the nipple.
  - **Microscopic Findings**: Histologically, within the dermis, there is a proliferation of curved, ductular structures lined by flattened-to-cuboidal cells, often with proteinaceous debris and keratin seen in their lumens, forming cysts. These ductules are often described as "comma shaped", "tear drop shaped" or "tadpole shaped". The comma-shaped ducts invade the smooth muscle bundles and nerves underneath the nipple-areola complex, simulating a malig-

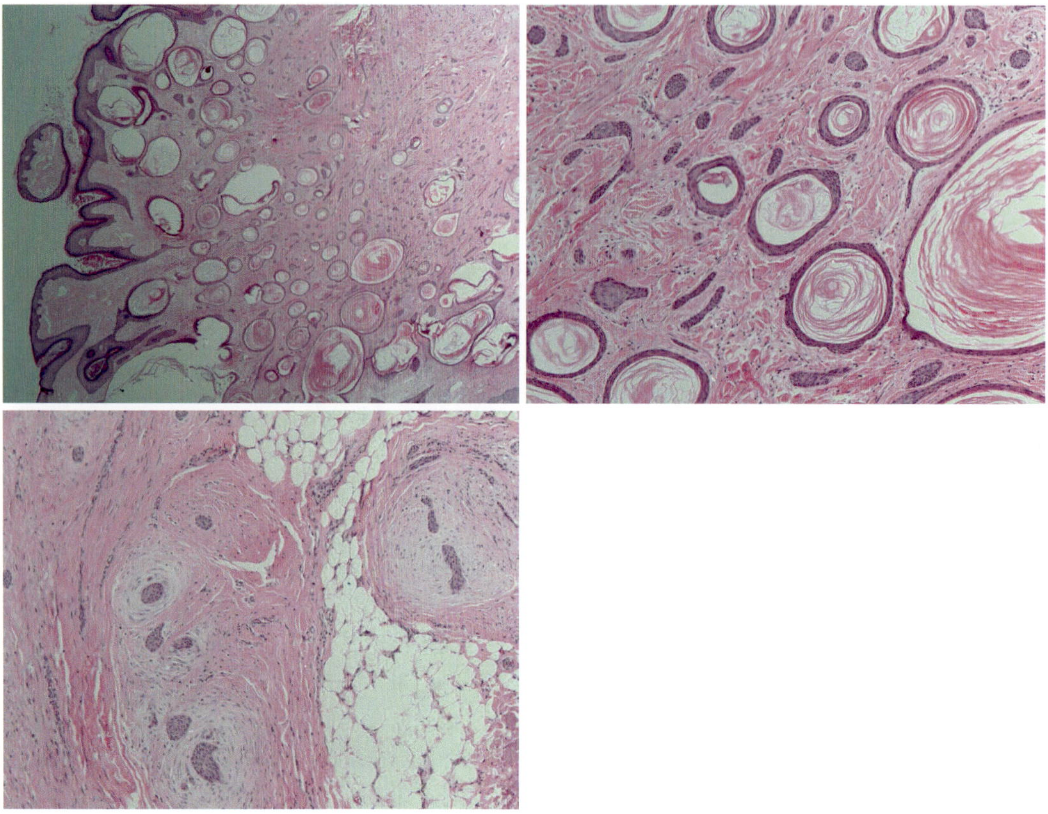

Figs. 10.26–10.28 Syringomatous adenoma of the nipple (H&E, 2×, 4×, and 10×). Subareolar tissue shows infiltrative solid nests with tails and angulated contours. Many nests have central keratinous material

nant mammary neoplasm. The proliferation and arrangement of the ducts may seem haphazard and infiltrative, but the myoepithelial cell layer is demonstrable by p63, smooth muscle myosin, high-molecular-weight cytokeratin 34bE12 or basal cytokeratin 5/6 immunostains. The overlying epidermis may show variable acanthosis and pseudo-epitheliomatous hyperplasia. The lesion may involve adjacent lactiferous ducts. The background stroma may be hyalinized or myxoid. In some cases, perineural invasion may also be seen.

- **Differential Diagnosis**: Nipple adenoma, low-grade adenosquamous carcinoma.
  - Nipple adenoma arises from lactiferous ducts. Nipple adenoma is non-infiltrative proliferation of glands and ducts with usual ductal hyperplasia.
  - Low-grade adenosquamous carcinoma can arise in nipple. The solid squamous nests and glands in adenosquamous carcinoma are variable in size and shape and accompanied by desmoplasia and tight lymphoid aggregate. Overt squamous differentiation and keratinous material may be present.

- **Management**: Complete surgical excision with negative margins as local recurrence is reported in as many as 30% cases (Figs. 10.26–10.28).

Paget Disease of Breast

Paget Disease of Breast: Mammary Paget disease (PD) is a unique type of breast adenocarcinoma which is characterized by intraepidermal proliferation of carcinoma cells. PD involves nipple and areolar skin. The PD is etiologically linked to in situ or invasive ductal carcinoma involving subareolar ducts or lobules.

- **Clinical Presentation**: PD affects both males and females over an age range of 27–88 years. PD is more common in postmenopausal women in the sixth decade; the mean age at diagnosis is 57 years. PD presents as erythematous crusted lesion of the nipple, which can form eroding and bleeding ulcer. The gross appearance can mimic that of an eczematous or inflammatory lesion sometimes associated with oozing. Pain and itching are frequently present. More advanced lesions may present as round, ovoid or eczema-like plaque with a pink or red hue that it is sharply demarcated from the adjacent normal skin.
- **Imaging Findings**:
  - **Mammogram**: The mammogram may be normal. Occasionally, thickening of the nipple and periareolar skin may be present. A suspicious mass and/or calcifications in the subareolar region or elsewhere in the breast may be present.
  - **US**: The affected nipple may be asymmetrically thickened and hypervascular. Dilated retroareolar ducts or a subareolar mass may be present.
  - **MRI**: The nipple may avidly enhance, with washout kinetics. MRI is recommended for patients presenting with Paget disease, to evaluate for mammographically/sonographically occult neoplasm [29, 30].
  - **BIRADS**: 1, 2, 3, 4, 5, depending on imaging findings. Paget disease may be an isolated clinical finding, in which case imaging may be BI-RADS 1 or 2.
  - **Differential Diagnosis**: Various benign dermatologic conditions (eczema, psoriasis, contact dermatitis), nipple adenoma, protruding intraductal papilloma, infection, locally advanced breast cancer involving the nipple, inflammatory breast cancer.
- **Pathology Findings**:
  - **Gross**: Nipple may appear normal. PD can present as redness, erosion, scaling and crusting of nipple and areolar skin.
  - **Microscopic Findings**: PD is characterized by presence of intraepidermal adenocarcinoma, also known as Paget cells. Paget cells are large cells with abundant, pale or clear cytoplasm and pleomorphic nuclei containing prominent nucleoli and mitoses. Paget cells are spread singly or clustered in small groups and rarely form glands. Intracytoplasmic mucin or melanin pigment can be present in the Paget cells. The underlying dermis shows reactive changes including variable degrees of telangiectasia and chronic inflammation, sometimes even appearing lichenoid. Dermal invasion by Paget cells is rare and reported in 4–8% of cases of PD [31, 32].
  - PD is associated with an underlying breast carcinoma, which is often a high-grade breast carcinoma of no special type. PD is associated with DCIS in 24–43% cases. PD without underlying carcinoma is rare, reported in 0–13% PD cases.
  - Immunohistochemically, the Paget cells are positive for low molecular weight keratins, like CK7, HER2 (80–90% cases) and GATA3. Paget cells are ER and PR positive in 40% and 30% of cases respectively. Paget cells are negative for melanoma markers (MITF, Melan A and HMB45). Mucicarmine can highlight intracytoplasmic mucin.
  - **Differential Diagnosis**: Toker cells, melanoma, clear cell change in keratinocytes, inflammatory changes such as atopic or contact dermatitis of the nipple, chronic eczema, psoriasis, squamous cell carcinoma in situ/Bowen disease, sebaceous carcinoma, breast carcinoma directly invading nipple skin.
    - Toker cells are cytologically bland and often ER and PR positive and HER2 negative.
    - Squamous cell carcinoma and melanoma of nipple and areola are rare. Squamous cell carcinoma is positive for high molecular weight keratin. Paget cells can contain melanin, and mimic melanoma. Paget cells are keratin posi-

tive and negative for melanoma markers (Melan A, MITF, and HMB 45). Paget cells can show IHC staining with S100 and SOX10 which are also positive in melanoma.

- **Management**: PD clinical presentation overlaps with inflammatory skin conditions, punch biopsy of the affected area of the nipple-areolar complex (NAC) should be performed for definite diagnosis. An associated breast cancer, either ductal carcinoma in situ (DCIS) or invasive cancer, is found within the breast in the majority of Paget cases. Thus, breast imaging, and subsequent core needle biopsy (CNB) of any suspicious lesions within the breast, needs to be performed. Magnetic resonance imaging (MRI) is recommended in the workup of patients so that the full extent of disease can be delineated. Mastectomy or lumpectomy can be used for surgical management of PD as long as the entire NAC and any underlying cancer are resected to appropriately negative margins. If lumpectomy is performed, this should be paired with adjuvant whole breast radiation. Even if mastectomy is performed for PD without evidence of invasive breast cancer, sentinel lymph node biopsy (SLNB) should be considered at the time of mastectomy in case an underlying cancer is found in the breast on final pathology. If there is an associated invasive cancer in the setting of PD then disease management should follow National Comprehensive Cancer Network (NCCN) guidelines for invasive breast cancer. If there is an associated DCIS in the setting of PD then disease management should follow NCCN guidelines for DCIS [33].

Case 1

Clinical Findings: A 62-year-old female presented with a scaly rash of her left nipple, with intermittent bleeding. She was seen by a dermatologist, who performed a punch biopsy of the nipple, establishing the diagnosis of Paget disease. She was subsequently referred for breast imaging (Figs. 10.29, 10.30, 10.31, 10.32, and 10.33).

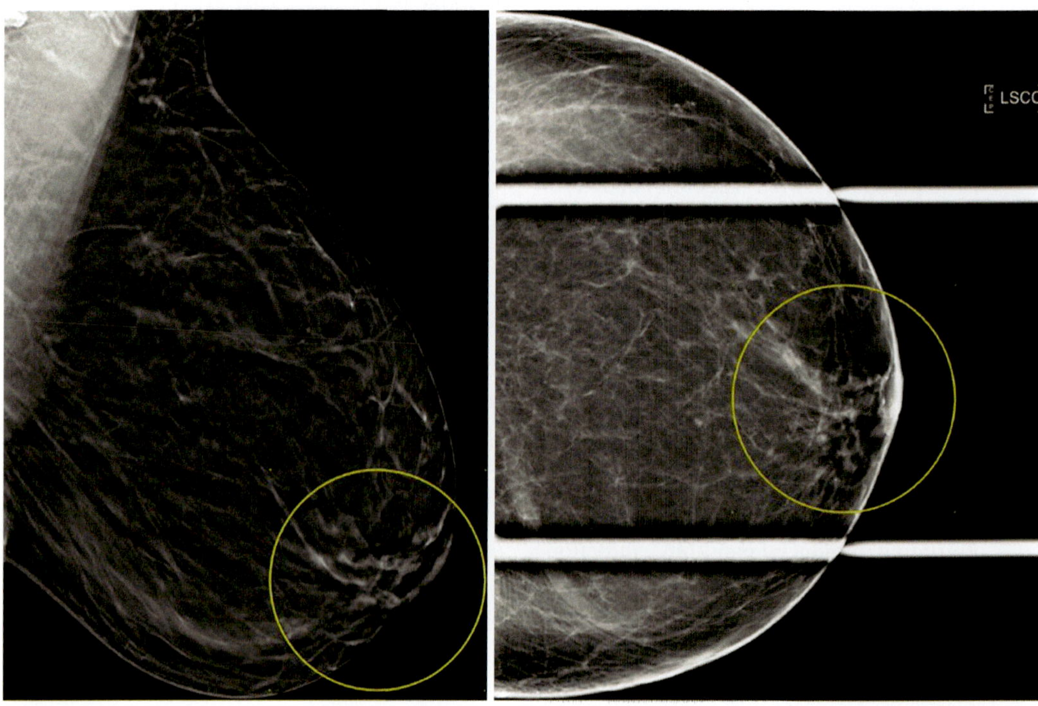

Figs. 10.29 and 10.30 **MMG findings**: Asymmetric, dilated ducts are noted in the left retroareolar region, but no other abnormalities are noted

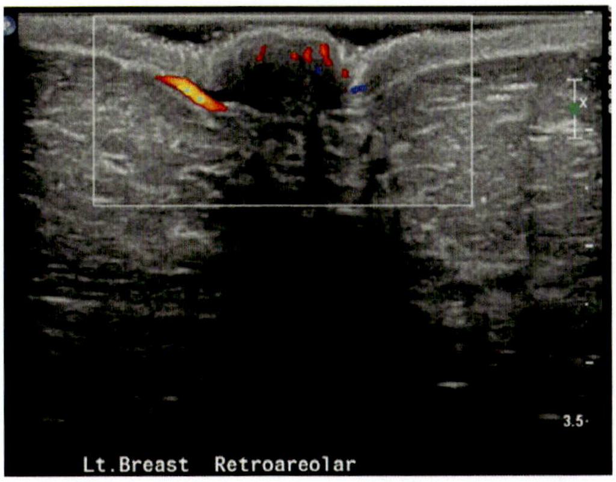

Fig. 10.31 **USG findings**: Asymmetric thickening and hypervascularity of the left nipple, without other suspicious findings

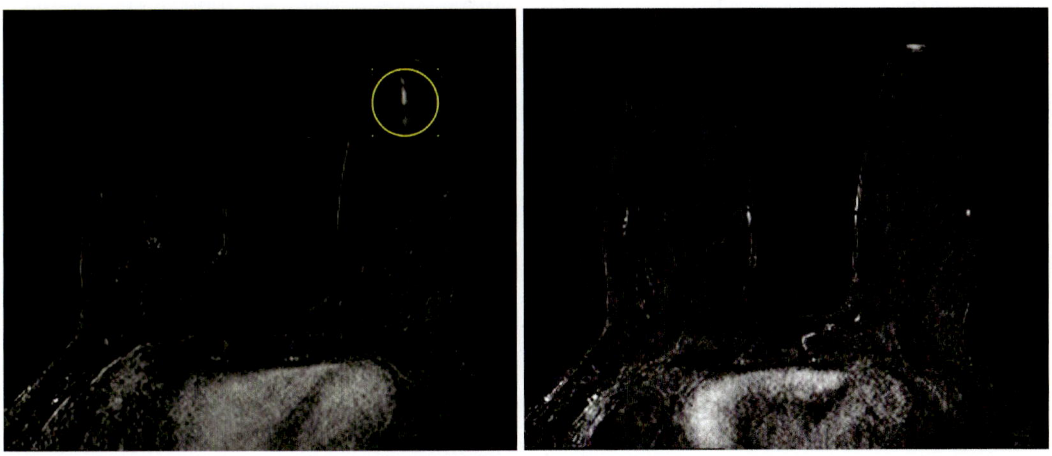

Figs. 10.32 and 10.33 **MRI findings**: An avidly enhancing left nipple, asymmetric when compared to the right breast, and abnormal linear non-mass enhancement in the left retroareolar region, corresponding to the mammographic finding of dilated ducts

BI-RADS: 4, suspicious findings.

An MRI-guided biopsy of the linear NME was performed, yielding DCIS (Figs. 10.34, 10.35, and 10.36).

Case 2

Clinical Findings: A 59-year-old female presenting with a palpable mass within the right nipple. No skin crusting or nipple discharge was reported (Figs. 10.37, 10.38, and 10.39).

BI-RADS: 4, suspicious findings.

The patient underwent a punch biopsy of the nipple, which demonstrated IDC. She subsequently underwent a central lumpectomy, which re-demonstrated IDC involving the nipple, including the dermis, but without evidence of PD. Additional findings in the lumpectomy were DCIS and LCIS (Figs. 10.40 and 10.41).

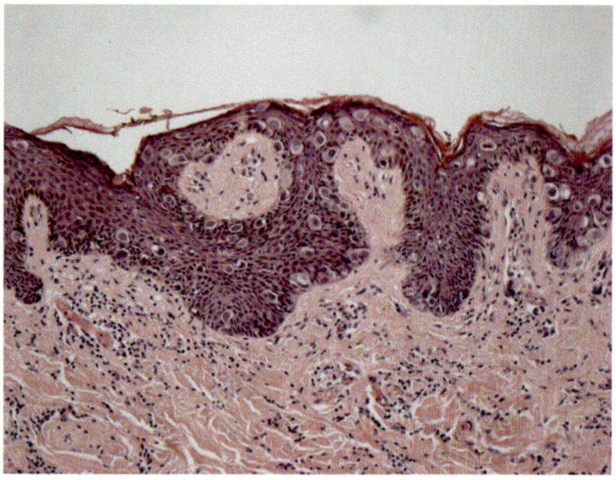

Fig. 10.34 Nipple skin biopsy showing Paget disease (H&E, 10×). Malignant epithelial cells are scattered in the nipple epidermis

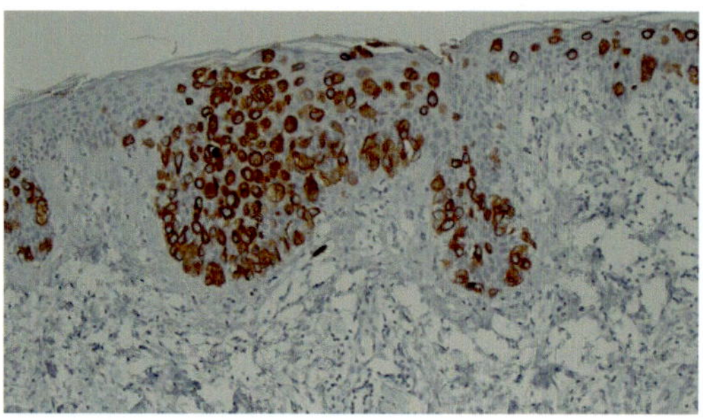

Fig. 10.35 Nipple skin biopsy showing Paget disease (keratin IHC). Keratin IHC highlights tumor cells in the epidermis

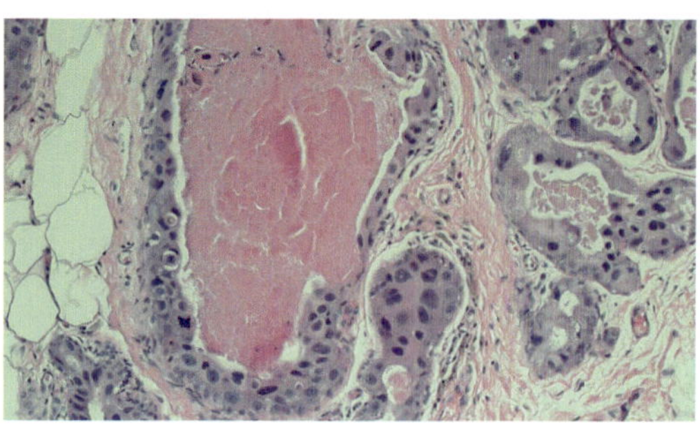

Fig. 10.36 Ductalc carcinoma in situ (H&E, 10×). High-grade DCIS in the separate breast biopsy shows a clinging pattern and comedo necrosis

Axillary Lesions

Abstract Axillary mass lesions can arise from soft tissue, lymph nodes, skin appendages, and axillary breast tissue. Axilla can be a site of peripheral nerve sheath tumors (schwannoma and neurofibroma), adipocytic tumors (lipoma, angiolipoma), myofibroblastic tumors (desmoid) and vascular lesion. The axillary soft tissue tumors are discussed elsewhere in other chapters. Other mass forming lesion in the axilla include ectopic/accessory breast tissue and inflammatory conditions involving axillary sweat glands. The ectopic breast tissue can occur anywhere along the milk line; it occurs most commonly in the axilla. Hidradenitis suppurativa is a chronic inflammatory condition of the cutis involving axilla or groin and it can form furuncles, fistulas, and abscesses.

With known breast cancer, palpable axillary lymph nodes are frequently worked up with imaging. The lymph nodes with abnormal imaging findings (thickened cortex, loss of fatty hilum) are sampled by image-guided fine needle aspiration or core needle biopsy to detect metastasis. Axillary lymph nodes may be enlarged due to reactive lymphadenopathy or by metastasis from breast carcinoma. Non-mammary carcinoma metastases can also involve axillary lymph nodes and should be considered as a possibility especially with normal breast imaging. Axillary lymph nodes can also be involved by lymphoproliferative disorders.

Keywords Axilla; Breast; Lymph node; Metastases; Reactive

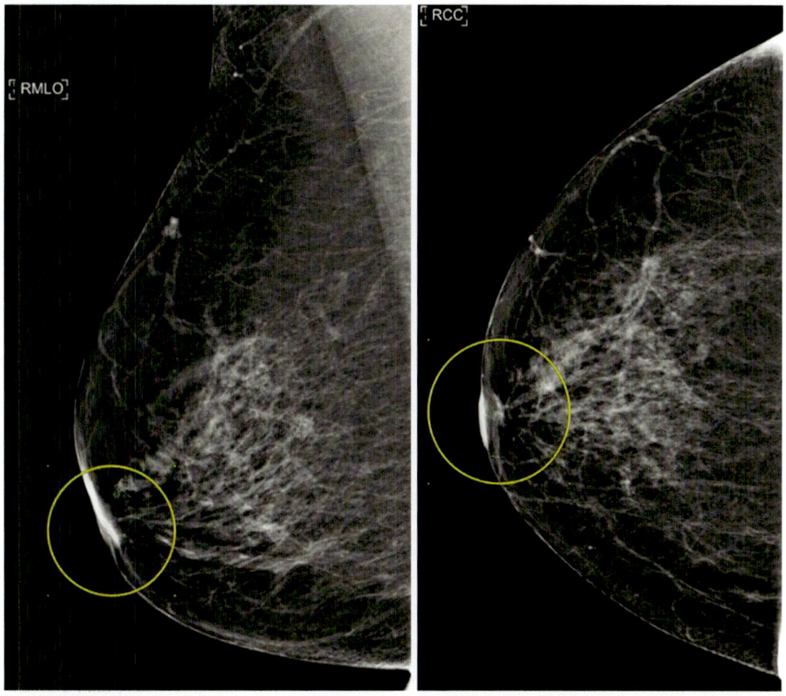

Figs. 10.37 and 10.38 MMG findings: The technologist had difficulty obtaining a view with the nipple in profile; the nipple is retracted and retroareolar architectural distortion is present

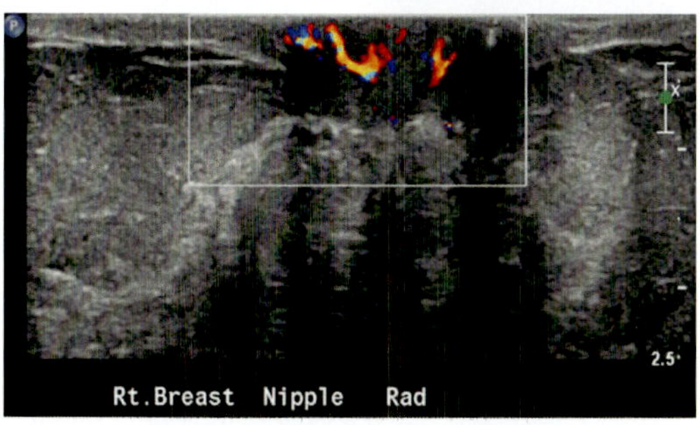

Fig. 10.39 USG findings: The right nipple is thickened, irregular, and hypervascular

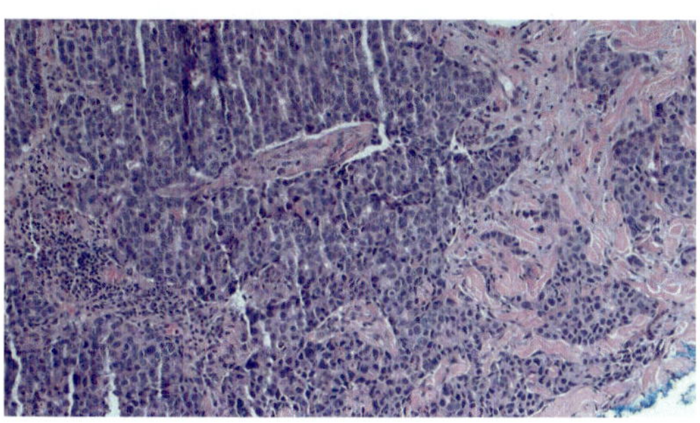

Fig. 10.40 Invasive ductal carcinoma (H&E 10×) involving subareolar breast tissue

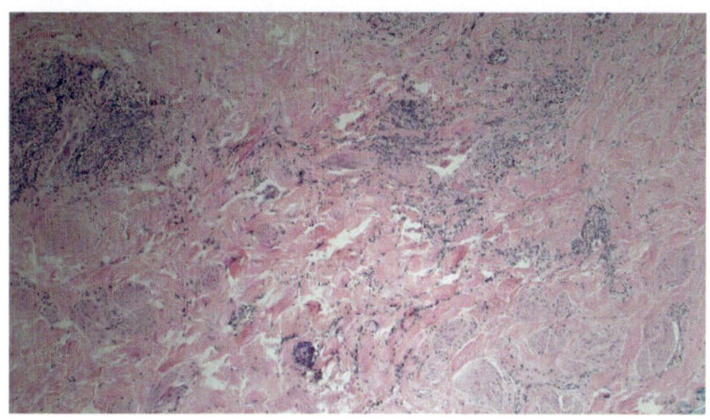

Fig. 10.41 Invasive ductal carcinoma (H&E 4×) involving subareolar breast tissue with lymphovascular invasion

Benign Reactive Lymph Node

Benign Reactive Lymph Node: Reactive lymphadenopathy is the most common etiology for enlarged and palpable axillary lymph nodes. The lymph node enlargement may be secondary to the skin condition, dermatopathic lymphadenopathy. Lymph nodes draining tumors can also show reactive enlargement without metastasis [34].

- **Clinical Presentation**: The reactive lymph nodes may be palpable or enlarged in radiology images.
- **Imaging Findings**: Ultrasound is the method of choice to assess axillary lymph nodes in the setting of known breast cancer.
  – **Mammogram**: Lymph nodes are seen as axillary densities. Because of limited spatial resolution and sometimes parts of the axillary area may not be visualized, the mammogram is not considered reliable for evaluating lymph nodes.
  – **US**: A normal axillary lymph node is characterized by a reniform shape, a maximal cortical thickness of 3 mm without focal bulging, smooth margins, and, depending on size, a discernable central fatty hilum. Morphologic characteristics predictive of malignancy are cortical thickness greater than 2.5–3.0 mm, focal cortical lobulation, loss of the fatty hilum, a round shape, and abnormal cortical blood flow.
  – **MRI**: MRI features suspicious for malignancy include cortical thickening, loss of fatty hilum, round shape, or a long axis to short axis ratio of less than 2. The presence of perifocal edema, defined as the area with marked T2 prolongation in the fat surrounding a node, has been shown to have the highest positive predictive value for malignancy.
  – **BIRADS**: Not applicable.
  – **Differential Diagnosis**: Reactive lymph node, lymphoma, metastasis.
- **Pathology Findings**: The reactive lymph node is tan-red in color and shows a smooth capsule and retained bean-shape.
  – **Gross**: The cut surface is smooth, homogeneous, and tan-brown in color.
  – **Microscopic Findings**: The capsule is smooth, and subcapsular sinuses are open. The reactive lymph node may show hyperplastic follicles, paracortical hyperplasia (T-cell zone), or both. Rarely, neutrophils and plasma cells may be prominent. In dermatopathic lymphadenitis, there is paracortical hyperplasia; melanin pigment containing histiocytes and dendritic cells are present.
  – **Differential Diagnosis**: Lymphoproplieraitve lesion, metastasis, especially lobular carcinoma.
- **Management**: Conservative management.

Case 1

Clinical Findings: A 48-year-old female with RA palpated an axillary mass (Figs. 10.42 and 10.43).

Core needle biopsy revealed a normal lymph node on biopsy (Figs. 10.44 and 10.45).

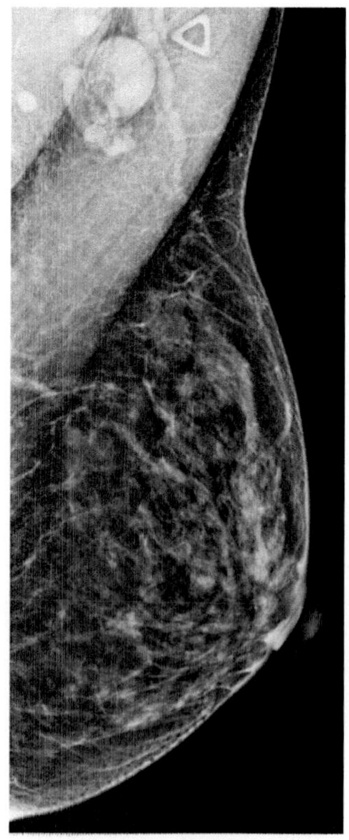

Fig. 10.42 **MMG findings**: Mammogram demonstrates an enlarged axillary lymph node

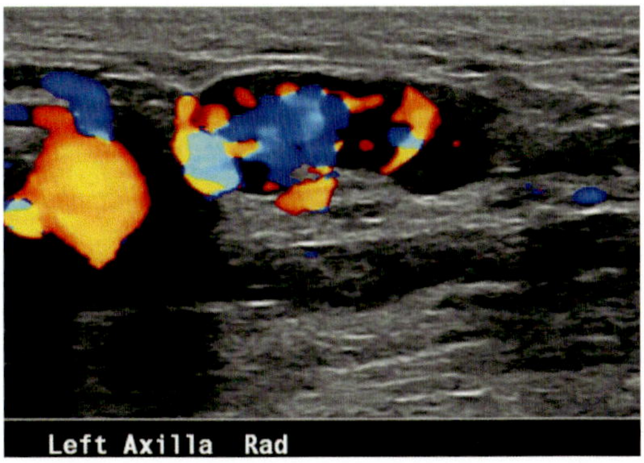

Fig. 10.43 **USG findings**: An enlarged lymph node with a concentrically thickened, hypervascular cortex. However, the lymph node maintains an oval shape and a fatty hilum is still visible

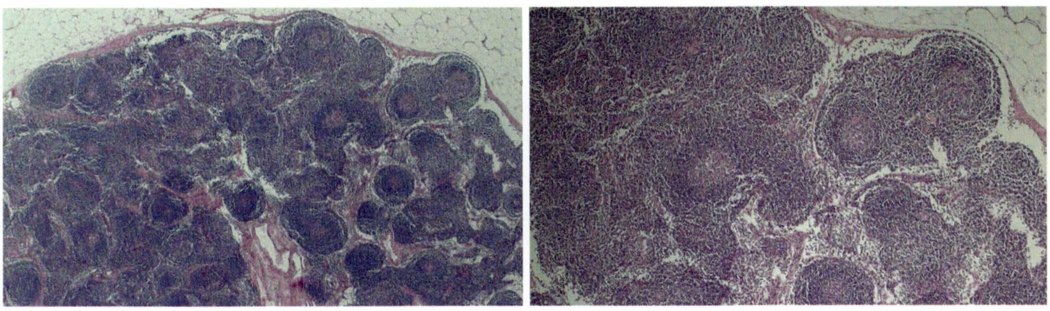

Figs. 10.44 and 10.45 Reactive lymph node (H&E, 4× and 10×). The reactive lymph node shows intact lymph node architecture with reactive follicles and open subcapsular sinuses

Accessory Breast Tissue in Axilla

Accessory Breast Tissue in Axilla: Axillary breast tissue can be present as a combination of adipose tissue, glandular tissue and nipple and areolae. Axillary breast tissue affects 2–6% of women and 1–3% of men. The chief complaints are functional and/or cosmetic concerns [35].

- **Clinical Presentation**: It can be asymptomatic or present with tenderness, swelling or irritation that worsens during puberty, menstruation, or pregnancy.
- **Imaging Findings**:
  - **Mammogram**: Islands of breast tissue of variable density within the axilla.
  - **US**: Ecogenic benign breast tissue with islands of breast tissue of variable echotexture.
  - **MRI**: Resembles normal breast tissue on all sequences.
  - **BIRADS**: 1 or 2.
  - **Differential Diagnosis**: Hamartoma, fat necrosis, fibroadenoma, and malignancy. Soft tissue tumors.
- **Pathology Findings**:
  - **Gross**: There are no specific gross findings for accessory breast tissue. The cut surface shows a variable degree of adipose tissue mixed with fibrous tissue.
  - **Microscopic Findings**: Benign breast lobules and ducts are identified in the fibrous

tissue. Larger ducts and prominent smooth muscle bundles may be present near skin, in a setting of accessory nipple.
  - **Differential Diagnosis**: Hamartoma, fat necrosis, fibroadenoma or malignancy. Soft tissue tumors.
- **Management**: Surgical or non-surgical removal of the accessory breast tissue.

Case 1

Clinical Findings: A 47-year-old female, palpable right axillary nodularity (Figs. 10.46, 10.47, 10.48, 10.49, and 10.50).

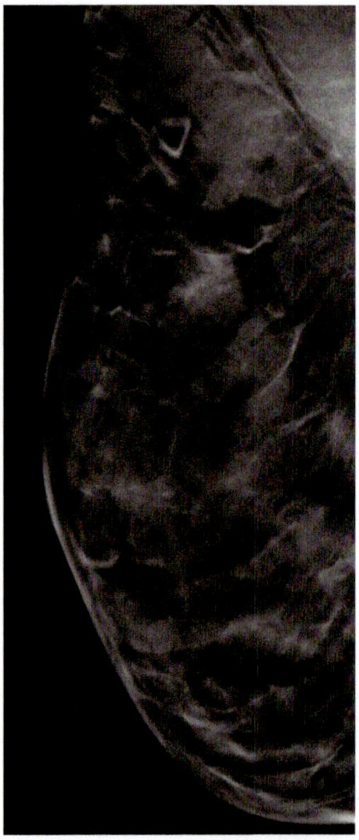

Fig. 10.46 MMG findings: Mammogram demonstrates a dense area of accessory axillary breast tissue

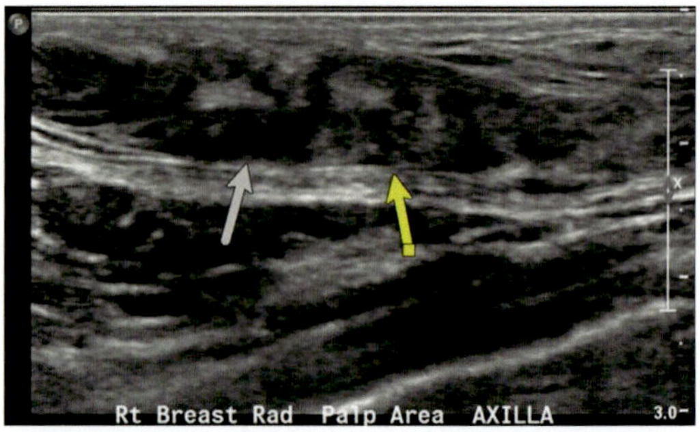

Fig. 10.47 USG findings: US confirms the presence of breast tissue without a focal lesion within the axilla

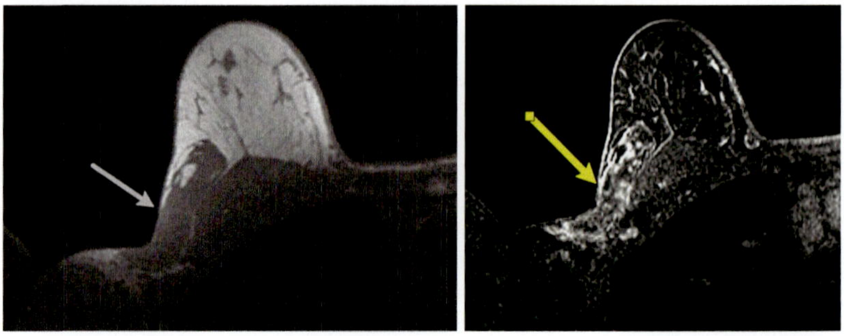

Figs. 10.48 and 10.49 MRI findings: MRI performed due to elevated risk of breast CA based on family history demonstrates axillary breast tissue without suspicious lesions

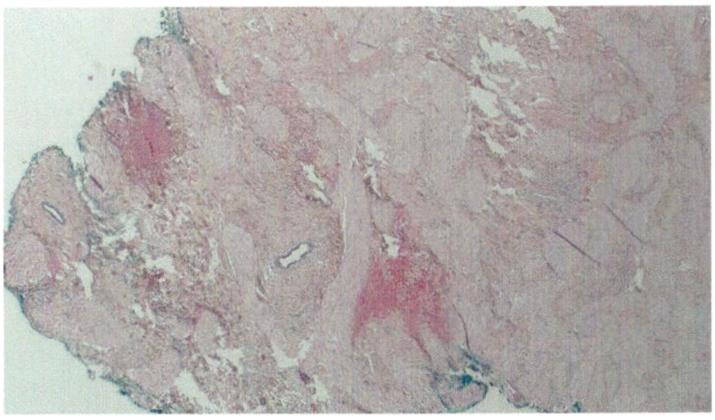

Fig. 10.50 Accessory breast tissue in the axilla (H&E, 4×) comprising of breast ducts and prominent smooth muscle bundles indicating accessory nipple

Hidradenitis Suppurativa

Hidradenitis Suppurativa: Hidradenitis suppurativa (HS) is an inflammatory skin condition of apocrine-gland bearing areas characterized by recurrent or chronic painful suppurative lesions.

- **Clinical Presentation**: Disease severity is traditionally classified according to the Hurley classification, which defines stage I as transient non-scarring inflammatory lesions; stage II as separate lesions consisting of recurrent abscesses with tunnel formation and scarring, and single or multiple lesions separated by normal-looking skin; and stage III as coalescent lesions with tunnel formation, scarring, and inflammation. HS lesions are very pruritic, painful, and located in the intertriginous areas and can be malodorous and have a purulent discharge [36, 37].
- **Imaging Findings**: The role of imaging in HS is to detect the actual type and extent of anatomic abnormalities by providing objective and precise information. Sonography supports early and more precise diagnosis and staging by providing critical objective information in real time. Color doppler ultrasound may support the management of HS.
  - **Mammogram**: Mammogram can demonstrate irregular masses focal asymmetries within the axilla.
  - **US**: The sonographic criteria for diagnosing HS are based on the following findings: widening of the hair follicles, dermal alterations, pseudocysts, fluid collections, and fistulae. The presence of three or more findings is the sonographic criteria for diagnosing HS. The sonographic scoring system for assessing severity in HS (SOS-HS) is based on anatomic alterations, such as dermal echostructural abnormalities, and the recognition of dermal and/or hypodermal fluid collections and fistulae.
  - **MRI**: MRI has been mainly used in some extensive and deep anogenital HS lesions.
  - **BIRADS**: Not applicable.
  - **Differential Diagnosis**: Furuncle, carbuncle, abscess, cutaneous Crohn's disease, and acne.
- **Pathology Findings**: HS is a disease of hair follicles characterized by a perifollicular lymphocytic infiltrate with subsequent sebaceous gland loss.
  - **Gross**: HS is characterized by inflamed nodules, abscesses, and pus-discharging tunnels. The inflammatory changes start around hair follicles. Persistent chronic immune response leads to pain, pus, tissue destruction, and scarring.
  - **Microscopic Finding**: The histological changes are variable and consists of inflammatory infiltrate involving hair follicles and apocrine glands. Histological findings include poral occlusion, simple folliculitis, sinus tract, epithelial cyst, abscess, diffuse dermal inflammation, pyogenic granuloma, and scarring.
  - **Differential Diagnosis**: Furuncle, carbuncle, abscess, cutaneous Crohn's disease, and acne.
- **Management**: Antibiotics, interleukin antibodies, tissue-sparing surgery, and carbon dioxide laser treatment.

Case 1

Clinical Findings: A 34-year-old female, has a family history of breast carcinoma, painful waxing, and waning dermal lesions in the axillae (Figs. 10.51, 10.52, 10.53, 10.54–10.56).

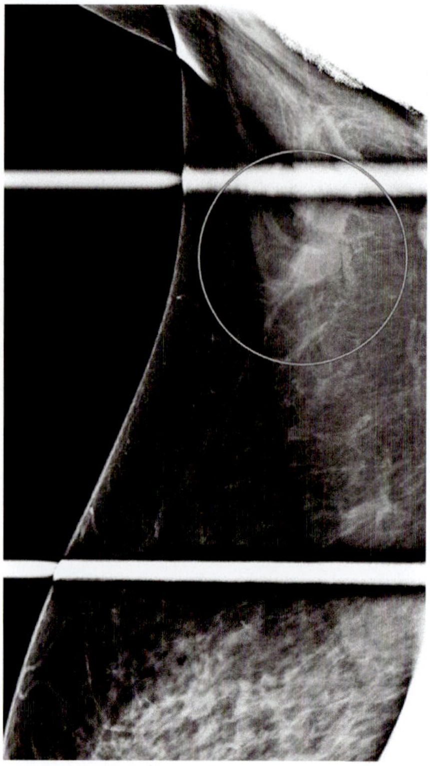

Fig. 10.51 **MMG findings**: The mammogram demonstrates an asymmetry with an irregular margin in the right axilla

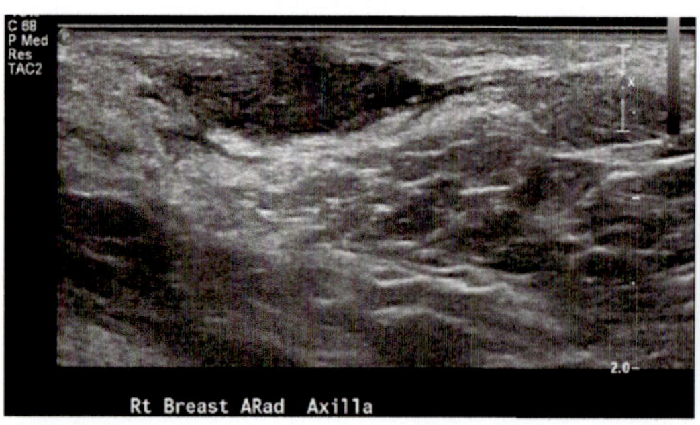

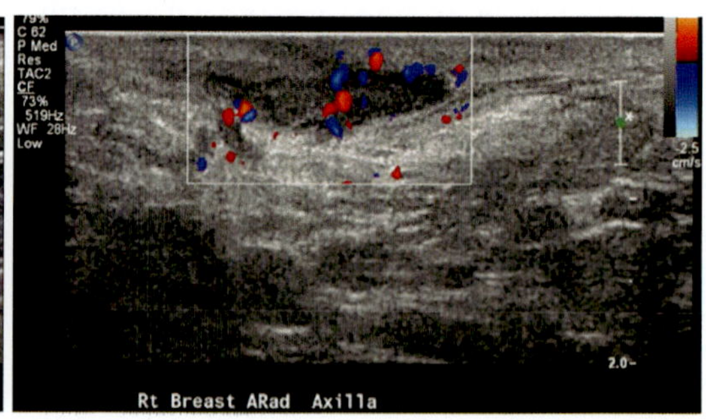

Figs. 10.52 and 10.53 **USG findings**: US demonstrates a vascular area of inflammation within the dermis, extending to the skin surface

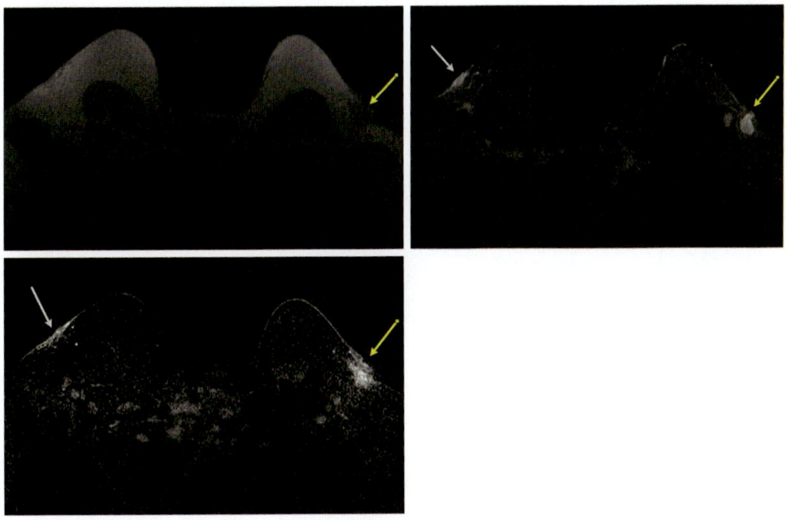

Figs. 10.54–10.56 MRI findings: MRI was performed due to elevated risk of breast CA due to family history, and demonstrates focal skin thickening with enhancement within the right axilla, and a small fluid collection with rim enhancement in the left axilla

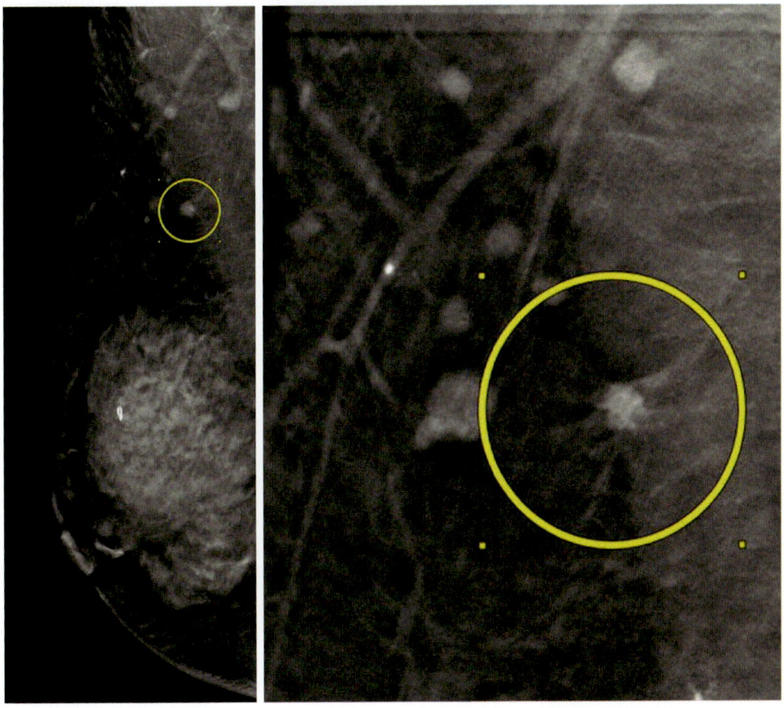

Figs. 10.57 and 10.58 MMG findings: A small, spiculated mass is noted in the right axilla, adjacent to normal axillary lymph nodes

Breast Carcinoma Presenting as Axillary Mass

Case 1

Clinical History: A 50-year-old female, presenting for screening mammography (Figs. 10.57, 10.58, 10.59, and 10.60).

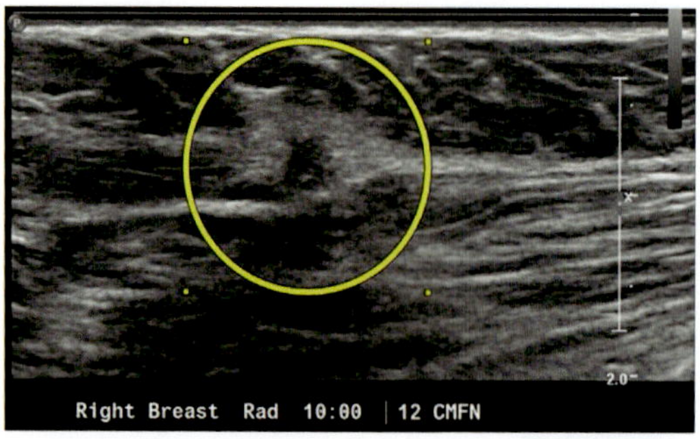

Fig. 10.59 **USG findings**: USG demonstrates a small, irregular hypoechoic mass with a hyperechoic halo

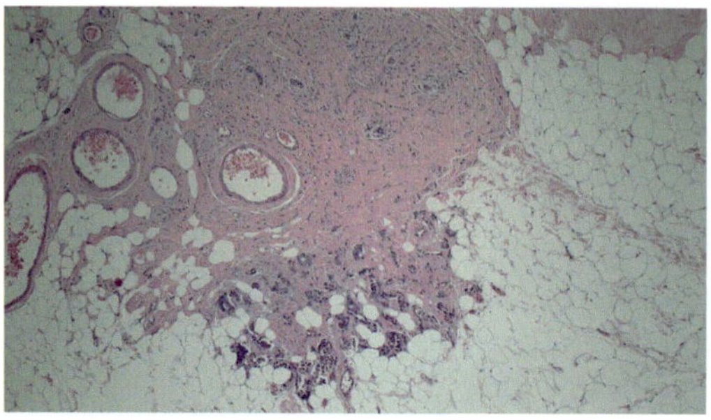

Fig. 10.60 Invasive ductal carcinoma histologic grade 2 (H&E, 4×). The tumor is located in the axilla adjacent to medium-sized vessels. No lymph node tissue is present

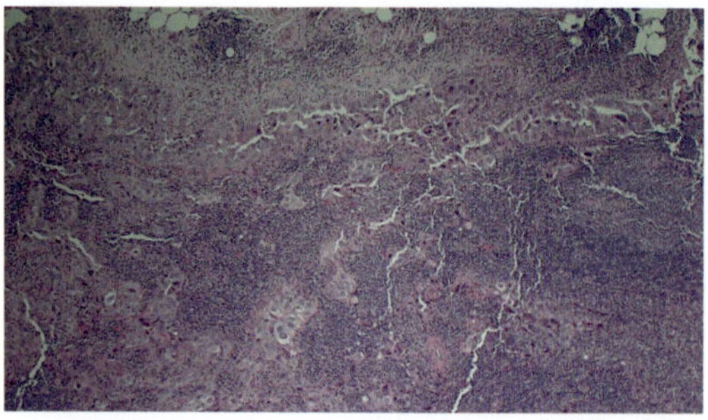

Fig. 10.61 Metastatic high-grade serous carcinoma involving axillary lymph node (H&E, 4×)

Non-Breast Lymph Node Metastasis

Case 1

A 72-year-old with a history of high-grade serous carcinoma of ovary presented with enlarged left axillary lymph node and elevated CA125 (Fig. 10.61).

References

1. Song HS, Jung SE, Kim YC, et al. Nipple eczema, and indicative manifestation of atopic dermatitis? A clinical, histological, and immunohistochemical study. Am J Dermatopathol. 2015;37(4):284–8.
2. Sweeney DJ, Wylie EJ. Mammographic appearances of mammary duct ectasia that mimic carcinoma in a screening programme. Australas Radiol. 1995;39(1):18–23. https://doi.org/10.1111/j.1440-1673.1995.tb00225.x. PMID: 7695522.
3. Allesio L, Maggi C, Savelli S, Angeletti M, Rabuffi P, Manganaro L, Porfiri LM. Adjunctive diagnostic value of ultrasonography evaluation in patients with suspected ductal breast disease. Radiol Med. 2007;112(3):354–65. https://doi.org/10.1007/s11547-007-0146-4. English, Italian. Epub 2007 Apr 20. PMID: 17440697.
4. Tso H, Yang WT. Duct ectasia. In: Berg WA, Leung JTW, editors. Diagnostic imaging: breast. 3rd ed. Amsterdam: Elsevier; 2019. p. 358–61.
5. Strachowski L, Berg WA. Mastitis. In: Berg WA, Leung JW, editors. Diagnostic imaging: breast. Philadelphia, PA: Elsevier; 2019. p. 900–3.
6. Dessauvagie B, Sterrett G, Bourke AG. Squamous metaplasia of lactiferous ducts (SMOLD). Clin Radiol. 2012;67:e42–6.
7. Lam E, Chan T, Wiseman SM. Breast abscess: evidence based management recommendations. Expert Rev Anti Infect Ther. 2014;12:753–62.
8. American Society of Breast Surgeons. Five things physicians and patients should question. 2018. https://www.choosingwisely.org/wp-content/uploads/2018/01/ASBrS_BenignBreastDisease-Choosing-Wisely-List.pdf.
9. Costanzo PR, Pacenza NA, Aszpis SM, Suárez SM, Pragier UM, Usher JGS, Cayoja MV, Iturrieta S, Gottlieb SE, Rey RA, Knoblovits P. Clinical and etiological aspects of gynecomastia in adult males: a multicenter study. BioMed Res Int. 2018;2018:8364824., 7 pages. https://doi.org/10.1155/2018/8364824.
10. Batteux B, Llopis B, Muller C, Khouri C, Moragny J, Liabeuf S, Masmoudi K, Gras V, French National Network of Pharmacovigilance Centres. The drugs that mostly frequently induce gynecomastia: a national case-noncase study. Therapie. 2020;75(3):225–38. https://doi.org/10.1016/j.therap.2019.06.001. Epub 2019 Jun 20. PMID: 31471065.
11. Lorek M, Tobolska-Lorek D, Kalina-Faska B, Januszek-Trzciakowska A, Gawlik A. Clinical and biochemical phenotype of adolescent males with gynecomastia. J Clin Res Pediatr Endocrinol. 2019;11(4):388–94. https://doi.org/10.4274/jcrpe.galenos.2019.2019.0027.
12. Acharya SV. Clinical features, presentation and hormonal parameters in patients with pubertal gynecomastia. J Fam Med Prim Care. 2021;10(2):648–51. https://doi.org/10.4103/jfmpc.jfmpc_1987_20.
13. Kornegoor R, Verschuur-Maes AHJ, Buerger H, van Diest PJ. The 3-layered ductal epithelium in gyneco-

mastia. Am J Surg Pathol. 2012;36(5):762–8. https://doi.org/10.1097/PAS.0b013e31824324e6.
14. Kanakis GA, Nordkap L, Bang AK, Calogero AE, Bártfai G, Corona G, Forti G, Toppari J, Goulis DG, Jørgensen N. EAA clinical practice guidelines-gynecomastia evaluation and management. Andrology. 2019;7(6):778–93. https://doi.org/10.1111/andr.12636. Epub 2019 May 16. PMID: 31099174.
15. Eghtedari M, Yang WT. Gynecomastia. In: Berg WA, Leung JTW, editors. Diagnostic imaging: breast. 3rd ed. Amsterdam: Elsevier; 2019. p. 958–63.
16. del Riego J, Pitarch M, Codina C, et al. Multimodality approach to the nipple-areolar complex: a pictorial review and diagnostic algorithm. Insights Imaging. 2020;11:89. https://doi.org/10.1186/s13244-020-00896-1.
17. Winkler NS, Yang WT. Tubular adenoma and nipple adenoma. In: Berg WA, Leung JW, editors. Diagnostic imaging: breast. Philadelphia, PA: Elsevier; 2019. p. 604–8.
18. Dillon DA, Lester SC. Lesions of the nipple. Surg Pathol Clin. 2009;2(2):391–412. https://doi.org/10.1016/j.path.2009.02.010. Epub 2009 Jun 2. PMID: 26838328.
19. Bonito MD, Cantile M, Collina F, et al. Adenoma of the nipple: a clinicopathological report of 13 cases. Oncol Lett. 2014;7(6):1839–42. https://doi.org/10.3892/ol.2014.2000.
20. Tatterton MR, Fiddes R. Nipple adenoma: a review of the literature. Ann Breast Surg. 2019;3:29.
21. Rosen PP. Rosen's breast pathology. 3rd ed. Philadelphia: Lippincott Williams & Wilkins (Wolters Kluwer); 2009.
22. Tavassoli FA, Devilee P, editors. Pathology and genetics of tumours of the breast and female genital organs, World Health Organization classification of tumors. Lyon: IARC Press; 2003.
23. Jorns JM. Papillary lesions of the breast: a practical approach to diagnosis. Arch Pathol Lab Med. 2016;140(10):1052–9. https://doi.org/10.5858/arpa.2016-0219-RA.
24. Lakhani SR, Ellis IO, Schnitt SJ, Tan PH, van de Vijver MJ, editors. WHO classification of tumours of the breast, World Health Organization classification of tumours, vol. 4. Lyon: IARC Press; 2012.
25. Strachowski L, Mercado CL. Papilloma, benign. In: Berg WA, Leung JW, editors. Diagnostic imaging: breast. Philadelphia, PA: Elsevier; 2019. p. 590–2.
26. Brookes MJ, Bourke AG. Radiological appearances of papillary breast lesions. Clin Radiol. 2008;63:1265–73.
27. Sarma DP, Stevens T. Infiltrating syringomatous eccrine adenoma of the nipple: a case report. Cases J. 2009;2:9118. https://doi.org/10.1186/1757-1626-2-9118.
28. Montgomery ND, Bianchi GD, Klauber-Demore N, Budwit DA. Bilateral syringomatous adenomas of the nipple: case report with immunohistochemical characterization of a rare tumor mimicking malignancy. Am J Clin Pathol. 2014;141(5):727–31. https://doi.org/10.1309/AJCPFJUZTLL0VGNX. PMID: 24713747.
29. Davis KM, Sobolewski RN, Berg WA. Paget disease of nipple. In: Berg WA, Leung JW, editors. Diagnostic imaging: breast. Philadelphia, PA: Elsevier; 2019. p. 896–8.
30. Lim HS, Jeong SJ, Lee JS, et al. Paget disease of the breast: mammographic, US, and MR imaging findings with pathologic correlation. Radiographics. 2011;31:1817–2114.
31. Dubar S, Boukrid M, Bouquet de Joliniere J, Guillou L, Vo QD, Major A, Ali NB, Khomsi F, Feki A. Paget's breast disease: a case report and review of the literature. Front Surg. 2017;4:51. https://doi.org/10.3389/fsurg.2017.00051. PMID: 29109950; PMCID: PMC5660109.
32. Karakas C. Paget's disease of the breast. J Carcinog. 2011;10:31. https://doi.org/10.4103/1477-3163.90676.
33. National Comprehensive Cancer Network. Breast cancer: special situations-Paget's disease (Version 5, 2020). 2021. https://www.nccn.org/professionals/physician_gls/pdf/breast.pdf.
34. Marino MA, Avendano D, Zapata P, Riedl CC, Pinker K. Lymph node imaging in patients with primary breast cancer: concurrent diagnostic tools. Oncologist. 2020;25(2):e231–42. https://doi.org/10.1634/theoncologist.2019-0427. Epub 2019 Oct 14. PMID: 32043792; PMCID: PMC7011661.
35. Yang WT, Suen M, Metreweli C. Mammographic, sonographic and histopathological correlation of benign axillary masses. Clin Radiol. 1997;52(2):130–5. https://doi.org/10.1016/s0009-9260(97)80106-7. PMID: 9043047.
36. Saunte DML, Jemec GBE. Hidradenitis suppurativa: advances in diagnosis and treatment. JAMA. 2017;318(20):2019–32. https://doi.org/10.1001/jama.2017.16691. PMID: 29183082.
37. Wortsman X. Imaging of hidradenitis suppurativa. Dermatol Clin. 2016;34(1):59–68. https://doi.org/10.1016/j.det.2015.08.003. PMID: 26617359.

Skin Thickening and Vascular Lesions

11

Liva Andrejeva, Sonali Lanjewar, Graham Woolf, Brigid Killelea, Kirstyn Brownson, Peter Podany, and Malini Harigopal

Skin Thickening Diffuse: Benign

Congestive Heart Failure (CHF)

***Congestive Heart Failure (CHF)*:** Congestive heart failure (CHF) is a relatively common disease which can lead to systemic venous congestion and diffuse edema. Imaging will show typical features of edema and volume overload, almost always bilaterally. These imaging findings are nonspecific and clinical correlation with physical exam findings and laboratory values is the key to diagnosis.

L. Andrejeva
Department of Radiology and Biomedical Imaging, Yale School of Medicine, New Haven, CT, USA
e-mail: liva.andrejeva@yale.edu

S. Lanjewar
Department of Pathology, Albert Einstein College of Medicine, Bronx, NY, USA

G. Woolf
Department of Radiology, Yale University, New Haven, CT, USA
e-mail: graham.woolf@yale.edu

B. Killelea
Department of Surgery, Brigham and Women's Hospital, Boston, MA, USA

K. Brownson
Department of Surgery, University of Utah, Salt Lake City, UT, USA
e-mail: Kirstyn.Brownson@hci.utah.edu

P. Podany · M. Harigopal (✉)
Department of Pathology, Yale University, New Haven, CT, USA
e-mail: peter.podany@yale.edu; malini.harigopal@yale.edu

- **Clinical Presentation:** In the setting of CHF patients may present with bilateral breast swelling and skin tightness in addition to other systemic signs of CHF such as dyspnea on exertion and orthopnea.
- **Imaging Findings:**
  - **Mammography**: CHF typically appears as bilateral interstitial edema of the breast as evidenced by trabecular thickening, thickening of Cooper's ligaments, and bilateral diffuse skin thickening [1, 2] (Fig. 11.1).
  - **US**: CHF will typically present on ultrasound as thickened skin, with heterogeneous echotexture, and may show thickening of the underlying glandular tissue [1, 2].
  - **MRI**: On MRI there will be bilateral, thickened, diffusely T2 hyperintense trabeculae and skin, reflecting edema.
  - **BI-RADS**: 2.
  - **Differential Diagnosis**: Inflammatory breast cancer, mastitis, superior vena cava syndrome, renal failure, liver failure (and other low protein states).
- **Pathology Findings:**
  - **Microscopic Histology:** Similar findings to lymphedema with increased spacing between collagen fibers, and no evidence of atypia.

M. Harigopal et al. (eds.), *Radiology Pathology Correlations of Breast Lesions*,
https://doi.org/10.1007/978-3-031-65711-5_11

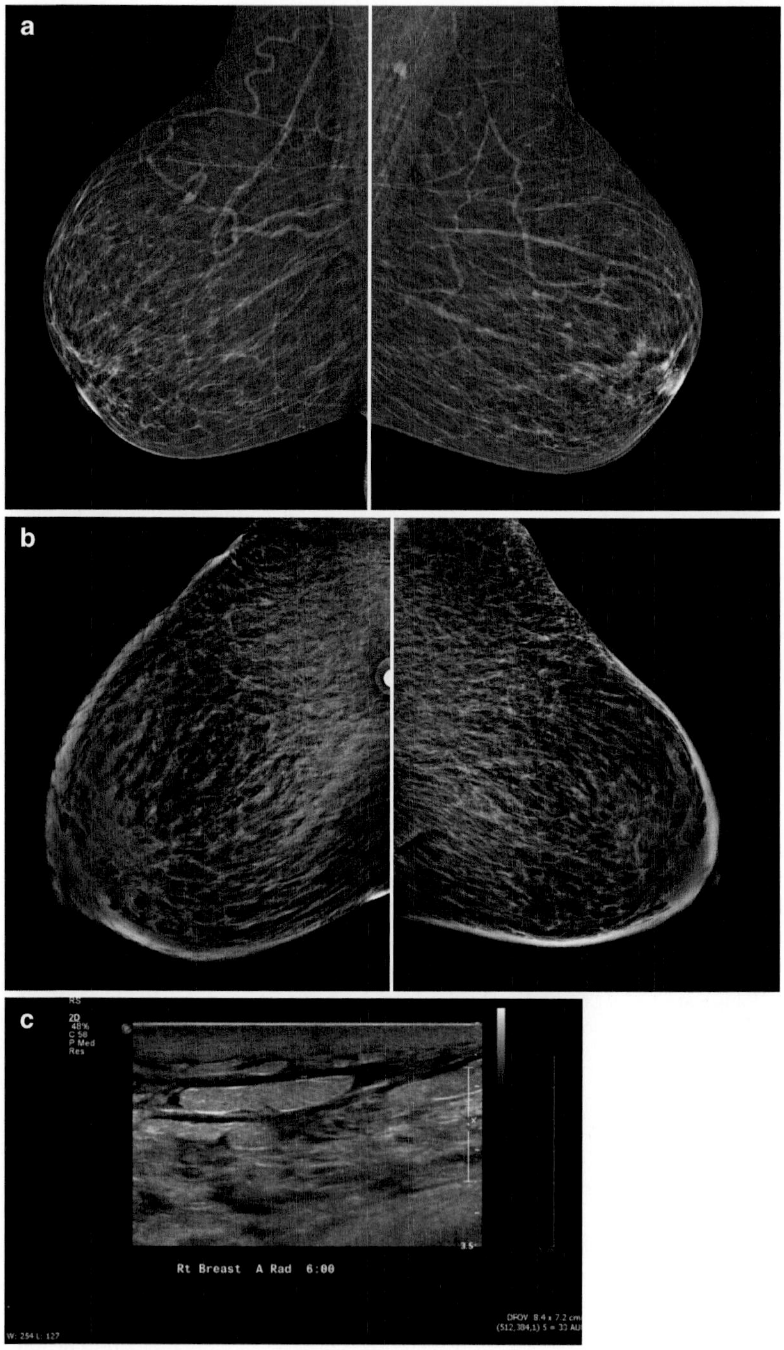

Fig. 11.1 Mammography imaging of a 72-year-old woman with CHF before (**a**) and after (**b**) progression of her congestive heart failure. After progression there is increased edema in the breast tissue as well as thickening of the skin noted. Ultrasound showed increased edema as well (**c**)

- **Differential Diagnosis:** Lymphedema.
- **Management:** Treatment is focused on medical management of the underlying CHF.

Lymphedema

***Lymphedema*:** Lymphedema is an often chronic condition that occurs due to accumulation of lymphatic fluid within the breast tissue, leading to inflammation. It is commonly seen secondary to breast cancer or breast cancer treatments. In breast cancer patients, postoperative edema can occur after axillary staging procedures at a rate up to 41% [3]. Skin thickening and edema are typically seen 6–12 months after the axillary surgery and resolve within 1–3 years [4]. The breast may show fibrosis and atrophy as a result of lymphatic obstruction and lymph stasis. Tumor can directly obstruct lymphatics, and both surgery and radiation therapy can damage lymphatics and lead to lymphedema. Other etiologies include trauma, infection, and congenital abnormalities. On imaging lymphedema will appear as unilateral breast edema. The imaging findings are nonspecific, and unilateral breast edema without an appropriate history to suggest lymphedema warrants a biopsy. In cases of persistent or increased breast edema, recurrent carcinoma should be considered [5].

- **Clinical Presentation:** Lymphedema will often present as unilateral upper extremity swelling, discomfort, and non-pitting edema.
- **Imaging Findings:**
  - **Mammography**: Lymphedema typically appears as unilateral increased density of the breast parenchyma, trabecular thickening, thickening of Cooper's ligaments, and unilateral diffuse skin thickening [6, 7] (Fig. 11.2).
  - **US**: Lymphedema will present on ultrasound as thickened skin with heterogeneous echotexture and may show increased echogenicity of the subcutaneous tissues.
  - **MRI**: On MRI there will be bilateral thickened, diffusely T2 hyperintense trabeculae and skin, reflecting edema [8].
  - **BI-RADS**: 2 or 4. Unilateral breast edema without an appropriate history to suggest a benign etiology warrants a biopsy.
  - **Differential Diagnosis**: DVT, breast cancer recurrence, metastatic disease, adenopathy secondary to cancer or infection.
- **Pathology Findings:**
  - **Microscopic Histology:** Lymphatic ectasia with edema between collagen fibers without evidence of atypia are the common findings [9] (Fig. 11.3).

    Fat necrosis may be present.

    Increased fibrosis extending into adipose tissue may be seen.

    May be associated with inflammation.

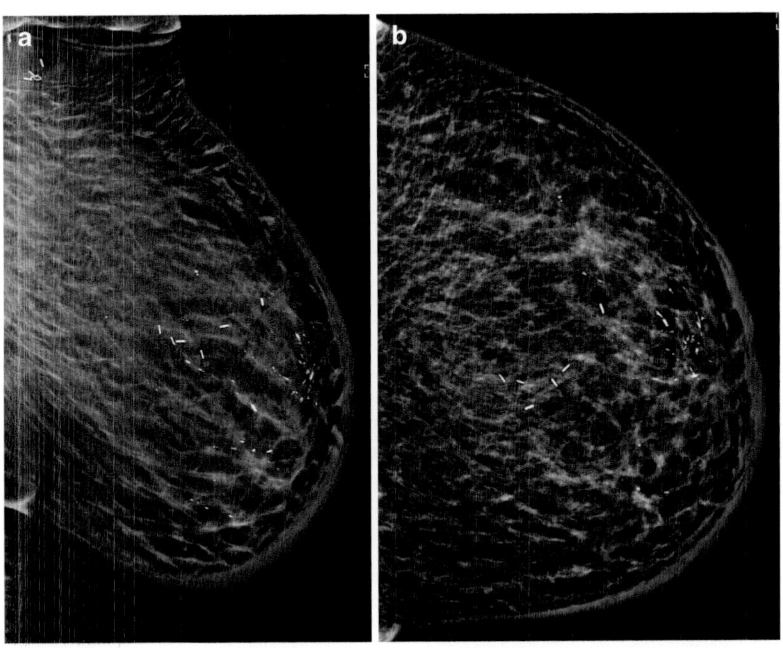

Fig. 11.2 A 74-year-old female status post-lumpectomy with axillary dissection and radiation. Mammogram of the left breast (**a, b**) demonstrates diffuse trabecular thickening, and skin thickening consistent with lymphedema

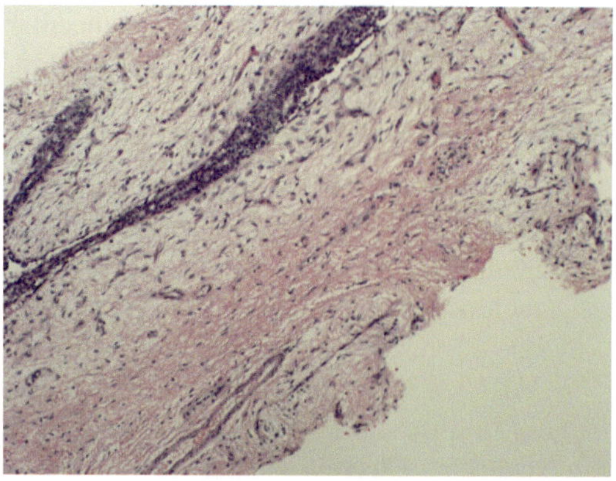

Fig. 11.3 A 50-year-old woman presented with a right breast mass. Ultrasound was performed and the lesion was moderately suspicious and called BIRADS 4. Core needle biopsy was performed revealing a fibroadenoma in edematous stroma. The collagen strands are loose and edema can be seen between the fibers

- **Differential Diagnosis:** Lipoma, mastitis if associated with inflammation, congestive heart failure.
- **Management:** Management for lymphedema is dependent on stage and consists of treatment options ranging from manual lymphatic drainage, progressive resistance training, use of compression garments, and intermittent pneumatic compression, to surgical interventions such as lymphovenous bypass and lymph node transfer [8, 10].

Breast Abscesses:

See Chap. 3.

Postradiation Change

***Postradiation Change*:** Radiation therapy to the breast and chest wall is often a part of breast cancer treatment strategies and can lead to radiation-induced changes in the breast. The pathophysiology involves radiation-induced inflammation to the breast parenchyma and vasculature potentially leading to fibrosis and/or necrosis. Skin findings can include erythema, induration, skin retraction, and ulceration. Breast tissue edema and skin thickening are also common findings. A potential late effect of radiation therapy to the breast is radiation-induced fibrosis, although the risk for fibrosis following conventional radiation therapy for breast cancer is low. Radiation-induced fibrosis can appear as architectural distortions, skin retraction, and even as spiculated masses within the treatment field, making differentiation from recurrent or residual malignancy difficult [11–13]. Features suggestive of benignity include changing appearances on different projections, thick spiculations, and central lucencies [14]. However, close attention on follow-up is necessary because decrease in size and prominence over time is the most reliable imaging finding of benignity [15, 16].

Biopsy is needed to establish diagnosis and rule out the presence of breast carcinoma.

- **Clinical Presentation:** Acute skin changes postradiation typically present within 90 days of radiation therapy, while chronic changes develop months to years later [17]. Risk factors for the development of postradiation cutaneous toxicity include, darker skin, large cumulative dose, smoking, obesity, and larger breast size [18–20]. Acute skin toxicity presents as a dry, erythematous patch at the site of radiation in the second week of radiotherapy. As the duration and dose of radiotherapy increases, patients may notice worsening edema, pruritus, tenderness, desquamation, and ulceration. In severe cases, fibrosis, necrosis, and skin ulceration also termed as radiation necrosis may occur [19]. Radiation changes can also result in Peau d'orange appearance of the skin due to lymphedema, which usually resolves within 1 year of treatment [21].

- **Imaging Findings:**
  - **Mammography**: On mammography post-radiation changes can have a variety of appearances and may show as skin thickening and breast tissue edema (Fig. 11.4).
    Radiation-induced fibrosis can appear as architectural distortions, skin retraction, heterogeneous or dystrophic calcifications and even as irregular, spiculated, soft-tissue density masses within the treatment field [12, 13].
  - **US**: Ultrasound may show a hypo or mixed echogenicity mass.
    Interspersed fat may be seen which can help identify the lesion as benign.
  - **MRI**: Will typically show trabecular and skin T2WI hyperintensity.
    Fibrosis may appear as a focal area of non-mass enhancement or as an irregular mass; usually displaying persistent kinetics on contrast-enhanced T1WI.
  - **BI-RADS**: 2–4. Fibrotic changes may appear similar to a new mass and biopsy may be warranted to rule out new or recurrent malignancy.
  - **Differential Diagnosis**: Recurrent breast cancer, inflammatory breast cancer, infection, and other causes of edema such as lymphedema and CHF.
- **Pathology Findings:**
  - **Microscopic Histology:** Atypical epithelial cells in lobules with large, hyperchromatic nuclei, and vacuolated cytoplasm (Fig. 11.5).
    Lobular sclerosis and atrophy may be present as well.
  - **Differential Diagnosis:** Residual tumor, atypical vascular lesions, angiosarcoma, lymphangioendothelioma.
  - **Management:** Treatment is primarily symptomatic. In rare cases of severe radiation-induced fibrosis, surgical excision has been effective.

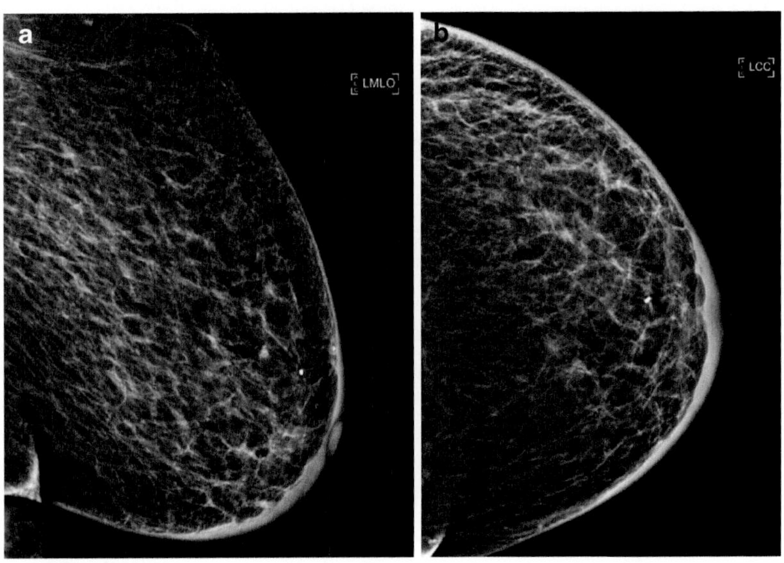

Fig. 11.4 A 76-year-old female presented status post left breast lumpectomy and radiation 9 months prior. Mammography was consistent with radiation changes, demonstrated skin thickening, and was called BI-RADS 2 (**a**, **b**)

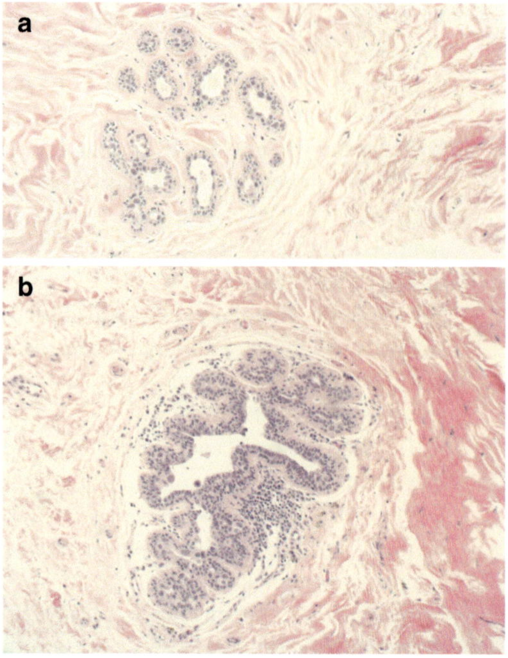

Fig. 11.5 Core needle biopsy from a 65-year-old woman with recent radiation therapy to the breast. In a background of sclerotic breast tissue the breast lobules and ducts demonstrate cellular atypia with nuclear pleomorphism, but retain normal overall architecture (**a**, **b**)

Mastitis: Acute and Chronic (Zuska's Disease)

Mastitis: Acute and Chronic (Zuska's Disease): Mastitis refers to inflammation of the breast tissue and has multiple different etiologies. Acute mastitis is most frequently secondary to a bacterial infection, commonly *Staphylococcus aureus* and Strep species [22, 23]. Diagnosis is clinical, although an ultrasound to rule out abscess is typically performed. Chronic mastitis can be caused by repeated infections, chronic inflammatory conditions such as Chronic Granulomatous Mastitis (CGM), or a combination thereof [22, 23]. Chronic mastitis may be complicated by recurrent abscesses, sinus tracks and fistulas (Zuska's disease). Imaging typically will show asymmetries or irregular masses, with or without associated adenopathy and abscesses [24]. Biopsy is necessary to exclude malignancy.

- **Clinical Presentation:** In acute mastitis, patients typically present with pain, focal swelling, and erythema. Chronic Granulomatous Mastitis may present as a single mass or multiple peripheral, tender masses.
- **Imaging Findings:**
  - **Mammography**: Acute mastitis is commonly subareolar.

    Focally increased breast density and skin thickening with or without dilated subareolar ducts is typically seen at the site of infection [25] (Fig. 11.6).

    CGM may present as asymmetries or irregular peripheral masses with indistinct margins, skin thickening, and adenopathy [26].
  - **US**: Sonographic findings of acute mastitis include skin thickening, focally increased echogenicity of the affected tissue due to edema, and increased vascularity on Doppler imaging [25], (Fig. 11.7).

    There may also be dilated, debris-filled ducts. Abscesses can be identified as focal thick walled, complex fluid collections.

    Adjacent reactive lymph nodes with diffusely thickened cortices may be present.

    Ultrasound in CGM will show irregular, hypoechoic masses with or without abscesses (complex fluid collections). Sinuses and fistulae may be seen as hypoechoic linear tracts [26].
  - **MRI**: On MRI acute mastitis will appear as a focal T2 hyperintensity. An abscess may appear as a rim-enhancing mass on contrast-enhanced T1 sequences [25].

    On MRI CGM will appear as non-mass enhancements or as masses with heterogeneous or rim-enhancement, and variable kinetics on contrast-enhanced T1. They are typically T2 hypointense.

- **BI-RADS**: Acute mastitis: 2–4. Mass-like, recurrent, or atypical imaging findings may warrant a biopsy to exclude malignancy.

  Chronic Mastitis: 2–4 typically warrants biopsy to exclude malignancy if the diagnosis is not known.
- **Differential Diagnosis**: Breast cancer, Paget's disease, superficial thrombophlebitis, radiation-induced dermatitis.

- **Pathology Findings:**
  - **Microscopic Histology:** A dense inflammatory infiltrate is characteristic.

    In acute mastitis the infiltrate is predominantly neutrophilic and abscess formation may be present.

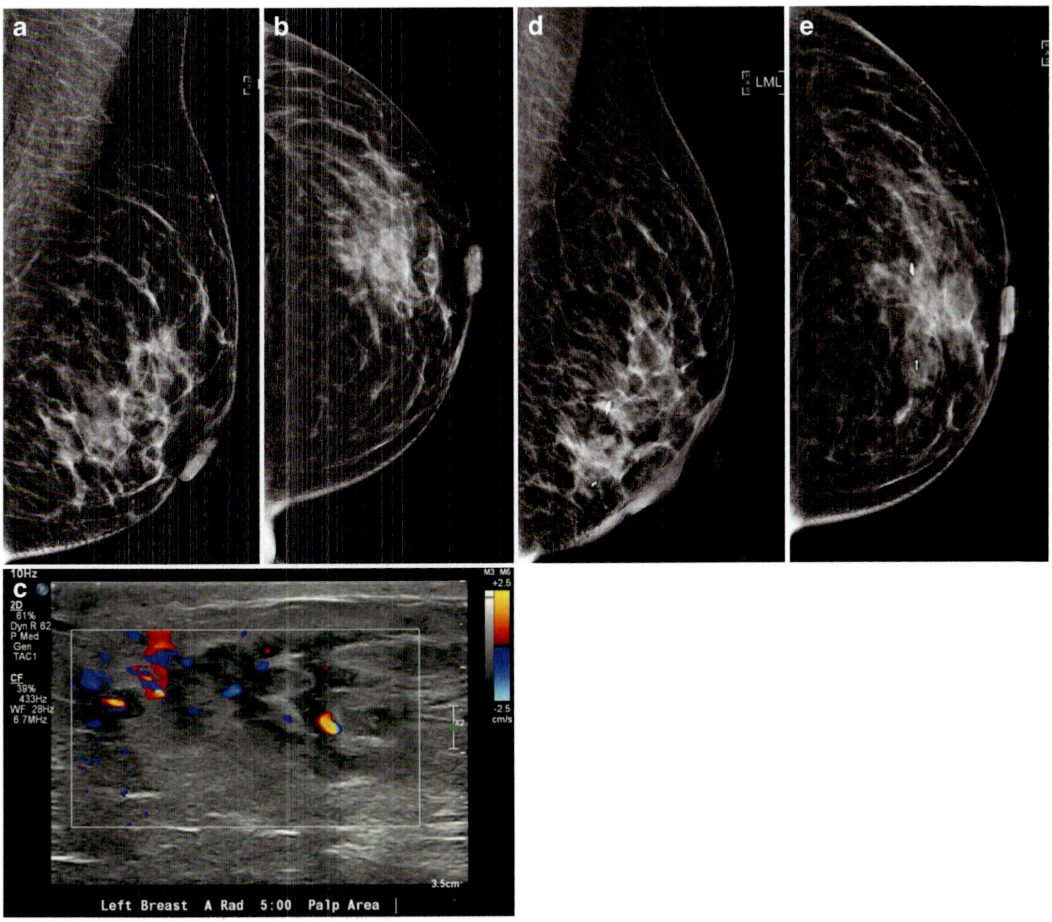

Fig. 11.6 A 22-year-old who presented with left breast pain. Mammogram (**a, b**) shows focal asymmetry with an indistinct margin in the left breast at 6:00 correlating to the area of reported pain. Ultrasound (**c**) showed an area in the left breast at 6 o'clock anterior depth with mixed echogenicity. This correlates as palpated to the reported pain and with mammography findings. Color flow imaging demonstrates that there is increased vascularity. These findings likely represent mastitis. The same 22-year-old on mammogram 4 months later showing increasing asymmetry with an indistinct margin in the left breast lower outer aspect anterior depth extending from 4 to 6 o'clock

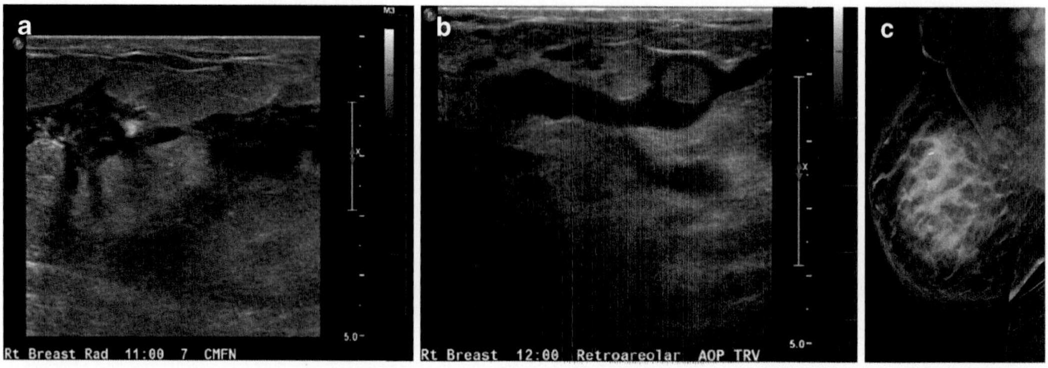

Fig. 11.7 A 29-year-old female, recently postpartum and breastfeeding, presents with a painful edematous right breast. Ultrasound showed an irregular hypoechoic mass and linear hypoechoic tracts suggestive of sinuses or fistulae tracts (**a**, **b**). Mammography also showed an irregular mass as well as skin thickening (**c**)

    - Necrosis may be present.
    - Normal breast tissue may be obscured.
    - Lymphocytic inflammation and granulation tissue may be seen as mastitis resolves (Fig. 11.8).

  In the case of cystic neutrophilic granulomatous mastitis there is lobulocentric mixed inflammation including neutrophils.

    - Lipid vacuoles may be present.
    - Non-necrotizing granulomas are generally found.
    - Gram stain may be positive for coryneform bacilli though molecular testing can also be used.

  Idiopathic granulomatous mastitis shares many features with cystic neutrophilic granulomatous mastitis with a lobulocentric granulomatous inflammation; however, microorganisms are not present (Fig. 11.9).

- **Differential Diagnosis:** Squamous metaplasia of lactiferous ducts, duct ectasia, fat necrosis, foreign body reaction.
- **Management:** Management of mastitis is dependent upon etiology. For acute mastitis, if cellulitis alone is present without accompanying abscess, then antibiotic coverage is sufficient [27]. If there is an associated abscess, drainage of this abscess is prudent. Per ASBrS Choosing Wisely® recommendations, percutaneous aspiration of the abscess should first be attempted prior to surgery in the form of incision and drainage [28]. However, there are instances, such as in the setting of devitalized tissue or abscess recalcitrant to repeat aspirations, where incision and drainage is required [28]. Chronic mastitis, like in the setting of periductal mastitis with fistulae, will require treatment with antibiotics, drainage of the abscess, and eventual excision of the fistulous tract and diseased duct(s) [29]. Antibiotic coverage for mastitis should target *Staphylococcus aureus* [30].

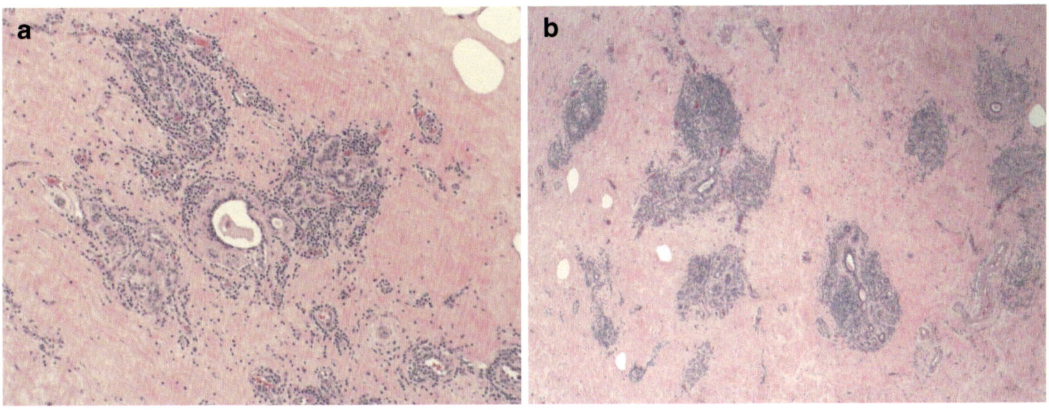

Fig. 11.8 Incidental mastitis seen on a resection specimen (**a**, **b**). There is lymphocytic inflammation with aggregate formation around the breast lobules and ducts

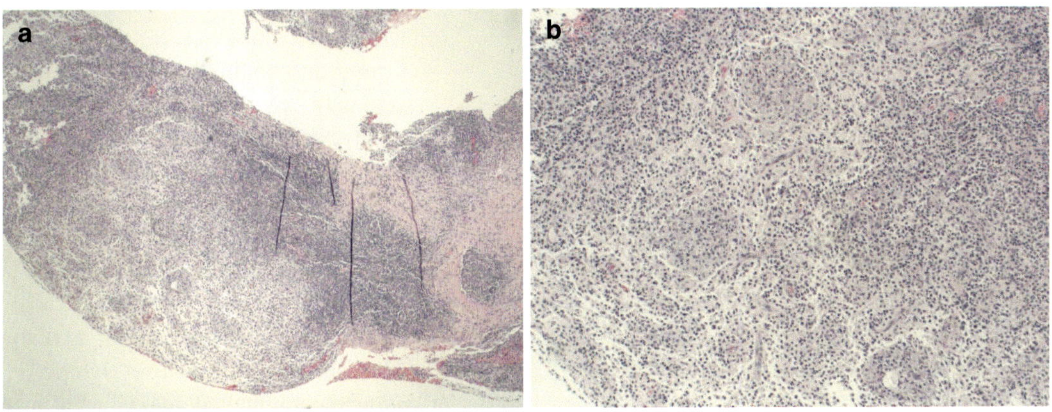

Fig. 11.9 Biopsy from a 35-year-old woman demonstrating chronic inflammation with granuloma formation consistent with chronic granulomatous disease (**a**, **b**)

Malignant

Invasive Ductal Carcinoma

See Chap. 7.

Inflammatory Breast Carcinoma

***Inflammatory Breast Carcinoma*:** Inflammatory breast carcinoma (IBC) is an extremely aggressive form of locally advanced breast cancer with a very poor prognosis. It is characterized by diffuse erythema, edema and involves more than 1/3rd of the breast skin with development of disease in a short span of time of less than 6 months [31]. It is characterized histologically by the presence of dermal lymphatic tumor emboli. Per AJCC staging criteria they are classified as T4d [32]. While any molecular subtype can present with IBC, the most common occurrence is with HER2+ and basal-like carcinoma. Increased angiogenesis and lymphangiogenesis has been noted to be associated with the classic clinical presentation in IBC [33]. Recent data suggests unknown alterations in the ALK pathway are found in IBC [34]. Typically, a skin punch biopsy is required to make a diagnosis.

- **Clinical Presentation:** Patients commonly experience tenderness and skin induration overlying an enlarging mass [31, 35]. However, in approximately 30% of patients, no palpable mass is evident [36]. The clinical picture is a result of lymphatic obstruction by dermal lymphatic tumor emboli. It affects younger women and the majority have local and/or distant metastases at the time of diagnosis [37].

- **Imaging Findings.**
  - **Mammography:** Mammographically, IBC will present as marked skin and trabecular thickening, often with axillary lymphadenopathy (Fig. 11.10).

    Masses may be radiographically occult or present as multiple, irregular masses.
  - **US:** Sonographically, IBC will demonstrate skin thickening, diffuse hyperechogenicity of the subcutaneous tissues with dilated lymphatics, and diffuse hypervascularity on Doppler imaging.

    Masses may present as multiple, irregular, hypoechoic masses with posterior acoustic shadowing.
  - **MRI:** Contrast-enhanced T1-weighted imaging typically shows skin thickening and enhancement and may show irregular masses or non-mass enhancements with rapid enhancement and washout kinetics.

    T2-weighted sequences will show diffuse edema.
  - **BI-RADS**: 5.
  - **Differential Diagnosis**: Other locally advanced breast cancer, metastatic disease, mastitis, postradiation changes, Paget's disease, lymphedema.
- **Pathology Findings**:
  - **Microscopic Histology**: Microscopic examination reveals the presence of tumor emboli in the dermal lymphovascular channels.

    Presence of dermal lymphovascular tumor emboli in the post excision specimen does not qualify for inflammatory breast carcinoma without the typical clinical findings.

    There is no desmoplastic response and no tumor infiltrating lymphocytes are identified (Fig. 11.11).

    Erythema does not represent a true inflammation.

    The tumor is generally high grade.

    IBC strongly expresses E-cadherin and seems to be associated with early metastasis.
  - **Differential Diagnoses:**

    Invasive or in situ carcinoma with retraction artifact. Use of myoepithelial markers such as P63, smooth muscle myosin and calponin along with endothelial markers like CD34, CD31, and D2-40 in combination with the clinical presentation can help establish the diagnosis.

    Mastitis: Clinical presentation and lactation history are important diagnostic clues favoring mastitis which responds favorably to antibiotics. Recurrent cases of mastitis should be further investigated with skin punch biopsy.

    Locally advanced cancers can cause ulceration and skin erythema. The characteristic clinical presentation is required for the diagnosis of inflammatory breast carcinoma.

    - Melanoma and lymphoma with extensive involvement of axillary lymphatics can cause lymphatic obstruction and edema. Clinical history with histomorphology and immunohistochemical markers for lymphoma and melanoma can help establish the diagnosis.
  - **Management**: Inflammatory breast cancer requires multi-modality therapy. Neoadjuvant chemotherapy is followed by surgery in the form of total mastectomy and level I and II axillary lymph node dissection if surgical resection to negative margins is anticipated [38, 39]. This is followed by adjuvant chest wall and comprehensive nodal basin radiation [38, 39]. If surgical resection to negative margins is thought to not be possible after chemotherapy, additional systemic chemotherapy and/or neoadjuvant radiation can be considered. Endocrine therapy should be administered in estrogen receptor (ER) and/or progesterone receptor (PR) positive patients [38, 39].

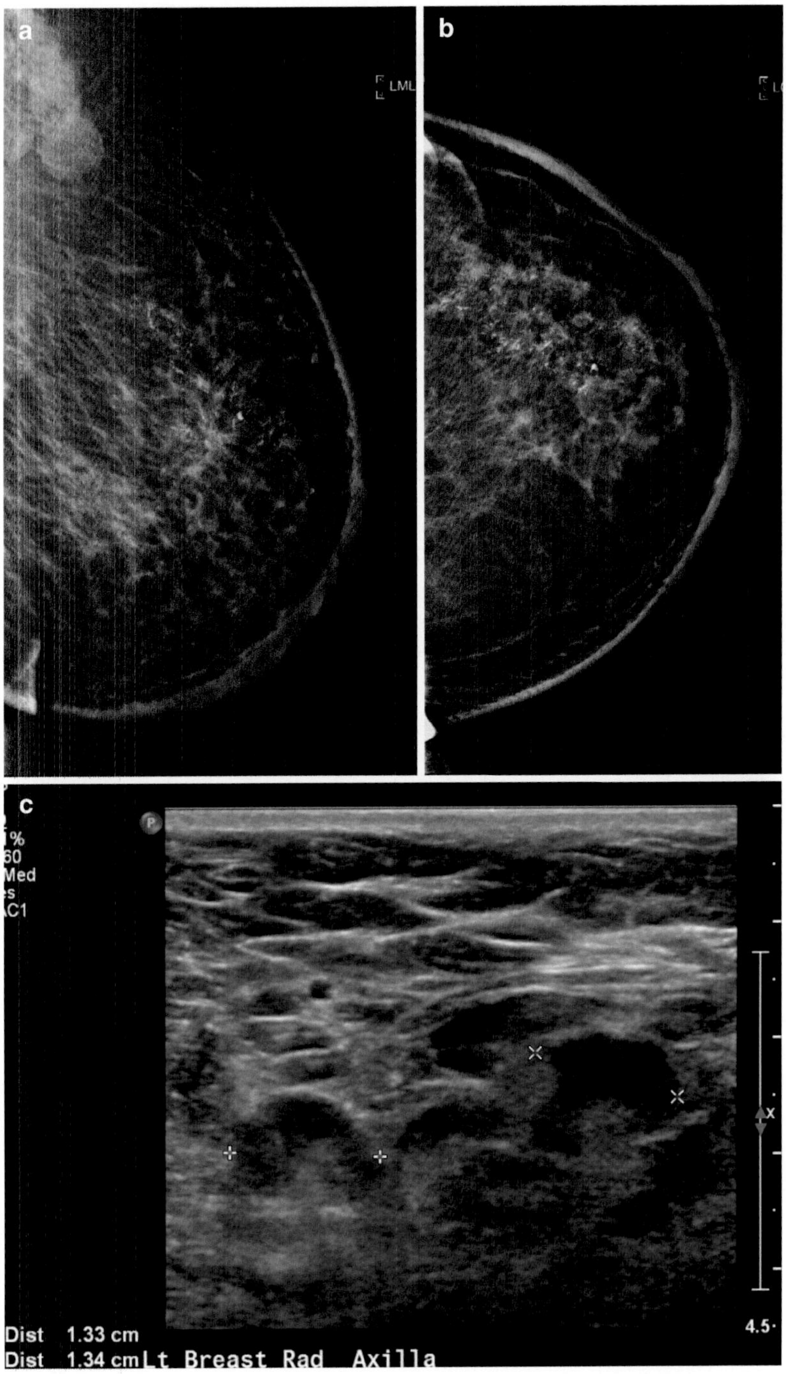

Fig. 11.10 A 58-year-old postmenopausal woman, noticed increasing redness in her left breast. Initially, this was attributed to a skin infection, and the patient took antibiotics for a few weeks, but the swelling and redness continued to progress and a diagnostic left breast skin biopsy and core needle biopsy of the breast showed invasive ductal carcinoma grade 2, ER and PR negative, HER-2 positive by FISH. Mammogram (**a**, **b**) shows linear and branching calcifications involving an area of at least 8 cm. There is diffuse skin thickening noted, suggestive of inflammatory breast cancer as well as prominent lymph nodes noted on MLO view. Ultrasound (**c**) also showed three separate enlarged left axillary lymph nodes

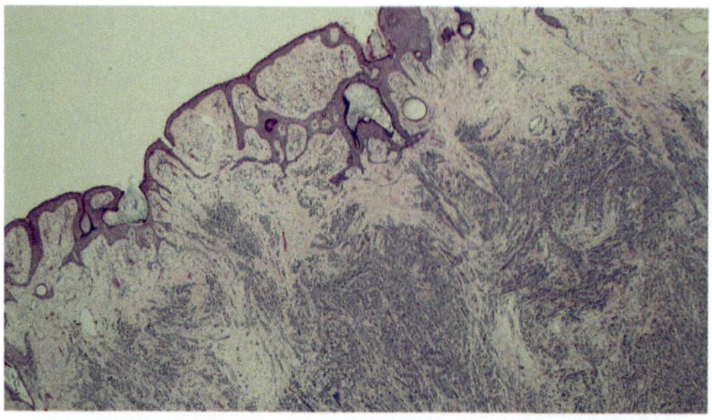

Fig. 11.11 Excisional specimen demonstrating inflammatory breast carcinoma on H&E (×200). There is a poorly differentiated tumor invading the tissue with minimal to no desmoplastic response. There is also an absence of tumor infiltrating lymphocytes

Locally Advanced Breast Carcinoma

***Locally Advanced Breast Carcinoma*:** Locally advanced breast carcinoma (LABC) represents bulky invasive disease involving breast skin, chest wall with or without extensive regional adenopathy and includes all primary inoperable nonmetastatic breast cancers, all T4 (a, b, c) breast cancers and inflammatory carcinoma (T4d) [40–43].

Tumors more than 5 cm in size with regional lymphadenopathy (N1–3), tumors of any size with direct extension to the chest wall, skin, or both (including ulceration or satellite nodules), regardless of regional lymphadenopathy, or tumors of any stage with the presence of regional lymphadenopathy (clinically fixed or matted axillary lymph nodes, or any of infraclavicular, supraclavicular, or internal mammary lymphadenopathy) are all included in locally advanced breast carcinomas [44]. Except for inflammatory breast carcinomas which are high grade, basal-like breast carcinomas and HER2-positive breast carcinomas, in most cases locally advanced breast cancers are heterogeneous with varying biological characteristics, and behaviors.

Most cases receive neoadjuvant chemotherapy due to inoperability at presentation and have poor prognosis. Around 2–3% invade skin without skin ulceration [45]. Presence of skin invasion is associated with higher nodal involvement [45]. Invasive lobular carcinomas rarely form a mass and can be missed on radiology and clinical examination resulting in a larger size at presentation. Even with combined modality treatment the medial survival ranges from 28 to 66 months [45–48].

- **Clinical Presentation:** In the United States, 10–15% of breast cancers present at a locally advanced stage [49]. Inflammatory breast carcinomas (IBC) typically occur at a younger age but when present in men are usually found at advanced ages [50]. T4a, b, and c stage locally advanced carcinomas are seen in older women [49].
- **Imaging Findings.**
  - **Mammography:** Mammography on locally advanced breast cancer will show a large mass, possibly associated with skin thickening and architectural distortion (Fig. 11.12).
  - **US:** Ultrasound typically shows a large, heterogeneous mass, sometimes with central necrosis, as well as skin thickening or ulceration.

    The mass will typically be hypervascular on Doppler imaging.
  - **MRI:** Contrast-enhanced T1 MRI will show a large, enhancing mass and will be the best imaging modality for evaluating extension into adjacent structures.
  - **BI-RADS**: 5.
  - **Differential Diagnosis**: Inflammatory breast carcinoma, mastitis, postradiation changes, metastatic disease.
- **Pathology Findings**:
  - **Gross:** Locally advanced breast carcinoma includes large bulky, fungating tumors, usually more than 5 cm in size. Due to the bulky nature of the tumor LABC can cause injury to breast skin, muscles, and lymph nodes [51].

    The tumors could be smaller with involvement of underlying chest wall or could cause extensive axillary lymphadenopathy, skin ulceration and form skin nodules.

    IBC, can cause swelling, redness, and by definition affects one third or more of

Fig. 11.12 A 64-year-old woman presented with a long-standing ulcerated mass in the medial aspect of the left breast. Mammography showed diffuse skin thickening and a large mass which was biopsied and found to be advanced involvement of the breast with carcinoma (**a**, **b**)

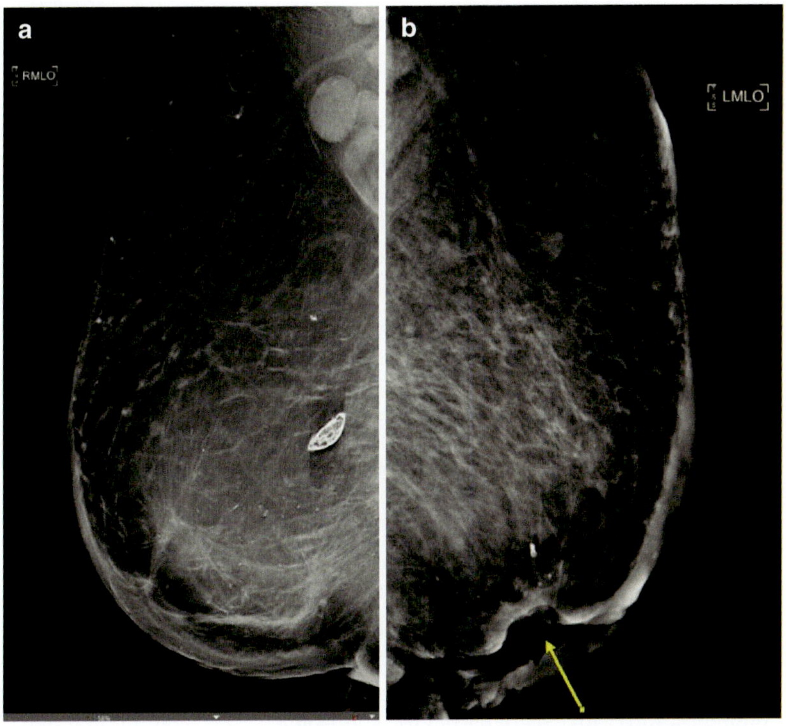

the breast with symptom development over a short time span (<6 months) [52].

- **Microscopic Histology**: Locally advanced breast carcinoma is a heterogeneous group of cancers with features that will vary from tumor to tumor (Fig. 11.13).
- **Management:** Neoadjuvant chemotherapy followed by surgical resection and radiotherapy is the preferred treatment modality. Overall, it has a poor prognosis with inflammatory breast cancers having worse survival [47, 48].

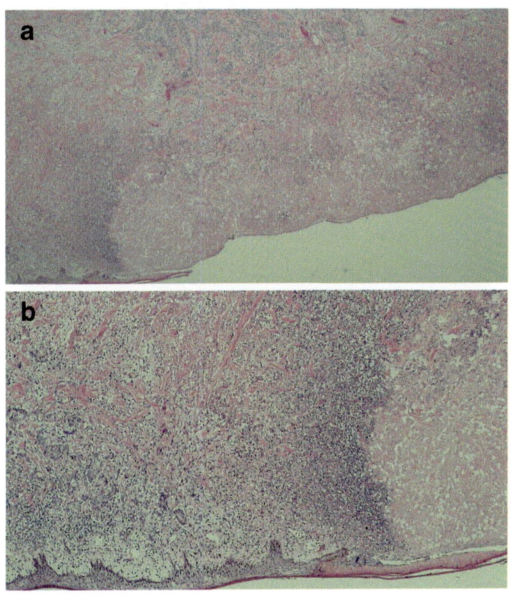

Fig. 11.13 An excisional biopsy demonstrating locally advanced breast cancer with ulceration and skin necrosis seen on low power (**a**). On higher power diffuse infiltration of the tissue by pleomorphic, discohesive tumor cells can be seen (**b**)

Diffuse Advanced ILC (Shrinking Breast with Skin Thickening):

***Diffuse Advanced ILC (Shrinking Breast with Skin Thickening)*:** Invasive lobular carcinoma (ILC) is the second most common type of invasive breast cancer accounting for 10–15% of cases [53]. The pathogenesis involves loss of normal cell adhesion and diffuse tumor infiltration in single-file columns of cells. It is associated with mutations in the CDH1 gene which encodes the E-cadherin cell adhesion protein [53]. ILC is typically larger than invasive ductal carcinoma at the time of diagnosis. Imaging may show a large, spiculated, mass, occasionally with associated architectural distortions. However, many ILC are mammographically occult, with sensitivity ranging from 57% to 81% and lower in women with dense breasts [54, 55]. In advanced disease, occasionally a shrinking breast may be the only mammographic finding [56]. See Chap. 5 for additional information on invasive lobular carcinoma.

- **Clinical Presentation:** If there is diffuse, advanced disease patients may present with an asymmetric, shrunken breast with areas of skin thickening and nipple retraction.
- **Imaging Findings:**
  - **Mammography**: Invasive lobular carcinoma can be difficult to detect mammographically as the lesions are often isodense to normal fibroglandular tissue and exhibit an infiltrative growth pattern.

    When seen, they can present as large, spiculated masses occasionally with associated architectural distortions. Advanced disease may display skin thickening, nipple retraction, and decreasing breast size (Fig. 11.14).
  - **US**: ILC will most commonly present as an irregular, hypoechoic mass with posterior acoustic shadowing on ultrasound.
  - **MRI**: Contrast-enhanced T1W1 MRI is the most sensitive imaging modality for ILC, which typically appears as an irregular, spiculated mass with heterogeneous enhancement.
  - **BI-RADS**: 5.
  - **Differential Diagnosis**: Invasive ductal carcinoma, radial scar, stromal fibrosis.
- **Pathology Findings:** See Chap. 5 for pathological findings in invasive lobular carcinoma (Fig. 11.15).
  - **Management:** Surgery followed by radiation, with endocrine therapy and/or chemotherapy.

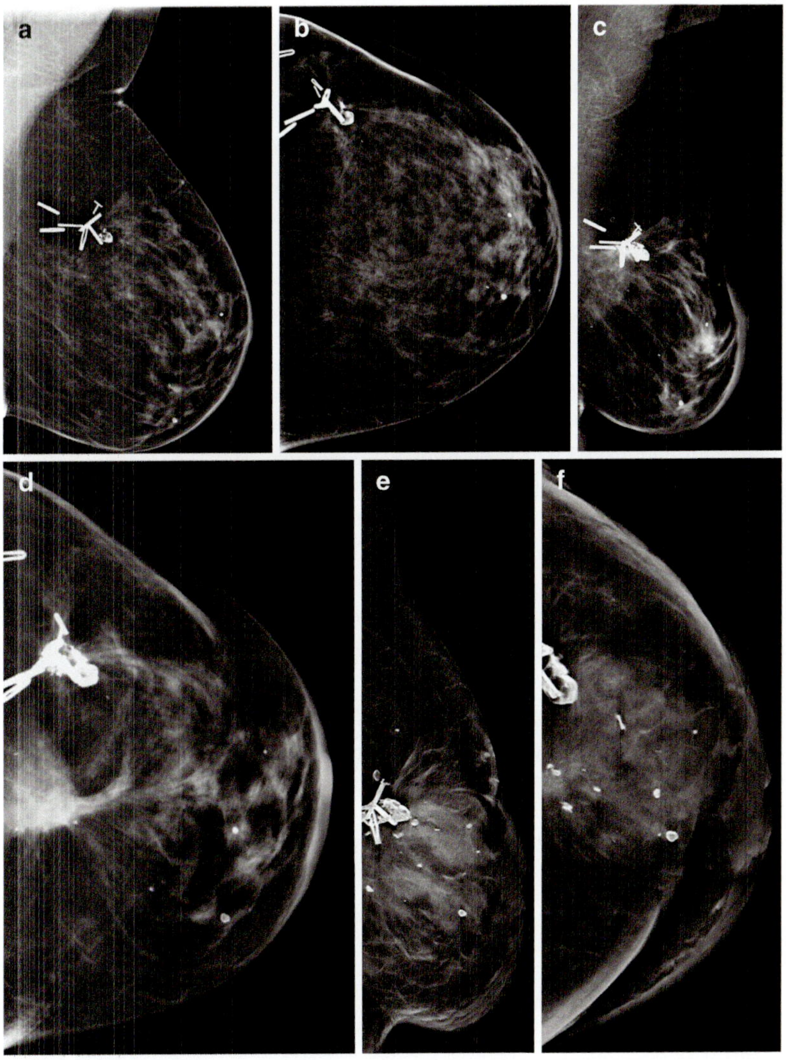

Fig. 11.14 A 57-year-old female with a history of diffuse invasive lobular carcinoma of the left breast, status post-lumpectomy. Mammogram in 2007 showed a breast with post-lumpectomy changes on LMLO (**a**) and amorphous calcifications in the medial left breast on LCC (**b**). LMLO and LCC in 2010 (**c, d** respectively) showed decreased breast size from the prior as well as postsurgical and postradiations changes. LMLO and LCC in 2018 (**e**, **f**) showed further decrease in size from the priors with postsurgical and postradiation changes

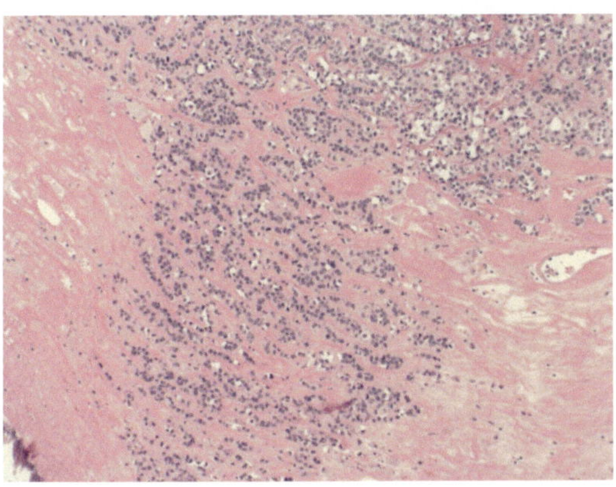

Fig. 11.15 A 63-year-old woman with history of diffuse invasive lobular breast cancer on excision which showed invasive lobular carcinoma with characteristic single filing tumor cells

Vascular Lesions, Benign

Papillomas

See Chap. 3.

Fibroadenomas

See Chap. 2.

Lymphangiomas

See Chap. 3.

Benign Vascular Malformations

***Benign Vascular Malformations*:** There is a spectrum of benign vascular malformations that can occur in the breast which are the result of the abnormal proliferation of vascular cells leading to a focal, disorganized collection of irregular vasculature. These include, arteriovenous malformations (AVMs), venous malformations, hemangiomas, and lymphangiomas. The majority are congenital; however, they can be the result of trauma or surgery [57, 58]. Primary, benign vascular tumors of the breast are relatively rare, and malignant neoplasms will need to be excluded on initial presentation. Lymphangiomas, for example, are exceedingly rare in the breast with only sporadic case reports in the literature [59]. They can however be associated with several genetic syndromes, including Klippel-Trenaunay-Weber syndrome, Turner syndrome, and Maffuci syndrome [57, 58]. Classic imaging findings are of superficial, well-circumscribed, lobulated masses that are T2WI hyperintense with variable enhancement patterns on contrast-enhanced T1WI [60, 61]. Treatment is only indicated if the lesion is causing the patient discomfort [57].

- **Clinical Presentation:** Most of these entities are diagnosed in childhood but may be seen incidentally on asymptomatic screening mammography.
- **Imaging Findings:**
  - **Mammography**: Commonly, benign vascular proliferations will appear as a round or irregular, often superficial, circumscribed mass on mammography (Fig. 11.16).
  - **US**: The ultrasound appearance of benign vascular proliferations can vary depending on the morphology of the abnormal vasculature.

    Typically, the lesions will appear as superficial, circumscribed masses.

    Malformations with large, cystic cavities (such as lymphangiomas) may appear hypoechoic.

    Those with numerous small cystic spaces and bridging septae (such as cap-

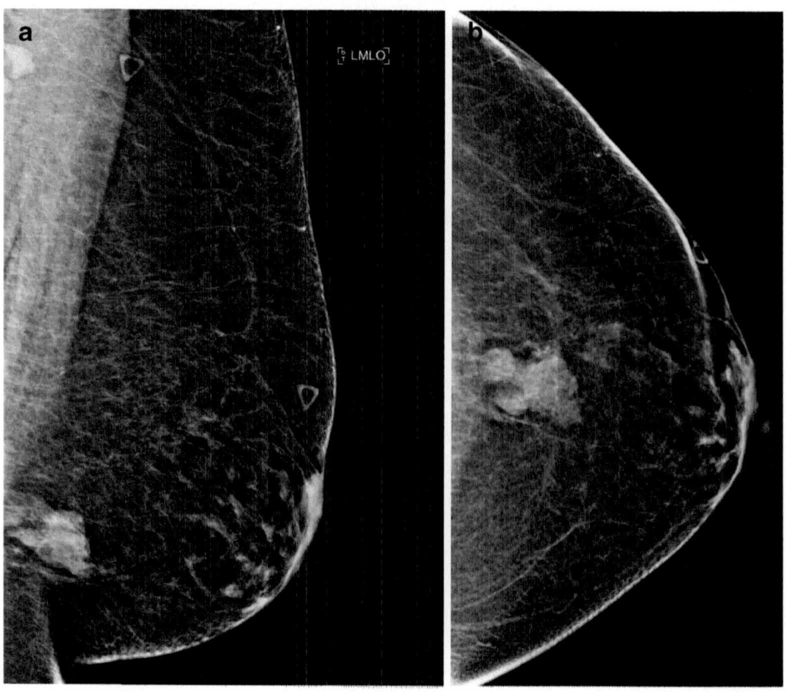

Fig. 11.16 A 42-year-old woman with history of reduction mammoplasty presents for diagnostic evaluation for a palpable mass. On mammography there is an irregular mass with a lobulated margin in the left breast (**a**, **b**). On ultrasound there is an anechoic mass with lobulated margins (**c**). The lesion was called BI-RADS 4. On biopsy the lesion was found to be an arteriovenous malformation

Fig. 11.16 (continued)

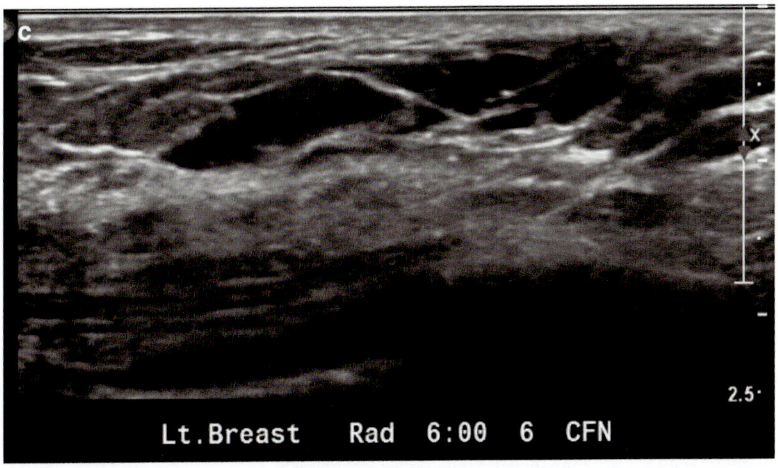

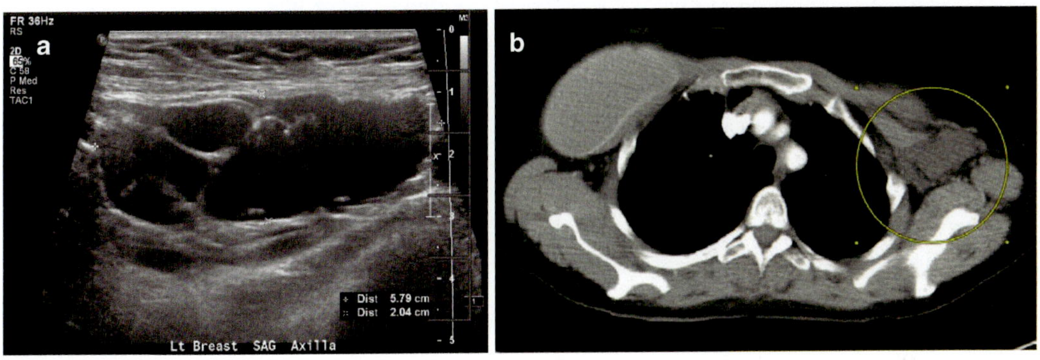

Fig. 11.17 A 48-year-old female with silicone breast implants, presented with an enlarging left axillary mass. Mammogram was unremarkable. On ultrasound there was a multiloculated cystic mass in the left axilla consisting of multiple tubular and cystic spaces separated by thickened septae (**a**). CT showed a multinodular large complex cystic mass in the left axilla (**b**). The lesion was called BI-RADS: 4. On biopsy the lesion was found to be a venous malformation

illary hemangiomas) may appear hyperechoic (Fig. 11.17).

- **MRI:** On MRI, benign vascular proliferations will commonly appear as superficial masses that are T2 hyperintense with variable enhancement patterns.
- **BI-RADS**: 2–4. Initial presentation of a mass without a known diagnosis may warrant a biopsy to exclude malignancy.
- **Differential Diagnosis**: Fibroadenoma, complicated cyst, hamartoma, angiosarcoma, breast cancer.

• **Pathology Findings:**

- **Microscopic Histology:** Well-differentiated proliferation of vascular or lymphatic vessels without atypia (Fig. 11.18).

  See lymphangioma (Chap. 3) for more information.

  See hemangioma (Chap. 11) for more information.
- **Differential Diagnosis:** Angiolipoma, angiosarcoma, atypical vascular lesion, lymphangioma.
- **Management:** No treatment is necessary; however, surgical excision may be performed if the lesion is large and bothers the patient [57].

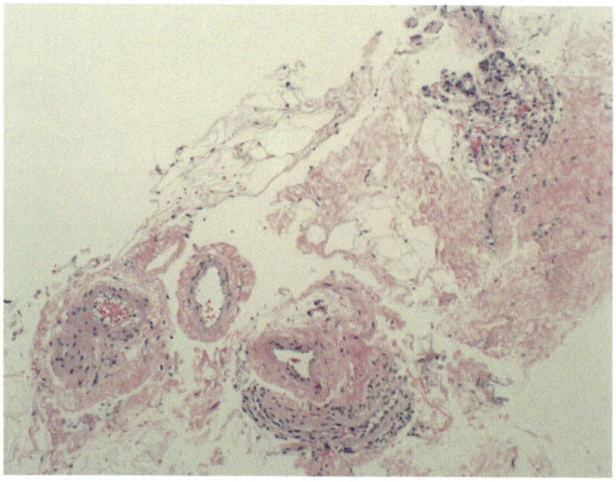

Fig. 11.18 A 75-year-old woman was found to have a suspicious mass at 9:00 in her right breast which was called BIRADS 4. On ultrasound-guided biopsy a benign vascular proliferation was seen with thick walled veins, capilaries and lymphatic channels. CD34 and CD31 highlighted the vascular structures. Ki-67 proliferative index was low and HHV8 was not expressed. WT-1 appeared lost or reduced in lesional endothelial cells suggesting a malformation. The lesion is compatible with a lymphatico-venous malformation

Hemangioma

Hemangioma: Hemangiomas are one of the most common benign vascular tumors of the breast. They can be classified as perilobular, capillary, or cavernous depending on the size of the blood vessels involved [2, 58]. They are usually superficially located and on imaging will present as a circumscribed mass that is hyperintense on T2WI and has a characteristic early peripheral and delayed central enhancement pattern on contrast-enhanced T1WI [61].

- **Clinical Presentation:** On occasion may present as a palpable lesion, but generally is an incidental finding.
- **Imaging Findings:**
  - **Mammography**: Hemangiomas will typically appear as a superficial mass often isodense to fibroglandular tissue, which may contain calcifications (Figs. 11.19 and 11.20).
  - **US**: Ultrasound will show a superficial, well-circumscribed, solid mass.
  - **MRI**: Hemangiomas will appear as a round or irregular mass that is T2WI hyperintense with an early peripheral and delayed central enhancement pattern on contrast-enhanced T1WI.
  - **BI-RADS**: 2–4. Initial presentation of a mass without a known diagnosis may warrant a biopsy to exclude malignancy.
  - **Differential Diagnosis**: Fibroadenoma, complicated cyst, hamartoma, other benign vascular proliferations, angiosarcoma, breast cancer.
- **Pathology Findings:**
  - **Microscopic Histology:** Generally, well-circumscribed vascular proliferations without endothelial cell atypia (Fig. 11.21).

    Cavernous hemangiomas are composed of a collection of larger dilated blood vessels.

    Capillary hemangiomas are composed of small blood vessels.

    Generally, the vascular proliferations are nonanastomosing.
  - **Differential Diagnosis:** Angiolipoma, angiosarcoma, atypical vascular lesion.
  - **Management:** No treatment is necessary; however, surgical excision may be performed if the lesion is large and bothers the patient.

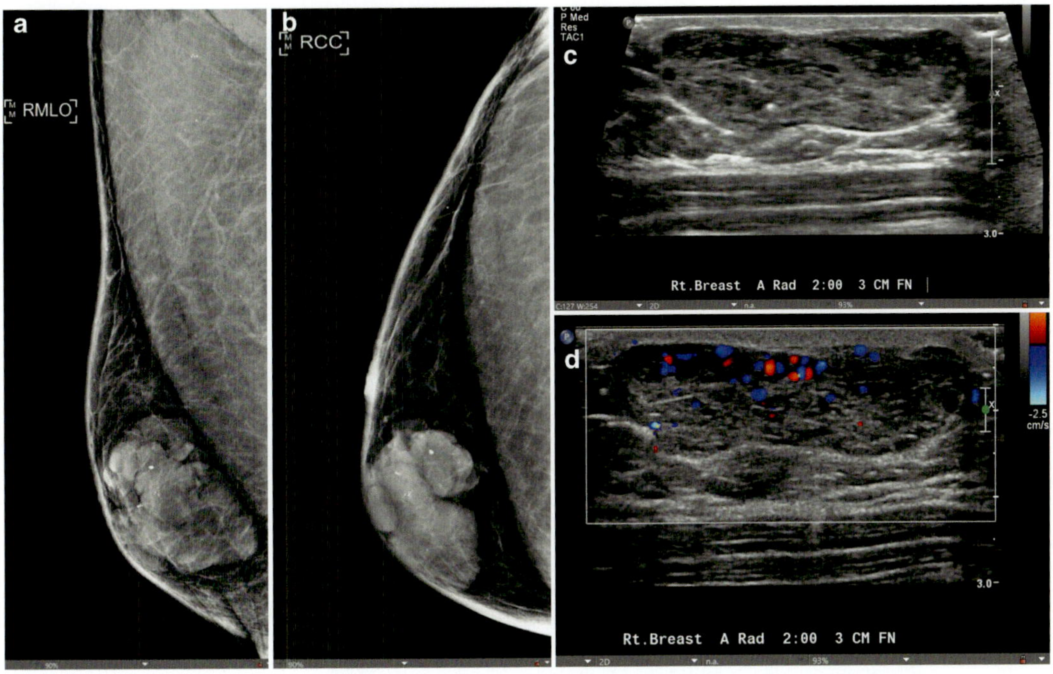

Fig. 11.19 A 60-year-old male who presented after a right breast lesion was incidentally noted on a Cardiac CT. Mammogram showed an irregular, circumscribed mass with associated calcifications (**a**, **b**). On ultrasound there was an oval, hypoechoic mass (**c**, **d**). The lesion was called BI-RADS 4. Biopsy confirmed the presence of a hemangioma

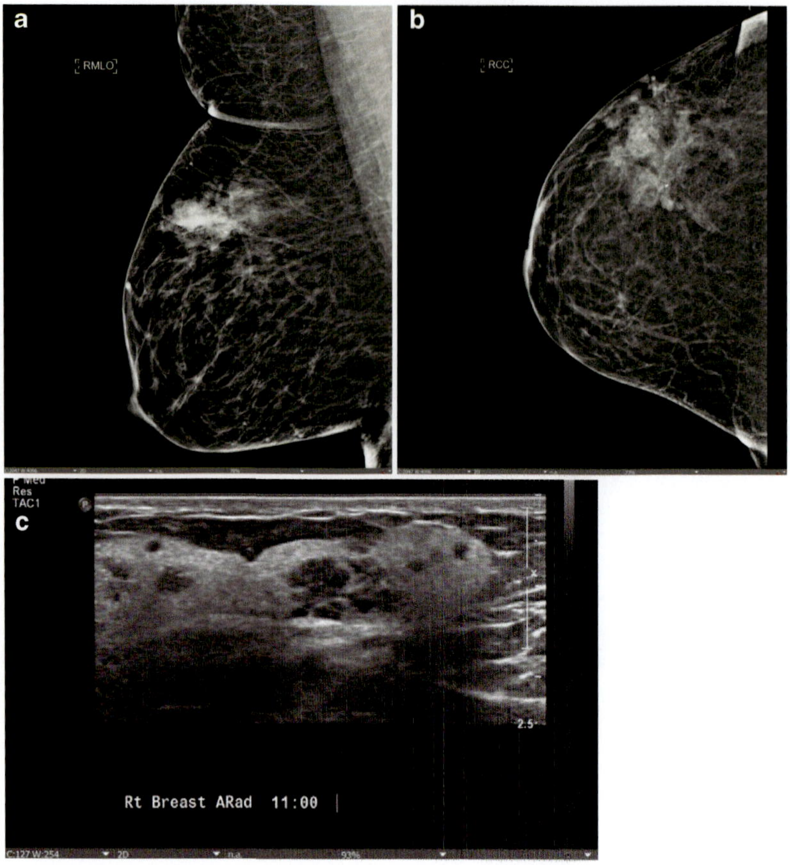

Fig. 11.20 A 37-year-old female who presented with left nipple changes underwent mammography on which an irregular, focal asymmetry with heterogeneous calcification in the right breast was incidentally noted (**a, b**). On ultrasound there was an indistinct mass with heterogeneous echogenicity (**c**). The lesion was called BI-RADS 4, and biopsy revealed a capillary hemangioma

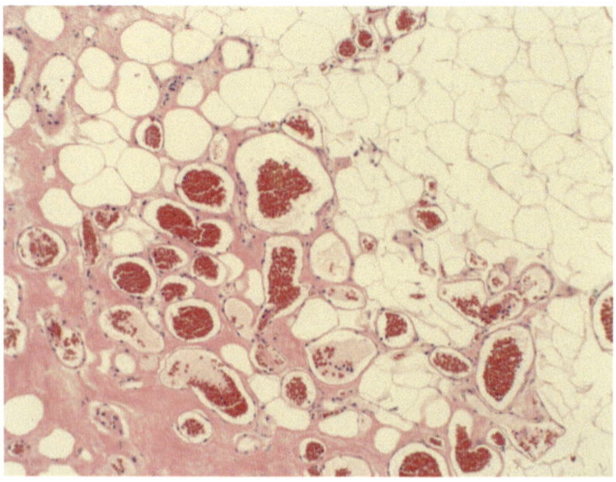

Fig. 11.21 A 42-year-old woman with a circumscribed mass on mammography underwent biopsy revealing a proliferation of benign blood vessels which was diagnosed as a hemangioma

Vascular Lesions, Malignant

Angiosarcoma

***Angiosarcoma*:** Angiosarcoma is a rare cancer in the breast, representing less than 1% of all breast malignancies [25]. It is caused by neoplastic transformation of endothelial cells. Prior radiation therapy is an important cause of secondary angiosarcoma, and another major risk factor is chronic lymphedema [62]. Primary angiosarcoma is typically diagnosed in women under 40, whereas secondary angiosarcoma has a median age of presentation in the 60s [63]. Patients will present with a large mass, which may have associated bluish discoloration of the overlying skin if superficial [64]. Imaging typically shows an ill-defined, infiltrative mass with overlying skin thickening. As compared with benign vascular tumors, angiosarcomas are characteristically hypervascular and will show significant, rapid enhancement with IV contrast administration [65].

- **Clinical Presentation:** Primary angiosarcoma typically presents in younger women (median age 35–40) as a palpable mass or breast swelling which in some cases may rapidly enlarge [63–66]. Secondary angiosarcoma on the other hand presents in older patients (median age 59–69) with a history of radiation therapy, is less likely to present as a mass, but more commonly presents as painless bruising that is often multifocal [63–66].
- **Imaging Findings:**
  - **Mammography**: Mammographic findings for angiosarcoma are nonspecific with the most common appearance being a mass or focal asymmetry.

    If the mass is superficial, there may be associated skin thickening and subcutaneous edema (Fig. 11.22).
  - **US**: Ultrasound findings are variable but may show a mixed echogenicity mass with increased vascularity.
  - **MRI**: Angiosarcoma can appear as a heterogeneous mass that is typically hyperintense on T2WI and displays avid enhancement following contrast administration.
  - **BI-RADS**: 4.
  - **Differential Diagnosis**: Inflammatory breast carcinoma, mastitis, invasive ductal carcinoma, metastases, Paget's disease.
- **Pathology Findings:**
  - **Microscopic Histology:** Based on histologic criteria angiosarcomas can be graded as low, intermediate or high grade [63, 64].

    Low-grade angiosarcomas have recognizable vascular channels with well-formed anastomosing channels and/or spaces lined by endothelial cells with hyperchromatic nuclei that are filled with varying numbers of red blood cells.
    - However, there is no increase in mitoses, no necrosis or solid growth pattern [63, 64].
    - The low-grade lesion is important to recognize on biopsy as it may sometimes be at the periphery of a higher-grade lesion not sampled in the biopsy.

    Intermediate-grade angiosarcomas have increased cellularity with focal papillary endothelial tufting of blood vessels and areas of solid growth with few or no vascular spaces.
    - Mitoses can be seen in cellular areas [63, 64].
    - Note that reparative and reactive vascular proliferations can resemble low-grade angiosarcoma in biopsy samples.

    High-grade angiosarcomas are composed of cytologically malignant cells with spindled and solid growth patterns with areas of hemorrhage, so called "blood lakes", mitoses, and necrosis (Fig. 11.23).
    - Some high-grade angiosarcomas have an epithelial/epithelioid appearance that resembles a poorly differentiated ductal carcinoma. This particular and rather unusual variant is the epithelioid variant and has the potential to be missed unless careful attention to histologic details and clinical history of radiation is noted [63].

    Angiosarcomas are notable for having variable areas of admixed high-grade and low-grade histology.

    Cases that are suspicious for angiosarcoma should be evaluated with appropriate immunohistochemical studies for vascular endothelial markers such as CD31, CD34, and ERG, as well as a cytokeratin stain (which should be generally negative with a few exceptions) [63, 64] (Fig. 11.24).

    Recent studies have shown that postradiation sarcomas commonly show MYC amplification and therefore an immunostaining for c-myc can also be performed [65].

Once the diagnosis for angiosarcoma is confirmed every attempt to conserve tissue for molecular studies such as tumor profiling should be made [65].

- **Differential Diagnosis:** Atypical vascular lesions, hemangioma, angiolipoma,
- **Management:** For both primary and secondary angiosarcoma of the breast, mastectomy is frequently performed given the importance of sufficient negative margins and considering that secondary angiosarcomas are usually the result of post-lumpectomy radiation [66–69]. Even with negative margins, recurrence is common and survival is poor [68]. Adjuvant radiation, when possible, has led to recurrence free survival benefit [69]. Chemotherapy may be recommended.

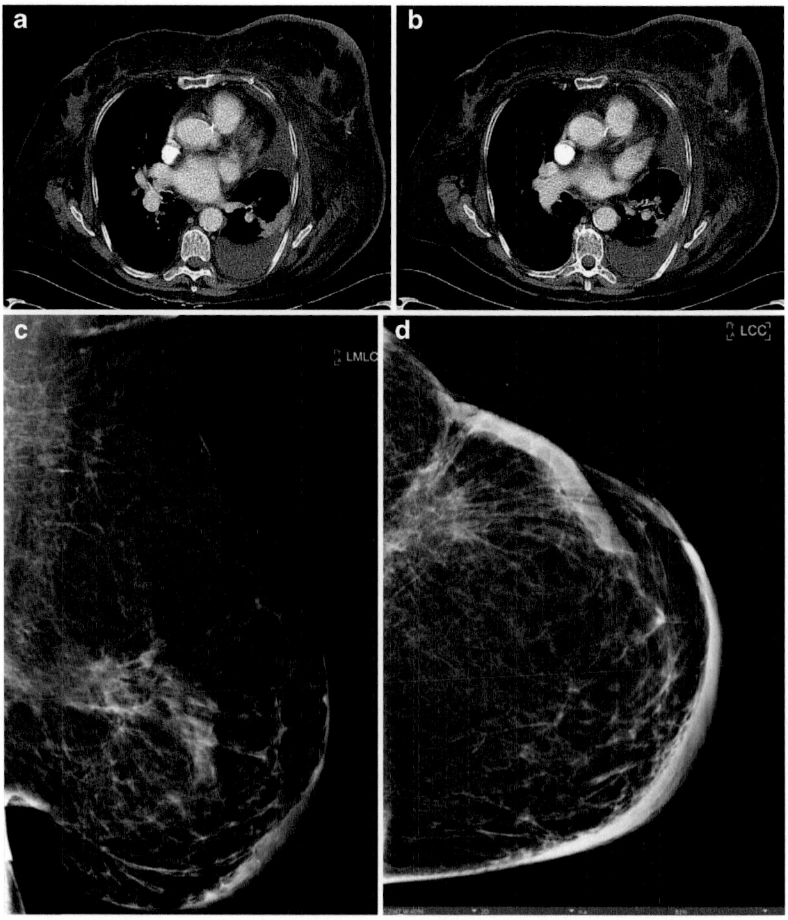

Fig. 11.22 An 87-year-old woman with remote history of left breast carcinoma status post-lumpectomy and radiation, presents with skin lesions and skin thickening of the left breast seen on CT (**a, b**), and LMLO and LCC views on mammography (**c, d**). A mastectomy specimen from the patient showed a postradiation angiosarcoma

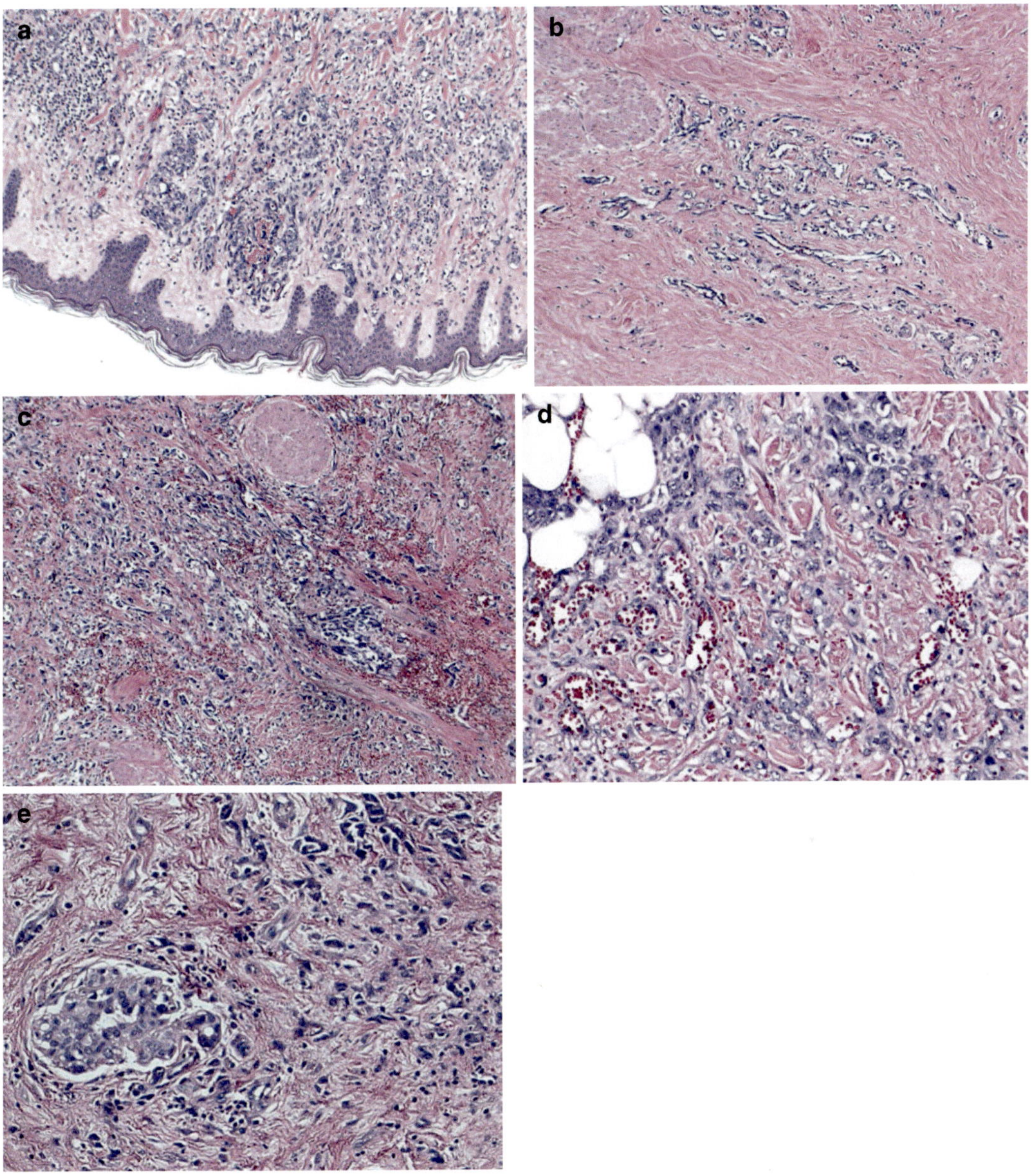

Fig. 11.23 A 76-year-old woman with history of right breast carcinoma treated with lumpectomy and radiation, now presents with skin thickening of the right breast. On mastectomy a postradiation angiosarcoma is diagnosed. H&E section shows tumor within the dermis with abnormal proliferation of blood vessels with infiltrative borders (**a**, **b**). Blood lakes can be visualized within the tumor (**c**). On higher magnification large pleomorphic malignant cells with high nuclear grade and increased mitoses are seen invading fibrous tissue (**d**). Vascular channels lined by cellular spindle cells and areas of papillary formations with marked nuclear atypia are appreciated (**e**)

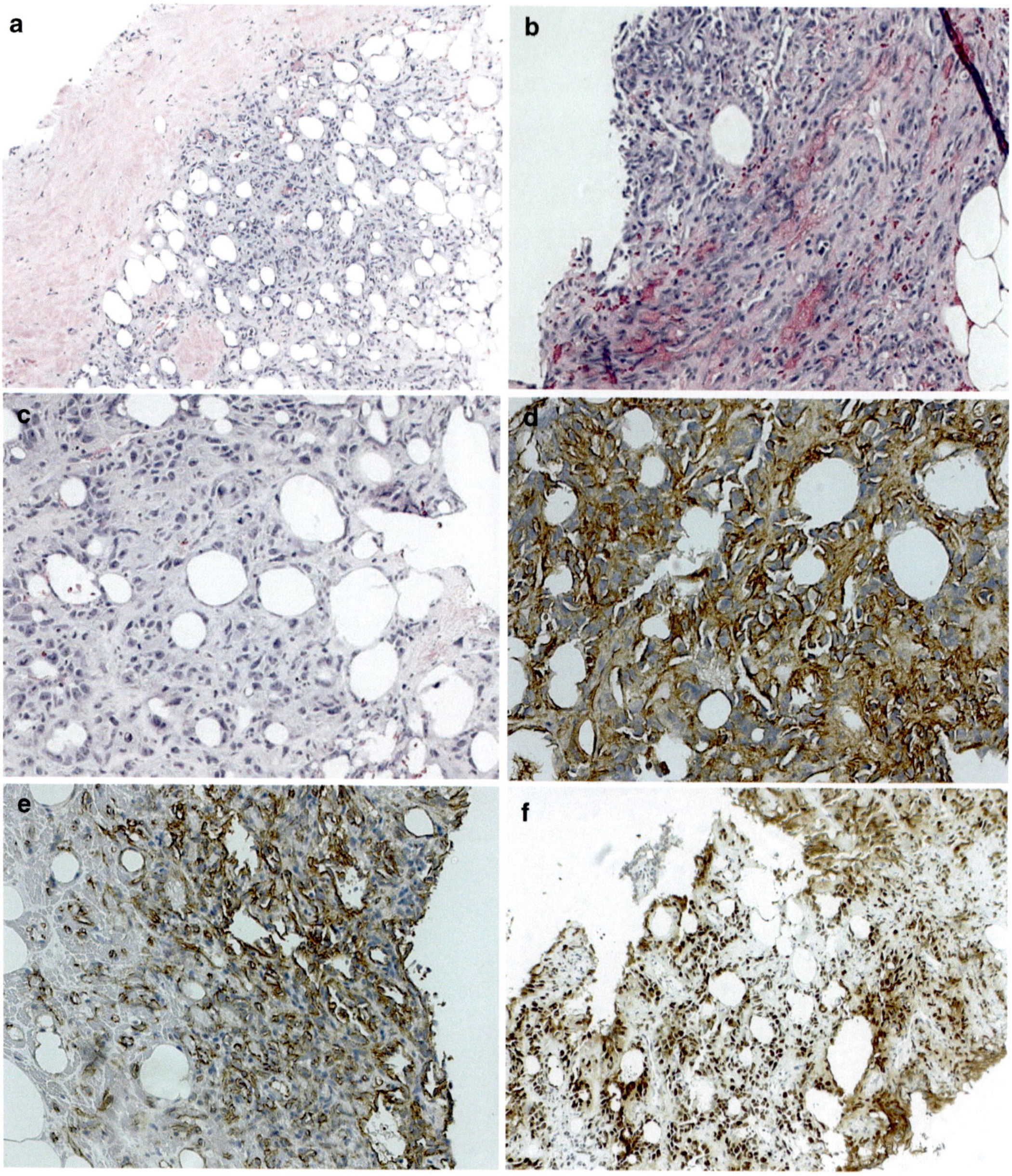

Fig. 11.24 Needle core biopsy showing predominantly spindle and epithelioid areas in fibrofatty tissue with no normal breast tissue (**a–c**). The spindle and epithelioid cells show diffuse staining for CD31 (**d**, **e**). Immunostains for c-Myc also shows strong diffuse staining in both epithelioid and spindle cells (**f**, **g**) supporting the diagnosis of angiosarcoma

g
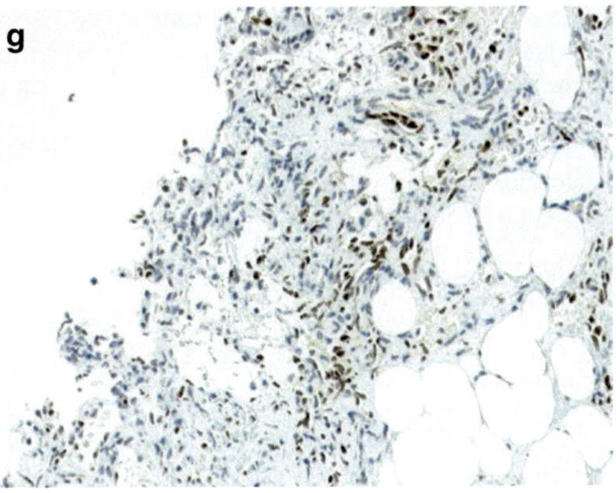

Fig. 11.24 (continued)

References

1. Cao MM, et al. Mammographic signs of systemic disease. Radiographics. 2011;31(4):1085–100.
2. Jesinger RA, et al. Vascular abnormalities of the breast: arterial and venous disorders, vascular masses, and mimic lesions with radiologic-pathologic correlation. Radiographics. 2011;31(7):E117–36.
3. Stolz JL, Friedman AK, Arger PH. Breast carcinoma simulation. Mammography in congestive heart failure mimics acute mastitis and advanced carcinoma. JAMA. 1974;229:682–3.
4. Gould D, Argiris A. Unilateral breast oedema as a manifestation of congestive heart failure. J Intern Med. 1998;243:328–9.
5. Oraedu CO, Pinnapureddy P, Alrawi S, Acinapura AJ, Raju R. Congestive heart failure mimicking inflammatory breast carcinoma: a case report and review of the literature. Breast J. 2001;7:117–9.
6. DiSipio T, et al. Incidence of unilateral arm lymphoedema after breast cancer: a systematic review and meta-analysis. Lancet Oncol. 2013;14(6):500–15.
7. McLaughlin SA, et al. Breast cancer-related lymphedema: risk factors, screening, management, and the impact of locoregional treatment. J Clin Oncol. 2020;38(20):2341–50.
8. National Comprehensive Cancer Network. Survivorship: lymphedema. (Version 1, 2021). 2021. https://www.nccn.org/professionals/physician_gls/pdf/survivorship.pdf.
9. Cormier JN, et al. Lymphedema beyond breast cancer: a systematic review and meta-analysis of cancer-related secondary lymphedema. Cancer. 2010;116(22):5138–49.
10. Patel KM, Manrique O, Sosin M, Hashmi MA, Poysophon P, Henderson R. Lymphatic mapping and lymphedema surgery in the breast cancer patient. Gland Surg. 2015;4(3):244–56.
11. Chansakul T, et al. The postconservation breast: part 1, expected imaging findings. AJR Am J Roentgenol. 2012;198(2):321–30.
12. Krishnamurthy R, et al. Mammographic findings after breast conservation therapy. Radiographics. 1999;19 Spec No:S53–62; quiz S262–3.
13. Neal CH, et al. Imaging of breast cancer-related changes after surgical therapy. AJR Am J Roentgenol. 2014;202(2):262–72.
14. Pierce SM, et al. Long-term radiation complications following conservative surgery (CS) and radiation therapy (RT) in patients with early stage breast cancer. Int J Radiat Oncol Biol Phys. 1992;23(5):915–23.
15. Revelon G, et al. Focal fibrosis of the breast: imaging characteristics and histopathologic correlation. Radiology. 2000;216(1):255–9.
16. van Geel AN, et al. Partial mastectomy and m. latissimus dorsi reconstruction for radiation-induced fibrosis after breast-conserving cancer therapy. World J Surg. 2011;35(3):568–72.
17. Mahoney MC, Ingram AD. Breast emergencies: types, imaging features, and management. AJR Am J Roentgenol. 2014;202:W390–9.
18. Trop I, Dugas A, David J, et al. Breast abscesses: evidence-based algorithms for diagnosis, management, and follow-up. Radiographics. 2011;31:1683–99.
19. Dener C, Inan A. Breast abscesses in lactating women. World J Surg. 2003;27:130–3.
20. Scott-Conner CE, Schorr SJ. The diagnosis and management of breast problems during pregnancy and lactation. Am J Surg. 1995;170:401–5.
21. Dabbas N, Chand M, Pallett A, Royle GT, Sainsbury R. Have the organisms that cause breast abscess changed with time? Implications for appropriate antibiotic usage in primary and secondary care. Breast J. 2010;16:412–5.
22. Angelopoulou A, et al. The microbiology and treatment of human mastitis. Med Microbiol Immunol. 2018;207(2):83–94.
23. Dixon JM, et al. Periductal mastitis and duct ectasia: different conditions with different aetiologies. Br J Surg. 1996;83(6):820–2.
24. Pluguez-Turull CW, et al. Idiopathic granulomatous mastitis: manifestations at multimodality imaging and pitfalls. Radiographics. 2018;38(2):330–56.
25. Rosen PP, et al. Rosen's breast pathology. Philadelphia: Wolters Kluwer Health; 2014.
26. Sabate JM, et al. Radiologic evaluation of uncommon inflammatory and reactive breast disorders. Radiographics. 2005;25(2):411–24.
27. Lam E, Chan T, Wiseman SM. Breast abscess: evidence based management recommendations. Expert Rev Anti-Infect Ther. 2014;12:753–62.
28. American Society of Breast Surgeons. Five things physicians and patients should question. 2018. https://www.choosingwisely.org/wp-content/uploads/2018/01/ASBrS_BenignBreastDisease-Choosing-Wisely-List.pdf.

29. Lannin DR. Twenty-two year experience with recurring subareolar abscess and lactiferous duct fistula treated by a single breast surgeon. Am J Surg. 2004;188(4):407.
30. Jahanfar S, Ng CJ, Teng CL. Antibiotics for mastitis in breastfeeding women. Cochrane Database Syst Rev. 2013;(2):CD005458.
31. Walshe JM, Swain SM. Clinical aspects of inflammatory of breast cancer. Breast Dis. 2005;22:35–44.
32. AJCC (American Joint Committee on Cancer) cancer staging manual. 8th ed. New York: Springer.
33. Vermeulen PB, van Golen KL, Dirix LY. Angiogenesis, lymphangiogenesis, growth pattern, and tumor emboli in inflammatory breast cancer: a review of the current knowledge. Cancer. 2010;116(Suppl 11):2748–54.
34. Robertson F, Petricoin EF, Van Laere SJ. Presence of anaplastic lymphoma kinase in inflammatory breast cancer. Springerplus. 2013;2:497.
35. van Uden DJ, Van Laarhoven HW, Westenberg AH. Inflammatory breast cancer: an overview. Crtit Rev Oncol Hematol. 2015;93(2):116–26.
36. Molckovsky A, Fitzegrald B, Freedman O, Haisey R, Clemons M. Approach to inflammatory breast cancer. Can Fam Physician. 2009;55(1):25–31.
37. Hance KW, Anderson WF, Devesa SS, Young HA, Levine PH. Trends in inflammatory breast carcinoma incidence and survival: the surveillance, epidemiology, and end results program at the National Cancer Institute. J Natl Cancer Inst. 2005;97(13):966–75.
38. Gonzalez-Angulo AM, Hennessy BT, Broglio K. Trends for inflammatory breast carcinoma: is survival improving? Oncologist. 2007;12(8):904–12.
39. National Comprehensive Cancer Network. Inflammatory breast cancer. (Version 4, 2021). 2021. https://www.nccn.org/professionals/physician_gls/pdf/breast.pdf.
40. Valero VV, Buzdar AU, Hortobagyi GN. Locally advanced breast cancer. Oncologist. 1996;1(1 and 2):8–17.
41. Perez EA, Foo ML, Fulmer JT. Management of locally advanced breast cancer. Oncology (Williston Park). 1997;11(9 Suppl 9):9–17.
42. Giordano SH. Update on locally advanced breast cancer. Oncologist. 2003;8:521–30.
43. Lee MC, Newman LA. Management of patients with locally advanced breast cancer. Surg Clin North Am. 2007;87:379–98; ix.
44. National Comprehensive Cancer Network (NCCN). NCCN clinical practice guidelines in oncology: breast cancer. Fort Washington, PA: NCCN; 2015. Ver. 2, 2015.
45. Gonzalez-Angulo AM, Hortobagyi GN. Inflammatory and locally advanced breast cancer. In: Management of breast diseases. Berlin: Springer; 2010.
46. Valagussa P, Zambetti M, Bignami P, et al. T3b-T4 breast cancer: factors affecting results in combined modality treatments. Clin Exp Metastasis. 1983;1:191–202.
47. Hortobagyi GN, Ames FC, Buzdar AU, et al. Management of stage III primary breast cancer with primary chemotherapy, surgery, and radiation therapy. Cancer. 1988;62:2507–16.
48. Bedwinek J, Rao DV, Perez C, et al. Stage III and localized stage IV breast cancer: irradiation alone vs irradiation plus surgery. Int J Radiat Oncol Biol Phys. 1982;8:31–6.
49. Simos D, Clemons M, Ginsburg OM, Jacobs C. Definition and consequences of locally advanced breast cancer. Curr Opin Support Palliat Care. 2014;8(1):33–8.
50. Anderson WF, Schairer C, Chen BE, Hance KW, Levine PH. Epidemiology of inflammatory breast cancer (IBC). Breast Dis. 2005;22:9–23.
51. Balogun OD, Formenti SC. Locally advanced breast cancer—strategies for developing nations. Front Oncol. 2015;5:89.
52. Chia S, Swain SM, Byrd DR, Mankoff DA. Locally advanced and inflammatory breast cancer. J Clin Oncol. 2008;26:786–90.
53. Dossus L, Benusiglio PR. Lobular breast cancer: incidence and genetic and non-genetic risk factors. Breast Cancer Res. 2015;17:37.
54. Brem RF, et al. Invasive lobular carcinoma: detection with mammography, sonography, MRI, and breast-specific gamma imaging. AJR Am J Roentgenol. 2009;192(2):379–83.
55. Johnson K, et al. Lobular breast cancer series: imaging. Breast Cancer Res. 2015;17(1):94.
56. Lopez JK, Bassett LW. Invasive lobular carcinoma of the breast: spectrum of mammographic, US, and MR imaging findings. Radiographics. 2009;29(1):165–76.
57. Donnelly LF, et al. Vascular malformations and hemangiomas: a practical approach in a multidisciplinary clinic. AJR Am J Roentgenol. 2000;174(3):597–608.
58. Glazebrook KN, et al. Vascular tumors of the breast: mammographic, sonographic, and MRI appearances. AJR Am J Roentgenol. 2005;184(1):331–8.
59. Chung SY, et al. Mammographic and sonographic findings of a breast cystic lymphangioma. J Ultrasound Med. 2003;22(3):307–9.
60. Ferru JM. Hemangioma of the breast: mammographic, sonographic and MRI features. J Radiol. 2011;92(5):441–5.
61. Mesurolle B, et al. Sonographic and mammographic appearances of breast hemangioma. AJR Am J Roentgenol. 2008;191(1):W17–22.
62. Seinen JM, Styring E, Verstappen V, et al. Radiation-associated angiosarcoma after breast cancer: high recurrence rate and poor survival despite surgical treatment with R0 resection. Ann Surg Oncol. 2012;19:2700.
63. Esposito E, Avino F, di Giacomo R, Donzelli I, Marone U, Melucci MT, Rinaldo C, Ruffolo F, Saponara R, Siani C, Tortoriello R, Botti G, Rinaldo M, Fucito A. Angiosarcoma of the breast, the unknown—a review of the current literature. Transl Cancer Res. 2019;8(Suppl 5):S510–7.

64. Arora TK, Terracina KP, Soong J, Idowu MO, Takabe K. Primary and secondary angiosarcoma of the breast. Gland Surg. 2014;3(1):28–34.
65. Nascimento AF, Raut CP, Fletcher CDM. Primary angiosarcoma of the breast: clinicopathologic analysis of 49 cases, suggesting that grade is not prognostic. Am J Surg Pathol. 2008;32(12):1896–904.
66. Abdou Y, Elkhanany A, Attwood K, Ji W, Takabe K, Opyrchal M. Primary and secondary breast angiosarcoma: single center report and meta-analysis. Breast Cancer Res Treat. 2019;178:523–33.
67. Von Mehren M, Kane JM, et al. NCCN guidelines version 4, 2019 soft tissue sarcoma, 2019.
68. Zelek L, Llombart-Cussac A, Terrier P, Pivot X, Guinebretiere JM, Le Pechoux C, Tursz T, Rochard F, Spielmann M, Le Cesne A. Prognostic factors in primary breast sarcomas: a series of patients with long-term follow-up. J Clin Oncol. 2003;21(13):2583–8.
69. Scow JS, Reynolds CA, Degnim AC, Petersen IA, Jakub JW, Boughey JC. Primary and secondary angiosarcoma of the breast: the Mayo Clinic experience. J Surg Oncol. 2010;101(5):401.

Changes Related to Breast Surgery and Neoadjuvant Therapy

12

Sunati Sahoo, Helena Hwang, and Stephen J. Seiler

Benign

Fat Necrosis with Scar (See Chaps. 5 and 7 for Additional Description)

Following surgical resection, imaging serves as an important surveillance tool. Edema and post-surgical fluid collections are the common findings in the first 6 months following resection. Over time, these changes are usually replaced by changes such as architectural distortion, oil cyst formation, dystrophic calcifications, and fat necrosis. Fat necrosis, in particular, can be difficult to distinguish from recurrent tumors by imaging alone, as it may display a variety of suspicious features on mammography, ultrasound, and MRI. Although temporal stability in the post-lumpectomy setting supports benignity, a developing mass or asymmetry usually requires biopsy.

Clinical features: Fat necrosis with associated scar appears after trauma to the breast, core biopsy, or surgical excision.

S. Sahoo (✉) · H. Hwang
Department of Pathology, University of Texas Southwestern Medical Center, Dallas, TX, USA
e-mail: sunati.sahoo@utsouthwestern.edu; helena.hwang@utsouthwestern.edu

S. J. Seiler
Department of Radiology, University of Texas Southwestern Medical Center, Dallas, TX, USA
e-mail: stephen.seiler@utsouthwestern.edu

Imaging Findings

Mammography: The mammographic appearance of fat necrosis with scar is variable.

- Tomosynthesis is better at demonstrating distortion that extends to skin, with central lucency.
- Coarse heterogeneous calcifications may develop along the lumpectomy bed and become coarser or more dystrophic over time. Calcifications can develop many years after surgery. Fine linear or pleomorphic calcifications are not typical and may require biopsy.
- Irregular spiculated mass or asymmetry usually remains stable or improves over time, although asymmetries may become denser over time with continuing fibrosis and contraction.
- Oil cysts present as round or oval circumscribed masses that may develop peripheral rim/eggshell calcifications.

Ultrasound: The sonographic appearance tends to evolve over time.

- *Acute*: Diffuse hyperechogenicity.
- *Subacute*: Complex cystic mass within edematous fat.
- *Remote*: Irregular mass with indistinct or angular margins and posterior acoustic shadowing.

M. Harigopal et al. (eds.), *Radiology Pathology Correlations of Breast Lesions*,
https://doi.org/10.1007/978-3-031-65711-5_12

- Oil cysts are typically anechoic or hypoechoic circumscribed masses that lack posterior acoustical features.
- Scar tissue can be tracked to the overlying skin incision and can cause posterior shadowing.

MRI: The MRI appearance is also variable and may overlap with recurrence.

- Postsurgical scar often enhances, particularly in the first 6–18 months, but it can enhance years after surgery.
- There is usually an internal signal that follows the fat signal on all MR sequences.
- A fluid-sensitive sequence (e.g., STIR) may have surrounding increased signal due to edema.
- Lesions can range from an oval circumscribed mass to an irregular spiculated mass.
- Masses may not enhance but most will demonstrate some degree of peripheral enhancement. Central enhancement is not common and may require biopsy.

BI-RADS:

- BI-RADS 2: Benign—Findings consistent with an oil cyst or fatty mass with rim calcifications.
- BI-RADS 3: Probably Benign—There is diagnostic uncertainty requiring short-interval follow-up.
- BI-RADS 4: Suspicious—Developing asymmetry, irregular mass or suspicious calcifications.

Differential Diagnosis:

- Fat-containing mass: Postsurgical fluid collection with fat, lipoma.
- Developing mass: Recurrent cancer.
- Suspicious calcifications: Ductal carcinoma in situ, invasive carcinoma.

Pathology Findings

Gross: Scars will manifest as irregularly shaped dense white fibrous tissue. Fat necrosis, depending on the age of the lesion, presents as bright yellow to yellowish-gray indurated fat with or without grittiness due to associated fine or coarse calcifications.

Microscopic Findings: Similar to imaging findings, the morphologic changes of the surgical site evolves with time. In the initial stage of healing, fat necrosis exhibits lipophages, small oil cyst, infiltration of the adipose tissue by mostly lymphocytes, plasma cells and giant cells, and variable degree of fibrosis. Over time, dense fibrosis or sclerosis with fewer inflammatory cells in the absence of glandular breast epithelium becomes the dominant finding. Foreign body multinucleated giant cells may persist for a long time. Calcifications if present, are usually granular early on and become dense, sometimes leading to osseous metaplasia.

Radiology Pathology Correlation: A patient history of prior surgery is extremely helpful.

Differential Diagnoses: Recurrent invasive carcinoma, reactive changes due to a ruptured cyst or duct ectasia.

Case Examples

See Fig. 12.1.

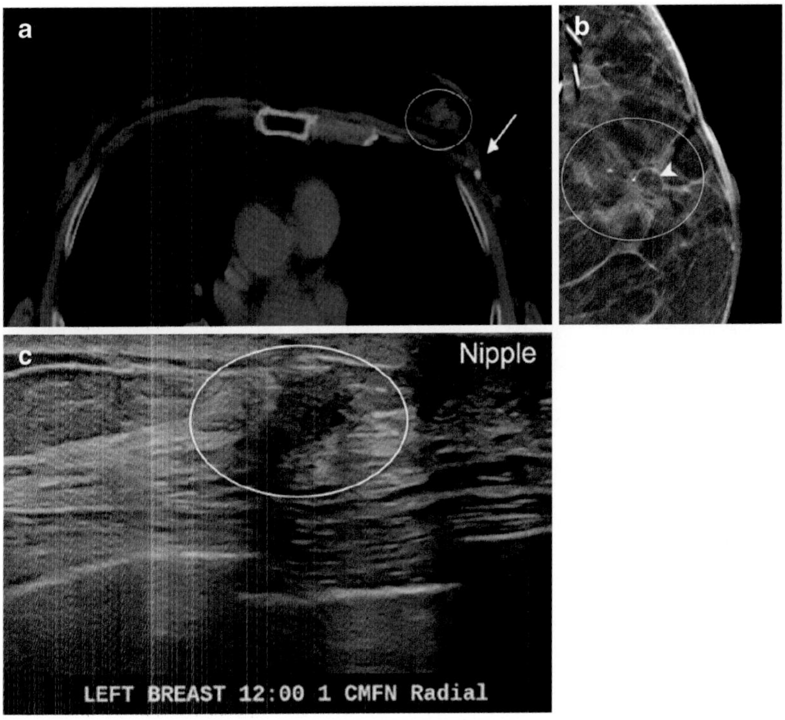

Fig. 12.1 A 68-year-old woman with a history of left breast IDC who underwent partial mastectomy 2 years ago underwent PET-CT imaging for re-staging and evaluation of new-onset weight loss. (**a**) A 1.3-cm area of increased FDG uptake (circled, SUV max 2.3) is identified in the retro-areolar region of the left breast adjacent to the lumpectomy bed (arrow). (**b**) Subsequent diagnostic tomosynthesis examination revealed a focal asymmetry and associated architectural distortion (circled) in the subareola. A small oil cyst (arrowhead) is seen within this region. (**c**) Ultrasound imaging confirms the presence of a 1.3-cm irregular hypoechoic mass (circled) with indistinct margins in the 12 o'clock left breast, located 1 cm from the nipple. An ultrasound-guided biopsy was performed with a 14-gauge needle and five cores were obtained. Pathology revealed fat necrosis with calcifications, scar tissue with multinucleated giant cells and rare breast ducts. No carcinoma identified

Case Examples

See Fig. 12.2.

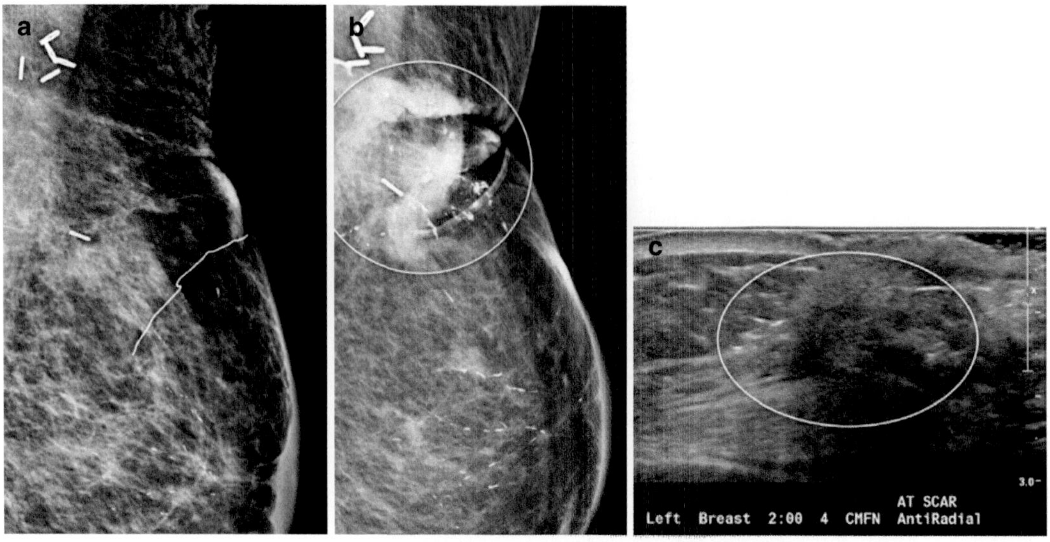

Fig. 12.2 An 82-year-old woman had undergone left partial mastectomy for IDC 1 year prior. (**a**) The diagnostic MLO mammogram performed for surveillance demonstrates multiple surgical clips in the superior aspect of the left breast as well as mild skin and trabecular thickening diffusely, related to edema and postradiation changes. (**b**) One year later, a diagnostic MLO mammogram shows development of a 3-cm asymmetry and coarse heterogeneous calcifications within the lumpectomy bed, associated with skin retraction. (**c**) A 1.8-cm solid heterogeneously hypoechoic mass with indistinct margins (circled) is seen on subsequent targeted ultrasound in the 2 o'clock left breast, at the site of the surgical scar. An ultrasound-guided biopsy was performed with a 14-gauge biopsy needle, taking three core samples. Pathology revealed fat necrosis with scar tissue and dystrophic calcifications

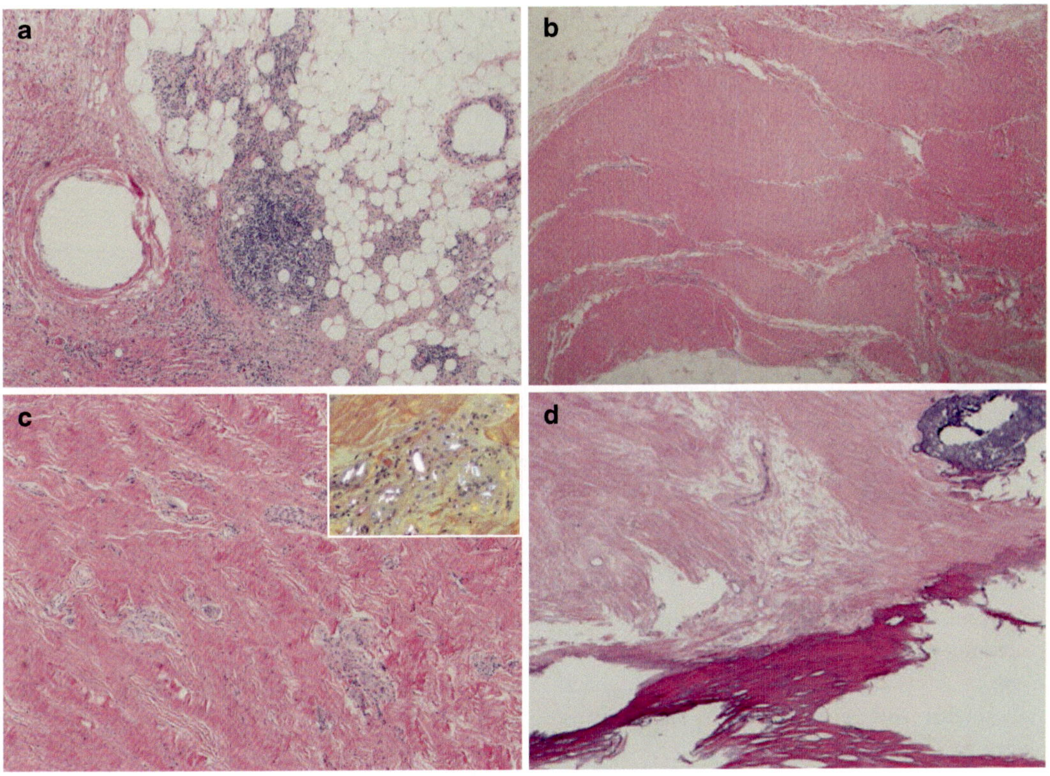

Fig. 12.3 A woman with prior lumpectomy for carcinoma underwent reconstruction for symmetry. (**a**) Some sections from the prior surgical site revealed fat necrosis with chronic inflammation and oil cysts. (**b**) Other areas revealed dense collagenous scar tissue. (**c**) The scar tissue contained a foreign body giant cell reaction with suture material, seen easily on polarized lens (inset). (**d**) In other areas the scar tissue showed focal calcifications (upper right) and osseous metaplasia seen in the lower half of the picture

Case Examples
See Fig. 12.3.

Malignant

Breast Carcinoma Treated with Neoadjuvant Chemotherapy

Neoadjuvant chemotherapy (NCT) is the most common form of neoadjuvant treatment for invasive breast carcinoma. The best response to NCT occurs in HER2-positive and triple-negative breast cancers. The radiologic assessment of response can be discrepant (under- or overestimation) from pathologic assessment. Irrespective of the types of response to treatment, surgical excision is currently a standard procedure after completion of neoadjuvant therapy.

Clinical Findings: Indications for NCT include locally advanced tumors, triple-negative breast cancers (TNBC), and HER2-positive tumors. Depending on the response of a tumor to NCT, the tumor may have markedly decreased in size or there may have been little to no appreciable effect. HER2-positive cancers and TNBC tend to show the best response to NCT while hormone receptor (HR)-positive/HER2-negative tumors are likely to exhibit partial response.

Imaging Findings

Radiologic imaging serves important purposes in the neoadjuvant setting [1]. The first step, prior to beginning neoadjuvant therapy, is to define the extent of disease in the ipsilateral breast, screen the contralateral breast and evaluate the regional lymph nodes for optimal clinical staging and surgical planning. During therapy, imaging may help identify nonresponders so the therapeutic regimen can be changed or discontinued to allow the patients to proceed with surgery. Lastly, at the conclusion of neoadjuvant therapy, imaging can evaluate the degree of response as well as aid in preoperative localization planning.

Currently, there are no established practice guidelines for assessment of treatment response by imaging. Conventional diagnostic imaging modalities such as digital mammography (with or without tomosynthesis) and ultrasound are routinely performed to supplement physical examination. However, the accuracy of mammography and ultrasound to determine tumor response is low and reported to be 74% and 79%, respectively [2]. Use of tomosynthesis may help improve the accuracy of mammography [3]. Ultrasound is better at predicting pathology tumor size and nodal response compared to mammography [4].

More advanced imaging techniques, specifically breast MRI, utilizes both anatomic and functional information for assessment of tumor response. MRI is currently the most accurate imaging modality, with a positive predictive value of 93%, negative predictive value of 65%, and an overall diagnostic accuracy of 84% [2]. This does vary by tumor subtypes, with the highest accuracy achieved in HER2-positive and triple-negative tumors [5]. Accuracy may also be affected by the type of chemotherapy regimen prescribed, since Taxanes and antiangiogenic drugs may alter contrast enhancement patterns due to their antivascular properties [6]. MRI might also underestimate the amount of residual disease in tumors that undergo fragmentation compared to those that remain intact and shrink concentrically. Conversely, MRI might overestimate residual disease if there is an exuberant fibrotic reaction or inflammatory response within the tumor bed [7]. Additionally, it is important to note that MRI may detect noninvasive disease.

Mammography: Imaging appearance of the carcinoma depends on the degree of response to treatment:

- The mass may not have changed in appearance or may be larger if there has been no response or progressive disease, respectively.
- The most common response to NCT is reduction in tumor size and decreased density of the mass lesion. The mass lesion may become a focal asymmetry as it shrinks and fragments.
- The lesion may no longer be visible if complete response has occurred.
- Calcifications may develop either as worsening of disease or as a response to treatment.

Ultrasound: Like mammography, the imaging is variable depending on response:

- Tumor size is the best indicator of response. The mass may be larger (progressive disease), stable (no response), smaller (partial response) or no longer visible (complete response).
- Ultrasound tends to be more accurate for detection of residual tumors than mammography, particularly for women with dense breast tissue.
- Echogenicity of the mass may increase, becoming more isoechoic, with treatment response and fibrosis.
- Treatment-related fibrosis may mimic residual tumors.

MRI: Tumoral size and assessment of residual tumor enhancement are the most important features for gauging NCT response using MRI.

- MRI is the most accurate imaging method for size/extent of residual tumor, especially for triple-negative and HER2-positive tumors (compared to luminal tumors).
- Concentric shrinkage of a tumor is easier to visualize and measure, although fragmentation occurs frequently as a manifestation of response with little concomitant change in overall tumor size.
- False-positive enhancement within the tumor bed may be due to fibrosis, necrosis, or inflammation.
- MRI can underestimate residual disease if treated with agents such as taxanes or antiangiogenic medications.
- Changes in diffusion-weighted imaging, with elevation of apparent diffusion coefficient values for responders, may be an early indicator of response before changes in tumor size.

PET/CT: Performed occasionally to assess response both mid therapy and post therapy.

BI-RADS: 6, known malignancy—appropriate management of the known malignancy is recommended.

Differential Diagnosis: Post-therapy fibrosis/tumor bed, residual viable tumor.

Pathology Findings

Gross: The term "tumor bed" was devised to describe the prior tumor site in the surgical specimen after NCT. Tumor bed is easier to identify on gross examination if there is minimal to no response to NCT, as the appearance of residual tumor is similar to untreated tumors. On the other hand, tumor bed may not be readily visible if a tumor had undergone complete pathologic response (PCR) to therapy. In the majority of cases of complete, almost complete and moderate partial response to NCT, the tumor bed appears as a vague fibrous area with a softer consistency. Therefore, deploying a biopsy clip or a marker at the time of core biopsy of the untreated tumor is crucial to identify the area of tumor bed after surgery. In many cases, radiographs of the specimen to locate the biopsy clip to locate the tumor bed ensures proper sampling of the tumor bed for microscopic examination.

Microscopic Histology: In PCR cases, the required element is microscopic confirmation of the tumor bed. An area of fibroelastotic or loose stroma due to edema and fragmentation of collagen characterizes the tumor bed. It appears paler than normal breast stroma and usually devoid of normal breast epithelium. The stroma may contain scattered lymphocytes, plasma cells, and hemosiderin-laden macrophages. In mucinous carcinoma, extracellular mucin remains in the tumor bed irrespective of the degree of response to therapy [8].

The microscopic appearance of residual tumor, when present, is variable. With minimal response, the tumor may not show any chemotherapy effect except a rim of tumor bed stroma at the periphery of the tumor. With partial response to therapy, the most common chemotherapy effect is loss of cellularity. In addition to loss of cellularity, in some cases cytological changes secondary to chemotherapy manifest as an increase in cytoplasmic volume, cytoplasmic vacuolization, enlarged and bizarre nuclei and lower mitotic activity. Necrosis in the tumor bed is not a common effect of chemotherapy. Distribution of residual tumor within the tumor bed varies from tumor to tumor, from scattered single cells to small clusters or larger nodules of tumor, as if the tumor fragmented with bits remaining. Not only does the size of the tumor decrease, but the density decreases due to loss of cellularity. When residual tumor is present primarily as single cells, it is possible for pathologists to overlook the tumor cells. In some instances, it is difficult to differentiate IC from DCIS or lymphovascular invasion (LVI) as tumor clusters appear circumscribed or have retraction artifact, respectively.

Axillary lymph nodes with metastatic carcinoma often mirror the changes seen in the breast specimen.

While there may be no residual IC present after chemotherapy, ductal carcinoma in situ (DCIS) and LVI tend to persist after NCT. As with IC, NCT tends to decrease mitosis and increase nuclear pleomorphism in DCIS. In HER2-positive tumors, prominent response in DCIS to chemotherapy and anti-HER2 therapy leads to ducts containing no or few residual neoplastic cells, and lumens filled with abundant macrophages with residual calcifications. The presence of residual DCIS does not change the classification of PCR.

Many classification systems are available to determine the response to therapy. However, the I-SPY NCT trial devised a web-based calculator called Residual Cancer Burden (RCB) to classify the response into four groups based on the estimated volume of residual tumor in the breast and regional lymph nodes [9]. The use of RCB systems in clinical trials has shown strong association between the different RCB class and patient outcome (disease-free survival) [10].

Differential Diagnoses: Residual invasive carcinoma vs. DCIS or LVI.

Management: Imaging surveillance after surgical treatment.

Case Examples

See Fig. 12.4.

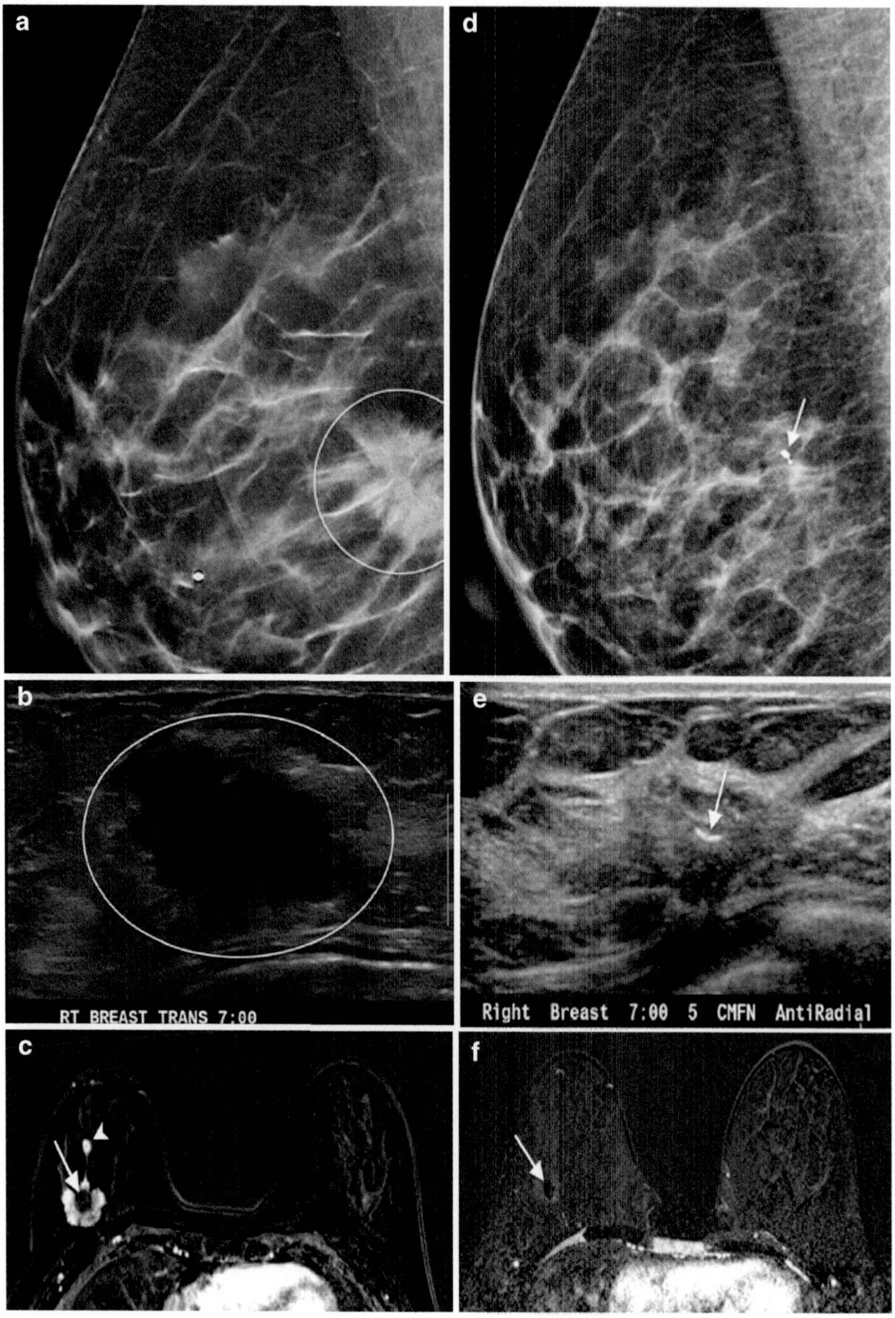

Fig. 12.4 A 35-year-old woman who was diagnosed with grade 3 IDC of the right breast (ER 70%, PR 2%, HER2 positive (FISH amplified with ratio of 3.3 and average Her2 copy number 6.26) and a high Ki-67 of 90%) underwent neoadjuvant chemotherapy with docetaxel, carboplatin, trastuzumab, and pertuzumab every 3 weeks for 6 cycles. (**a–c**) A 3-cm irregular mass (circled) with indistinct margins is identified in the 7 o'clock right breast. MRI also demonstrates a satellite nodule anteriorly (**c**, arrowhead). (**d–f**) The mass has resolved on subsequent imaging following neoadjuvant chemotherapy. The biopsy clip seen is on all three modalities (arrows) without a visible surrounding mass (complete response). The satellite mass on MRI has also resolved

Case Examples

See Fig. 12.5.

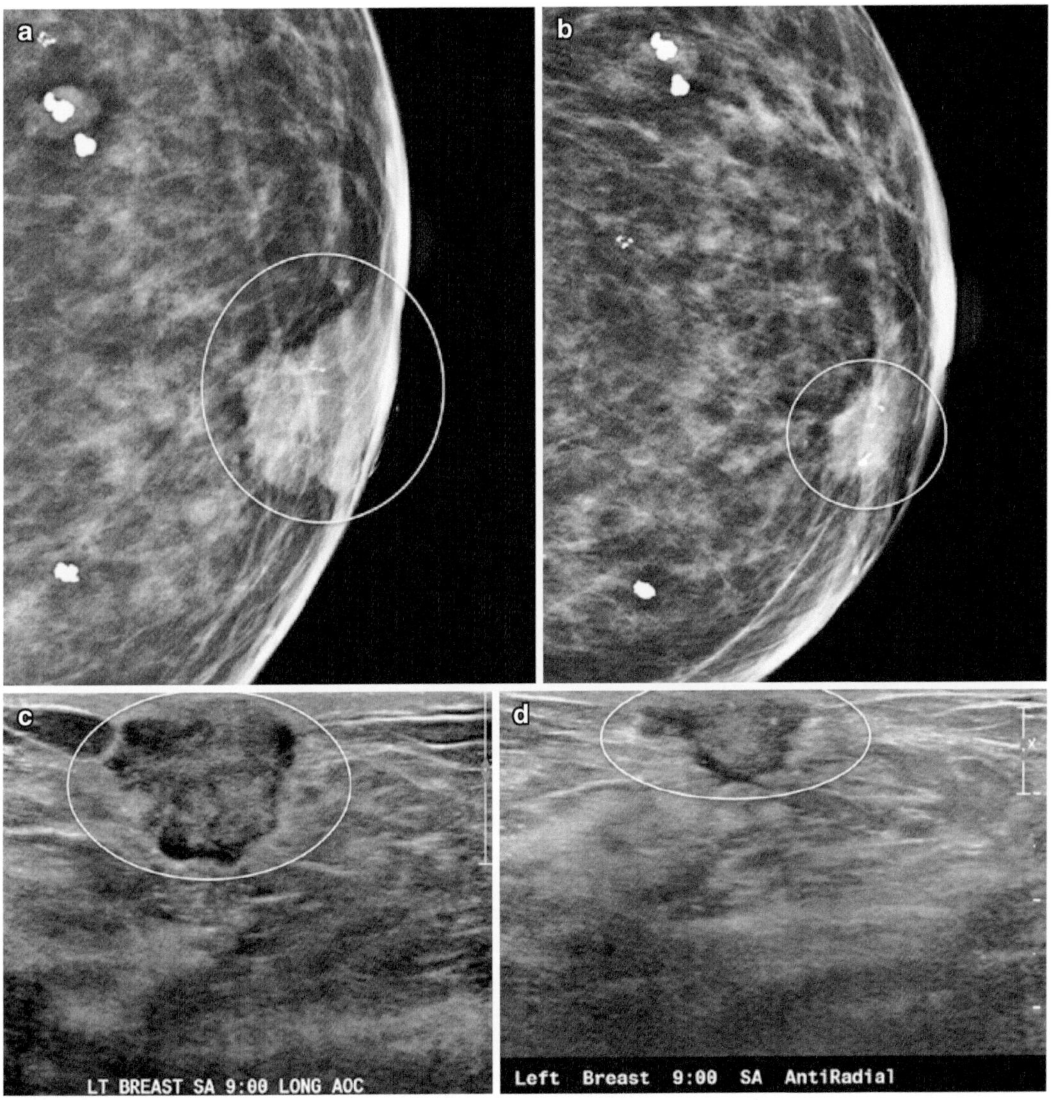

Fig. 12.5 A 65-year-old woman who was diagnosed with grade 3 IDC of the right breast (ER 100%, PR 100%, HER2 negative, Ki-67 40–55%) underwent neoadjuvant endocrine therapy with Arimidex daily followed by chemotherapy. (**a**, **b**) Initial mammogram and ultrasound imaging reveals a superficial subareolar irregular hypoechoic mass extending into the overlying dermis. (**c**, **d**) Follow-up imaging taken 5 months later and 4 months after initiation of therapy demonstrates partial response, with the mass decreasing in volume by approximately 80% mammographically and 70% sonographically

Case Examples

See Fig. 12.6.

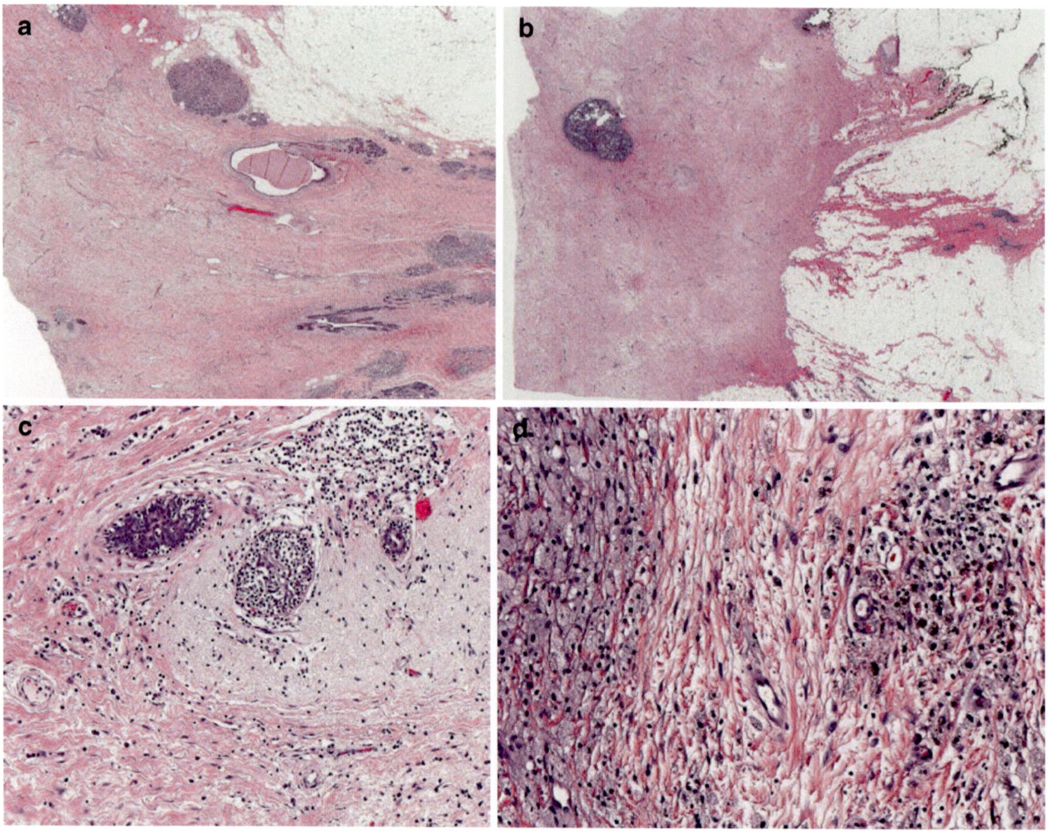

Fig. 12.6 Microscopic appearance of "tumor bed". (**a**) Scanning view of a section taken from the tumor bed area depicts pale stroma rimmed by normal breast ducts and lobules. (**b**) Section from a different case shows tumor bed area with core biopsy clip site at the upper left corner. (**c**) Medium power view of the tumor bed reveals edematous loose stroma with elastosis and scattered inflammatory cells. (**d**) Tumor bed with sheets of foamy histiocytes and hemosiderin-laden macrophages

Case Examples

See Fig. 12.7.

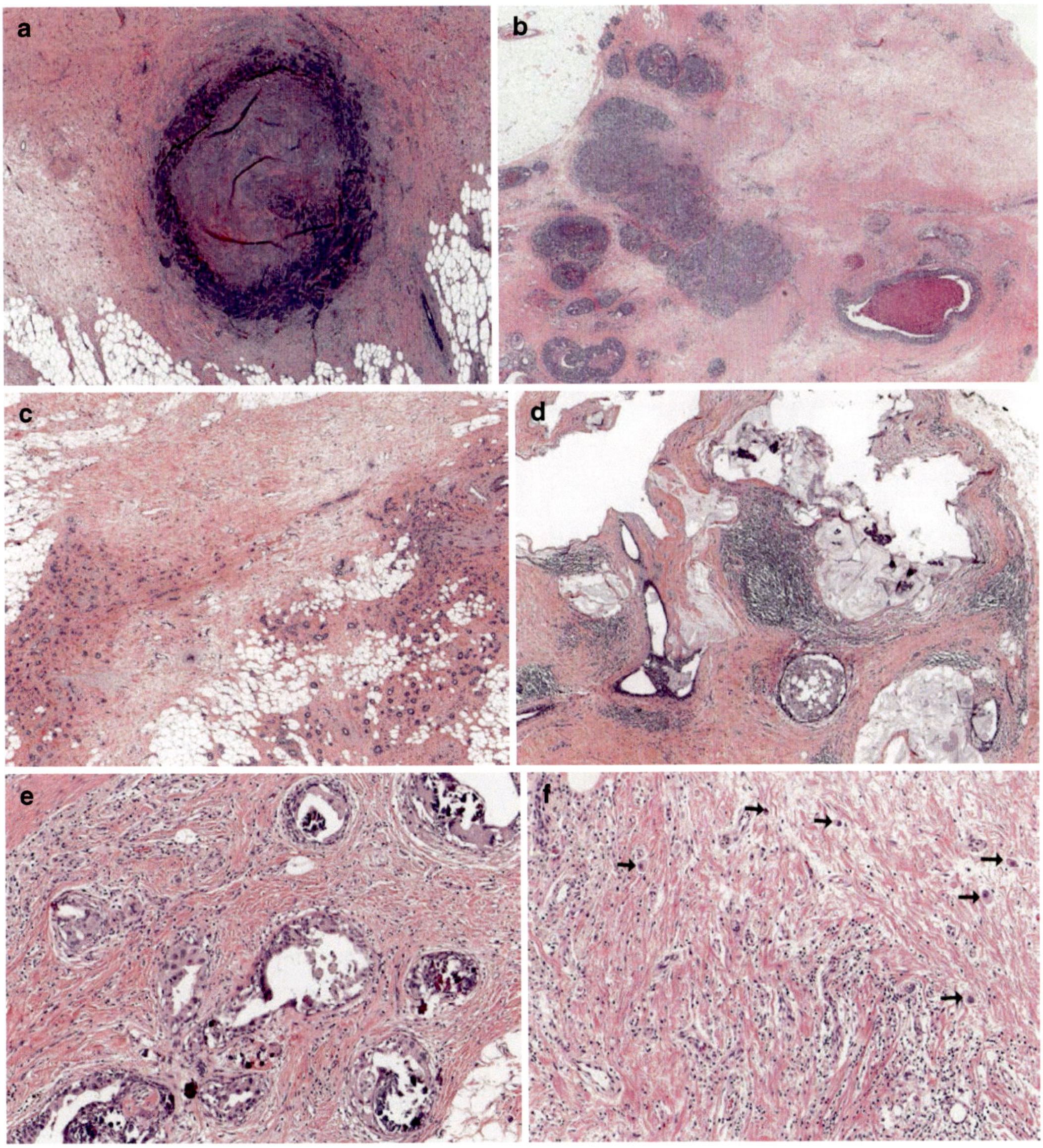

Fig. 12.7 Microscopic appearance of tumor bed with partial response to therapy. (**a**) Tumor bed with a single residual nodule of residual tumor. (**b**) Partial response with right half of the tumor bed with loss of tumor cells (60% viable cells). (**c**) Multiple patches of residual tumor cells with intervening stroma without tumor cells. (**d**) High-grade mucinous carcinoma with few clusters of tumor cells with abundant extracellular mucin in the stroma. (**e**) Tumor bed with predominantly residual ductal carcinoma in situ with associated calcifications. (**f**) Scattered single tumor cells (arrows) in a fibro-inflammatory tumor bed can be easily overlooked unless examined carefully

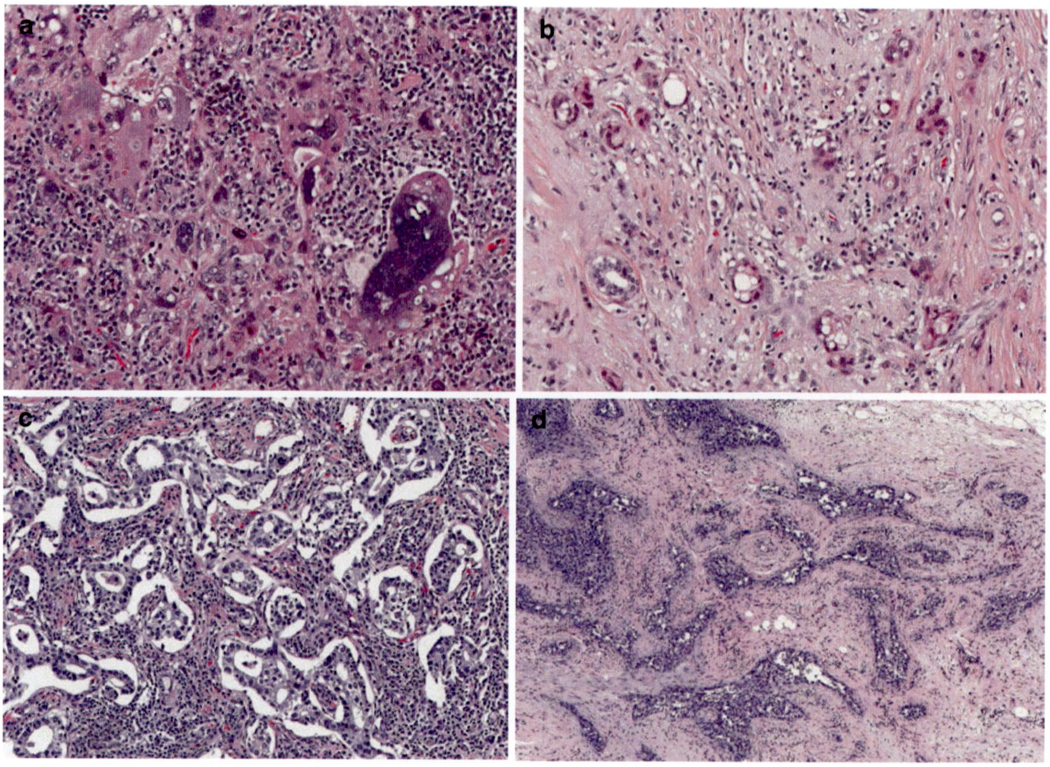

Fig. 12.8 Cytologic alteration due to therapy. (**a**) Residual tumor cells with marked nuclear enlargement and pleomorphism. (**b**) Residual tumor cells with cytoplasmic vacuolization. (**c**) Tumor nests with prominent retraction artifact. (**d**) Residual entrapped DCIS with distorted outlines mimicking invasion

Case Examples
See Fig. 12.8.

Breast Carcinoma Treated with Neoadjuvant Endocrine Therapy

Endocrine therapy is a standard treatment for hormone receptor (HR)-positive breast carcinomas. Unlike NCT where the agents are cytotoxic, with neoadjuvant endocrine therapy (NET), the goal of the treatment is to stop further growth and proliferation, thus PCR is rare. NET tends to show minimal to partial response and the tumor bed changes are not prominent. However, in the majority of cases, the proliferation index, as measured by Ki-67, decreases markedly after NET [11, 12].

Clinical features: Neoadjuvant endocrine therapy is offered to patients with locally advanced strongly HR-positive, HER2-negative IC with a low proliferative index (Ki67 <15%). It is also an option for patients who are unable to tolerate chemotherapy or are enrolled in clinical trials for HR-positive tumors. During the COVID pandemic, many breast cancer patients received endocrine therapy while awaiting for surgery, leading to a temporary increase in NET cases [13].

Imaging Findings

Multimodality imaging findings for NET response assessment are somewhat different to that of NCT, in that response to therapy is usually more gradual and less often results in complete response.

BI-RADS: 6, known malignancy—appropriate management of the known malignancy is recommended.

Differential Diagnosis: Post-therapy fibrosis/tumor bed, residual viable tumor.

Pathology Findings

Gross: As NET usually shows mild to partial response, tumor is evident grossly and looks similar to untreated IC. Classically, IC appears as a stellate tan-white lesion with infiltrative borders that cuts with a gritty sensation.

Microscopic histology: Unlike NCT, with NET, it is less common for the tumor to show fragmentation, loss of cellularity or cytologic effect due to therapy. In most cases, a tumor bed with characteristic fibroelastosis or loose stroma may not be appreciable. The tumor may appear histologically identical to an untreated tumor. As tumor bed changes are usually minimal, significant decrease in size of the tumor is not common. In cases with pronounced response, tumor bed changes as seen in NCT may be present with a decrease in cellularity and size of the tumor. Irrespective of change in size or morphology of the tumor, the only objective way to evaluate response in NET setting is to assess the proliferative index in the residual tumor. Tumors that respond to NET often have a dramatic decrease in the Ki-67 index to a very low level, for example 1–2% or less. Additional changes seen after NET include reduced or loss of expression of progesterone receptor (more common) and estrogen receptor (less common) in the tumor.

Differential Diagnoses: Untreated tumor.

Management: Imaging surveillance after surgical treatment.

Case Examples
See Fig. 12.9.

Case Examples
See Fig. 12.10.

Case Examples
See Fig. 12.11.

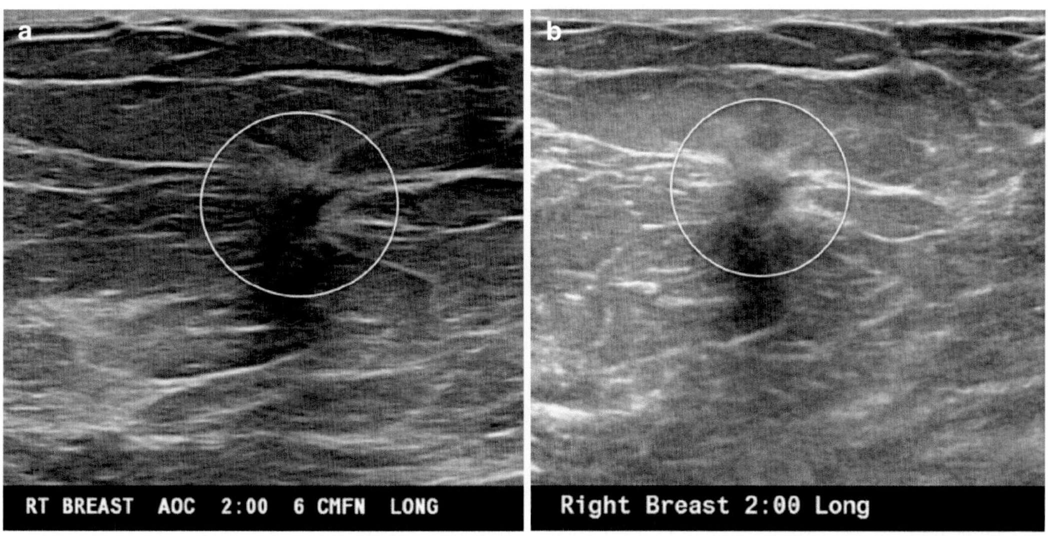

Fig. 12.9 A 55-year-old woman with grade 2 IDC of the right breast (ER 100%, PR 80%, HER2 negative, Ki-67 15%) underwent neoadjuvant endocrine therapy with letrazole. (**a**) Initial ultrasound imaging reveals an irregular hypoechoic mass (circled) with spiculated margins, measuring up to 9 mm. (**b**) Follow-up ultrasound imaging taken 22 days later demonstrates partial response, with the mass (circled) measuring up to 8 mm and a decreased tumor volume by approximately 24%

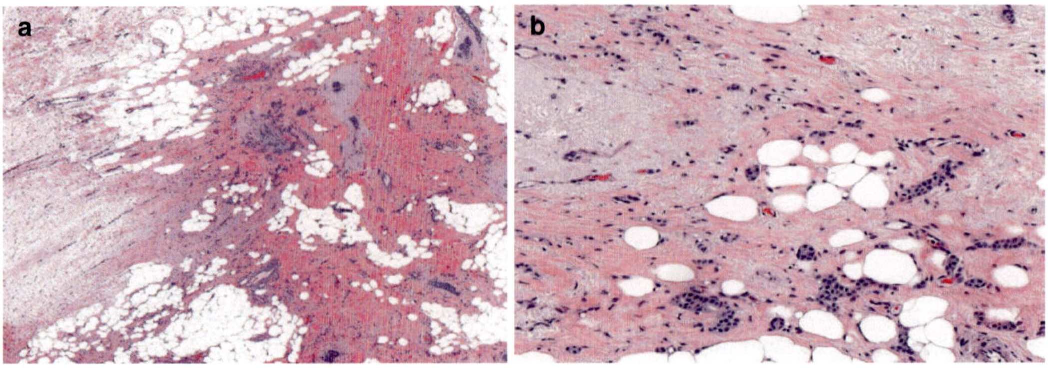

Fig. 12.10 Invasive lobular carcinoma treated with neoadjuvant endocrine therapy. (**a**) Low power view reveals partial response to therapy with patchy loss of tumor cells, most prominent on the left half. (**b**) Medium power view reveals vascularized elastotic stroma and fewer residual tumor cells (the Ki-67 dropped from pretreatment value of 10% to below 1% after therapy)

Recurrent Tumor

Clinical features: Recurrent breast cancer may manifest as IC or DCIS. Depending on the surgery previously performed, recurrent malignancy may be located in the residual breast tissue or prior surgical site or in the chest wall after total mastectomy. Factors associated with increased risk of loco-regional recurrence include young age at diagnosis, advanced tumor size, involvement of regional lymph nodes, high grade, vascular invasion, and omitting any indicated adjuvant radiotherapy [14]. The prognosis of local recurrent tumor also depends if the recurrent tumor is a true recurrence vs. new primary tumor [15].

Imaging Findings

Mammography: While recurrent invasive carcinoma often presents as a developing asymmetry or mass, recurrent DCIS presents as new suspicious pleomorphic or fine linear branching calcifications.

- Findings that increase or worsen over time are suspicious for recurrence. Changes related to fat necrosis with scar will remain stable or improve over time.
- New or developing asymmetry or mass with or without calcifications at or near the lumpectomy scar should often prompt biopsy.
- Tomosynthesis improves sensitivity of mammography for the detection of recurrence.

Ultrasound: Recurrent invasive carcinoma often presents as an irregular hypoechoic mass within or in close proximity to the surgical bed and often possesses demonstrable internal blood flow on Doppler analysis.

- Recurrent DCIS is typically occult on sonography.

MRI: A recurrent invasive carcinoma often presents as an irregular enhancing mass while recurrent DCIS presents as clumped linear or clustered ring non-mass enhancement.

- Absence of enhancement near the surgical bed is a reassuring finding.

BI-RADS: 4, suspicious for malignancy, biopsy is recommended for histologic confirmation.

Differential Diagnosis: Scar, fat necrosis, postsurgical fluid collection, second new primary cancer, radiation-induced sarcoma.

Pathology Findings

Gross: Recurrent invasive breast cancer has a similar appearance to de novo invasive carci-

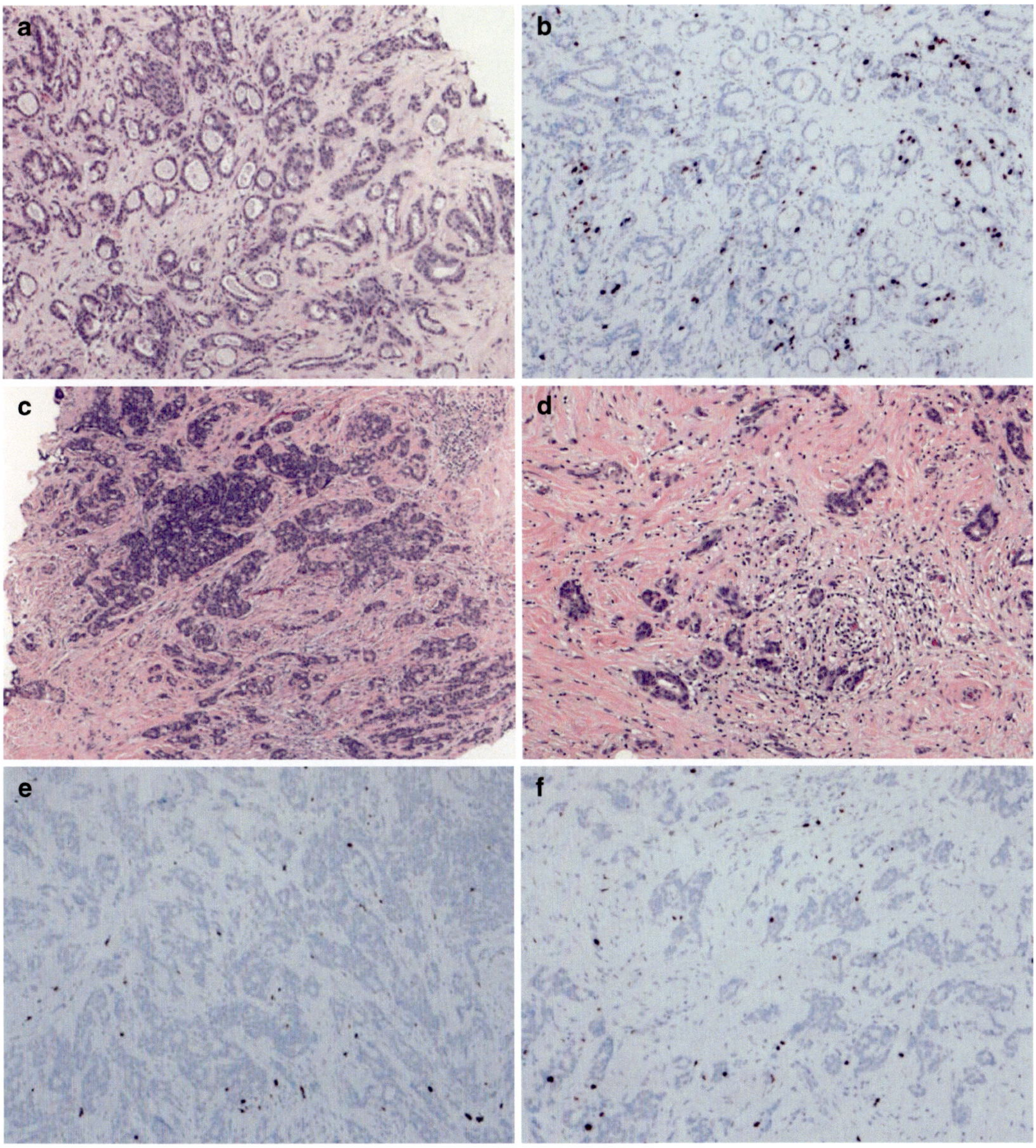

Fig. 12.11 Invasive ductal carcinoma treated with neoadjuvant endocrine therapy. (**a**) Medium power view of the pretreatment core biopsy revealing a grade 1 invasive ductal carcinoma. (**b**) Corresponding Ki-67 stain on the core biopsy shows approximately 15% cells positive. (**c**) Medium power view of the post treatment excisional biopsy with areas of high cellularity. (**d**) Other areas of the post-treated tumor showing partial response in the form of loss of cellularity. (**e**, **f**) Immunostain for Ki-67 in the cellular and less cellular areas of the tumor reveals low Ki-67 level (1%)

noma. When it involves the scar site, it may be difficult to differentiate the tumor from the surgical scar; however, the area of invasive carcinoma may appear softer and fleshy while the scar is more fibrotic. As in de novo DCIS, recurrent DCIS will not be grossly evident.

Microscopic histology: The morphology of the recurrent invasive carcinoma and recurrent

DCIS is usually similar to that of the initial tumor, unless the ipsilateral tumor is a new primary.

Management: Individualized based on the diagnosis and prior treatments.

Case Examples
See Fig. 12.12.

Case Examples
See Fig. 12.13.

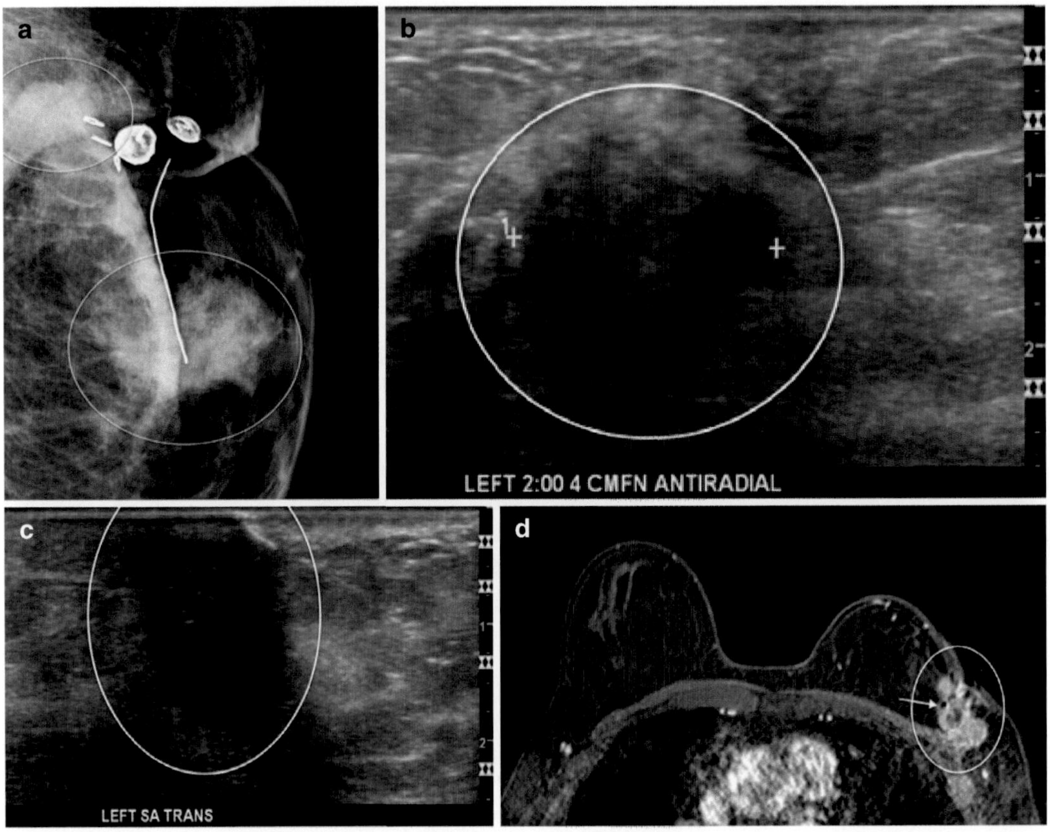

Fig. 12.12 A 60-year-old woman who presents with new left periareolar skin changes. She underwent prior left partial mastectomy. (**a**) A left diagnostic MLO mammogram image demonstrates post-lumpectomy changes in the superior aspect of the left breast as well as two new focal asymmetries (circled) and an intervening area of skin thickening along the surgical scar (wire marker). (**b**, **c**) Targeted ultrasound of the left breast demonstrates a 2.5-cm irregular hypoechoic mass in the 2 o'clock left breast (circled, **b**) and a 3-cm mass in the subareolar left breast (circle, **c**). Both were biopsied, yielding grade 2 invasive lobular carcinoma at both locations. (**d**) Subsequent MR imaging to evaluate extent of disease demonstrates an irregular heterogeneously enhancing mass in the upper outer left breast that extends from the retracted skin surface to the pectoralis muscle

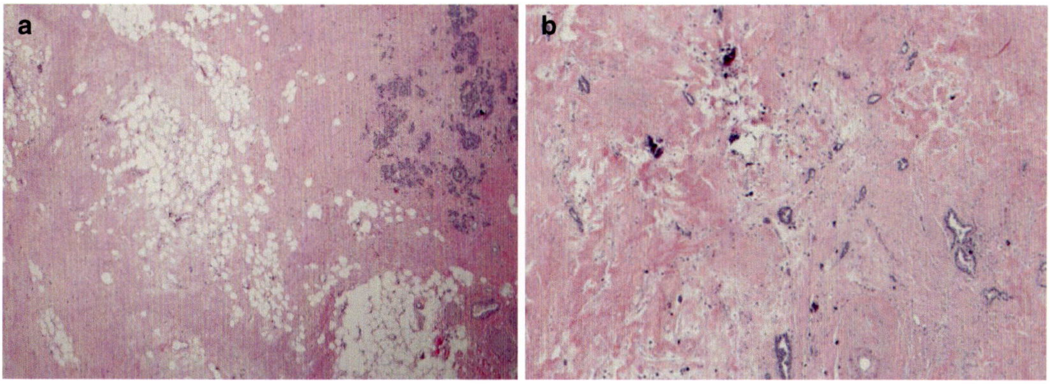

Fig. 12.13 Recurrent grade 2 invasive ductal carcinoma in a prior lumpectomy scar. (**a**) Low power view of the carcinoma in the upper right corner and extensive scarring seen in the left half of the picture. (**b**) Medium power view of another area of the tumor with sclerotic stroma with dystrophic calcification and residual tumor (patient was treated with neoadjuvant chemotherapy due to extensive disease)

References

1. Fowler AM, Mankoff DA, Joe BN. Imaging neoadjuvant therapy response in breast cancer. Radiology. 2017;285(2):358–75.
2. Croshaw R, Shapiro-Wright H, Svensson E, Erb K, Julian T. Accuracy of clinical examination, digital mammogram, ultrasound, and MRI in determining postneoadjuvant pathologic tumor response in operable breast cancer patients. Ann Surg Oncol. 2011;18(11):3160–3.
3. Förnvik D, Zackrisson S, Ljungberg O, et al. Breast tomosynthesis: accuracy of tumor measurement compared with digital mammography and ultrasonography. Acta Radiol. 2010;51(3):240–7.
4. Keune JD, Jeffe DB, Schootman M, Hoffman A, Gillanders WE, Aft RL. Accuracy of ultrasonography and mammography in predicting pathologic response after neoadjuvant chemotherapy for breast cancer. Am J Surg. 2010;199(4):477–84. https://doi.org/10.1016/j.amjsurg.2009.03.012. PMID: 20359567; PMCID: PMC3252889.
5. Mukhtar RA, Yau C, Rosen M, et al. Clinically meaningful tumor reduction rates vary by prechemotherapy MRI phenotype and tumor subtype in the I-SPY 1 TRIAL (CALGB 150007/150012; ACRIN 6657). Ann Surg Oncol. 2013;20(12):3823–30.
6. Bahri S, Chen JH, Mehta RS, et al. Residual breast cancer diagnosed by MRI in patients receiving neoadjuvant chemotherapy with and without bevacizumab. Ann Surg Oncol. 2009;16(6):1619–28.
7. Wasser K, Sinn HP, Fink C, et al. Accuracy of tumor size measurement in breast cancer using MRI is influenced by histological regression induced by neoadjuvant chemotherapy. Eur Radiol. 2003;13(6):1213–23.
8. Sahoo S, Krings G, Chen Y-Y, et al. Standardizing pathologic evaluation of breast carcinoma after neoadjuvant chemotherapy: recommendations from the I-SPY Pathology Working Group. Arch Pathol Lab Med. 2022;147:591. https://doi.org/10.5858/arpa.2022-0021-EP.
9. Symmans WF, Peintinger F, Hatzis C, et al. Measurement of residual breast cancer burden to predict survival after neoadjuvant chemotherapy. J Clin Oncol. 2007;25(28):4414–22. https://doi.org/10.1200/JCO.2007.10.6823.
10. Yau C, Osdoit M, van der Noordaa M, et al. Residual cancer burden after neoadjuvant chemotherapy and long-term survival outcomes in breast cancer: a multicentre pooled analysis of 5161 patients. Lancet Oncol. 2022;23(1):149–60. https://doi.org/10.1016/S1470-2045(21)00589-1. Epub 2021 Dec 11. PMID: 34902335; PMCID: PMC9455620.
11. Martí C, Yébenes L, Oliver JM, et al. The clinical impact of neoadjuvant endocrine treatment on luminal-like breast cancers and its prognostic significance: results from a single-institution prospective cohort study. Curr Oncol. 2022;29(4):2199–210. https://doi.org/10.3390/curroncol29040179. PMID: 35448153; PMCID: PMC9026529.
12. Ellis MJ, Tao Y, Luo J, A'Hern R, Evans DB, Bhatnagar AS, Chaudri Ross HA, von Kameke A, Miller WR, Smith I, Eiermann W, Dowsett M. Outcome prediction for estrogen receptor-positive breast cancer based on postneoadjuvant endocrine therapy tumor characteristics. J Natl Cancer Inst. 2008;100(19):1380–8. https://doi.org/10.1093/jnci/djn309. Epub 2008 Sep 23. PMID: 18812550; PMCID: PMC2556704.

13. Martí C, Sánchez-Méndez JI. Neoadjuvant endocrine therapy for luminal breast cancer treatment: a first-choice alternative in times of crisis such as the COVID-19 pandemic. Ecancermedicalscience. 2020;14:1027. https://doi.org/10.3332/ecancer.2020.1027.
14. Wallgren A, Bonetti M, Gelber RD, Goldhirsch A, Castiglione-Gertsch M, Holmberg SB, Lindtner J, Thurlimann B, Fey M, Werner ID, et al. Risk factors for locoregional recurrence among breast cancer patients: results from international breast cancer study group trials I through VII. J Clin Oncol. 2003;21:1205–13.
15. Komoike Y, Akiyama F, Iino Y, et al. Analysis of ipsilateral breast tumor recurrences after breast-conserving treatment based on the classification of true recurrences and new primary tumors. Breast Cancer. 2005;12(2):104–11. https://doi.org/10.2325/jbcs.12.104. PMID: 15858440.

13 Rare Breast Tumors

Malini Harigopal, Peter Podany, Liva Andrejeva, and Kamaljeet Singh

Mucocele-Like Lesion (MLL)

Mucocele-Like Lesion (MLL): Mucocele-like lesion of the breast is a recently recognized breast lesion. They are relatively uncommon, but can occur in women of all ages, often presenting with calcifications seen on screening. Histologically an MLL is characterized by focally dilated ducts that are filled with mucin and may rupture, producing acellular extracellular mucin in the breast parenchyma [1]. Calcifications are frequently found in association with the stromal mucin and adjacent ducts. MLL in core needle biopsy is frequently associated with proliferative epithelial changes, which can be atypical, leading to follow-up excision. MLL with non-atypical epithelial proliferative changes, after radiology-pathology correlation, can be followed up conservatively [2].

M. Harigopal · P. Podany
Department of Pathology, Yale University, New Haven, CT, USA
e-mail: malini.harigopal@yale.edu; peter.podany@yale.edu

L. Andrejeva
Department of Radiology and Biomedical Imaging, Yale School of Medicine, New Haven, CT, USA
e-mail: liva.andrejeva@yale.edu

K. Singh (✉)
Department of Pathology and Laboratory Medicine, Brown University and Women and Infants Hospital of RI, Providence, RI, USA
e-mail: kamaljeet_singh@brown.edu

- **Clinical Presentation**: The incidence of MLL is 0.2% in core needle biopsies (CNB) with a mean age of presentation of 54 years (range 27–82 years) [1, 3]. Calcifications are the most frequent target lesion in MLL (83–95%), followed by a mass (5–18%) [3]. MLL is associated with a spectrum of ductal epithelial proliferation that can be further categorized as benign or atypical. In CNB, atypical ductal proliferation or MLL with atypia is identified in 36–66% of cases [3].
- **Imaging Findings**:
  - **Mammography**: Coarse heterogeneous calcifications, but may also present as pleomorphic calcifications.
    Associated mass or asymmetry may be present.
  - **US**: May be negative, or demonstrate a complicated cyst, complex cystic and solid mass, clustered cysts, or even a solid appearing mass with associated calcifications.
  - **MRI**: T2 hyperintense mass with variable degree of enhancement.
  - **BI-RADS**: 4, suspicious of malignancy.
  - **Differential Diagnosis**: These may mimic common benign lesions, such as degenerating fibroadenomas, or malignant lesions, such as DCIS.
- **Pathology Findings**:

M. Harigopal et al. (eds.), *Radiology Pathology Correlations of Breast Lesions*,
https://doi.org/10.1007/978-3-031-65711-5_13

- **Gross Description**: Macroscopic appearance of MLL is not known. The lesion is grossly inconspicuous.
- **Microscopic Histology**: The MLL is characterized by acellular stromal mucin in perilobular, periductal or fibroadipose stromal tissue. The mucin has a viscid appearance. On hematoxylin and eosin, mucin shows variable light to moderate basophilic staining. Mucin is often associated with large chunky phosphate-type calcifications and is present as variable-sized gelatinous blobs embedded in or dissecting through the stroma. Dislodged and misplaced microscopic blobs of mucin can be present. Mucin in the stroma may or may not show continuity with mucin in ducts and lobules.
  - MLL associated with ruptured benign ducts and lobules and benign proliferative changes is categorized as MLL without atypia (Fig. 13.22).
  - MLL arising in a setting of atypical intraductal epithelial proliferation, like flat epithelial atypia and atypical ductal hyperplasia is classified as MLL with atypia. MLL may be seen with DCIS, which may raise concern for microinvasion.
- **Differential Diagnosis**: Mucinous carcinoma, disrupted cyst.
  - In an MLL with free-floating epithelial fragments, mucinous carcinoma is in the differential diagnosis.
  - Demonstration of myoepithelial cells by IHC excludes mucinous carcinoma.
    - However, in MLL associated with DCIS, the epithelial fragments in the mucin can be myoepithelial deficient. Pathologists should exercise caution before labeling myoepithelium-depleted epithelium in the mucin as invasive. Disrupted mucinous DCIS with dislodged epithelium should be excluded. A comment explaining the uncertainty regarding invasion and follow up with an excision to exclude invasion is a pragmatic approach.
- **Management**: Excision has been traditionally recommended for all MLL; however, conservative management may be considered for MLL without atypia that reveal concordant radiology and pathology findings. MLL with large extent of calcifications, residual calcifications after CNB and mass lesion should be excised. MLL with atypia is managed by surgical excision.
  - A careful radiology-pathology correlation is required for all MLL.

Case

Clinical History: A 50-year-old female was recalled from screening mammography due to new grouped left breast calcifications (Figs. 13.1 and 13.2).

BI-RADS: 4, suspicious of malignancy.

A stereotactic biopsy was recommended and performed yielding a mucocele-like lesion with atypia (Figs. 13.3 and 13.4).

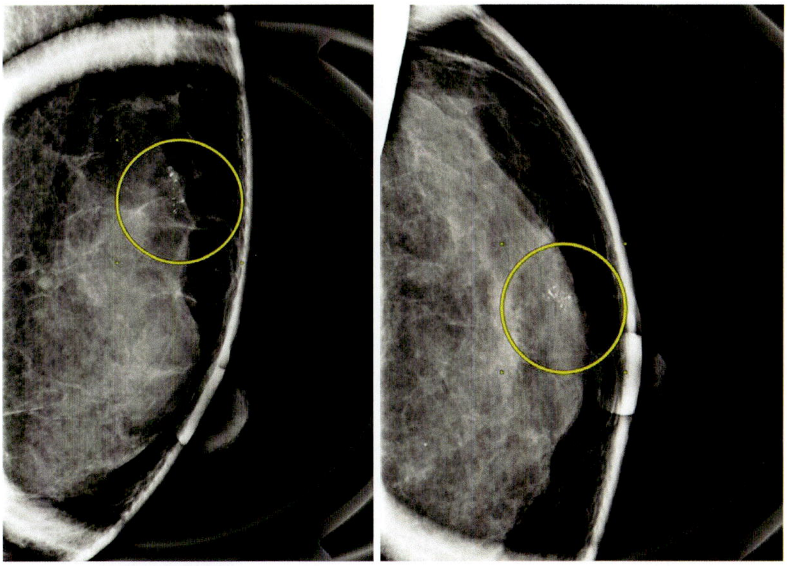

Figs. 13.1 and 13.2 **MG findings**: Magnification views on mammogram demonstrate grouped coarse heterogeneous calcifications

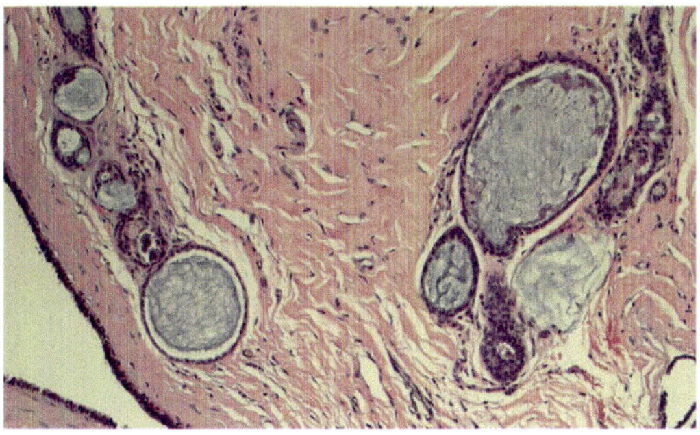

Fig. 13.3 A benign mucocele-like lesion (H&E, 20×) with benign mammary ducts and lobules distended with pale blue mucin. An extravasated mucin pool is present in the stroma

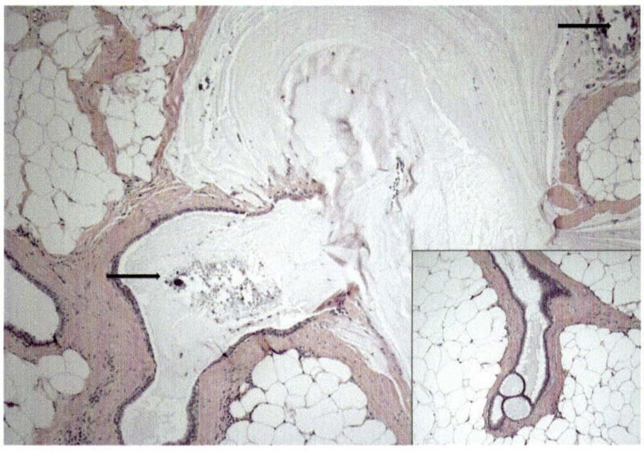

Fig. 13.4 A mucocele-like lesion with atypia (H&E, 10×). The breast ducts are distended with mucin and associated stromal mucin pools and calcifications (arrow) are present. The inset shows a focus of atypical ductal hyperplasia in the mucin-filled ducts

Myofibroblastoma

Myofibroblastoma: A myofibroblastoma is a rare, benign mesenchymal spindle cell tumor of the breast, which occurs with similar frequency in women and men, usually at middle age (50–75), but has been occasionally reported in adolescents [4]. It is a well-circumscribed, lobulated, homogeneous, solid mass without calcifications.

- **Clinical Presentation**: Myofibroblastoma usually presents as a slow-growing, painless, non-tender mobile mass in postmenopausal women, but may occur in men as well. It may be palpable or screening detected (in women).
- **Imaging Findings**:
  - **Mammography**: Oval or round mass with circumscribed margins, usually without calcifications.
  - **US**: Oval or round, usually circumscribed hypoechoic or mixed echogenicity mass, with or without vascularity.
  - **BI-RADS**: 3 or 4, as this lesion may mimic probably benign lesions such as a fibroadenoma or papilloma, particularly if screening detected.
  - **Differential Diagnosis**: Benign: Fibroadenoma, PASH, papilloma, epider-

moid inclusion cyst. Malignant: IDC, DCIS, primary breast sarcoma, lymphoma, metastatic lesion.

- **Pathology Findings**:
  - **Gross Description**: A myofibroblastoma is well circumscribed often round to oval solid mass. The cut surface is tan white to tan yellow.
  - **Microscopic Histology**: The mass consists of bland, spindled cells with pale eosinophilic cytoplasm arranged haphazardly or in intersecting fascicles with interspersed variably hyalinized collagen globules.
    - Nuclei may show grooves and pseudo inclusions without mitosis.
    - A range of unusual cytological features and metaplastic changes have been described, which can complicate the histological diagnosis [5].
    - Extreme epithelioid cytology of the cells may lead to confusion with an epithelial lesion-like lobular carcinoma.
    - Has circumscribed pushing borders.
    - The tumor cells express myofibroblastic markers (desmin) and hormonal receptors (ER and PR) [6]. They are also CD34 positive and show loss of RB1 expression in the majority of cases.
  - **Differential Diagnosis**: Spindle cell lesions, metaplastic carcinoma, fibromatosis, pseudoangiomatous stromal hyperplasia (PASH).
  - **Management**: Conservative excision.

Case

Clinical History: A 47-year-old female presented with a screening detected left breast mass (Figs. 13.5, 13.6, 13.7, and 13.8).

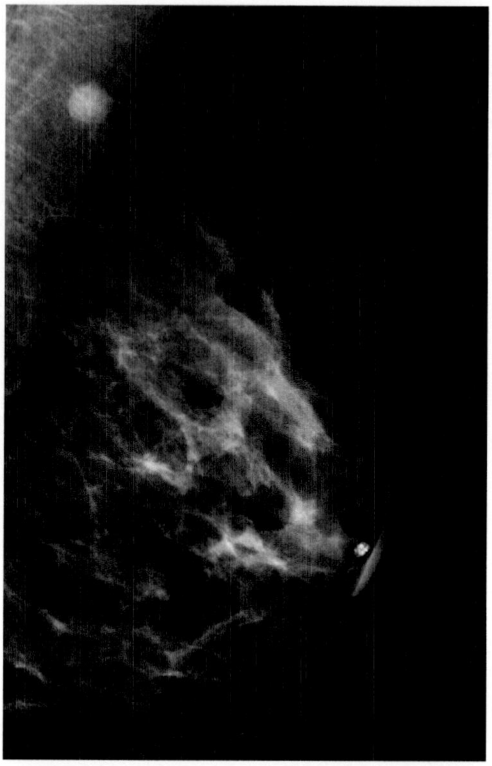

Fig. 13.5 MG findings: On mammogram there is a round mass with an indistinct margin in the upper aspect of the left breast, seen on the MLO view only due to its extreme posterior location

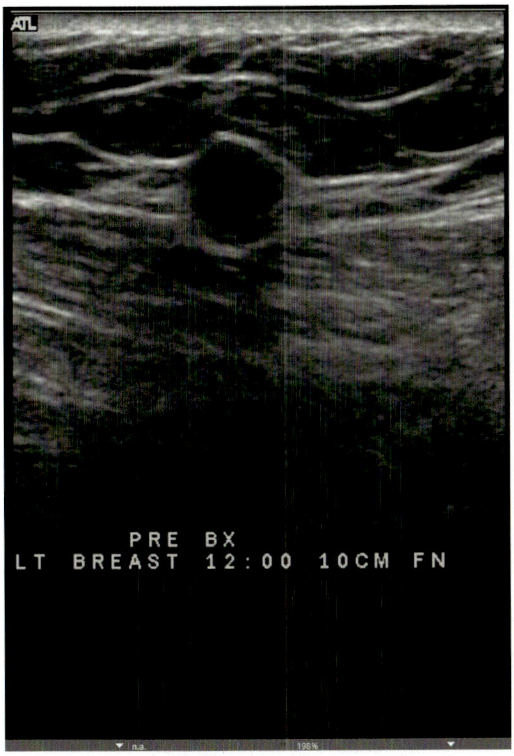

Fig. 13.6 **USG Findings**: Ultrasound showed a round, hypoechoic mass with an indistinct margin, posterior acoustic shadowing, and no demonstrable internal vascularity. The mass was called BI-RADS 4, suspicious for malignancy, and an US-guided biopsy was recommended and performed revealing a myofibroblastoma

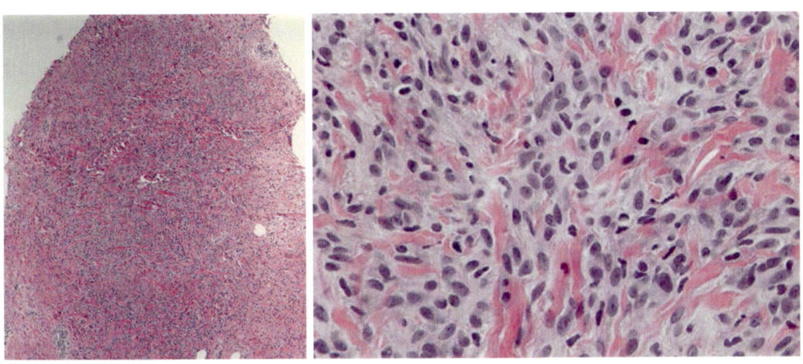

Figs. 13.7 and 13.8 Myofibroblastoma (H&E, 2× and 20×) Core needle biopsy from a 56-year-old woman comprised of sheets of plump spindle cells spread in collagenous stroma. The tumor cells have bland, pale chromatin and absent mitotic activity. The lesion was diagnosed as a myofibroblastoma

Malignant

Adenoid Cystic Carcinoma

Adenoid Cystic Carcinoma (ADCC): Adenoid cystic carcinoma of breast is a salivary gland-type primary breast tumor. ADCC is a rare tumor in the breast representing only 0.1% of all breast cancers [7]. Despite being triple negative, unlike salivary gland tumors, ADCC of breast has an excellent prognosis. This invasive carcinoma is composed of a mixture of epithelial and myoepithelial neoplastic cells. Tumor cells harbor the *MYB-NFIB* gene fusion.

- **Clinical Presentation**: ADCC of breast usually presents as a mass lesion that can be palpable or screening-detected. Axillary nodal metastases and distant metastases are rare. Although mostly diagnosed in women during the fifth and sixth decade of life, there is a wide age range from the second to the eighth decade [7, 8].
- **Imaging Findings**:
  - **Mammography**: Round, oval, or irregular, with margins ranging from circumscribed to indistinct, occasionally with associated architectural distortion. Calcifications are uncommon.
  - **US**: Oval, round, solid hypoechoic mass with irregular, or microlobulated margins, with variable internal vascularity.
  - **BI-RADS**: 4, suspicious of malignancy.
  - **Differential Diagnosis**: When circumscribed it may mimic benign lesions such as fibroadenomas.
- **Pathology Findings**:
  - **Gross Description**: ADCC presents as a well-circumscribed nodule with pushing borders.
  - **Microscopic Histology**: Adenoid cystic carcinoma (ADCC) of the breast is composed of epithelial and myoepithelial cells entwined with basophilic stroma and basement membrane material, arranged in cribriform, tubular, and solid patterns.
    - ADCC of the breast is histologically similar to ADCC of salivary glands.
    - Classic ADCC histology shows varying patterns including cribriform, tubular or glandular, reticular, basaloid, and solid.
    - Focal sebaceous and adenosquamous differentiation can be seen.
    - True lumens lined by epithelial cells with eosinophilic cytoplasm are admixed with pseudo lumens filled with myxoid or pale blue material surrounded by myoepithelial/basaloid cells that show scant cytoplasm and dark hyperchromatic nuclei.
    - The epithelial and myoepithelial components stain differentially with keratin immunohistochemical stains. Immunostains are particularly useful as true lumens are outlined by cytokeratin 7-positive epithelial cells and basaloid myoepithelial cells are demonstrated by cytokeratin 5/6, 14, myoepithelial markers like p63, S100, and CD10.
    - c-KIT (CD117) is positive in the luminal cells, but not specific to ADCC.
    - The genetic changes reported in ADCC include the MYB-NFIB fusion gene, MYBL1 rearrangements, and MYB amplification [8].
    - The solid basaloid subtype of ADCC is characterized by solid nests of basaloid cells that show marked nuclear atypia, high mitotic count, and necrosis [9, 10].
    - The ADCC can be present in association with high-grade breast carcinoma, a setting described as ADCC with high-grade transformation.
    - The ADCC are triple-negative, i.e., they lack ER, PR, and HER2.
    - Unlike salivary gland ADCC, mammary ADCC has an excellent prognosis.
    - Although lymph node metastases are rare it has been reported more frequently in the solid variant of ADCC.
  - **Differential Diagnosis**:
    - Collagenous spherulosis is a benign proliferation of epithelial and myoepithelial cells with basement membrane-like material and a cribriform pattern. Collagenous spherulosis is an incidental

microscopic finding, often measuring <0.5 cm in size.
  - Invasive cribriform carcinoma can show histologically similar architecture; however, cribriform carcinoma lacks myoepithelial cells and is strongly ER positive.
  - Adenomyoepithelioma is composed of epithelial and myoepithelial cells and can be confused with ADCC on core biopsy. Matrix formation is minimal in adenomyoepithelioma.
  - Skin adnexal lesions can mimic ADCC, especially in a small limited sample. Clinical correlation and information regarding location of lesion (proximity to skin) can help.
- **Management**: ADCC, classic type is considered a favorable histologic subtype [11].
  - Treated with partial mastectomy and lymph node sampling.

Case

Clinical History: A 43-year-old female palpated a left breast mass (Figs. 13.9 and 13.10).

The lesion was called BI-RADS 4, suspicious for malignancy.

An US-guided biopsy was recommended and performed, yielding an adenoid cystic carcinoma (Figs. 13.11, 13.12, 13.13, and 13.14).

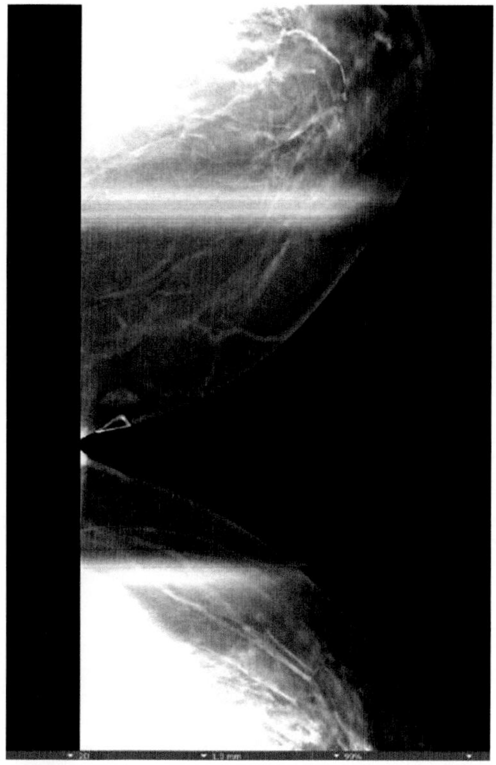

Fig. 13.9 **MG findings**: On mammography there was an oval, circumscribed mass in the subcutaneous tissues of the left breast

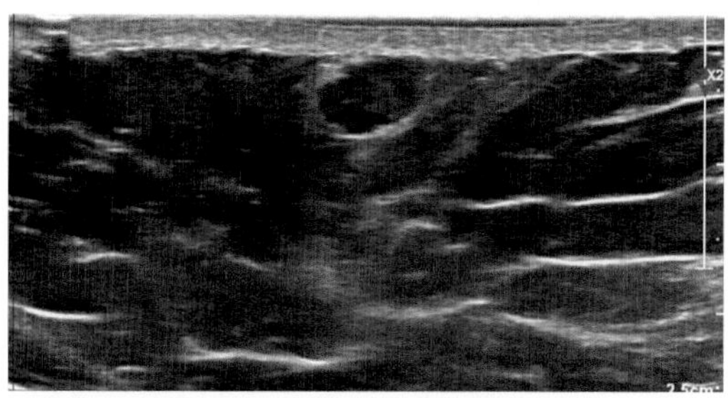

Fig. 13.10 **USG findings**: Ultrasound demonstrated an oval, hypoechoic mass with microlobulated margins, and markedly increased vascularity

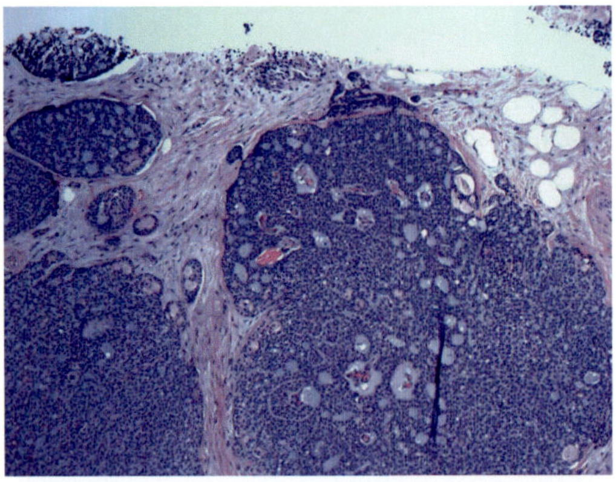

Fig. 13.11 Classic adenoid cystic carcinoma (H&E, 10×) of breast on excision. Cribriform, solid, and papillary architecture with basaloid appearance. Blue matrix fills the cribriform spaces. Classic ADCC cells display minimal mitotic activity and moderate nuclear atypia

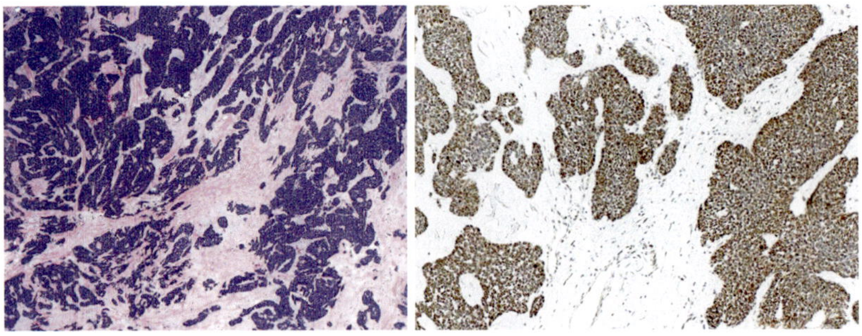

Figs. 13.12 and 13.13 Solid basaloid ADCC (H&E, 4×) with high-grade nuclei and brisk mitoses. Immunostaining for MYB demonstrates strong nuclear expression

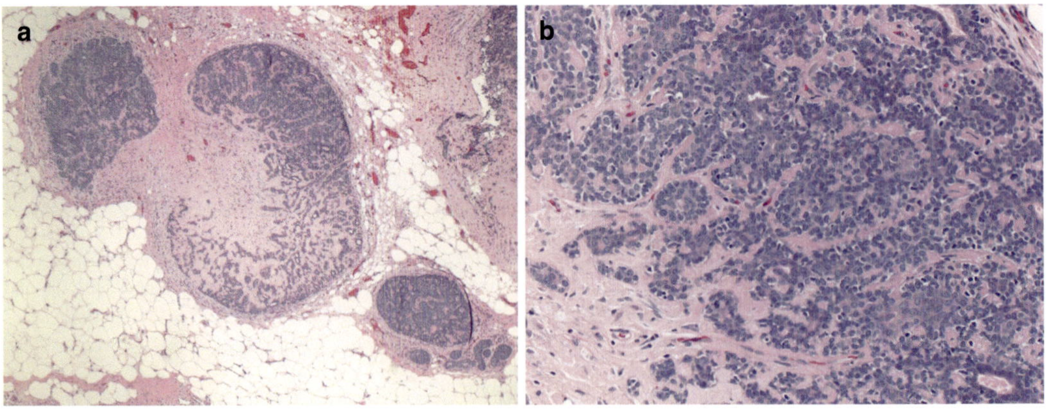

Fig. 13.14 A 48-year-old woman was found to have a solid mass in the subcutaneous location in the breast which on biopsy showed histology suspicious of adenoid cystic carcinoma. She then underwent resection revealing a benign skin adnexal tumor with well-circumscribed nodules of basaloid cells embedded in an eosinophilic collagenous matrix (**a**). The adnexal tumor is composed of a dual population of cells—elongated dark nuclei at the periphery of the nests and plump epithelioid luminal cells (**b**). Lesion was present in dermis and diagnosed as an eccrine spiradenoma

Carcinoma with Apocrine Differentiation

Carcinoma with Apocrine Differentiation: Carcinoma with apocrine differentiation (CAAD) is a rare breast tumor, comprising <1% of breast cancers. CADD is characterized by large neoplastic cells resembling apocrine glands—large polygonal cells with abundant eosinophilic cytoplasm, round nucleus with vesicular chromatin, and a nucleolus. CAAD is ER-negative and androgen receptor-positive with either an overall triple-negative or HER2-positive biomarker profile.

- **Clinical Presentation**: CAAD presents as palpable mass and may be associated with bloody nipple discharge or Paget disease of the nipple. CAAD may also be screening-detected. Although usually occurring in older, postmenopausal women, there is a wide age range, from late teenage years to the ninth decade [12]. It may be associated with apocrine ductal carcinoma in situ (ADCIS).
- **Imaging Findings**:
  - **Mammography**: Irregular mass with or without calcifications (which may represent the ADCIS component).
    - May have associated architectural distortion.
  - **US**: Irregular mass with a non-circumscribed margin. May appear as a complex solid and cystic mass.
  - **BI-RADS**: 4, suspicious of malignancy. However, when there is a large cystic component, the findings may be interpreted as benign fibrocystic changes.
  - **Differential Diagnosis**: Invasive ductal carcinoma NOS, invasive lobular carcinoma, metaplastic carcinoma, fibrocystic change, fat necrosis, abscess, fibroadenoma, granulomatous mastitis.
- **Pathology Findings**:
  - **Gross Description**: CAAD does not have a distinct macroscopic appearance. The tumors are of variable size and often form tan white solid lesions.
  - **Microscopic Histology**: Breast carcinomas with apocrine differentiation are invasive carcinomas with >90% of the tumor cells having cytological features of apocrine differentiation, which is similar to apocrine sweat glands.
    - The tumor cells are large and display abundant eosinophilic granular cytoplasm, large usually round nuclei, thick nuclear membrane, vesicular chromatin, and often central prominent nucleoli.
    - Tumor cells often grow in solid sheets.
    - CAAD is estrogen receptor negative, androgen receptor-positive and HER2-positive in 30–60% of cases [13].
    - CAAD is frequently positive for alpha-methylacyl-CoA racemase (AMACR), and GCDFP-15 [14].
  - **Differential Diagnosis**: Invasive ductal carcinoma NOS, invasive lobular carcinoma, metaplastic carcinoma, granular cell tumor.
  - **Management**: Same as invasive carcinoma, no special type.

Case

Clinical History: A 77-year-old female presented with a palpable mass in the right breast, which she had for years with no significant changes of late (Figs. 13.15 and 13.16).

The findings were thought to represent fibrocystic changes and a 6-month follow-up was recommended. The patient returned for a 6-month follow-up, at which point the findings were deemed stable and probably benign. The patient was asked to return for imaging in another 6 months.

On a 6-month follow-up (Figs. 13.17, 13.18, and 13.19):

The lesion was now called BI-RADS 4, suspicious for malignancy.

An US-guided biopsy was recommended and performed, yielding invasive mammary carcinoma with apocrine features, necrosis, and associated calcifications.

The patient subsequently underwent a simple mastectomy, which also yielded invasive carcinoma with apocrine differentiation (Figs. 13.20 and 13.21).

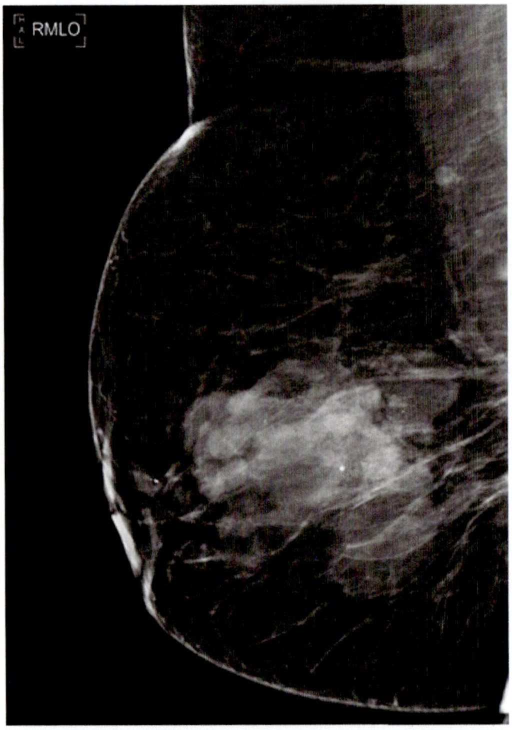

Fig. 13.15 **MG findings**: On mammography there was a large, circumscribed mass with amorphous calcifications

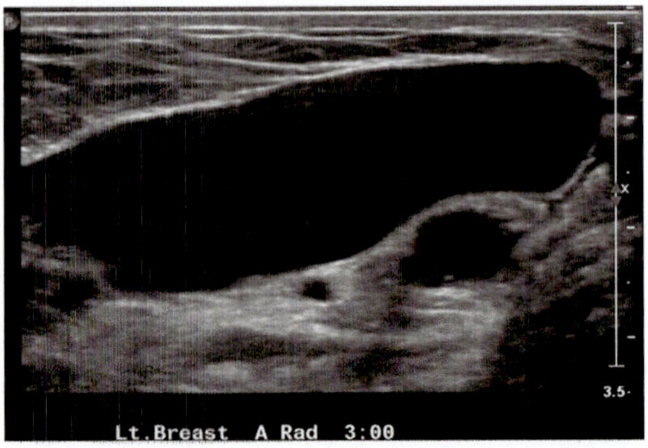

Fig. 13.16 **USG findings**: Ultrasound showed large cysts and clusters of cysts. The mass was called BI-RADS 3, probably benigns

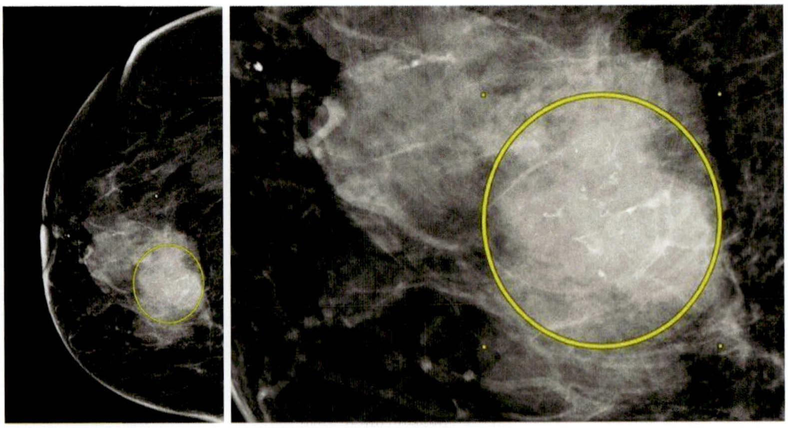

Figs. 13.17 and 13.18 **MG findings**: Mammogram showed that the large, circumscribed mass had not changed in size, but the calcifications had increased in number and now appear heterogeneous with a linear distribution

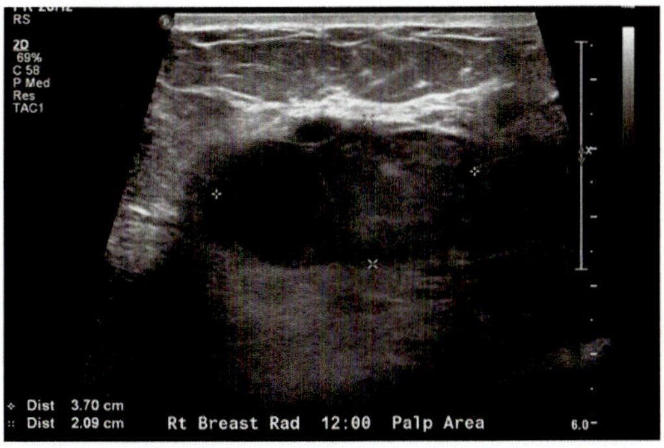

Fig. 13.19 **USG findings**: On ultrasound a solid component was now identified within the areas of cysts, which now appeared as a complex cystic and solid mass

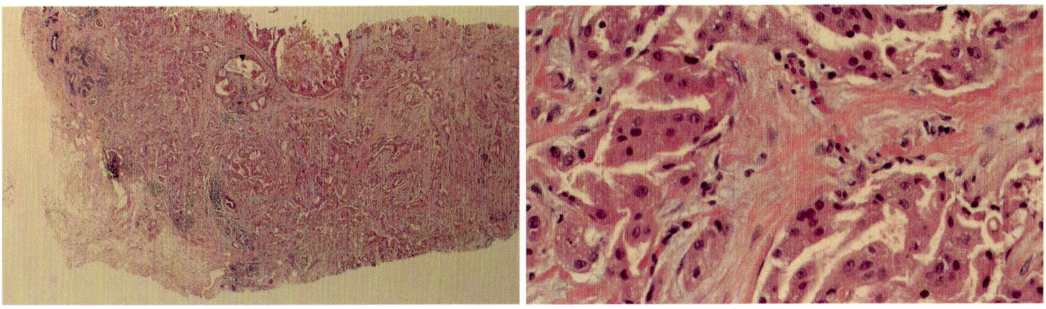

Figs. 13.20 and 13.21 **(H&E, 2× and 20×)** Core biopsy from a 54-year-old woman demonstrating invasive carcinoma with apocrine differentiation associated with DCIS. The tumor cell cytomorphology is similar to apocrine glands—large polygonal cells with abundant granular to foamy cytoplasm, central round nucleus with thick nuclear membrane and prominent nucleolus

Secretory Carcinoma

Secretory Carcinoma: Secretory carcinoma is salivary gland-type primary breast carcinoma which is a favorable histologic subtype of triple-negative breast carcinomas. Secretory carcinoma is rare and comprises <0.05% of breast cancers [15, 16]. Neoplastic epithelial cells show intra- and extracytoplasmic eosinophilic secretions and these tumors are frequently associated with *ETV6-NTRK3* fusions.

- **Clinical Presentation**: Most secretory carcinomas arise near the nipple or in the upper outer quadrant of the breast, but any breast location can be involved. Secretory carcinoma has been described in males as well. It usually presents as a slow-growing palpable mass. Due to its circumscribed appearance on imaging, clinically it can be confused with other benign breast masses, like a fibroadenoma. Traditionally it was described in children, however, the mean age of presentation is 53 years (range: 3–87 years) [16]. In men, secretory carcinoma usually arises in the subareolar location.
- **Imaging Findings**:
  - **Mammography**: Lobulated mass, with circumscribed or irregular margins.

- **US**: Oval or round, hypoechoic or isoechoic mass with circumscribed or microlobulated margins.
- **BI-RADS**: 3 or 4, as these may mimic benign lesions such as fibroadenomas, when presenting as circumscribed, oval masses, particularly when presenting in young women.
- **Differential Diagnosis**: Benign: fibroadenoma, lactating adenoma. Malignant: medullary carcinoma, papillary carcinoma, mucinous carcinoma.

- **Pathology Findings**:
  - **Gross**: Secretory carcinoma is usually a single mass that is firm, often circumscribed with a tan-white to yellowish-white cut surface. Reported tumor size ranges from 0.5 cm to up to 16 cm.
  - **Microscopic Histology**: Secretory carcinoma is composed of apocrine-type cells, displaying moderate to abundant eosinophilic granular cytoplasm.
    - Tumor cells form microcystic, solid, or papillary patterns.
    - Intracytoplasmic and extracellular eosinophilic secretions are present.
    - Microcystic spaces with pink colloid-like eosinophilic secretions can mimic thyroid-like follicles.
    - Nuclei are intermediate size with mild to moderate pleomorphism and inconspicuous mitosis.
    - The tumor-associated stroma is often hypocellular and sclerotic.
    - An associated in situ component, sometimes with a papillary pattern, may be identified.
    - By immunohistochemistry, the tumor cells express mammary differentiation markers (mammaglobin, GATA3, and SOX10).
      - S100 can be diffuse and strong.
    - Basal markers like keratin 5/6 are expressed and can be focal.
    - Most cases are triple-negative for ER, PR, and HER2. The KI-67 expression is low, often <20% [15].
    - Secretory carcinoma belongs to the TRK fusion carcinoma family. A t(12;15)(p13;q25) translocation, which results in ETV6-NTRK3 fusion gene, is specific for secretory carcinoma [16].
    - Pan-TRK IHC is sensitive and specific for breast carcinoma [17].
  - **Differential Diagnosis**: Invasive ductal carcinoma NOS, carcinoma with apocrine differentiation, acinic cell carcinoma, and fibroadenoma.
    - Documentation of ETV6-NTRK3 fusion can be used to support the diagnosis.
  - **Management**: Secretory carcinoma is classified as a favorable histology among triple-negative breast tumors. Excision with negative margins is the mainstay of treatment. Limited available data support local therapy with consideration of systemic therapy in nodal disease.

Case

Clinical History: A 63-year-old female presented with a screening detected right breast mass (Figs. 13.22, 13.23, 13.24, and 13.25).

The lesion was graded as BI-RADS 4, suspicious of malignancy.

An US-guided biopsy yielded a secretory carcinoma (Figs. 13.26 and 13.27).

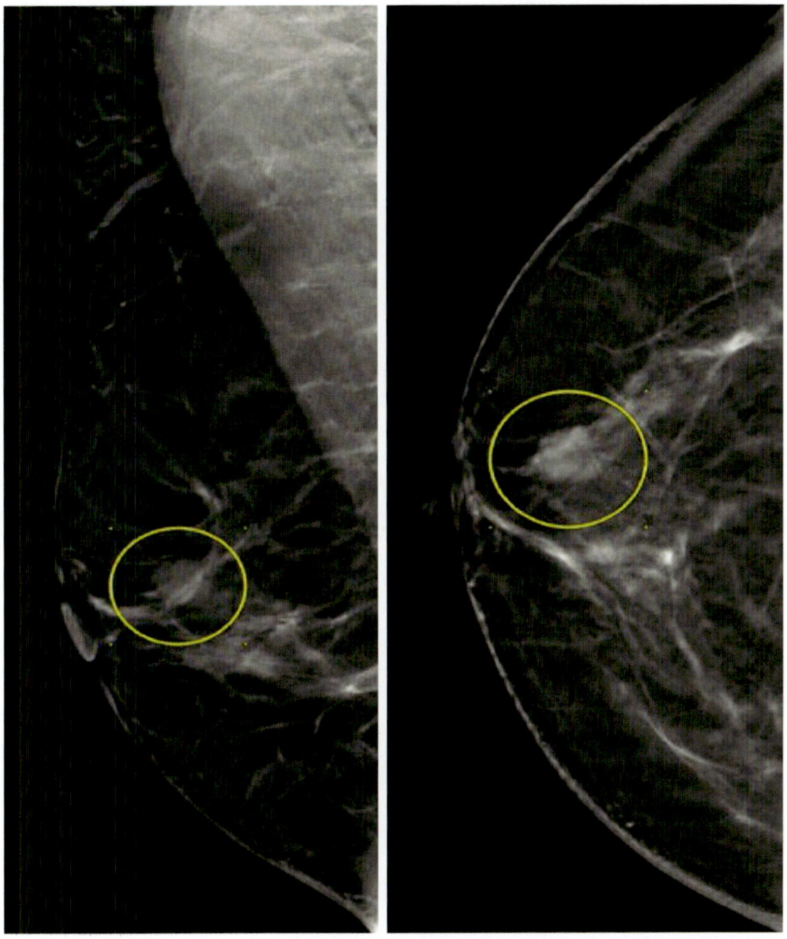

Figs. 13.22 and 13.23 **MG findings**: On mammography there was a round mass with an indistinct margin in the right retroareolar region

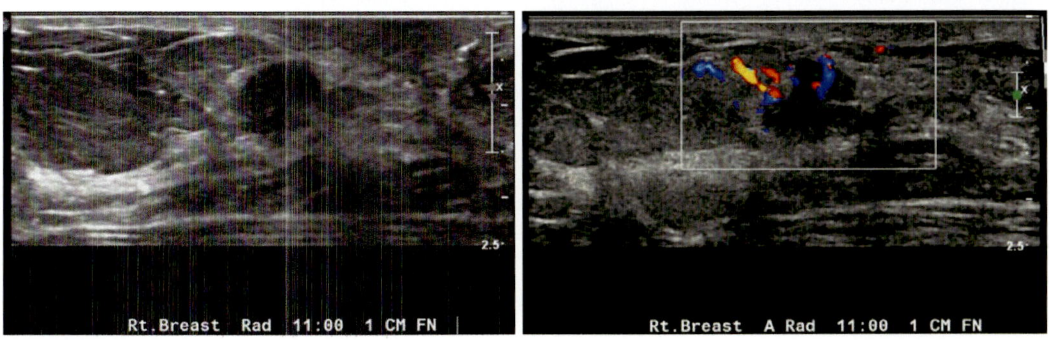

Figs. 13.24 and 13.25 **USG findings**: Ultrasound showed a round, hypoechoic mass with a microlobulated margin and internal vascularity

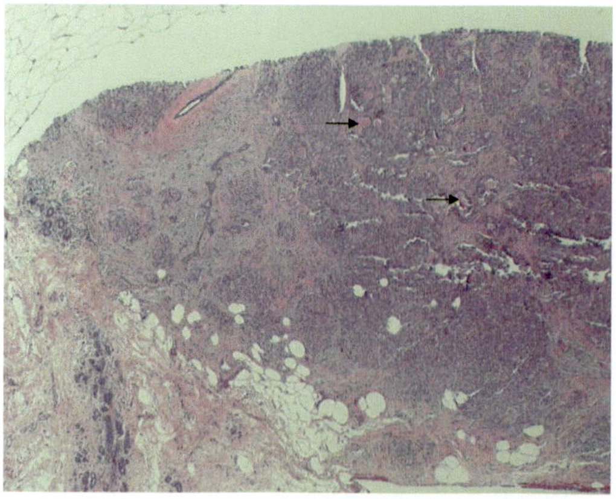

Fig. 13.26 Secretory carcinoma (H&E, 2×). Poorly circumscribed infiltrative lesion with solid, papillary, and microcystic architecture. Pale eosinophilic colloid-like secretory material fills the glandular microcystic spaces (arrows)

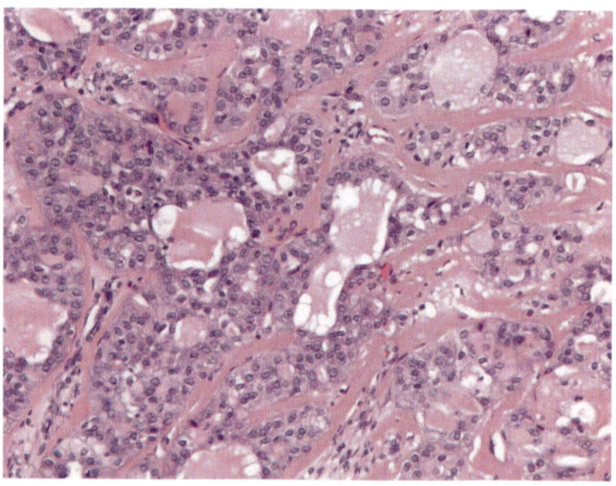

Fig. 13.27 Secretory carcinoma (H&E, 20×) cells have vague apocrine cytomorphology. The microcystic spaces are filled with colloid-like secretory material

Tall Cell Carcinoma with Reverse Polarity

Tall Cell Carcinoma with Reverse Polarity (TCCRP): Tall cell carcinoma with reverse polarity (TCCRP) is a recently described rare invasive breast tumor [18, 19]. TCCRP is a papillary carcinoma that histologically resembles the tall cell variant of papillary thyroid carcinoma and shows distinct *IDH2 R172* hotspot mutations [18–21].

- **Clinical Presentation**: It usually presents as a small palpable mass or a screening-detected mass lesion. Axillary nodal metastases and distant metastases are extremely rare. The median age of diagnosis is 64 years [18–20].
- **Imaging Findings**:
  - **Mammography**: This is a rare lesion, which radiographically does not have distinctive features.
    - This lesion presents as a solid mass or a focal asymmetry on screening mammography, with a median size of 0.9 cm, and may mimic more common benign and malignant lesions.
  - **US**: Oval, hypoechoic mass. May have a focally irregular margin.
- **Pathology Findings**:
  - **Gross Description**: TCCRP most often presents as a poorly circumscribed, firm, tan-white mass. The tumor ranges in size from 0.5 to 5 cm.
  - **Microscopic Histology**: Histologically the TCCRP is composed of circumscribed round nodules of polygonal or columnar epithelial cells that are arranged in papillary patterns.
    - Tumor islands are often embedded in eosinophilic fibrous stroma without any overt or minimal desmoplastic response.
    - Many tumor papillae are lined by a distinctive double layer of tall columnar epithelial cells with fibrovascular cores that may be distended by aggregates of foamy histiocytes.
    - The most characteristic feature of this tumor is the low to intermediate grade nuclei with occasional grooves being in the apical rather than in the basal location giving the reverse polarity appearance.
    - Amphophilic colloid-like secretions are also described.
    - By immunohistochemistry complete absence of myoepithelial cells confirms the invasive categorization.

- The majority of these tumors reported in the literature are triple-negative lacking ER, PR, and HER2 and with few cases showing some hormone receptor expression.
- Cytokeratin 5/6 may be strongly expressed though, some have shown a complete absence of CK 5/6.
- The *IDH2 R172* hotspot mutations have been described in 77–100% of tumors. *PRUNE2* and *TET2* mutations have also been described in TCCRP [20, 21].
- IDH2 immunostain shows strong cytoplasmic staining in 93% of cases [21].

– **Differential Diagnosis**: Invasive ductal carcinoma NOS, DCIS, solid papillary carcinoma, encapsulated papillary carcinoma. Benign lesions: fibroadenoma, papilloma.

– **Management**: Surgical excision is the mainstay of treatment. Although triple-negative, these tumors have favorable outcomes. Therefore, adjuvant treatment may be deferred in a low stage setting.

Case

Clinical History: A 68-year-old female was recalled from screening ultrasound due to a 1.4-cm mass seen in the right breast on screening ultrasound.

MG Findings: Her screening mammogram was negative, but she had dense breast tissue, which likely obscured the lesion (Fig. 13.28).

An US-guided biopsy was performed, yielding a tall cell carcinoma with reverse polarity (Figs. 13.29, 13.30, 13.31, and 13.32).

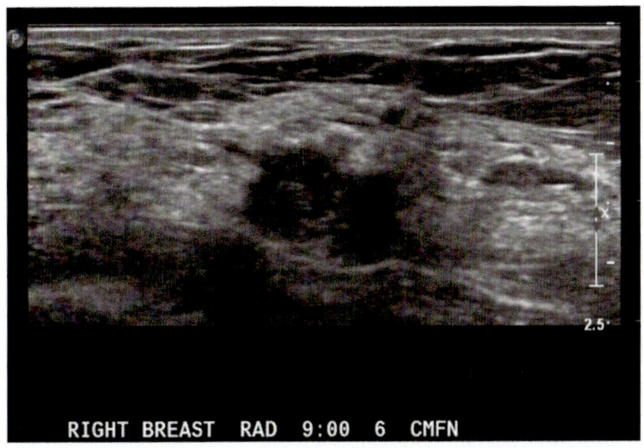

Fig. 13.28 **USG findings**: On ultrasound there was an oval, hypoechoic mass with a focally irregular margin which was called BI-RADS 4, suspicious for malignancy

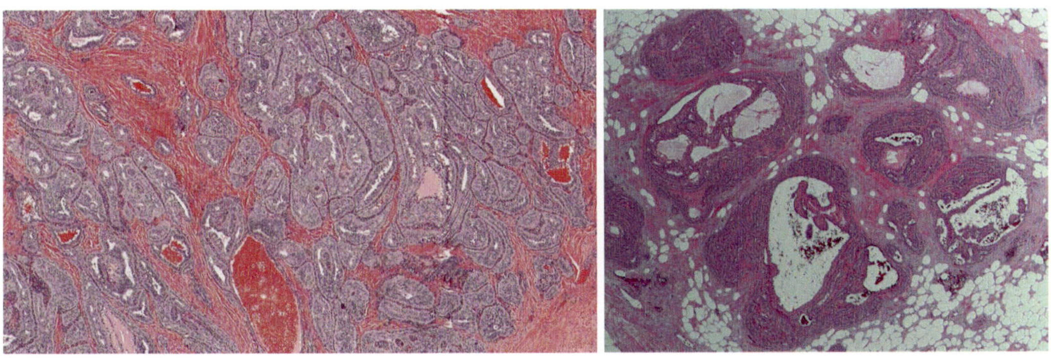

Figs. 13.29 and 13.30 Tall cell carcinoma with reverse polarity (H&E, 2× and 4×) demonstrating rounded papillary nests embedded in fibrous stroma. Cystic spaces often filled with colloid-like material are present

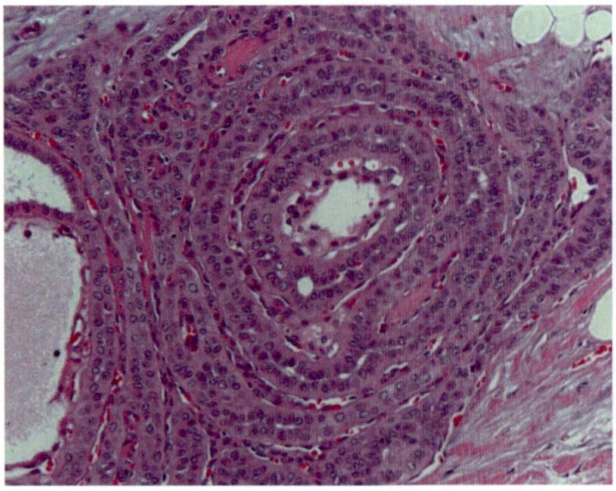
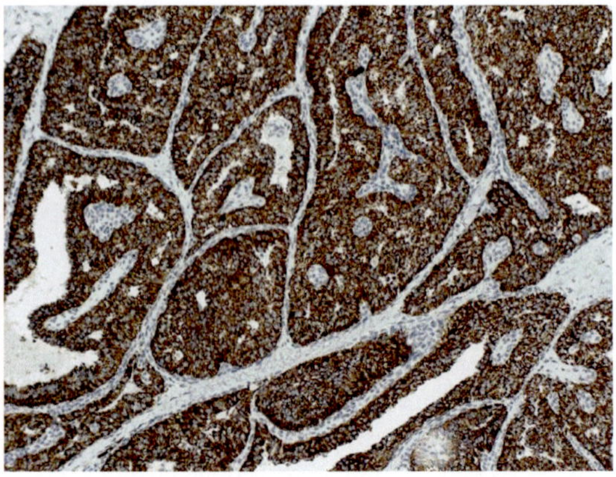

Figs. 13.31 and 13.32 (H&E, 10× and IDH2 IHC) Tall columnar cells with nuclei lifted up away from the stromal pole of the cell giving an impression of reverse polarity in a case of tall cell carcinoma with reverse polarity. Tumor cells of TCCRP demonstrate diffuse strong immunostaining with IDH2 antibody

Acinic Cell Carcinoma

Acinic Cell Carcinoma (ACC): Acinic cell carcinoma (ACC) is a rare salivary gland-type primary breast carcinoma [22, 23]. ACC is a malignant epithelial neoplasm composed of tumor cell nests and glands with intracytoplasmic serous (zymogen) granules. Some cases of ACC have been reported to arise in a setting of microglandular adenosis (MGA) and atypical MGA [24].

- **Clinical Presentation**: The clinical presentation is similar to invasive ductal carcinoma, NOS.
- **Imaging Findings**: Palpable, poorly definable lump/mass with microcalcifications; occasionally, other clinical and radiologic appearances may occur (e.g., lesion without a mass, radiologically hidden cancer, or small oval radiopaque mass).
- **Pathology Findings**:
  - **Gross Description**: There are no distinct gross findings reported for ACC. The tumor is macroscopically similar to invasive ductal carcinoma, NOS.
  - **Microscopic Histology**: The tumor is composed of infiltrative solid nests as well as small glands.
    - The unique histological finding of ACC is polygonal tumor cells with abundant granular cytoplasm (Figs. 13.33 and 13.34).
      - The granules are often plump and chunky and the staining of granules can be variable, ranging from bright eosinophilic to basophilic.
    - Cytoplasmic clearing can be present.

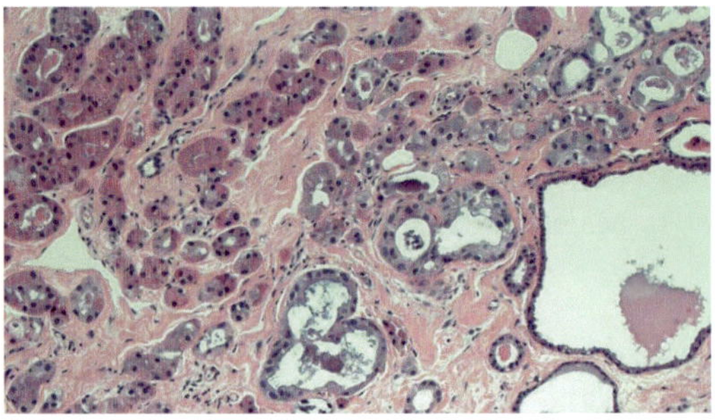

Fig. 13.33 (H&E, 20×) Acinic cell carcinoma arising in a background of microglandular adenosis. The tumor cells are large and polygonal in shape and the cytoplasm contains abundant serous granules

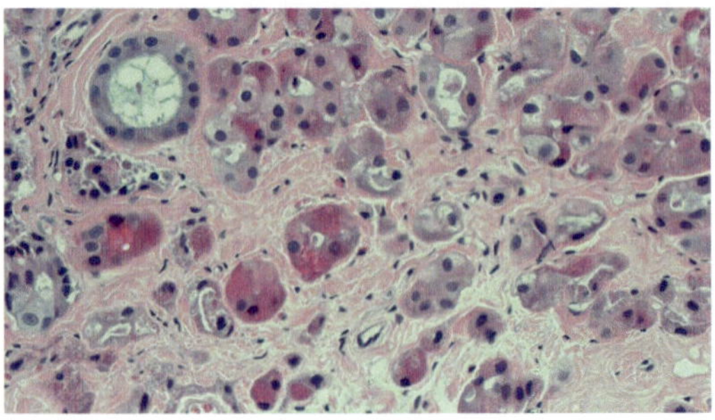

Fig. 13.34 Infiltrating glands and small solid nests of tumor cells with abundant granular cytoplasm can be seen on high power magnification

  - o Mitotic activity is prominent in solid areas.
  - o Serous differentiation can be confirmed by IHC for lysozyme and alpha-chymotrypsin.
  - o ACC is negative for estrogen receptor, progesterone receptor and HER2 (triple negative).
  - o The granules are positive for PAS (with diastase).
- – **Differential Diagnosis**: Secretory carcinoma, invasive ductal carcinoma, NOS.
  - o Secretory carcinoma. ACC is negative for t(12:15) *ETV6-NTRK3.*
  - o High-grade invasive ductal carcinoma, NOS. Intracytoplasmic coarse granules indicate acinic differentiation. IHC for lysozyme and alpha-chymotrypsinogen confirms the diagnosis.
- – **Management**: ACC is managed similar to triple-negative invasive breast carcinoma.

Primary Breast Neuroendocrine Neoplasms

Neuroendocrine Neoplasm (NEN): Breast NENs are defined as breast carcinomas with more than 90% of the tumor demonstrating histological features of neuroendocrine differentiation, which is confirmed by diffuse immunohistochemical expression of neuroendocrine markers (chromogranin, synaptophysin, and INSM1). Solid papillary carcinoma and hypercellular mucinous carcinoma are not included in breast NEN. Both of these lesions are distinct breast neoplasms that can express neuroendocrine markers, but these should not be classified as NEN. The rarity of primary neuroendocrine neoplasms in the breast and limited literature has led to poor consensus on defining features of NEN of the breast. The recent WHO classification of breast tumors classifies NEN of breast into two groups: (1) Neuroendocrine tumors (low to intermediate grade) and (2) Neuroendocrine carcinoma (small cell and large cell neuroendocrine carcinoma) [25–27].

Primary neuroendocrine carcinoma (NEC) of the breast is a rare type of breast cancer that accounts for 2–5% of all breast cancers. NEC originates from neuroendocrine cells that are present throughout the body. The clinical outcome of NEC of the breast is poor compared to IDC. It tends to present in somewhat older patients (mean age at diagnosis: 63 years).

- **Clinical Presentation**: Similar clinical features to invasive ductal carcinoma NOS. Patients may present with complaints including palpable mass, focal pain, nipple discharge or nipple retraction, or it may be detected on screening mammography.
- **Imaging Findings**:
  - – **Mammography**: Appearance is variable, but a mass is most common.
    - o The shape of the mass is frequently round, oval or lobulated, and less frequently irregular. The margins are most commonly circumscribed, obscured or indistinct, and less commonly speculated.
    - o Calcifications are associated with a minority of cases (26%).
  - – **US**: Most commonly, these tumors are irregular, hypoechoic, and vascular. Axillary lymph node metastasis is frequently found at the time of diagnosis.
  - – **BI-RADS**: 4.
  - – **Differential Diagnosis**: Fibroadenoma, complicated cyst, papilloma, invasive ductal carcinoma.
- **Pathology Findings:**
  - – **Gross**: There are no distinct gross features of breast NEN.
  - – **Microscopic Histology**: The histological features of breast NEN are similar to neuroendocrine tumors of other organs, like lung and intestine.
    - o The NEN of the breast consists of cellular solid nests of plasmacytoid to polygonal cells with moderate to abundant eosinophilic granular to cleared cytoplasm.
    - o The tumor cell nuclei are low to intermediate grade and mitoses are incon-

spicuous. Overall histologic grade is 1–2.

- o Metastatic well-differentiated NENs (carcinoids) from lung or gastropancreatic origin should be excluded before making a diagnosis of primary breast NEN.
- o Neuroendocrine carcinoma (NEC, small cell or large cell) is an invasive carcinoma characterized by high-grade neuroendocrine histomorphology.
  - Small cell neuroendocrine carcinoma (SCNEC) is characterized by sheets of small dark hyperchromatic cells with high N:C ratio, scant cytoplasm, minimal cytoplasm, inconspicuous nucleoli and nuclear molding.
  - Large cell NEC cells contain appreciable cytoplasm and coarse chromatin. Necrosis and high mitotic activity is characteristic.

- **Differential Diagnosis**: Metastatic NEC (small cell and large cell) of non-mammary origin, metaplastic carcinoma, solid basaloid adenoid cystic carcinoma, invasive ductal carcinoma NOS with basaloid cells and melanoma should be considered in differential diagnosis.
  - o Presence of in situ carcinoma or a conventional IDC supports primary nature of the NEC.
- **Management**: SCNEC is associated with worse prognosis than NEN. Management of localized SCNEC is similar to IDC, NOS. In a metastatic setting, regimens targeting small cell lung cancer are usually employed.

Case

Clinical History: A 76-year-old female presented with a palpable mass near the nipple and bloody nipple discharge (Figs. 13.35, 13.36, and 13.37).

The mass was called BI-RADS 4, suspicious and an US-guided core needle biopsy was recommended and performed revealing a neuroendocrine tumor (Figs. 13.38, 13.39, 13.40, and 13.41).

Metastases

Metastasis: Metastases to the breast from other sites are uncommon, comprising 2–3% of breast malignancies [28]. Cancers that may metastasize

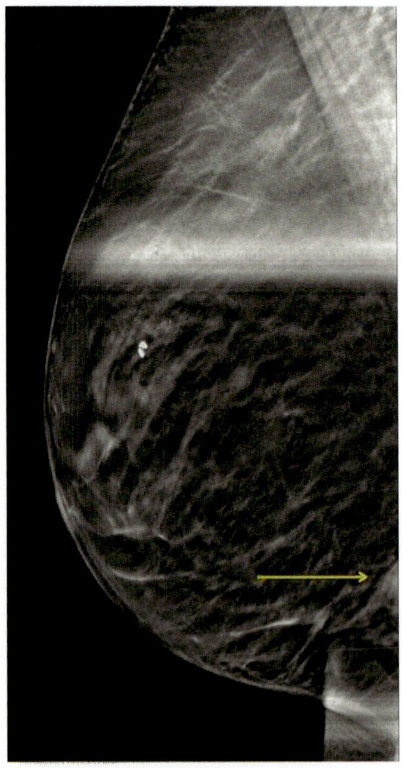

Fig. 13.35 **MMG findings**: Mammogram found a small, oval mass with an obscured margin in the left breast, retroareolar position

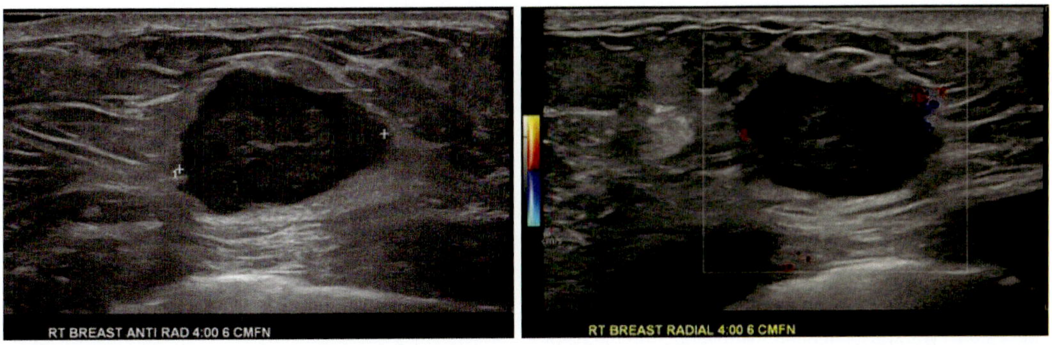

Figs. 13.36 and 13.37 **USG findings**: On ultrasound there was a round, hypoechoic mass with an angular margin and adjacent vascularity. Incidentally noted was an adjacent, oval, hypoechoic mass with an angular margin. No posterior acoustic features are demonstrated

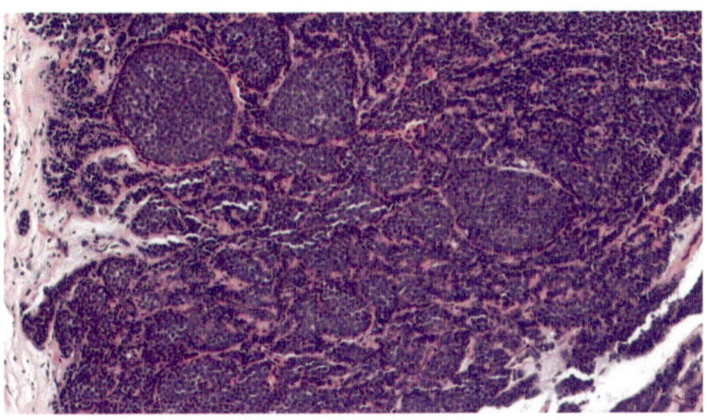

Fig. 13.38 Infiltrating epithelial cells arranged in solid nests and anastomosing trabeculae. The tumor has a "small round blue cell" morphology with minimal cytoplasm and hyperchromatic nuclei

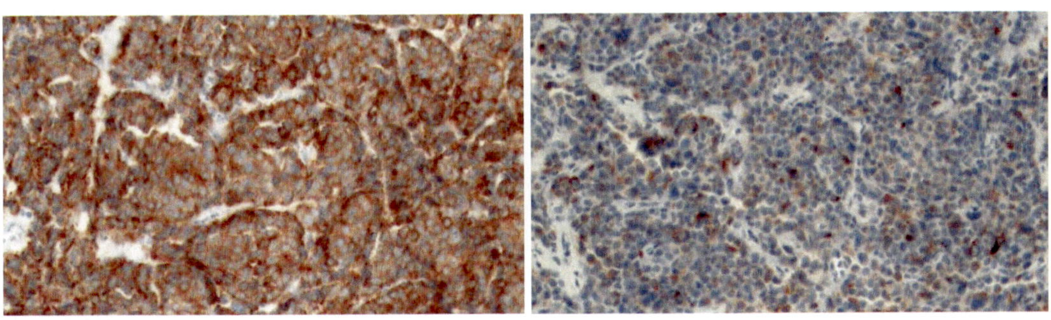

Figs. 13.39 and 13.40 On immunohistochemistry the tumor shows strong and diffuse synaptophysin staining (left), and scattered strong chromogranin immunostaining confirming neuroendocrine differentiation (right)

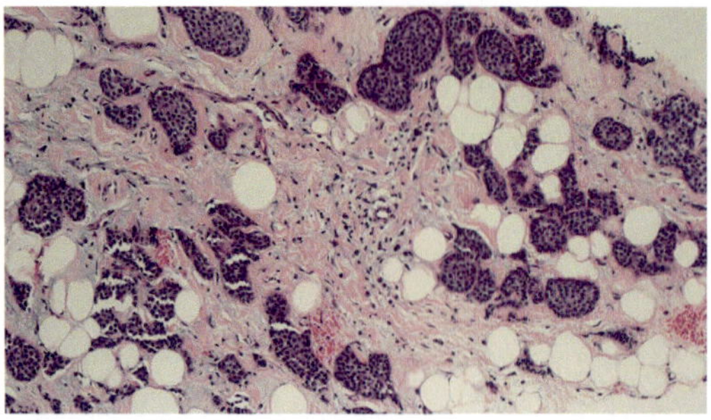

Fig. 13.41 Well-differentiated neuroendocrine tumor of breast (H&E, 10×). Nests and cords of tumor cells with low to intermediate nuclear grade

to the breast include melanoma, lymphoma, lung cancer, ovarian/peritoneal cancers, sarcomas, GI tract malignancies, and prostate cancer [28, 29]. In most cases of detected metastasis to the breast, a history of a known extramammary malignancy exists. However, a breast lesion could be the initial presentation of a systemic malignancy, and small cell carcinoma of the lung is most common. Most systemic malignancies typically spread to the breast via the hematogenous route, but some may do so via the lymphatic route. These may present clinically as palpable masses, or be screening detected. Most patients are diagnosed in the sixth decade of life, and prognosis is poor, with life expectancy of less than a year from the time of diagnosis [28, 29].

- **Clinical Presentation**: Metastases to breast frequently present as multiple unilateral or bilateral masses. Rarely metastases can present as a single mass or an asymmetry similar to a primary breast lesion. Mass lesions can involve breast parenchyma, skin and subcutaneous tissue or the chest wall. Metastases are often present in older postmenopausal women or older males.
- **Imaging Findings:**
  - **Mammography**: Metastases to the breast are more commonly round masses, with circumscribed to indistinct margins.
    - These are typically noncalcified, although calcifications can be present in some ovarian, GI and thyroid malignancies.
    - Most metastases are solitary, but multiple and/or bilateral masses or diffuse involvement can occur.
    - The most common location is the upper outer quadrant, relatively close to skin.
  - **US**: Round, hypoechoic masses with circumscribed or microlobulated margins, sometimes appearing as complex cystic masses, with posterior acoustic enhancement frequently noted.
    - Melanoma and lymphoma may appear anechoic and resemble cysts.
    - Internal hypervascularity is noted in 39% of cases.
  - **MRI**: Enhancing, T2 hyperintense masses, with plateau or washout kinetic curves, although persistent enhancement can occur.
  - **BI-RADS**: 4 or 5, suspicious or highly suspicious for malignancy.
    - Although most masses will have suspicious features, some may be mistaken for benign lesions of the breast, such as fibroadenomas, phyllodes tumors, papillomas, complicated cysts or clusters of cysts.
  - **Differential Diagnosis**: Invasive ductal carcinoma NOS, poorly differentiated invasive ductal carcinoma, malignancies that may present as circumscribed masses: medullary, mucinous, encapsulated papillary carcinoma; primary lymphoma (if solitary mass); benign breast lesions: fibroadenoma, phyllodes, papilloma, cysts.
- **Pathology Findings**: The pathology findings depend on the primary site of the tumor. The breast lesions are often multiple with no specific gross feature. The lesions can be solid to cystic and show areas of hemorrhage and necrosis.
  - **Gross**: There are no specific features of metastases. The gross appearance can vary based on the primary site. Grossly, metastasis from colon and lung carcinomas can be stellate solid lesions and mimic a breast primary. The cut surface can be necrotic in metastasis from colon, and mucinous and shiny in those from lung. Melanoma may show discoloration and variable black-brown pigmentation.

- **Microscopic Histology**: In the absence of appropriate clinical history, histological diagnosis of metastasis to breast can be extremely challenging. A high index of suspicion is needed to identify a metastasis to breast. Unusual location in the breast, absence of in situ component, prominent lymphovascular invasion, and unusual histological features are often present in metastatic lesions to breast.
  - Metastatic serous carcinoma: Serous carcinomas often show prominent micropapillary architecture and abrupt nuclear pleomorphism. Positivity for estrogen and progesterone receptor can be confusing; breast markers (GATA3 and SOX10) will clarify the definite diagnosis.
  - Metastatic lung adenocarcinoma: Often hypercellular, lacks desmoplastic reaction and frequently shows disparity in extent of gland formation and nuclear atypia.
  - Metastatic carcinoid tumor: Shows histological overlap with breast neuroendocrine tumor. Carcinoid metastatic deposits are often multiple and lack an in situ component.
  - Melanoma: Melanoma deposit in the breast can be seen in relatively younger patients. Tumor cells can show nested architecture and display epithelioid to spindle cell cytomorphology. Tumor nuclei are hyperchromatic and often contain prominent central nucleoli. Identification of melanin pigment will help in determining the correct diagnosis.
- **Differential Diagnosis**: Primary breast carcinoma, neuroendocrine tumor, breast carcinoma with signet-ring cell morphology, metaplastic carcinoma, breast micropapillary carcinoma.
  - Metastatic tumors can mimic the various histologic subtypes of breast carcinoma making the histological diagnosis difficult.
  - Immunohistochemical panels containing breast markers (GATA3, GCDFP15, Mammaglobin, SOX10, Keratin, ER, and PR) and suspected primary site (TTF-1, PAX8, CDX2, Melan-A) are needed for definite diagnosis.
- **Management**: The management rests on the primary tumor site and stage. Oligometastatic disease with an isolated breast lesion can be managed with excision.

Case

Clinical History: A 74-year-old female palpated a right breast mass, located near the inframammary fold (Figs. 13.42 and 13.43).

A right axillary lymph node with uniform thickening of the cortex was also noted.

The lesion was called BI-RADS 4, suspicious for malignancy.

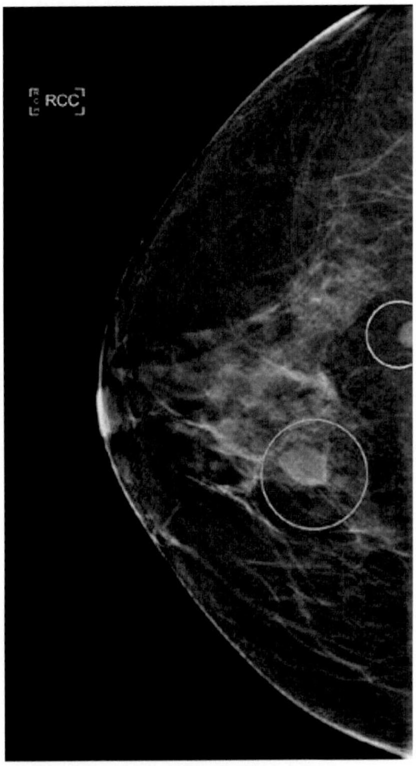

Fig. 13.42 MMG findings: Mammography showed a partially visualized asymmetry with an indistinct margin, seen on the MLO view only, near the inframammary fold

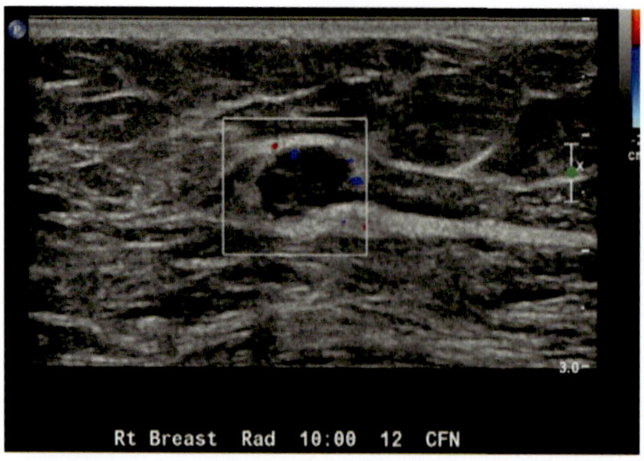

Fig. 13.43 **USG findings**: On ultrasound there was an oval, hypoechoic mass with focally microlobulated margins, with posterior acoustic enhancement

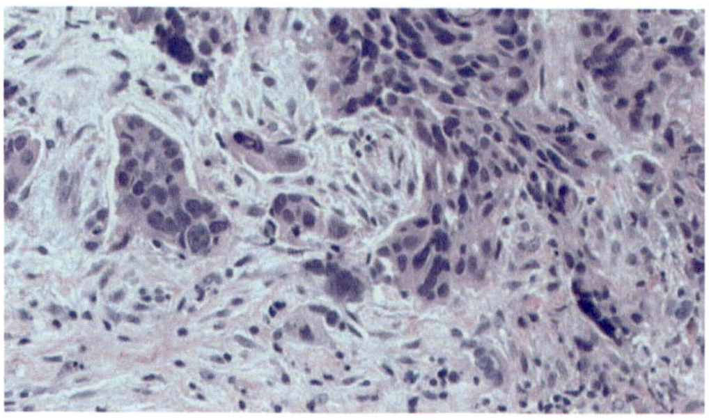

Fig. 13.44 High-grade serous carcinoma metastatic to breast. The carcinoma cells show micropapillary morphology and marked nuclear pleomorphism (H&E, 20×)

An US-guided biopsy of the palpable mass and the right axillary lymph node was recommended and performed.

Pathologic diagnosis yielded a high grade carcinoma of mullerian origin. The biopsy of the axillary lymph node yielded benign lymphoid tissue. Subsequently they received a diagnosis of malignant ascites with high-grade serous carcinoma (Figs. 13.44, 13.45, 13.46, and 13.47).

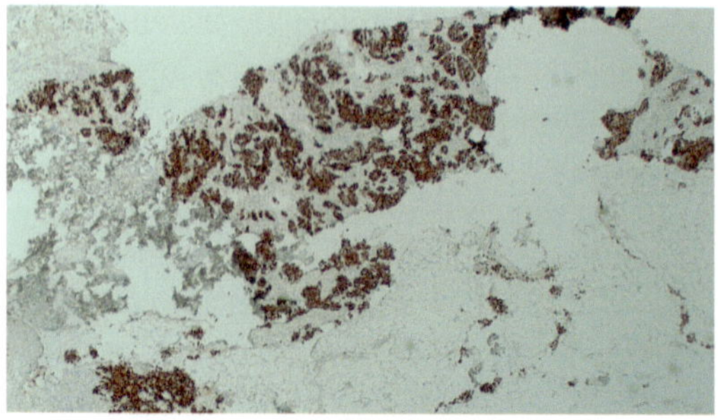

Fig. 13.45 Strong nuclear PAX8 staining confirms the mullerian origin of the carcinoma (PAX8 IHC)

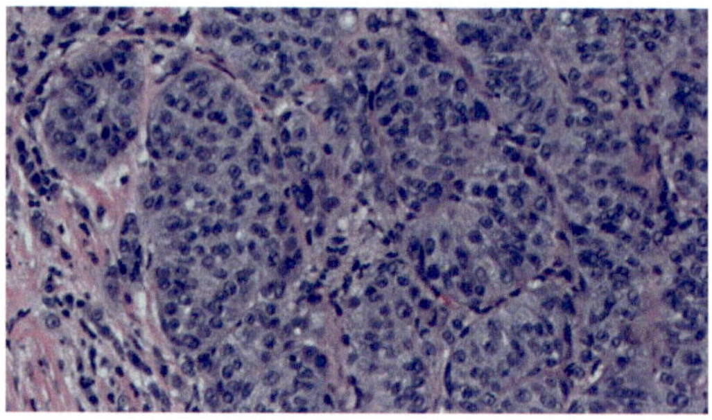

Fig. 13.46 Melanoma metastasis to breast. Nests of cohesive tumor cells with epithelioid morphology mimicking carcinoma (H&E, 20×)

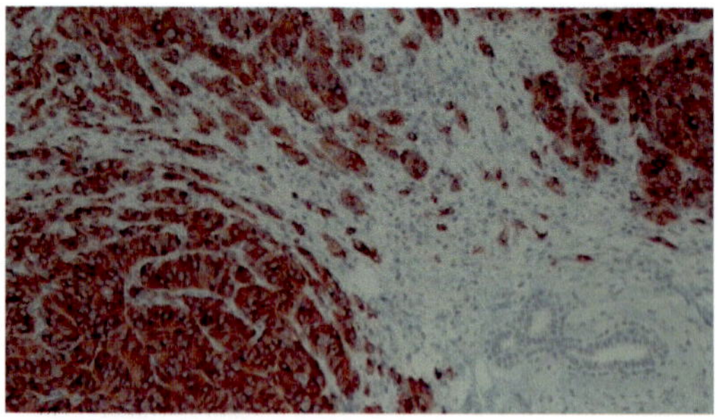

Fig. 13.47 Cytoplasm contains faint dusty brown melanin pigment. Diffuse strong melan-A immunostaining confirms melanoma (Melan-A IHC). Benign breast tissue in the section is negative for melan-A

Lymphoma

Lymphoma: Primary breast lymphoma (PBL) is less common than lymphoma secondarily involving the breast, with the B-cell types more common than T-cell types. Primary lymphoma of the breast is confined to one or both breasts and/or regional lymph nodes, without any previous history of lymphoma. Breast lymphoma is rare and comprises 2% of all extranodal lymphomas [30, 31]. Diffuse large B-cell lymphoma (DLBCL), extranodal marginal zone lymphoma and follicular lymphoma account for most breast lymphomas [31]. Breast-implant associated anaplastic lymphoma arises in a setting of a breast implant and is specific to the breast. Breast is also a distinct site for Burkitt lymphoma.

The median age of presentation is in the fifth decade, with ages at diagnosis ranging widely from teenage years to the ninth decade [30].

- **Clinical Presentation**: PBL may present as a painless, palpable, rapidly enlarging mass. Rarely, it may present with diffuse breast swelling and/or peau d'orange, thus mimicking inflammatory breast carcinoma. Axillary adenopathy is present in 30–50% of patients at the time of diagnosis.
- **Imaging Findings**
  - **Mammography**: Noncalcified, usually solitary, round mass with circumscribed to indistinct margins.
    - May also present as a global asymmetry.
    - Skin and trabecular thickening may also be present.
  - **US**: Oval or irregular mass hypoechoic with indistinct margins, which may be hypervascular and demonstrate an echogenic rim.
    - Skin thickening and edema may also be present.
  - **BI-RADS**: 4, suspicious of malignancy.
  - **Differential Diagnosis**: Primary breast cancer, particularly mucinous, papillary, medullary, poorly differentiated IDC, TNBC, inflammatory breast cancer (particularly when presenting with breast edema and global asymmetry), secondary lymphoma, benign processes such as: fibroadenoma, phyllodes, abscess, granulomatous mastitis, diabetic mastopathy, benign-dependent edema (due to heart failure or venous obstruction).
- **Pathology Findings:**
  - **Gross**: Grossly lymphoma can present as a well-defined or a poorly defined infiltrative lesion.
  - **Microscopic Histology:**
    - Diffuse large cell lymphoma: Primary DLBCL of breast is composed of sheets of large lymphoma cells. The tumor cells infiltrate breast parenchyma and the lymphoma cells can resemble centroblasts or immunoblasts. The IHC profile of breast DLBCL is similar to DLBCL elsewhere and is positive for B-cell markers.
    - Extranodal marginal zone lymphoma (MALToma): The lymphoma cells are present in close proximity to the mammary epithelium. The histological features of MALT lymphoma of breast are similar to MALT lymphoma of other sites. Tumor cells are centrocyte-like marginal zone cells of small to medium size with slightly irregular nucleus and scant to abundant pale cytoplasm. Reactive follicles, plasma cells and amyloid deposition can be present. Large cell transformation to DLBCL can occur. Monotypic immunoglobulin expression by IHC or flow cytometry is present.
    - Follicular lymphoma: The histology of breast follicular lymphoma is similar to nodal and other extranodal sites. Tumor cells can show follicular of diffuse growth pattern and histologic grade 1 or 2 are more common than grade 3 lesions.
  - **Differential Diagnosis**: Lymphoma of breast needs to be differentiated from reactive lesions and secondary involvement of breast by lymphomas arising in extramammary locations. Correlation with clinical findings is a must before diagnosing a primary breast lymphoma.

  - Mastitis: Infectious and noninfectious etiology-related inflammatory infiltrates in the breast can mimic lymphoma especially in a chronic setting. Assessment for nuclear atypia in the lymphoid population, polymorphous infiltrate with granulation tissue, and granulomas indicate reactive inflammatory process.
  - Ruptured cyst/ducts can be associated with mass formation and chronic inflammation.
  - Flow cytometry and IHC studies can be performed to exclude a monotypic nature of the inflammatory infiltrate.
- **Management**: Management depends on the lymphoma histology and staging. Most lymphomas are treated by systemic immunochemotherapy with or without radiation. Localized lesions in MALT lymphoma can be treated with excision.

Case

Clinical History: An 83-year-old female with history of left breast IDC status post-lumpectomy and radiation therapy 7 years ago presents with a palpable lump and skin thickening of the left breast (Figs. 13.48, 13.49, and 13.50).

The mass was called BI-RADS 4, suspicious for malignancy and an US-guided biopsy was recommended and performed, yielding diffuse large cell lymphoma (Figs. 13.51, 13.52–13.54).

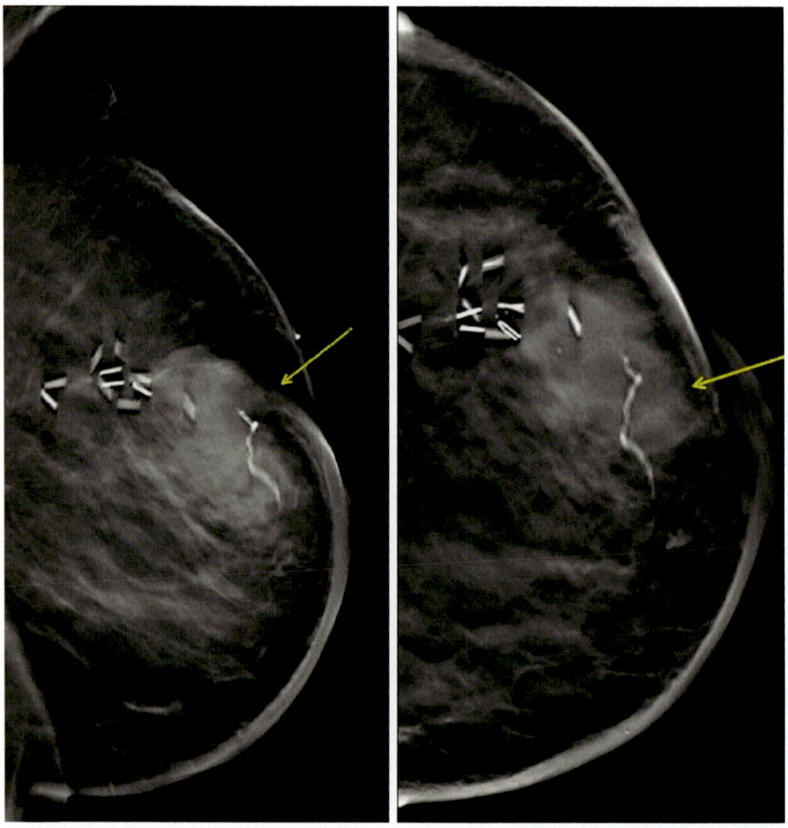

Figs. 13.48 and 13.49 MMG findings: Mammogram reveals an oval left breast mass with an indistinct margin that correlates with the palpable finding

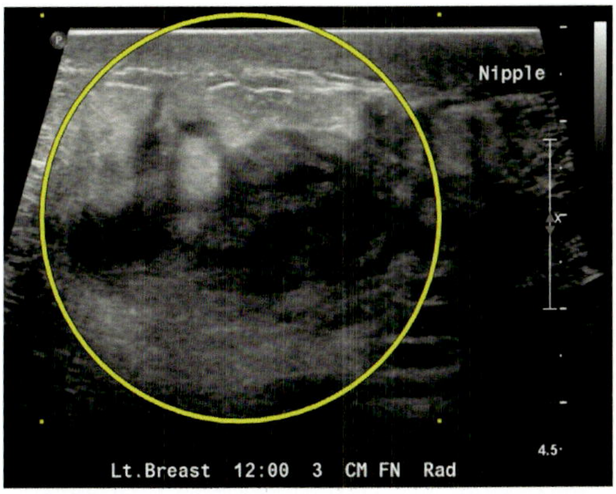

Fig. 13.50 **USG findings**: Ultrasound shows an irregular mass with an indistinct margin, with heterogeneous echotexture, without increased internal vascularity

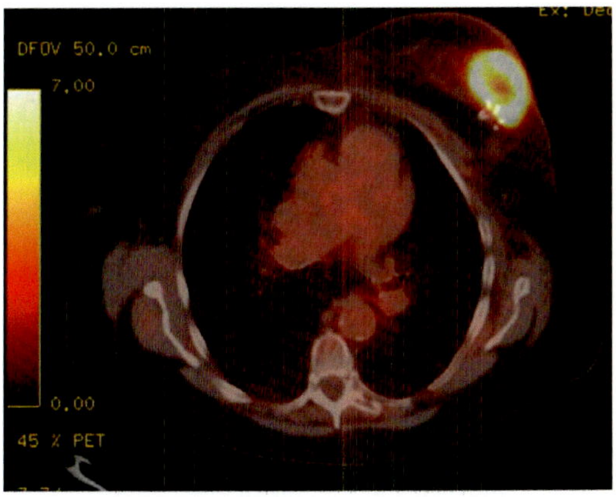

Fig. 13.51 The patient subsequently underwent a body PET/CT scan for staging, which demonstrated the large hypermetabolic left breast mass, but no additional suspicious lesions

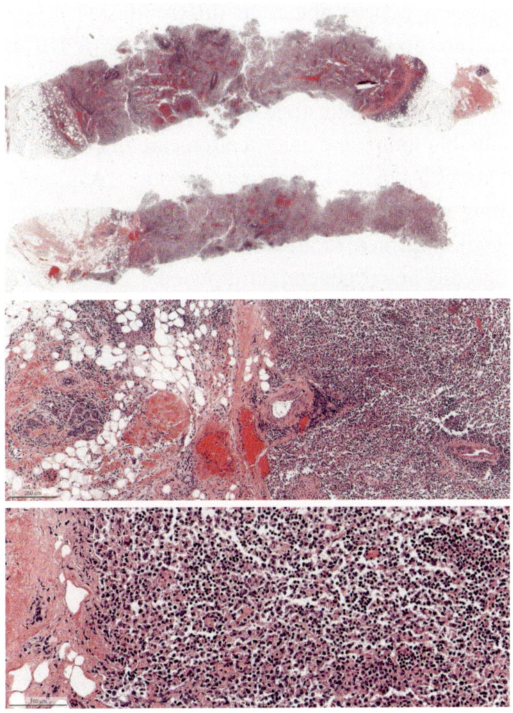

Figs. 13.52–13.54 Diffuse large B-cell lymphoma (DLBCL) of breast (H&E, low power, 10× and 20×). Sheets of large atypical lymphoid cells can be seen infiltrating the breast parenchyma in core needle biopsy. A lobule is present to the left of the atypical lymphoid cells

Metaplastic Carcinoma

Metaplastic Carcinoma: Metaplastic carcinomas are a heterogeneous group of invasive breast carcinomas where the tumor cells display squamous, spindle and or mesenchymal differentiation. Metaplastic carcinomas can present with a single pure histologic pattern, however, more often, these tumors contain a mixture of squamous, mesenchymal or glandular differentiation. They are rare and account for less than 1% of IBCs. Metaplastic carcinomas are more likely to present at an advanced stage. Most cases present as a palpable lump, and calcifications are uncommon. Although metaplastic carcinomas frequently show morphologic heterogeneity, genetic studies have confirmed monoclonal origin of the histologically heterogeneous components. Metaplastic carcinomas are frequently triple negative (ER−, PR−, and HER2−) and are relatively chemoresistent.

- **Clinical Presentation**: The patient may present with a large, rapidly growing, palpable mass, frequently with involvement of axillary lymph nodes at the time of diagnosis.
- **Imaging Findings:**
  - **Mammography**: A large mass that may be round or irregular, which may have a circumscribed or partially circumscribed margin. It may contain coarse heterogeneous calcifications.
  - **US**: Hypoechoic mixed cystic and solid mass with internal vascularity.
  - **MRI**: A large, rapidly enhancing mass that may demonstrate rim enhancement that is T2 hyperintense due to internal necrosis.
  - **BI-RADS**: 4 or 5, suspicious or highly suspicious.
  - **Differential Diagnosis**: Malignant phyllodes tumor, invasive ductal carcinoma, mucinous carcinoma, primary breast sarcoma, metastasis to breast.
- **Pathology Findings:**
  - **Gross**: There is no distinct gross appearance of metaplastic carcinoma. As compared to IDC, NOS metaplastic carcinomas are larger in size at presentation, often more than 2 cm.
    - Cystic degeneration can be seen in metaplastic carcinoma with squamous cell carcinoma.
    - The cut surface of metaplastic carcinoma can be sarcoma-like with soft tan white fleshy appearance and areas of hemorrhage and necrosis.
    - Pearly white and firm to gritty consistency is seen with mesenchymal differentiation to chondroid and osseus areas.
  - **Microscopic Histology**: Metaplastic carcinomas constitute a heterogeneous group of histologically distinct patterns with different outcomes. Metaplastic carcinoma is named descriptively based on the type and proportion of the histopathological patterns [32–34]. It can be comprised of one pure histopathologic pattern or contain two or more components. The two or more components can all be metaplastic (squamous, spindle or mesenchymal) or a metaplastic histologic pattern can be present with an adenocarcinoma. Metaplastic carcinomas can be classified as one of the following types:
    - Low-grade adenosquamous carcinoma (LGASC): This histopathologic pattern is often present as a pure component, and it has a favorable prognosis. The tumor is composed of glands and tubules (adeno component) as well as solid squamous cell nests (squamous component) that are intimately mixed and present in a desmoplastic spindle cell background. The tumor is infiltrative and often shows dense clusters of lymphocytes at the periphery.
    - Fibromatosis-like metaplastic carcinoma: This is another favorable histologic pattern of metaplastic carcinoma. The tumor is characterized by an infiltrative lesion composed of plump myofibroblastic-like cells spread in a collagenous connective tissue. Tumor cells express keratins and p63, by immunohistochemistry.
    - Spindle cell carcinoma: Spindle cell carcinomas are characterized by malignant spindle-shaped tumor cells embedded in a variable amount of fibrous tissue. The spindles are arranged in a variety of architectural patterns: storiform, fascicles, or herringbone. The tumor cells show moderate to high nuclear grade and often contain foci of

epithelioid cells displaying overt squamous differentiation. The epithelial nature of the spindle cells can be confirmed by keratin immunostains (heavy molecular weight keratins).

- Squamous cell carcinoma: Pure metaplastic squamous cell carcinoma usually presents a cystic lesion lined by layers of atypical squamous cells with often moderate to high-grade nuclear atypia. A squamous cell carcinoma component is often intermixed with spindle cell carcinoma or an adenocarcinoma (IDC, NOS).
- Metaplastic carcinoma with mesenchymal differentiation: These metaplastic carcinomas are characterized by carcinoma foci admixed with malignant chondroid, osteoid, rhabdomyoid or neuroglial differentiation. Traditionally this group of metaplastic carcinomas was labeled as matrix-producing carcinomas. Extensive sampling may be required in some of these cases to identify carcinomatous areas and to distinguish these cases from bone and soft tissue sarcomas. p63 and keratin expression can help to distinguish metaplastic carcinoma with mesenchymal differentiation from a malignant phyllodes tumor.
- Mixed metaplastic carcinoma: A large proportion of metaplastic carcinomas are composed of a variable mixture of aforementioned histology's with conventional IDC (NOS).

– **Differential Diagnosis**: Diagnosis of a metaplastic carcinoma can be challenging, especially in a limited sample-like core needle biopsy. The differential diagnosis of a spindle cell proliferation of breast includes a variety of benign and malignant lesions (see below) and the definite diagnosis rests on meticulous histological evaluation, judicious use of an IHC panel and correlation with clinical findings.

- Benign spindle cell lesions.
  - Myofibroblastoma: Well-circumscribed lesion in a postmenopausal woman. No entrapped lobules/ducts. Benign spindled cells with negative p63 and keratin stains.
  - Nodular fasciitis: Tissue culture-like myofibroblastic proliferation. No entrapped lobules/ducts. Negative p63 and keratin IHC.
  - Fibromatosis: Negative p63 and keratins. Positive myofibroblastic IHC (desmin, vimentin, and SMA). Abnormal beta-catenin [35].
  - Fibrous scar: Negative keratin and p63 IHC.
- Malignant phyllodes tumors: The stomal component of phyllode tumor (benign and borderline) is CD34 positive and negative for p63 and keratins. Because of the overlap of IHC features, malignant phyllode tumor stroma can be very difficult to distinguish from metaplastic spindle cell carcinoma, especially in small needle biopsies. In this setting it is best to defer a definite diagnosis to the excisional tissue.
- Pleomorphic adenoma: Lacks the malignant histological features.
- Angiosarcoma: Positive vascular markers (ERG).

– **Management**: Metaplastic breast carcinoma is staged similarly as other types of IBCs. Lymph node metastases are found significantly less frequently in metaplastic carcinoma as compared to size and grade matched IBC, NST. Distant metastasis can be present in the absence of lymph node metastasis. LGASC and fibromatosis-like metaplastic carcinoma have a more indolent behavior and favorable outcomes [36]. Radiotherapy provides survival benefits and as a group metaplastic carcinomas have lower response rate with chemotherapy.

Case

Clinical Findings: A 67-year-old female palpated a left breast mass. Her prior screening mammogram 16 months ago was negative (Figs. 13.55, 13.56, 13.57, and 13.58).

The lesion was called BI-RADS 5, highly suspicious for malignancy.

An US-guided biopsy of the mass and a representative axillary lymph node were performed revealing a metaplastic carcinoma (Figs. 13.59, 13.60, 13.61, 13.62, 13.63, 13.64, and 13.65).

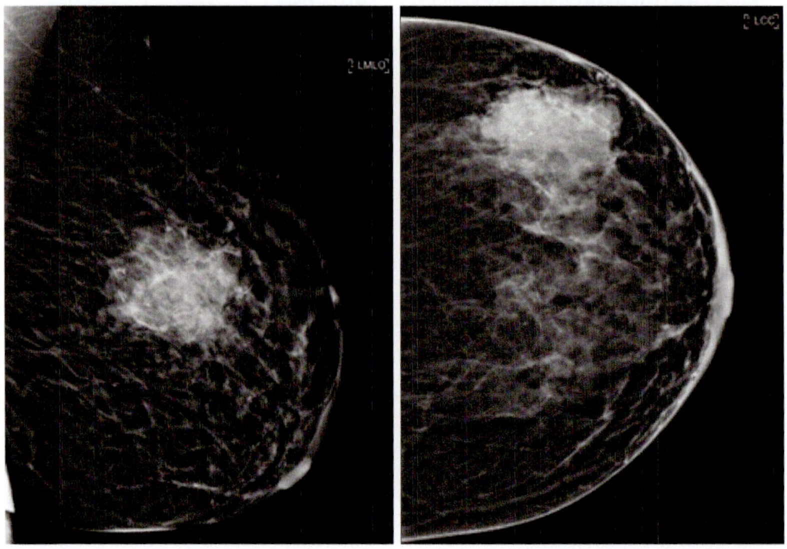

Figs. 13.55 and 13.56 **MMG findings**: Mammogram now reveals a large, irregular mass with a microlobulated margin and associated coarse heterogeneous calcifications. Enlarged left axillary lymph nodes were also noted

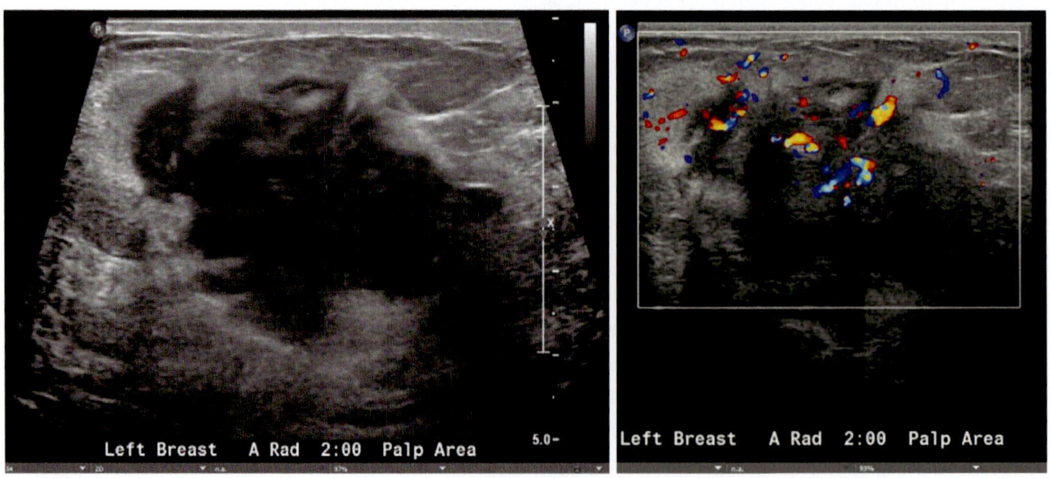

Figs. 13.57 and 13.58 **USG findings**: Ultrasound showed an irregular mass with a microlobulated margin, with internal vascularity and a hyperechoic rim. Enlarged left axillary lymph nodes were also noted

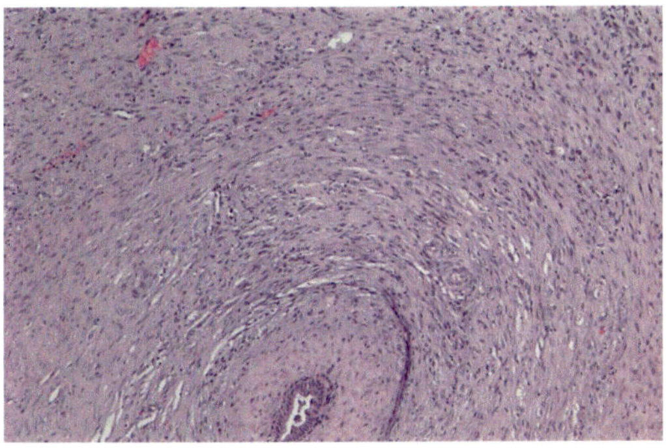

Fig. 13.59 Spindle cell carcinoma (H&E, 4×). The metaplastic carcinoma cells have elongated spindled nuclei with rare scattered epithelioid tumor cells

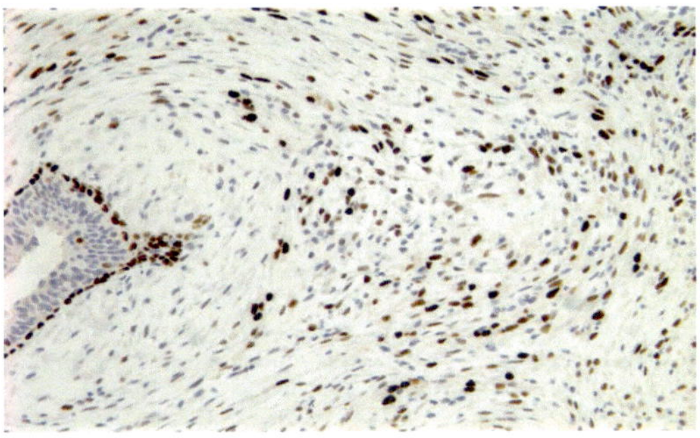

Fig. 13.60 (p63 IHC, 20×) Strong nuclear p63 immunostaining in tumor cells support the diagnosis of a metaplastic carcinoma. Myoepithelial cells in entrapped benign ducts also show nuclear p63 staining

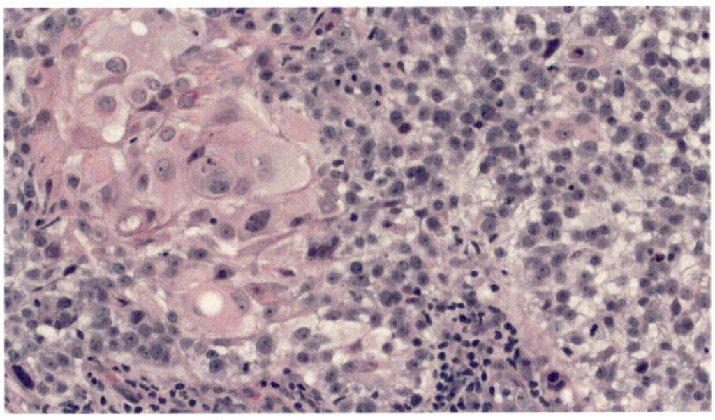

Fig. 13.61 Metaplastic carcinoma with squamous differentiation (H&E, 20×). The tumor cells (left side) show abundant eosinophilic cytoplasm, thick cell membrane, and intercellular bridges— consistent with squamous differentiation

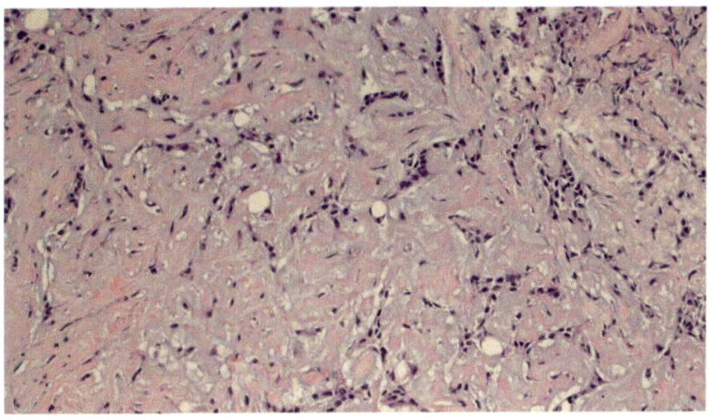

Fig. 13.62 Carcinoma with mesenchymal differentiation (aka matrix producing carcinoma; H&E, 10×). Carcinoma cells form anastomosing cords that are embedded in pale blue myxoid stroma. Some tumor cells have tapered ends and show spindled morphology

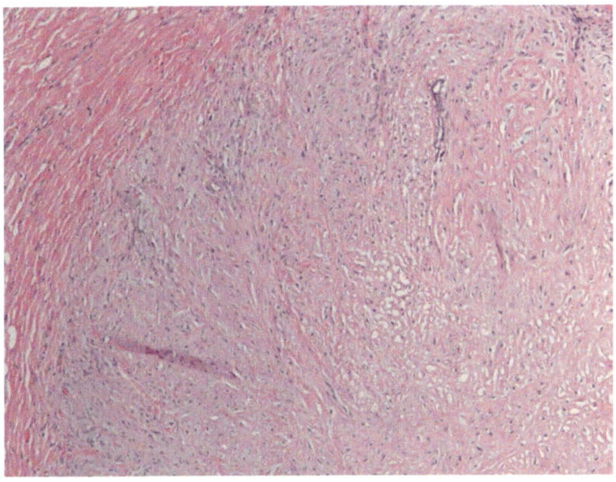

Fig. 13.63 Low-grade fibromatosis-like metaplastic carcinoma (H&E, 10×). The tumor is overall hypercellular with spindled carcinoma cells embedded in fibromyxoid stroma. Tumor cells show fibroblastic cytomorphology

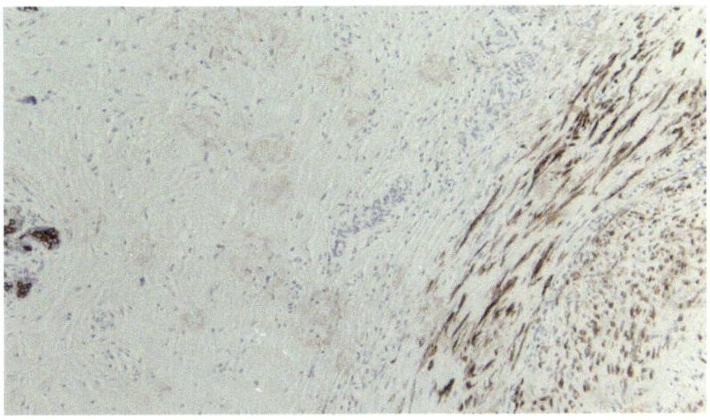

Fig. 13.64 Cytoplasmic keratin expression (IHC, 10×) in the spindled carcinoma cells support the diagnosis of low-grade fibromatosis-like carcinoma

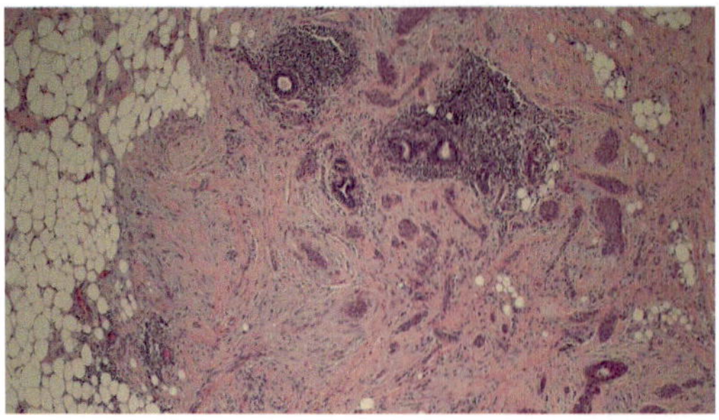

Fig. 13.65 Low-grade adenosquamous carcinoma (H&E, 4×). The carcinoma is comprised of solid round and angulated squamous nests mixed with glands. Desmoplastic response and lymphoid infiltrate are also present

References

1. Harrison BT, Dillon DA. An update of mucinous lesions of the breast. Surg Pathol Clin. 2018;11:61–90.
2. Gibreel WO, Boughey JC. Mucocele-like lesions of the breast: rate of upstaging and cancer development. Ann Surg Oncol. 2016;23:3838–42.
3. Singh K, Karamchandani D. Mucinous lesions of the breast: potpourri of old and new. Diagn Histopathol. 2019;26:69–75.
4. Magro G. Mammary myofibroblastoma: a tumor with a wide morphologic spectrum. Arch Pathol Lab Med. 2008;132(11):1813–20.
5. Magro G. Mammary myofibroblastoma: an update with emphasis on the most diagnostically challenging variants. Histol Histopathol. 2016;31(1):1–23. Epub 2015 Sep 2. PMID: 26328916.
6. Lee AH, Sworn MJ, Theaker JM, Fletcher CD. Myofibroblastoma of breast: an immunohistochemical study. Histopathology. 1993;22(1):75–8. https://doi.org/10.1111/j.1365-2559.1993.tb00074.x. PMID: 8382185.
7. Slodkowska E, Xu B, Kos Z, Bane A, Barnard M, Zubovits J, Iyengar P, Faragalla H, Turbin D, Williams P, Barnes PJ, Mulligan AM. Predictors of outcome in mammary adenoid cystic carcinoma: a multi-institutional study. Am J Surg Pathol. 2020;44(2):214–23.
8. Persson M, Andrén Y, Mark J, Horlings HM, Persson F, Stenman G. Recurrent fusion of MYB and NFIB transcription factor genes in carcinomas of the breast and head and neck. Proc Natl Acad Sci U S A. 2009;106(44):18740–4. https://doi.org/10.1073/pnas.0909114106. Epub 2009 Oct 19. PMID: 19841262; PMCID: PMC2773970.
9. Schwartz CJ, Brogi E, Marra A, Da Cruz Paula AF, Nanjangud GJ, da Silva EM, Patil S, Shah S, Ventura K, Razavi P, Norton L, D'alfonso T, Weigelt B, Pareja F, Reis-Filho JS, Wen HY. The clinical behavior and genomic features of the so-called adenoid cystic carcinomas of the solid variant with basaloid features. Mod Pathol. 2022;35(2):193–201. https://doi.org/10.1038/s41379-021-00931-6. Epub 2021 Oct 1. PMID: 34599282; PMCID: PMC9197148.
10. Fukuoka K, Hirokawa M, Shimizu M, Sadahira Y, Manabe T, Kurebayashi J, Sonoo H. Basaloid type adenoid cystic carcinoma of the breast. APMIS. 1999;107(8):762–6. https://doi.org/10.1111/j.1699-0463.1999.tb01470.x. PMID: 10515126.
11. Cima L, Kaya H, Marchiò C, Nishimura R, Wen HY, Fabbri VP, Foschini MP. Triple-negative breast carcinomas of low malignant potential: review on diagnostic criteria and differential diagnoses. Virchows Arch. 2022;480(1):109–26. https://doi.org/10.1007/s00428-021-03174-7. Epub 2021 Aug 30. PMID: 34458945; PMCID: PMC8983547.
12. Vranic S, Gatalica Z. An update on the molecular and clinical characteristics of apocrine carcinoma of the breast. Clin Breast Cancer. 2022;22(4):e576–85.
13. Niemeier LA, Dabbs DJ, Beriwal S, Striebel JM, Bhargava R. Androgen receptor in breast cancer: expression in estrogen receptor-positive tumors and in estrogen receptor-negative tumors with apocrine differentiation. Mod Pathol. 2010;23(2):205–12. https://doi.org/10.1038/modpathol.2009.159. Epub 2009 Nov 6. PMID: 19898421.
14. Lerner G, Tang H, Singh K, Golestani R, St Claire S, Humphrey PA, Lannin D, Janostiak R, Harigopal M. AMACR expression is a potential diagnostic marker in apocrine lesions of breast, and is associated with high histologic grade and lymph node metastases in some invasive apocrine breast cancers. Clin Breast Cancer. 2023;23(2):199–210. https://doi.org/10.1016/j.clbc.2022.11.012. S1526-8209(22)00268-3. PMID: 36577560.
15. Vasudev P, Onuma K. Secretory breast carcinoma: unique, triple-negative carcinoma with a favorable prognosis and characteristic molecular expression. Arch Pathol Lab Med. 2011;135(12):1606–10.
16. Hoda RS, Brogi E, Pareja F, Nanjangud G, Murray MP, Weigelt B, Reis-Filho JS, Wen HY. Secretory carcinoma of the breast: clinicopathologic profile of 14 cases emphasizing distant metastatic potential. Histopathology. 2019;75(2):213–24.
17. Harrison BT, Fowler E, Krings G, Chen YY, Bean GR, Vincent-Salomon A, Fuhrmann L, Barnick SE, Chen B, Hosfield EM, Hornick JL, Schnitt SJ. Pan-TRK immunohistochemistry: a useful diagnostic adjunct for secretory carcinoma of the breast. Am J Surg Pathol. 2019;43(12):1693–700. https://doi.org/10.1097/PAS.0000000000001366. PMID: 31498178.
18. Chiang S, Weigelt B, Wen HC, Pareja F, Raghavendra A, Martelotto LG, Burke KA, Basili T, Li A, Geyer FC, Piscuoglio S, Ng CK, Jungbluth AA, Balss J, Pusch S, Baker GM, Cole KS, von Deimling A, Batten JM, Marotti JD, Soh HC, McCalip BL, Serrano J, Lim RS, Siziopikou KP, Lu S, Liu X, Hammour T, Brogi E, Snuderl M, Iafrate AJ, Reis-Filho JS, Schnitt SJ. IDH2 mutations define a unique subtype of breast

cancer with altered nuclear polarity. Cancer Res. 2016;76(24):7118–29. https://doi.org/10.1158/0008-5472.CAN-16-0298. Epub 2016 Oct 20. PMID: 27913435; PMCID: PMC5502804.

19. Bhargava R, Florea AV, Pelmus M, Jones MW, Bonaventura M, Wald A, Nikiforova M. Breast tumor resembling tall cell variant of papillary thyroid carcinoma: a solid papillary neoplasm with characteristic immunohistochemical profile and few recurrent mutations. Am J Clin Pathol. 2017;147(4):399–410. https://doi.org/10.1093/ajcp/aqx016. PMID: 28375433.
20. Lozada JR, Basili T, Pareja F, Alemar B, Paula ADC, Gularte-Merida R, Giri DD, Querzoli P, Cserni G, Rakha EA, Foschini MP, Reis-Filho JS, Brogi E, Weigelt B, Geyer FC. Solid papillary breast carcinomas resembling the tall cell variant of papillary thyroid neoplasms (solid papillary carcinomas with reverse polarity) harbour recurrent mutations affecting IDH2 and PIK3CA: a validation cohort. Histopathology. 2018;73(2):339–44.
21. Pareja F, da Silva EM, Frosina D, Geyer FC, Lozada JR, Basili T, Da Cruz PA, Zhong E, Derakhshan F, D'Alfonso T, Wen HY, Giri DD, Hayes MM, Krings G, Bhargava R, Palazzo JP, Rakha EA, Hoda SA, Sanders ME, Collins LC, Schnitt SJ, Chen YY, Weigelt B, Jungbluth AA, Reis-Filho JS, Brogi E. Immunohistochemical analysis of IDH2 R172 hotspot mutations in breast papillary neoplasms: applications in the diagnosis of tall cell carcinoma with reverse polarity. Mod Pathol. 2020;33(6):1056–64.
22. Ajkunic A, Skenderi F, Shaker N, Akhtar S, Lamovec J, Gatalica Z, Vranic S. Acinic cell carcinoma of the breast: a comprehensive review. Breast. 2022;66:208–16. https://doi.org/10.1016/j.breast.2022.10.012. Epub 2022 Oct 28. PMID: 36332545; PMCID: PMC9636467.
23. Cserni G, Quinn CM, Foschini MP, Bianchi S, Callagy G, Chmielik E, Decker T, Fend F, Kovács A, van Diest PJ, Ellis IO, Rakha E, Tot T, European Working Group for Breast Screening Pathology. Triple-negative breast cancer histological subtypes with a favourable prognosis. Cancers (Basel). 2021;13(22):5694. https://doi.org/10.3390/cancers13225694. PMID: 34830849; PMCID: PMC8616217.
24. Geyer FC, Berman SH, Marchiò C, Burke KA, Guerini-Rocco E, Piscuoglio S, Ng CK, Pareja F, Wen HY, Hodi Z, Schnitt SJ, Rakha EA, Ellis IO, Norton L, Weigelt B, Reis-Filho JS. Genetic analysis of microglandular adenosis and acinic cell carcinomas of the breast provides evidence for the existence of a low-grade triple-negative breast neoplasia family. Mod Pathol. 2017;30(1):69–84. https://doi.org/10.1038/modpathol.2016.161. Epub 2016 Oct 7. PMID: 27713419; PMCID: PMC5221420.
25. Tsang JY, Tse GM. Breast cancer with neuroendocrine differentiation: an update based on the latest WHO classification. Mod Pathol. 2021;34(6):1062–73. https://doi.org/10.1038/s41379-021-00736-7. Epub 2021 Feb 2. PMID: 33531618.
26. Metovic J, Cascardi E, Uccella S, Maragliano R, Querzoli G, Osella-Abate S, Pittaro A, La Rosa S, Bogina G, Cassoni P, Marchiò C, Sapino A, Castellano I, Papotti M. Neuroendocrine neoplasms of the breast: diagnostic agreement and impact on outcome. Virchows Arch. 2022;481(6):839–46. https://doi.org/10.1007/s00428-022-03426-0. Epub 2022 Oct 15. PMID: 36243799; PMCID: PMC9734208.
27. Bean GR, Najjar S, Shin SJ, Hosfield EM, Caswell-Jin JL, Urisman A, Jones KD, Chen YY, Krings G. Genetic and immunohistochemical profiling of small cell and large cell neuroendocrine carcinomas of the breast. Mod Pathol. 2022;35(10):1349–61. https://doi.org/10.1038/s41379-022-01090-y. Epub 2022 May 19.
28. Lee AHS, Hodi Z, Soomro I, Sovani V, Abbas A, Rakha E, Ellis IO. Histological clues to the diagnosis of metastasis to the breast from extramammary malignancies. Histopathology. 2020;77(2):303–13. https://doi.org/10.1111/his.14141. Epub 2020 Jul 23. PMID: 32396659.
29. DeLair DF, Corben AD, Catalano JP, Vallejo CE, Brogi E, Tan LK. Non-mammary metastases to the breast and axilla: a study of 85 cases. Mod Pathol. 2013;26(3):343–9. https://doi.org/10.1038/modpathol.2012.191. Epub 2012 Nov 23. PMID: 23174933.
30. Topalovski M, Crisan D, Mattson JC. Lymphoma of the breast. A clinicopathologic study of primary and secondary cases. Arch Pathol Lab Med. 1999;123(12):1208–18. https://doi.org/10.5858/1999-123-1208-LOTB. PMID: 10583925.
31. Lalani N, Winkfield KM, Soto DE, Yeap BY, Ng AK, Mauch PM, Jimenez RB. Management and outcomes of women diagnosed with primary breast lymphoma: a multi-institution experience. Breast Cancer Res Treat. 2018;169(1):197–202. https://doi.org/10.1007/s10549-018-4671-8. Epub 2018 Jan 22. PMID: 29356916.
32. Carter MR, Hornick JL, Lester S, Fletcher CD. Spindle cell (sarcomatoid) carcinoma of the breast: a clinicopathologic and immunohistochemical analysis of 29 cases. Am J Surg Pathol. 2006;30(3):300–9. https://doi.org/10.1097/01.pas.0000184809.27735.a1. PMID: 16538049.
33. Van Hoeven KH, Drudis T, Cranor ML, Erlandson RA, Rosen PP. Low-grade adenosquamous carcinoma of the breast. A clinocopathologic study of 32 cases with ultrastructural analysis. Am J Surg Pathol. 1993;17(3):248–58. https://doi.org/10.1097/00000478-199303000-00005. PMID: 8434705.
34. Gobbi H, Simpson JF, Borowsky A, Jensen RA, Page DL. Metaplastic breast tumors with a dominant fibromatosis-like phenotype have a high risk of local recurrence. Cancer. 1999;85(10):2170–82. https://doi.org/10.1002/(sici)1097-0142(19990515)85:10<2170::aid-cncr11>3.0.co;2-x. PMID: 10326695.
35. Han M, Zhang H, Dabbs DJ. Best practice (efficient) immunohistologic panel for diagnosing metaplas-

tic breast carcinoma. Appl Immunohistochem Mol Morphol. 2021;29(4):265–9. https://doi.org/10.1097/PAI.0000000000000873. PMID: 32858538.

36. Tadros AB, Sevilimedu V, Giri DD, Zabor EC, Morrow M, Plitas G. Survival outcomes for metaplastic breast cancer differ by histologic subtype. Ann Surg Oncol. 2021;28(8):4245–53. https://doi.org/10.1245/s10434-020-09430-5. Epub 2021 Jan 2. PMID: 33389291.

14 Discordances Between Radiology and Pathology

Malini Harigopal, Anuj Verma, Liva Andrejeva, and John Lewin

Examples of Radiology-Pathology Discordances

Case 1

A 72-year-old female undergoing screening mammography. New linearly distributed calcifications are identified in the upper-outer left breast (Fig. 14.1a). The patient is recalled for magnification views, which confirm the calcifications and show them to be heterogeneous and therefore suspicious of malignancy (Fig. 14.1b). The patient undergoes stereotactic vacuum-assisted biopsy with successful retrieval of calcifications by specimen radiography. Pathology reveals multifocal atypical lobular hyperplasia (Fig. 14.1c). Calcifications are identified in dense hyalinized nodular stroma suggestive of a fibroadenoma. Because the ALH diagnosis was both high-risk and discordant (i.e., it does not explain the calcifications), surgical excision was performed. The surgical specimen contains numerous calcifications. The surgical excision showed ALH and ADH, as well as high-grade DCIS (Fig. 14.1d). The calcifications were in the ALH and in fibrous stroma. The DCIS was not associated with calcifications.

M. Harigopal (✉) · A. Verma
Department of Pathology, Yale University, New Haven, CT, USA
e-mail: malini.harigopal@yale.edu; anuj.verma@yale.edu

L. Andrejeva · J. Lewin
Department of Radiology and Biomedical Imaging, Yale School of Medicine, New Haven, CT, USA
e-mail: liva.andrejeva@yale.edu; John.Lewin@yale.edu

M. Harigopal et al. (eds.), *Radiology Pathology Correlations of Breast Lesions*, https://doi.org/10.1007/978-3-031-65711-5_14

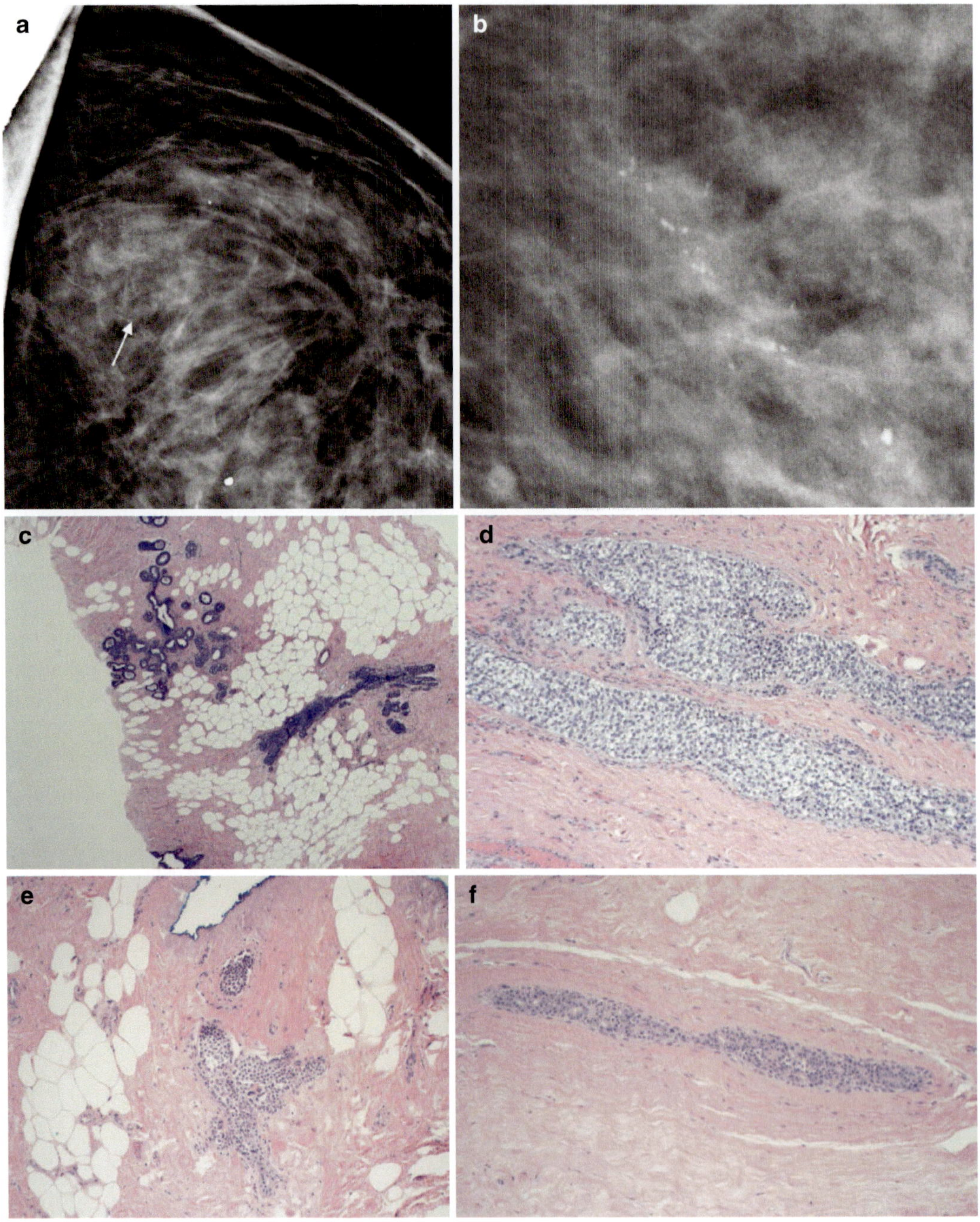

Fig. 14.1 Screening mammogram in a 72-year-old woman. (**a**) Left MLO mammographic view shows linearly distributed calcifications (arrow). (**b**) Magnification view shows the calcifications to be heterogeneous. (**c**) H&E slide of the core biopsy shows multifocal atypical lobular hyperplasia with associated calcifications. (**d**) H&E slide of the excision shows grade-3 DCIS without calcifications. (**e**) The excisional showed more ALH with calcifications as well as calcifications in an area of fibrotic stroma/scar suggesting a prior surgical procedure at that site. (**f**) ADH was also seen

Educational Note

The core biopsy findings of atypical lobular hyperplasia did not correlate with imaging findings of branching linear calcifications which are regarded as suspicious findings. The patient underwent an excisional biopsy as the biopsy findings were considered discordant with imaging. Atypical lobular hyperplasia is usually an incidental finding in breast biopsies for calcifications [1]. High-grade DCIS seen on excisional biopsy is usually seen as a mammographically detected linear branching and pleomorphic calcification.

Therefore suspicious calcifications seen on mammogram are a common presentation of DCIS and not ALH.

In this unusual case, the calcifications were mostly in benign ducts. Both the ALH and the DCIS were apparently incidental to the mammographic finding (although the ALH did have some calcifications in it). Having ALH and ADH raises the overall risk for cancer, so in that sense it is less surprising that cancer (in the form of DCIS) was found in the adjacent tissue.

Case 2

A 46-year-old female undergoing screening mammography with tomosynthesis. Architectural distortion is identified in the left breast on the standard 2D mammography (Fig. 14.2a) and is better seen with tomosynthesis (Fig. 14.2b). Stereotactic biopsy is performed, with a result of sclerosis adenosis and nodular adenosis involved by atypical apocrine adenosis (Fig. 14.2c). Surgical excision is performed both because of the atypia and because the architectural distortion was not explained. The excision showed a radial scar/complex sclerosing lesion with prior biopsy site changes (Fig. 14.2d) and, in the adjacent tissue, intermediate-grade DCIS (Fig. 14.2e). Note that the RS/SCL is concordant with the architectural distortion.

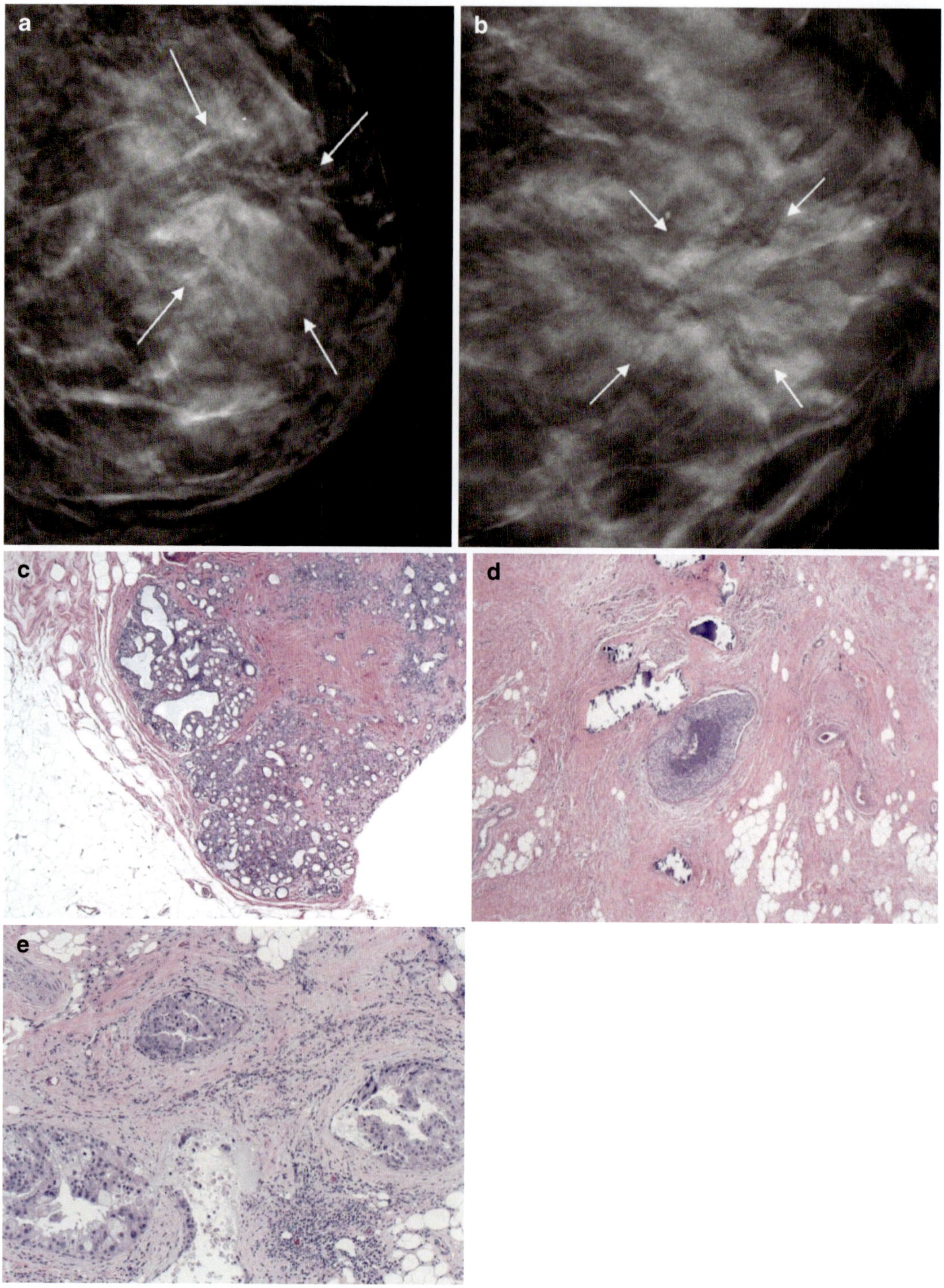

Fig. 14.2 Screening mammogram in a 46-year-old woman. (**a**, **b**) Architectural distortion seen in the left breast at 11 o'clock middle depth on screening mammography. (**c**) Core biopsy showed nodular adenosis involved by atypical apocrine adenosis with central sclerosis. (**d**) The excision biopsy showed a radial scar/complex sclerosing lesion. Changes from the prior percutaneous biopsy are identified. (**e**) Grade-2 DCIS was noted away from the biopsy site

Educational Note

Radial scars/complex sclerosing lesions (RS/CSL) are associated with malignancy (typically DCIS or low-grade IDCA) at surgical excision 15–40% of the time depending on the type of percutaneous biopsy (core vs. vacuum-assisted) and whether or not the lesion was identified with tomosynthesis, as opposed to standard mammography [2–4]. The cancer is usually at the periphery. Even without cancer found in the lesion, the presence of an RS/CSL increases the patient's overall risk.

Adenosis is a benign proliferative lesion which can present as a mammographic abnormality either as a mass when there is florid adenosis or is referred to as a nodular adenosis. The epithelium within the adenosis glands exhibit apocrine metaplasia with enlarged cells with large nuclei, prominent nucleoli, and abundant eosinophilic granules. Varying degrees of cytologic atypia can be seen where the atypia can be particularly difficult to distinguish from apocrine DCIS. In a core biopsy a conservative approach is preferred in equivocal cases. When the atypical cells show a threefold increase in nuclei with nuclear pleomorphism without the complex architectural pattern and glandular expansion seen in apocrine DCIS it is prudent to call the lesion atypical apocrine adenosis. These lesions should be excised as areas of DCIS may be present on excision as illustrated in this case.

Case 3

A 50-year-old female with bloody left nipple discharge. MRI was performed showing an extensive dilated duct system in the lateral breast containing multiple enhancing foci and 3–6 mm masses (Fig. 14.3a, b). Ultrasound of the subareolar breast showed multiple circumscribed masses suggestive of papillomas (Fig. 14.3c). The largest mass was 1.5 cm. Biopsies of the masses showed intraductal papillomas with usual ductal hyperplasia (Fig. 14.3d, e). Because of the multiplicity, an excisional biopsy was performed which showed intermediate grade DCIS within a papilloma (Fig. 14.3f, g). Additional stains confirmed the DCIS and showed it to be ER-positive (Fig. 14.3h, i).

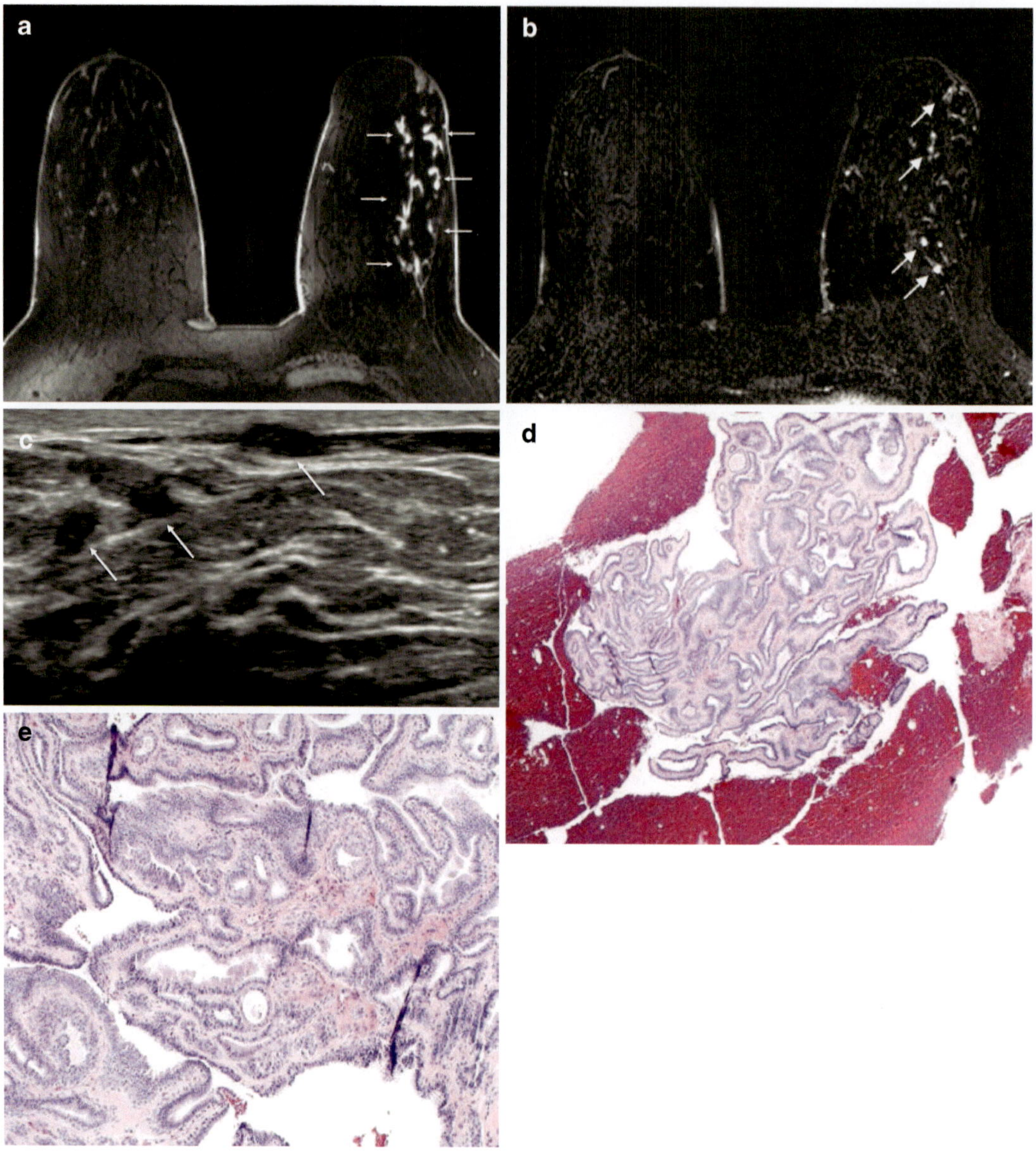

Fig. 14.3 (**a**) Pre-contrast T1-weighted fat suppressed axial MRI showing 8 cm of dilated ducts containing proteinaceous or bloody fluid in the lateral left breast (arrows). (**b**) Post-contrast subtraction image at the same level showing scattered enhancing foci and small masses within the ducts (arrows). (**c**) Left breast ultrasound showing multiple intraductal masses in the subareolar region. (**d, e**) A core biopsy from the region showed features of intraductal papilloma with focal features of usual ductal hyperplasia. (**f, g**) H&E slides from the resection showed an intraductal papilloma involved by a grade-2 DCIS. (**h**) CK 5/6 immunohistochemistry showing loss of staining within the DCIS. (**i**) ER immunohistochemistry showing strong and diffuse staining

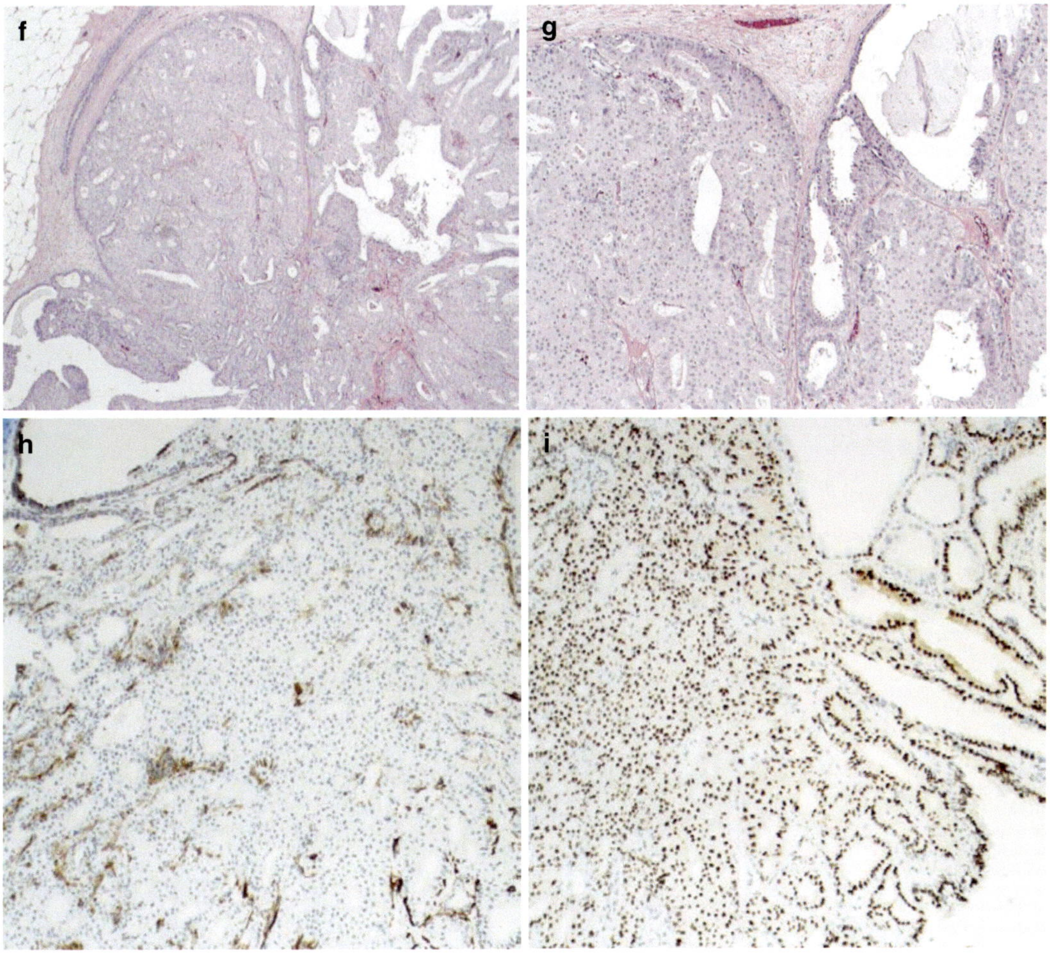

Fig. 14.3 (continued)

Educational Note

The biopsy showed portions of intraductal papilloma. A solitary papilloma without atypia does not generally require excision [5]. In this case, however, because the presence of multiple intraductal masses increases the likelihood of atypia or cancer being present in one of them, an excision was performed. The excision confirmed the presence of DCIS grade 2 with a solid growth pattern involving the papilloma. The diagnosis was supported by immunostains which showed absence of high molecular weight keratins (CK5/6) and diffuse expression of ER in the in situ component.

Case 4

A 58-year-old female with asymmetry in the superolateral right breast on screening mammography (Fig. 14.4).

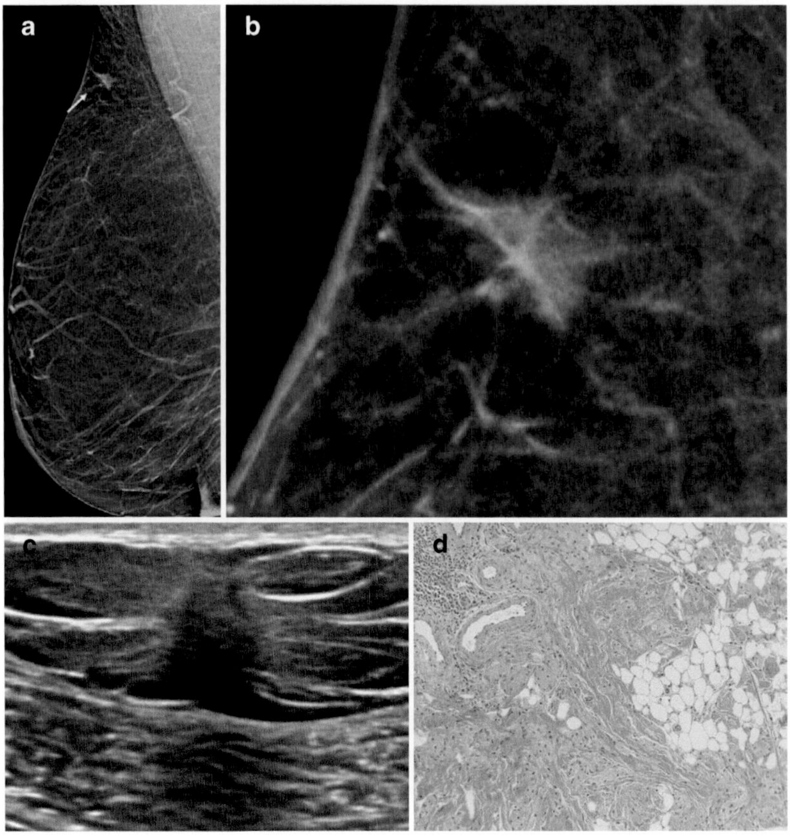

Fig. 14.4 (**a**) Mammogram showing an irregular mass with a spiculated margin in the right breast posterior depth superior region (arrow). (**b**) Digital zoom of the mammographic lesion. (**c**) Targeted ultrasound shows an irregular hypoechoic mass with an indistinct margin and posterior shadowing. (**d**) Biopsy of the mass showed fibroadipose tissue with benign granular cell tumor characterized by proliferation of cells with abundant eosinophilic granular cytoplasm and a small nucleus

Educational Note

This example of a granular cell tumor was included in this chapter to illustrate that granular cell tumors mimic breast cancers on clinical, radiologic, and gross examination.

The suspicion for malignancy is high based on the mammographic findings of a spiculated lesion and clinically can be associated with a palpable hard mass with skin retraction or fixed to chest wall due to infiltration into the skeletal muscle. Classical findings of tumor cells with granular cytoplasm and small nuclei infiltrating into adjacent stroma is sufficient for a diagnosis of a granular cell tumor but confirmatory immunostains such as CD68, S100, and keratins, such as AE1/AE3, are often performed [6, 7]. The CD68 and S100 will show strong and diffuse staining, and the keratins will be negative, supporting a neural origin and helping to exclude apocrine or variant forms of lobular carcinoma, especially the histiocytoid variant, which can mimic granular cell tumors. This case is not a true discordance since the appearance of the mammographic lesion is concordant with the final diagnosis on pathology. It is a surprising but concordant benign result.

Case 5

A 68-year-old female with history of right breast invasive ductal carcinoma with incidentally detected soft tissue density in the reconstructed left breast on surveillance chest CT (Fig. 14.5).

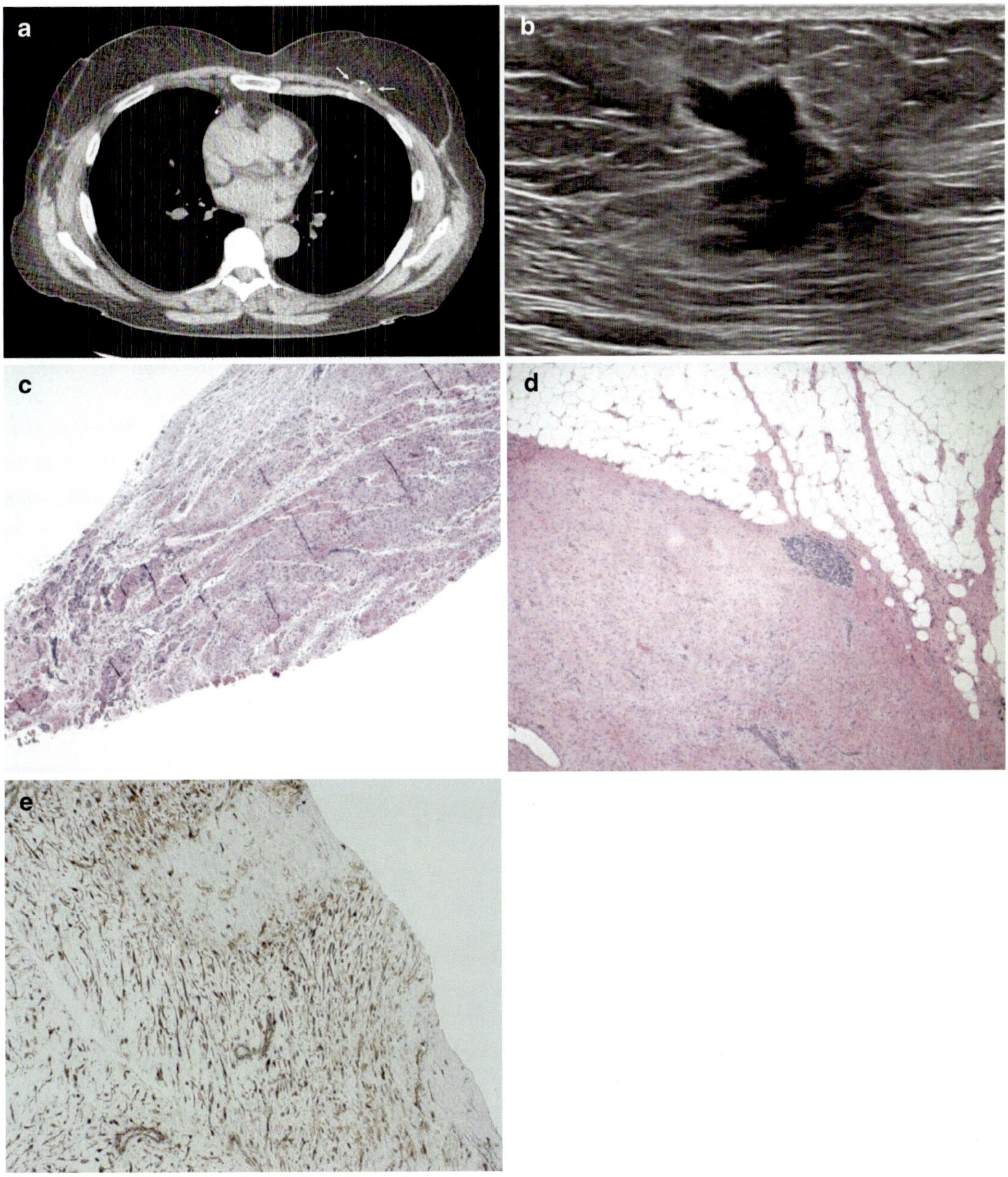

Fig. 14.5 (**a**) Ultrasound showed an irregular complex and solid and cyst mass in the left reconstructed breast at 12 o'clock at middle depth. (**b**, **c**) Biopsy of the lesion showed a scar and degenerating skeletal muscles. (**d**) Excision showing spindle cell proliferation infiltrating the adipose tissue and lymphoid aggregate. (**e**) Spindle cells showing nuclear beta catenin staining by immunohistochemistry confirming the diagnosis of mammary fibromatosis

Educational Note

Mammary desmoid fibromatosis is a rare locally aggressive disease accounting for <0.2% of all breast tumors. It is seen predominantly in middle-aged patients but can occur in patients from 13 to 83 years. The disease presents with firm palpable nodules, ranging in size from a few mm to over 10 cm. The nodules can be attached to the skin or pectoral fascia, resulting in skin or nipple retraction. Fibromatosis of the breast is highly suspicious on clinical and radiologic presentation. Although locally aggressive, it does not metastasize. Most reported cases are unilateral. The local recurrence rates following surgery is between 18% and 29% [8]. Recurrence can occur despite achieving a clear margin on excision.

On mammography breast fibromatosis usually appears as a high density irregular or spiculated mass. On ultrasound it is usually an ill-defined hypoechoic mass with a thick echogenic rim and posterior shadowing. The appearance is usually indistinguishable from cancer.

In this case, due to the radiologic-pathologic discordance on the ultrasound-guided biopsy, which showed only fibrous scar, an excisional biopsy was performed. The excisional biopsy showed a spindle cell proliferation with long sweeping bundles of interlacing spindle cells, positive for smooth muscle actin and beta catenin diagnostic of fibromatosis.

On pathology from a core needle biopsy, it is important to differentiate fibromatosis from a low-grade fibromatosis-like metaplastic carcinoma or a low-grade fibrosarcoma. Benign spindle cell entities that enter the differential include nodular fasciitis, schwannoma, leiomyoma, solitary fibrous tumor, myofibroblastoma, myoepithelioma, and fibrous scar [9].

Case 6

A 52-year-old female with new calcifications on screening mammography (Fig. 14.6).

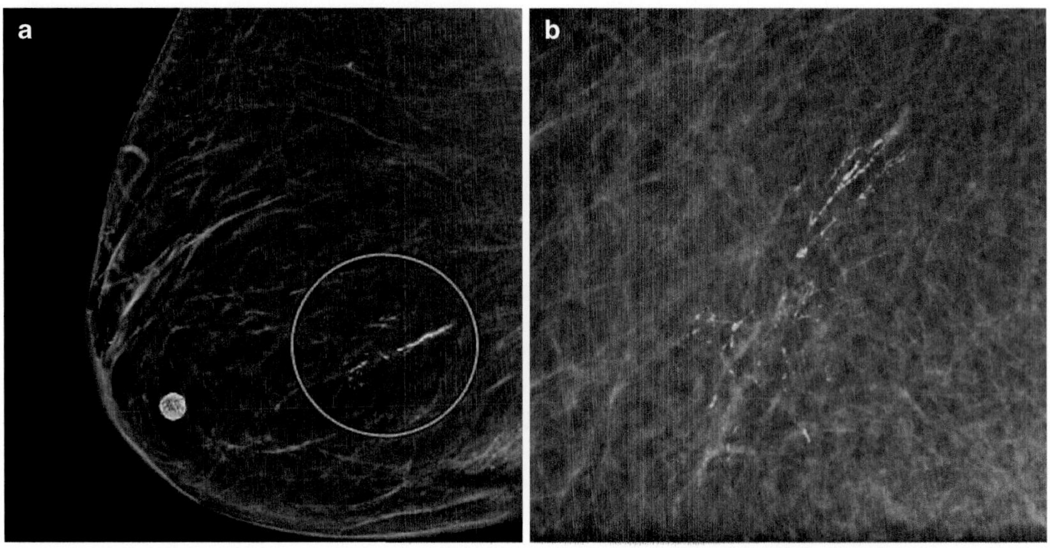

Fig. 14.6 (**a**) Screening mammogram showing a new area of linear distributed calcifications in the inferior right breast. (**b**) Magnification view of the calcifications show them to be linear branching and highly suspicious of malignancy. (**c**) Biopsy of the calcified area revealed grade 2–3 DCIS. (**d**) Specimen radiograph from the partial mastectomy shows linearly distributed calcifications. (**e, f**) Pathology from the partial mastectomy showed fibrosis, inflammation, suture granuloma and no residual DCIS. (**g**) Mammography 1 year later shows linear branching calcifications at the surgical site, as evidenced by the surgical clips. (**h**) Core biopsy then showed grade-3 DCIS involving 2 duct spaces. (**i**) A subsequent resection showed grade-3 DCIS

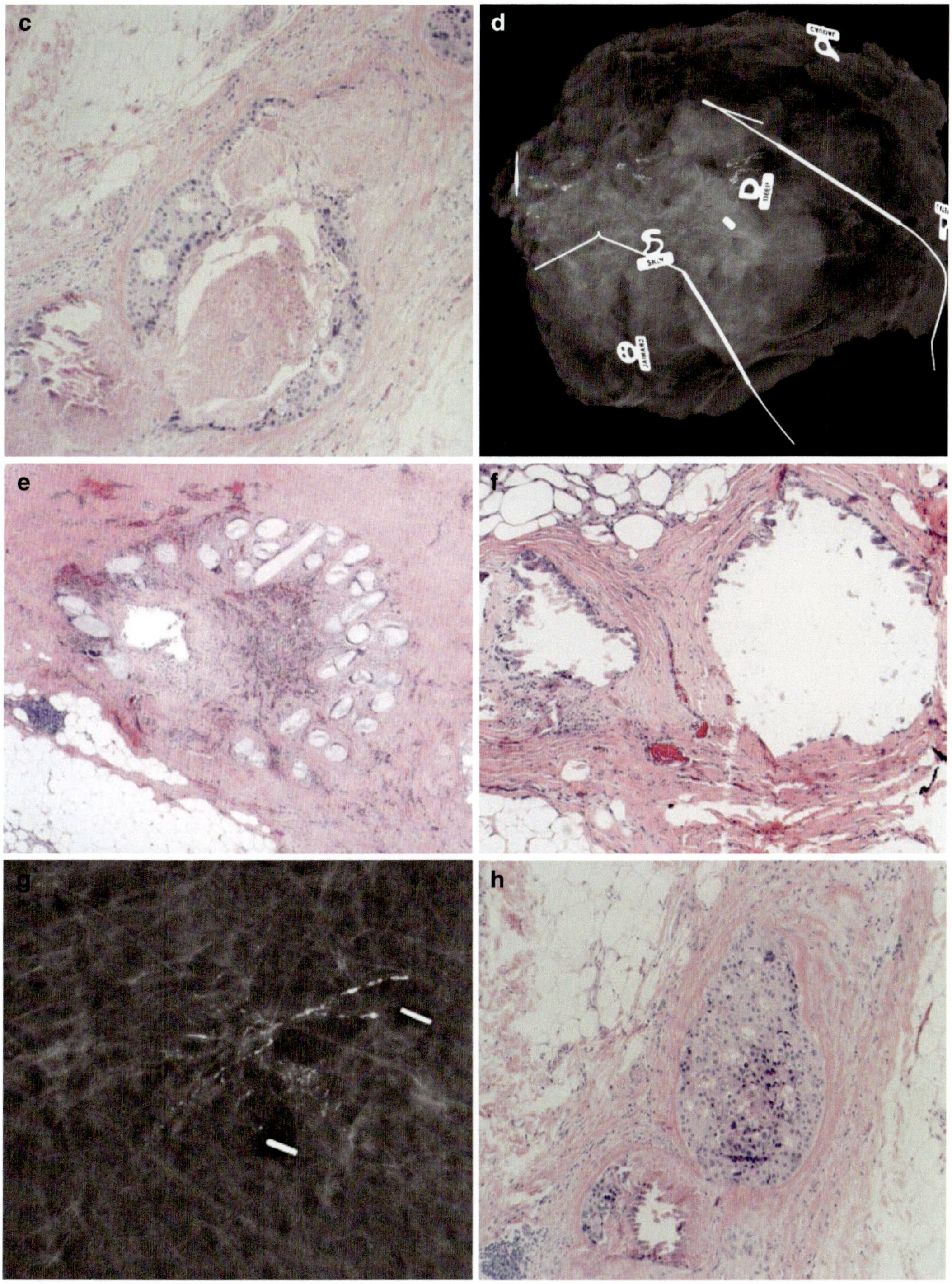

Fig. 14.6 (continued)

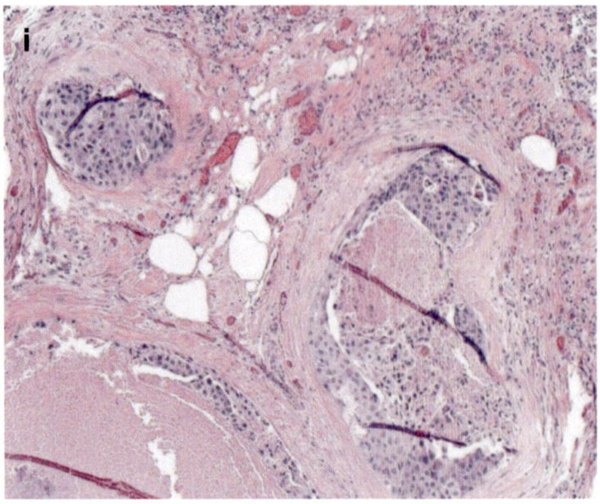

Fig. 14.6 (continued)

Educational Note

In this case the right partial mastectomy showed ducts with no lining DCIS epithelium but abundant abnormal calcifications which was noted by the pathologist in the final report stating that although no DCIS was seen, calcifications similar to that seen in the initial core biopsy with DCIS was present. Additional deeper H&E recuts would be helpful as some DCIS can be "regressing" without residual lining epithelium but have suspicious calcifications. The pathologist should indicate that these calcifications are abnormal and although no DCIS is visualized despite additional workup.

It appeared that all the calcifications were removed at surgical excision but given the unexpected pathology result, a mammogram should have been performed to evaluate for residual calcifications, prior to starting radiation. In this case, the patient did not have radiation after the initial diagnosis, in part because of the unclear final pathology and in part because of institutional guidelines and patient choice to defer treatment during the height of the COVID pandemic.

In the end the patient remained at stage 0 (DCIS only) so the 1-year delay in definitive treatment is unlikely to affect her survival. Because she did not have radiation therapy after her first diagnosis, she was eligible to receive it after the second partial mastectomy. Note that, although surgery is considered the gold standard for diagnosis, like percutaneous biopsy it is imperfect, especially for non-palpable lesions. Radiology-pathology correlation is critical to guide appropriate management.

Case 7

A 17-year-old female presents with palpable right breast mass at 5:00 (Fig. 14.7).

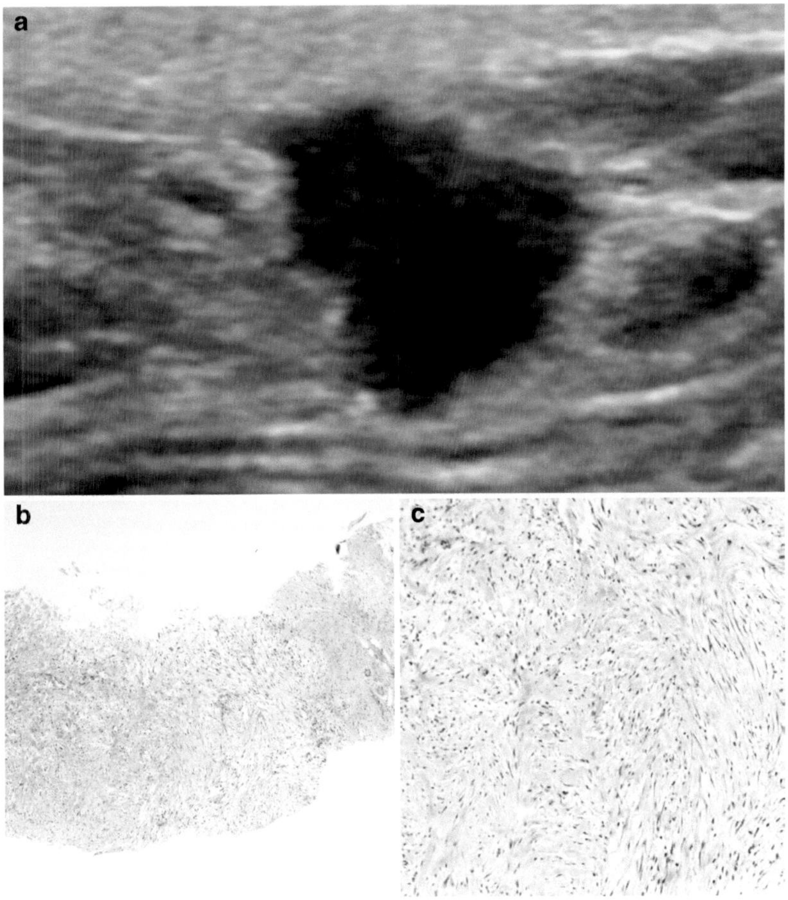

Fig. 14.7 (**a**) Ultrasound of the palpable mass shows a 0.9-cm irregular hypoechoic mass with a microlobulated margin, just deep to the skin. (**b**, **c**) Core biopsy of the mass shows a nodular fasciitis characterized by cellular proliferation of spindle cells focally in fascicles on a myxoid to collagenous background with scattered inflammatory cells and extravasated RBCs

Educational Note

Nodular fasciitis can present as a painful mass in the subcutaneous tissue, muscle or within the breast parenchyma. On imaging they have an irregular shape and mimic carcinoma. On microscopic examination the lesion has a variable appearance depending on the age of the lesion. The clue to the diagnosis is when the short spindle cells are loosely arranged in a myxoid stroma. The spindle cells have small regular nuclei with prominent nucleoli and mitoses are frequent. The spindle cells do not infiltrate around ducts and lobules like in fibromatosis. Stroma can have granulation tissue-like areas with increased number of delicate vessels with extravasation of red blood cells. Lymphocytes and plasma cells are distributed throughout the stroma. In older lesions the stroma is more collagenized. The differential diagnosis includes spindle cell carcinoma. Immunostains for keratins and CD34 is absent. Immunostains for muscle markers smooth muscle actin, desmin, and calponin may be positive. On core biopsy the diagnosis can be particularly challenging due to limited sampling. Clinical presentation of a rapidly growing tender mass in a superficial location is helpful. Although accurate diagnosis on core biopsy can be challenging, excluding other lesions using a panel of immunohistochemical stains is important as these lesions regress over time and surgery can be avoided [10, 11].

Case 8

A 28-year-old female presents with 3 weeks of left breast pain and nipple discharge. Physical examination shows skin thickening and *peau d'orange* changes inferolaterally. Ultrasound elsewhere is suggestive of mastitis. MRI is performed (Fig. 14.8).

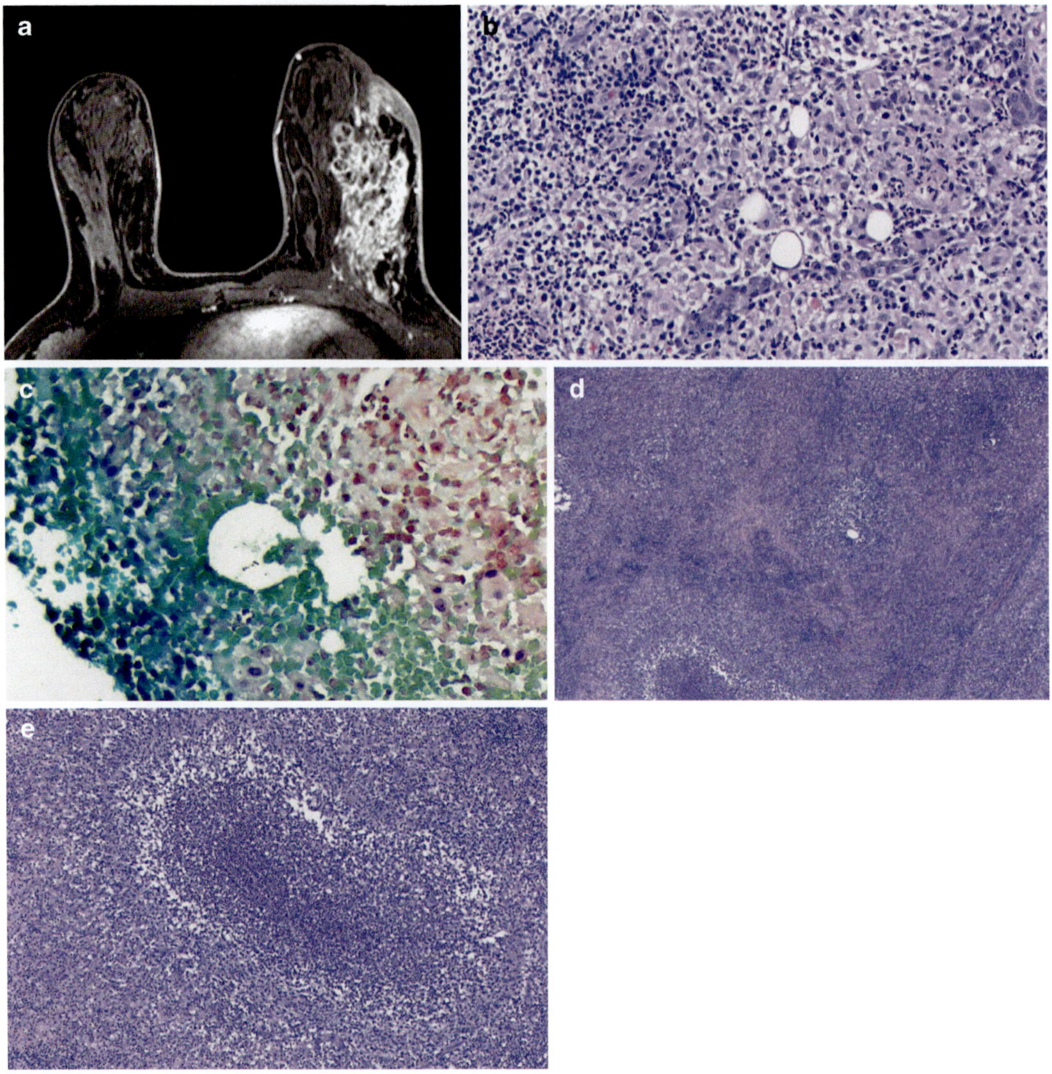

Fig. 14.8 (**a**) Breast MRI with contrast showing a 13-cm region of clumped non-mass enhancement with a ring enhancing pattern, as well as marked focal skin thickening. (**b**) Breast ultrasound-guided core biopsy from the abnormal region showing inflammatory cells composed of mononuclear cells and neutrophils with scattered microcystic spaces surrounded by neutrophils and giant cells. (**c**) Gram stain on breast biopsy few cystic spaces showed gram-positive bacteria. (**d, e**) Mastectomy specimen showing extensive histiocytic, neutrophilic and granulomatous inflammation involving ducts and lobules with scattered characteristic neutrophil-lined cysts

Educational Note

Cystic neutrophilic granulomatous mastitis is a relatively recent entity described in the pathology literature caused by bacterial infection. There are few reported cases in the literature with an incidence of <1% of all breast specimens [12]. The mean patient age was 35 years. Patients are women who present with a painful mass in the breast and associated fever and can mimic malignancy. Usually, have a history of pregnancy or are currently pregnant. Clinically the most common presentation is a unilateral breast mass. Nipple inversion and sinus formation and breast pain with abscess formation can be seen. The presentation on imaging is variable. The disease can present as a mass, asymmetry, dilated ducts and fluid collections. Histology shows a mixed inflammatory infiltrate with neutrophils and lymphocytes and giant cells. Imaging findings can mimic malignancy on all modalities.

The histologic hallmark of the disease is the presence of lipid vacuoles which are seen as clear spaces rimmed by neutrophils. Another useful feature that is helpful is that on occasional cases bacteria can be seen within the lipid vacuoles and may require a gram stain to reveal gram-positive rod-shaped organisms. Some studies have shown a strong association with corynebacterium species. Although, there are no established diagnostic criteria for diagnosis of cystic neutrophilic mastitis a possibility of this diagnosis can be raised based on the histologic features and presence of gram positive. Ultimately, microbiologic culture studies and 16S rRNA sequencing may be helpful in identifying the specific organisms which are mostly corynebacterium species. The differential diagnosis is broad including granulomatous mastitis, lactational abscess, tuberculosis, and sarcoidosis [13].

Although infectious in etiology, the patients require prolonged treatment with antibiotics and/or corticosteroids and may still not respond. In addition to unremitting pain and deformity, complications can include non-healing, draining wounds.

In this case, the patient had continued pain after 4 months of treatment with both antibiotics and corticosteroids and elected to undergo mastectomy for treatment.

Case 9

A 70-year-old male with a palpable mass behind the left nipple (Fig. 14.9).

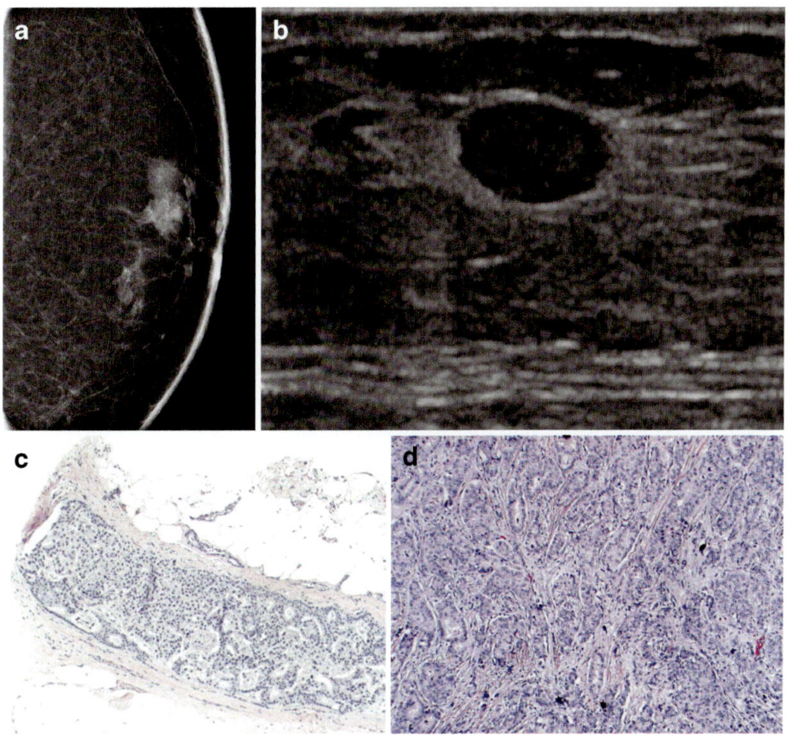

Fig. 14.9 (**a**) Mammogram showing an oval mass with fine pleomorphic calcification in the retroareolar region. (**b**) The ultrasound demonstrates a lesion with 1 cm oval component and adjacent irregular indistinct component central to the nipple. (**c**) Core biopsy of the mass showed an atypical intraductal papillary proliferation and focal calcification. (**d**) Mastectomy of the mass showed an invasive ductal carcinoma, grade 2 with focal cribriform features and calcifications

Educational Note

Male breast cancer accounts for less than 1% of all breast cancers and <0.1% of all male cancer deaths. The majority of breast cancers in male are invasive ductal carcinoma presenting usually as a solitary mass and 5% of male breast cancers are purely intraductal lesions [14]. An intraductal component is found in up to 50% of male patients versus 75% in female patients. Approximately 15–20% of patients have a family history of breast or ovarian cancer with increased risk for BRCA 1 and BRCA 2 mutation carriers. Patients present with a palpable mass or nipple discharge. The differential diagnosis clinically is gynecomastia, myofibroblastoma, and metastases.

Breast cancers in males are mostly luminal subtype with ER and PR positivity and less frequently are HER2-positive or basal or triple-negative subtypes [15, 16].

Imaging findings are similar to female breast cancers. On histology IDC, NST is similar to cancers seen in female patients with grade 2 and 3 tumors predominantly. Among the special subtypes papillary carcinomas are the most common although other subtypes such as mucinous and tubular have been reported. On histology the most important differential to exclude is a metastatic carcinoma which can present as breast mass before the primary is detected. Metastatic prostate cancer can mimic breast cancer and ancillary studies such as CK7, PSA, PAP, and ER are helpful to exclude a breast primary. The presence of an intraductal component such as in this case is convincing evidence that this is a primary in the breast.

This case is unusual in that the patient presented with nipple discharge with a palpable mass. He was found to have a BRCA mutation variant of uncertain significance. He had a history of nephrectomy for a renal mass but no history of prostate cancer. His father had a history of lung cancer but his mother and sisters do not have a history of cancer. He underwent bilateral mastectomy with bilateral sentinel axillary lymph node dissection. The lymph nodes were negative. Postoperatively he was treated with tamoxifen, leuprolide, and anastrozole. The patient is currently alive with no evidence of disease.

References

High-Risk Lesions (ADH/LCIS)

1. Elfgen C, Leo C, Kubik-Huch RA, et al. Third international consensus conference on lesions of uncertain malignant potential in the breast (B3 lesions). Virchows Arch. 2023;483(1):5–20. https://doi.org/10.1007/s00428-023-03566-x.

Radial Scar/Complex Sclerosing Lesion

2. Quinn EM, Dunne E, Flanagan F, et al. Radial scars and complex sclerosing lesions on core needle biopsy of the breast: upgrade rates and long-term outcomes. Breast Cancer Res Treat. 2020;183(3):677–82. https://doi.org/10.1007/s10549-020-05806-z.
3. Ha SM, Cha JH, Shin HJ, et al. Radial scars/complex sclerosing lesions of the breast: radiologic and clinicopathologic correlation. BMC Med Imaging. 2018;18(1):39. Published 2018 Nov 3. https://doi.org/10.1186/s12880-018-0279-z.
4. Patterson JA, Scott M, Anderson N, Kirk SJ. Radial scar, complex sclerosing lesion and risk of breast cancer. Analysis of 175 cases in Northern Ireland. Eur J Surg Oncol. 2004;30(10):1065–8. https://doi.org/10.1016/j.ejso.2004.08.004.

Multiple Papillomas

5. Rella R, Romanucci G, Arciuolo D, et al. Multiple papillomas of the breast: a review of current evidence and challenges. J Imaging. 2022;8(7):198. Published 2022 Jul 13. https://doi.org/10.3390/jimaging8070198.

Granular Cell Tumor

6. Meani F, Di Lascio S, Wandschneider W, et al. Granular cell tumor of the breast: a multidisciplinary challenge. Crit Rev Oncol Hematol. 2019;144:102828. https://doi.org/10.1016/j.critrevonc.2019.102828.

7. Corso G, Di Nubila B, Ciccia A, et al. Granular cell tumor of the breast: molecular pathology and clinical management. Breast J. 2018;24(5):778–82. https://doi.org/10.1111/tbj.13036.

Fibromatosis/Desmoid Tumor of the Breast

8. Boland MR, Nugent T, Nolan J, et al. Fibromatosis of the breast: a 10-year multi-institutional experience and review of the literature. Breast Cancer. 2021;28(1):168–74. https://doi.org/10.1007/s12282-020-01145-5.
9. Rakha EA, Brogi E, Castellano I, Quinn C. Spindle cell lesions of the breast: a diagnostic approach. Virchows Arch. 2022;480(1):127–45. https://doi.org/10.1007/s00428-021-03162-x.

Nodular Fasciitis

10. Paliogiannis P, Cossu A, Palmieri G, et al. Breast nodular fasciitis: a comprehensive review. Breast Care (Basel). 2016;11(4):270–4. https://doi.org/10.1159/000448185.
11. Shimizu TK, Gibbs P, Orrison S, Ma A. Nodular fasciitis of the breast. Breast J. 2020;26(5):1054–5. https://doi.org/10.1111/tbj.13734.

Cystic Neutrophilic Granulomatosis

12. Wu JM, Turashvili G. Cystic neutrophilic granulomatous mastitis: an update. J Clin Pathol. 2020;73(8):445–53.
13. Turashvili G, Li X. Inflammatory lesions of the breast. Arch Pathol Lab Med. 2023;147(10):1133–47.

Male Breast Carcinoma

14. Anderson WF, Jatoi I, Tse J, Rosenberg PS. Male breast cancer: a population-based comparison with female breast cancer. J Clin Oncol. 2010;28(2):232–9.
15. Deb S, Lakhani SR, Ottini L, Fox SB. The cancer genetics and pathology of male breast cancer. Histopathology. 2016;68(1):110–8.
16. Hill A, Yagmur Y, Tran KN, Bolton JS, Robson M, Borgen PI. Localized male breast carcinoma and family history. An analysis of 142 patients. Cancer. 1999;86(5):821–5.

Correction to: Radiology Pathology Correlations of Breast Lesions

Malini Harigopal, Liva Andrejeva,
Kamaljeet Singh, and John Lewin

Correction to:
M. Harigopal et al. (eds.), Radiology Pathology Correlations of Breast Lesions, https://doi.org/10.1007/978-3-031-65711-5

The original version of this book has been revised to reflect an update in the affiliation of Editor Dr. Kamaljeet Singh, which has been updated throughout the book.

The updated version of this book can be found at https://doi.org/10.1007/978-3-031-65711-5

M. Harigopal et al. (eds.), *Radiology Pathology Correlations of Breast Lesions*,
https://doi.org/10.1007/978-3-031-65711-5_15

Index

M. Harigopal et al. (eds.), *Radiology Pathology Correlations of Breast Lesions*,
https://doi.org/10.1007/978-3-031-65711-5

GPSR Compliance

The European Union's (EU) General Product Safety Regulation (GPSR) is a set of rules that requires consumer products to be safe and our obligations to ensure this.

If you have any concerns about our products, you can contact us on ProductSafety@springernature.com

In case Publisher is established outside the EU, the EU authorized representative is:

Springer Nature Customer Service Center GmbH
Europaplatz 3
69115 Heidelberg, Germany

Batch number: 10756384

Printed by Printforce, the Netherlands